Intellectual Disability in Health and Social Care

Many practitioners in health and social care come into contact with people with intellectual disabilities and want to work in ways that are beneficial to them by making reasonable adjustments in order to meet client needs and expectations. Yet the health and wellbeing of people with learning disabilities remains a neglected area, where unnecessary suffering and premature deaths continue to prevail.

This text provides a comprehensive insight into intellectual disability healthcare. It is aimed at those who are training in the field of intellectual disability nursing and also untrained practitioners who work in both health and social care settings. Divided into five parts, it explores how a wide range of biological, health, psychological and social barriers impact upon people with a learning disability, and includes:

- six guiding principles used to adjust, plan and develop meaningful and accessible health and social services
- assessment, screening and diagnosis of intellectual disability across the life course
- addressing lifelong health needs
- psychological and psychotherapeutic issues, including sexuality, behavioural and mental health needs, bereavement, and ethical concerns
- the changing professional roles and models of meeting the needs of people with intellectual and learning disabilities.

Intellectual Disability in Health and Social Care provides a wide-ranging overview of what learning disability professionals' roles are and offers insight into what health and social care practitioners might do to assist someone with intellectual disabilities when specific needs arise.

Stacey Atkinson is a Senior Lecturer of Learning Disability Nursing and Field Leader for Learning Disability Nursing in the Department of Human and Health Sciences at the University of Huddersfield, UK.

Joanne Lay is a Learning Disability Nurse currently working as a Nurse Lecturer in the School of Healthcare, University of Leeds, UK.

Su McAnelly is a Registered Nurse for people with learning disabilities who now works in the Higher Education sector as a Director of Programmes at Northumbria University, UK.

Malcolm Richardson is a Learning Disabilities Nurse and Principal Lecturer (Learning Disabilities) in the Faculty of Health and Wellbeing at Sheffield Hallam University, UK.

Intellectual Disability in Health and Social Care

**Edited by Stacey Atkinson, Joanne Lay,
Su McAnelly and Malcolm Richardson**

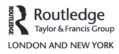

Routledge
Taylor & Francis Group

LONDON AND NEW YORK

First published 2015
by Routledge
2 Park Square, Milton Park, Abingdon, Oxon OX14 4RN

and by Routledge
711 Third Avenue, New York, NY 10017

Routledge is an imprint of the Taylor & Francis Group, an informa business

British Library Cataloguing in Publication Data
A catalogue record for this book is available from the British Library

Library of Congress Cataloging-in-Publication Data
Intellectual disability in health and social care / edited by Stacey Atkinson,
Joanne Lay, Su McAnelly, and Malcolm Richardson.
    p. ; cm.
Includes bibliographical references.
I. Atkinson, Stacey, editor.   II. Lay, Joanne, editor.   III. McAnelly, Su,
editor.   IV. Richardson, Malcolm, 1953- editor.
[DNLM: 1. Intellectual Disability–nursing.   2. Learning
Disorders–nursing.   3. Mental Health Services.   4. Nurse's
Role–psychology.   5. Psychiatric Nursing–methods. WY 160]
RC440
616.89'0231—dc23

                                                                2014006117

ISBN: 978-0-415-73389-2 (hbk)
ISBN: 978-0-273-76387-1 (pbk)
ISBN: 978-1-315-81912-9 (ebk)

Typeset in Bembo
by RefineCatch Limited, Bungay, Suffolk

Printed and bound in the United States of America by
Edwards Brothers Malloy on sustainably sourced paper

Contents

Figures

Tables

Contributors

Editors

Stacey Atkinson is a learning disability nurse who presently works as a senior lecturer of Learning Disability nursing and field leader for learning disability nursing in the department of Human and Health Sciences at the University of Huddersfield. She has vast experience of working with adults and children with a learning disability. Her particular areas of interest are the needs of people with behaviours which challenge and those with Autistic Spectrum Disorder (ASD), the needs of children, psychotherapeutic approaches, ethics and sexuality education and support. Stacey's previous sexuality work has resulted in her receiving national accolade and an MBE for services to children with disabilities. Stacey has had experience of providing nursing care to people with complex needs, including those with behaviours that challenge and people with mental health needs. She has worked in multi-disciplinary teams and has also been involved in producing and facilitating inter-professional education around the communication needs of people with ASD. She is an advisor for the Learning Disability Practice journal and is widely involved in educating about the needs of people with a learning disability within mainstream settings.

Joanne Lay is a learning disability nurse currently working as a Nurse Lecturer in the School of Healthcare, University of Leeds. Jo has many years of experience working in learning disability services, particularly within the voluntary sector. She is passionate about person-centred approaches to support and is a person-centred planning facilitator. Jo developed an innovative 'accessible CV' project to enhance communication between service users and students in practice placement settings. Jo received a developmental University Student Education Fellowship from Leeds in 2013 in recognition of excellence in learning and teaching. She is using this award to improve the learning experience of disabled students in the School of Healthcare. Jo is a facilitator for the Positive Choices Network which promotes networking for student nurses undertaking the learning/intellectual disability field. She is committed to the long-term future of the profession and holds a Conduct and Competence Panellist role with the Nursing and Midwifery Council.

Su McAnelly is Registered Nurse for people, with learning disabilities who now works in the Higher Education sector. Su has spent the last 30 years engaging with issues of care for people with learning disability. Her doctoral research study focused upon the social constructions of clients with learning disability by professionals and she has continued this interest in her teaching and academic support of students studying for professional qualifications in health and social care. Su has worked for health authorities in Halifax, and Doncaster, and also University of Huddersfield, the University of Sheffield and Northumbria University. Su is on the editorial advisory board for *Learning Disability Practice* (RCN pubs) and peer reviews for *British Journal of Learning Disability*. She has reviewed numerous publications, conference submissions and text books.

Malcolm Richardson is a learning disabilities nurse and Principal Lecturer (Learning Disabilities) in the Faculty of Health and Wellbeing at Sheffield Hallam University. His doctoral research involved the participation of a group of people with learning disabilities as co-researchers of their own life experiences. Currently his role includes working strategically within the Faculty and with the Faculty's external partners to promote education about learning disabilities and the inclusion of people with learning disabilities in the delivery of programmes leading to professional awards in areas of health and social care.

Contributors

Paul Armitage is a counsellor and counselling supervisor for Mental Health Access Team, NHS South West Yorkshire Mental Health Trust.

Helen Atherton is a Lecturer in Nursing for the School of Healthcare, University of Leeds.

David Atkinson is an Independent Consultant Nurse. Dave has worked as a learning disability nurse for 22 years in a variety of specialist roles and service settings. He has a strong background in developing and delivering specialist services for people with challenging needs, as well as more recently developing initiatives to address the health inequalities experienced by people with learning disabilities and to measure the outcomes of effective service delivery.

Lyndsey Charles is an Allied Health professional Lead for Learning Disabilities. She is employed by Leeds and York Partnership Foundation Trust.

Debbie Crickmore is a Lecturer in Learning Disability with the Faculty of Health and Social Care at the University of Hull.

Dan Dearden is a Learning Disability Nurse and Senior Mental Health Practitioner with the mental health liaison team at Barnsley District General Hospital.

Mary Dearing is a Lecturer in Learning Disability in the Faculty of Health and Social Care at the University of Hull.

Shaun Derry is a Registered Nurse in Learning Disabilities who currently works for the Leeds and York Partnership Foundation Trust.

Catherine Dunne is a Practising Learning Disability Nurse and Ward Manager for the South West Yorkshire Partnership Foundation Trust.

Kaydii Inglis is an (RNLD) Primary Care Liaison Nurse educated at Northumbria University. She currently work in health facilitation and part of the role is to liaise with, educate and advise primary care practitioners, such as GPs and practice nurses on the health needs of people with learning disabilities. She also runs joint clinics for annual health checks within GP surgeries and provides health promotion, education and practical support with physical health.

Pamela Inglis is a Learning Disability Nurse and academic. She is currently the Director of Programmes for Learning Disability Nursing, Mental Health Nursing and Occupational Therapy at Northumbria University. Her professional doctoral studies centred on the discourses surrounding forensic practice for people with a learning disability. She is a member of the steering group for the academic network for learning disability nurses, a member of the editorial board for the *Journal of Intellectual Disability and Offending Behaviour* and reviews for several other journals.

Sheena Kelly is a Learning Disability Nurse and a Clinical Services Manager for learning disabilities services for Leeds, York and Selby community services. She is employed by Leeds and York Partnership Foundation Trust.

Helen Laverty is a Learning Disability Nurse and Senior Lecturer at the University of Nottingham.

Anne Lyons is a Chartered Paediatric Physiotherapist. She helped established the Regional Postural Wheelchair and Seating for Children and Young People with Complex Disabilities in the North-East of England in 1978, and for many years co-ordinated and advanced this service. She is currently employed as a Senior Lecturer at Northumbria University. For her doctoral research she explored comfort and discomfort among children and young people with severe physical, learning and communication difficulties who depend on postural management equipment.

Dorothy Matthews works for Macmillan CNS Learning Disabilities. Her career spans many years within learning disability services, and her current post of Macmillan Nurse for people with learning disabilities was developed in partnership with Macmillan and Northumberland Tyne and Wear NHS Foundation Trust (formerly Northgate and Prudhoe NHS Trust) in 2004.

Alex McClimens is a Senior Research Fellow at the Centre for Health and Social Care Research at Sheffield Hallam University.

Nigel McLoughlin is a Clinical Services Manager in learning disability services for South West Yorkshire Partnership Trust.

Sheena Miller is a Senior Lecturer in learning disability nursing at the University of Huddersfield, with a particular interest in person-centred approaches to care. Her background is in community nursing for adults with learning disabilities.

Lesley Montesci is a Registered Learning Disability Nurse with considerable experience as a community nurse and nurse consultant. She is now Deputy Director of Enable Care and Home Support and is nominated individual for Care Quality Commission. Lesley has a long-standing association with the RCN and served as an elected committee member on the National Learning

Disability Nurses Forum. She has also participated in numerous regional and national groups to promote learning disability nursing and address the specific needs of service users.

Gwen Moulster has recently moved to South Staffordshire and Shropshire NHS Foundation Trust as Clinical Director/Consultant Nurse (Learning Disabilities) where her role is focused on ensuring high quality services and best practice. Gwen has extensive experience of working with people who have learning disabilities and their families. She is part of the team who developed the Health Equalities Framework (HEF) outcome measurement tool, and has presented this with colleagues at conferences across the UK and in Australia and Finland.

Monica Murphy is a Lecturer and Student Education Fellow at the School of Healthcare, the University of Leeds.

Isabel Quinn is a Senior Lecturer in palliative and end of life care at Northumbria University. She worked as National Programme Manager for End of Life Care and has produced a range of guidance around improving palliative and end of life care delivery for people with conditions other than cancer. Isabel began her nursing career working with people with learning disabilities and continues to maintain an interest in this specialism.

Angela Ridley is a Senior Lecturer and Programme Leader for learning disability nursing at Northumbria University.

Bronwyn Roberts is a Senior Lecturer and Course Leader at the University of Huddersfield. She has worked with people with a learning disability, their family and friends since 1976. She worked within the NHS for 25 years, has been a third sector director and worked in integrated services before becoming a nurse lecturer. She is also a governor for Calderstones Learning Disability Trust. Her main interests are effective healthcare for people with complex needs.

Andrew Stafford has been in The Lawnmowers Independent Theatre Company for 28 years, and is a senior core member of the company. His role over the years has involved union representation, outreach work, mentoring younger members, Board presentations and presentations at many events and conferences and to hundreds of networks. Andy is an established, professional actor and Equity member who has appeared in film and TV programmes.

Anne Todd is an Advanced Nurse Practitioner and Senior Clinical Practitioner in learning disabilities, South West Yorks Partnership Foundation Trust.

Mick Wolverson is a Lecturer in learning disability nursing at the University of York.

Foreword

We are a group of people with learning disabilities who are members of various self-advocacy groups and are also Partners In Learning at Sheffield Hallam University.

We would like to begin by welcoming you, the reader, and shaking your hand because that is how one human being should be towards others. We know we cannot do this in person. But maybe some day our paths will cross.

We want you to read this book because we are experts in living with a learning disability, we have lots of friends and acquaintances who have learning disabilities and we are very good at supporting each other, for example, in recognising when we are unwell, happy or sad and helping each other to remain positive and well. We are members of peer buddying and advocacy schemes to support each other.

We want you to be at least as good as we are at supporting people with learning disabilities. This book will help you do that.

Too often people do not see us, they only see our disability and dismiss us. Sometimes they see we can walk, so dismiss our difficulties and call us scroungers. But many of our difficulties are hidden, significant, even life-threatening. This book will help you to see 'us' so that when we do meet, you will understand better how to greet us, how to 'shake our hands', demonstrate your respect and ensure that we are not ignored, neglected or fobbed off, like these examples:

I wrote to the Cabinet Office and was ignored.

The bus driver told me to order a taxi, I showed my pass, he implied I was a scrounger.

This is what Part I of this book is all about, how to make sure people with learning disabilities are treated with dignity and respect.

Part II looks at what you can do if you are involved in assessments related to people with learning disabilities at various times from birth throughout life.

Part III is all about the lifelong health of people with learning disabilities. Sometimes we are born with these and at other times we develop them. But they do not always get recognised or treated correctly and that can lead to premature deaths. This part of the book will help you to see beyond the person's learning disability, to recognise and support their health and well-being.

Part IV covers a range of support issues including: psychological, sexual, challenging behaviour, mental health, criminal justice, bereavement and ethics.

Finally, Part V considers inter-professional working, health promotion and third sector services.

So, welcome, enjoy your reading and should you need any support or reasonable adjustments, please let us know. We respect your difference.

Partners in Learning members:
Jonno, Jodie, Barry, James, David, Darren,
Graham, Billy, Kevin, Michael and Robert

Note on terms

The terms 'intellectual disability' and 'learning disability' have been used interchangeably throughout this book. Both terms are problematic as neither learning disabilities nor intellectual disabilities are terms that are universally approved by the people to whom these terms are applied and nor are there any accepted alternatives terms that are used for this purpose.

In the United Kingdom, learning disabilities has been in use for several decades and is the term used by the Department of Health and many agencies and providers of services as well as within the field of Learning Disabilities Nursing. However, the term intellectual disability is becoming increasingly common internationally, where the term learning disabilities may not be recognised or in common use. For this reason the authors have used both terms throughout, with the intention that their meaning is equivalent.

Introduction

Stacey Atkinson, Joanne Lay, Su McAnelly and Malcolm Richardson

> *Jonno:*   I'd like to register with a GP please.
> *Receptionist:*   I'm sorry, we don't deal with people like you here.
>
> The above is a synopsis of what happened to Jonno when he tried to register with a GP. Jonno has a learning disability associated with his autistic spectrum disorder.

Much of the health deficit that people with a learning disability experience is attributable to avoidable causes and the reduced socio-economic circumstances in which many find themselves (Robertson *et al.*, 2010).

Some people with learning disabilities do not readily attempt to use healthcare facilities. The reasons for this are varied and often include factors such as communication difficulties and the presence of disabling barriers, such as Jonno encountered above. Therefore, people with learning disabilities who do make the effort to access health support services are often thwarted by the disabling barriers that they encounter. Consequently, many people with learning disabilities need appropriate assistance and a service ready and able to make 'reasonable adjustments' to enable proper access and benefit from health services. In the absence of appropriate assistance and reasonable adjustments, their healthcare needs too often remain significantly unmet.

The aim of this book, therefore, is to enable you, in whatever role or capacity you meet and engage with people who have learning disabilities, to deliver appropriate support. To do so, the book explores a wide range of biological, health, psychological and social barriers that impact upon people with learning disabilities. The book provides examples of how to support access to services and the attainment of appropriate health–related outcomes.

In the UK in recent years, government policy has driven a range of initiatives to improve access to health services and the health of people with learning disabilities (e.g. Scottish Executive, 2000; DH, 2001; Welsh Office, 2001; DHSSPS, 2005). These policies give particular emphasis to the human rights of each person with a learning disability living within an inclusive society. Emphasis is also placed upon the personalisation of support, by locating the individual at the centre of decision-making and choice.

Recent years bear witness to the introduction of annual health checks for people with learning disabilities (Disability Right Commission, 2006; Michael, 2008; Robertson *et al.*, 2010). A review of the evidence arising from these annual health checks (Robertson *et al.*, 2010) clearly demonstrates that they have frequently resulted in the detection of unmet, unrecognised and potentially treatable health conditions, including those which are serious such as cancer, heart disease and dementia.

The health and well-being of people with learning disabilities remain an important but neglected area where high incidences of unnecessary suffering and premature deaths continue to prevail (Mencap, 2007, 2012; Michael, 2008; CIPOLD, 2013). This book will assist its readers to play their part, as a health or social care practitioner, in ensuring that people with learning disabilities are supported to access and engage with health services, their health needs recognised, reasonable adjustments put in place and appropriate health outcomes pursued.

Reader Activities

You will be encouraged throughout the book to develop your insight by engaging in reader activities. Whilst there are no set answers for these activities, they are designed to enable deeper thinking around the points raised. As your career progresses and you revisit these exercises your answers to the questions raised will no doubt become more detailed and insightful. You may like to debate the answers to the questions with your colleagues or with people with learning disabilities themselves. Whatever way you wish to consider the issues raised.

References

CIPOLD (2013) *Confidential Inquiry into Premature Deaths of People with Learning Disabilities (CIPOLD): Final Report*. Available at: http://www.bris.ac.uk/cipold/ (accessed 25 Nov. 2013).

DH (Department of Health) (2001) *Valuing People: A New Strategy for Learning Disabilities for the 21st Century*. London: HMSO.

DH (Department of Health) (2010) *Health Action Plans – What Are They? How Do You Get One? A Booklet for People with Learning Disabilities*. Available at: http://www.easyhealth.org.uk/sites/default/files/health%20action%20plans.pdf (accessed 26 June 2013).

DHSSPS NI Direct (Northern Ireland Department of Health, Social Services and Public Safety) (2005) *Equal Lives 2005*. Available at: http://www.dhsspsni.gov.uk/annex_d_-_equal_lives_review__2005__core_values.pdf (accessed 26 June 2013).

Mencap (2007) *Death by Indifference: Following up the Treat Me Right! Report*. Available at: www.mencap.org.uk.

Mencap (2012) *Death by Indifference: 74 Deaths and Counting: A Progress Report 5 Years On*. Available at: www.mencap.org.uk.

Michael, J. (2008) *Healthcare for All: Report of the Independent Inquiry into Access to Healthcare for People with Learning Disabilities*. London: Independent Inquiry into Access to Healthcare for People with Learning Disabilities.

Robertson, J., Roberts, H. and Emerson, E. (2010) *Health Checks for People with Learning Disabilities: A Systematic Review*. Durham: Improving Health and Lives: Learning Disability Observatory. Available at: http://www.improvinghealthandlives.org.uk/uploads/doc/vid_7646_IHAL2010-04HealthChecksSystemticReview.pdf (accessed 27 June 2013).

Scottish Executive (2000) *Same As You? A Review of the Services for People with Learning Disabilities*. Edinburgh: Scottish Executive.

Welsh Office (2001) *Fulfilling the Promises*. Cardiff: the Welsh Assembly.

Part I

The six guiding principles

We have a duty to challenge ourselves and each other on behalf of our patients.

(DH, 2013)

This statement was made in the Foreword to *Patients First and Foremost: The Initial Government Response to the Mid-Staffordshire NHS Foundation Trust Public Inquiry* in 2013 as a result of the Francis Inquiry (2012), reporting on poor quality and neglectful care in Britain in the twenty-first century. Many of the shocking revelations were attributed to a lack of consideration by professionals of the needs of vulnerable clients and patients.

Many people with intellectual or learning disabilities are vulnerable and inarticulate in the presence of professionals and service providers (DH, 2012). Their carers may also struggle to present their needs accurately. As a result, this client group who suffer from greater health needs than the general population often experience inappropriate treatment, ineffective care and consequently even poorer health (Emerson and Baines, 2010).

Part I introduces the six guiding principles which can be used to adjust, plan and develop meaningful and assessable health and social services for adults and children with intellectual/learning disabilities. These principles have been developed from the personal experiences of life (both living with disability and also living alongside those with disabilities), the professional experience of caring, and the empirical research of the contributors.

These six principles are integrated within the philosophy and content of this book and the contributors believe them to be at the forefront when considering how best to meet the needs of people with intellectual or learning disabilities. We aim to enable you to consider these principles in your own actions and in those of others in your daily contacts with your clients and patients.

The six guiding principles presented and chapters in Part I are:

Chapter 1 Guiding principle 1: Ensuring dignity and respect
Chapter 2 Guiding principle 2: The importance of providing accessible information for people with learning disabilities

References

DH (Department of Health) (2012) *Transforming Care: A National Response to Winterbourne View Hospital*, London: Department of Health.

DH (Department of Health) (2013) *Patients First and Foremost: The Initial Government Response to the Mid Staffordshire NHS Foundation Trust Public Inquiry*. London: Department of Health.

Emerson, E. and Baines, S. (2010) *Health Inequalities and People with Learning Disabilities in the UK*. Available at: www.improvinghealthandlives.org.uk.

Francis, R. (2013) *Mid Staffordshire NHS Foundation Trust Public Inquiry*. Available at: www.midstaffspublic-inquiry.com/report.

1 Guiding principle 1: Ensuring dignity and respect

Su McAnelly and Dorothy Matthews

Learning outcomes

After reading this chapter you will be able to:

- identify and consider your own skills and abilities in caring for all people
- consider ways in which dignity and respect can be assured within good health and social care practice
- apply the principles of holism to working with people with learning disabilities.

Introduction

> Every life deserves a certain amount of dignity, no matter how poor or damaged the shell that carries it.
>
> (Bragg 1998).

This chapter gives an introduction to the overall guiding principles and is intended to enable you to think and develop ideas about your own development needs. The section offers reader activity boxes which are designed to provoke ideas and discussion around the complexities of working with people with learning disabilities who have health and social needs. In addition, the chapter refers to a case study featuring a real scenario based upon a person with a learning disability. Additional reference material and fast fact boxes offer further reading or access to on-line materials, fact sheets and reports.

This chapter looks at the many issues and complexities of working with people who are vulnerable. The reflection that you will be asked to undertake in it will be based upon the values and attitudes you have towards other people in general, but you may become more acutely aware of these beliefs as you come to deal with more challenging situations.

The chapter focuses upon a case story about a man named Colin and covers the following topics:

- human drives
- motivations

- dignity
- respect
- confusion and misunderstandings.

Human drives

As human beings, our behaviour is influenced by many things; our environment, our social relation-ships, our biological make-up and also our internal drives. For many people, internal drives relate to psychological motivations, emotional histories or even genetic precedents. However, it is perhaps most important for health and social care workers to attempt to understand the reasons for their own behaviour towards others and vice versa.

Abraham Maslow (1943) is most famously known for a set of universal ideas which have been used as a framework to explain the inter-relationships between our motivations to meet our various unsat-isfied needs. Figure 1.1 explains his theory that humans are driven to satisfy their most basic needs in hierarchical order. This theory helps us understand that human drives are based upon many variants and that we are all striving for similar human goals but with differing degrees of success.

Physiological needs

The drives to meet our basic physical survival are considered the strongest and the most obvious. A threat to these needs, which include the human need to eat and to stay warm, will probably override the need for friendship or learning, for example.

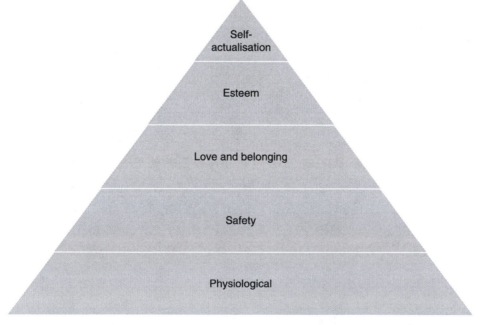

Figure 1.1 Maslow's hierarchy of needs

Source: Maslow (1943).

Safety needs

When physical needs are being met, Maslow argues that a desire to be safe and secure follows. These needs may consist of personal safety, financial safety, health and well-being. These drives are complex and are dependent upon the person's perceived situation. For many vulnerable people, these drives are the most complex and can result in psychological problems such as post-traumatic illness and phobias.

Love and belonging

When a person begins to feel physiologically sound and perceives their situation as safe, the most compelling drive may be to be loved and to be cherished. The need for love and friendship can be overwhelmed by isolation or incarceration during events such as hospital stays or severe rejection.

Esteem

All humans have a need to be respected and recognised for their own worth. The search for esteem and belonging can be on two levels: first, to be happy with one's image of oneself, and, second, to be well received by others. It is believed by Maslow that the former (being happy with one's self) is essential to becoming recognised by others. The strong desire for recognition leads people to aim for previously unobtainable goals, For example, to be famous, to be a winner or to be known more widely.

Self-actualisation

As a relatively comfortable human being, the desire turns to meeting an additional need; to be what you want to be or be the ideal! To reach your full potential. This desire to meet a need is intrinsic (known from within) and for many people this goal is not achieved. This is mainly because other needs may re-emerge and must be mastered before the desire for self-actualisation can become a drive to achieve an internal goal.

Reader activity 1.1 Our drives and other people's drives

- Think about your own motivations based on Maslow's hierarchy of needs, for food, to be safe, to have friends, to learn.
- Do you think these are the same as your colleagues?
- How do we differ from each other?
- How are we the same?

Motivations

The science of psychology attempts to explain why we as human beings are motivated to behave as we do in relation to other people and situations. Theories of motivation are heavily debated and tend to focus upon particular aspects of human behaviour, for example, the theory of physical motivation to eat or the theory of the motivation to make money. For those of us working in health and social care for vulnerable clients, it is right to examine the theories which motivate people to care for others.

We can be motivated by money or rewards

This theory attempts to explain the reasons why people will be motivated to behave or act towards others because they will receive an external reward. This reward could be a salary/wage or a bonus or other treat (see Beck, 2003). Studies have shown that there is relationship between a worker's motivation to achieve goals (to earn more money, to achieve higher status/promotion) and their rate of performance and the quality of their work (see Herzberg, 1968; Locke, 1997).

The idea that health and social care workers should and could be motivated by incentives (such as bonus and rewards) has worried researchers and also patient/client groups who argue that good standards of care work cannot be motivated by incentives alone even if these were intrinsic – that is, internally set by the person themselves (see Wilson, 1989). But what should motivate health and social care work?

> ### Reader activity 1.2   What motivates you to work where you do?

List the five key factor/reasons which helped you decide to work in the caring field (be honest!):

1.
2.
3.
4.
5.

Individual differences in personality are important

The type of person you are and how you react in situations, with problems and with people, are determined by many factors, and it is difficult to determine and even harder to assess and predict. However, the ability to show care and compassion to our clients is paramount to the roles we occupy in health and social care; how much can we predict in ourselves and others?

The *Big 5 factors* of personality are universally accepted to be a model when discussing the ranges and extremes in behaviour that people exhibit and that can be attributed to their personality, which is a result of both their environment and biological/hereditary factors. The Big 5 factors are explained below. These sets of theories suggest that the type of personality a care worker possesses can influence the way they relate to their clients and other colleagues (see Goldberg, 1991).

The Big 5 factors are:

1. *extroversion*: to be excitable and seek social contact with others. The tendency to be talkative.
2. *agreeableness*: the extent to which a person can show a high degree of trust and kindliness and affection;
3. *conscientiousness*: a tendency to high levels of goal-driven behaviour and self-control;
4. *neuroticism*: refers to the ability to control the level of personal stability and anxiety management. The extent to which a person can feel emotions (both negative and positive).
5. *openness*: has a high level of interest and imagination and the scope to show good insight.

Reader activity 1.3   How does personality affect health and social work?

Take each personality trait from the list above and write a short description of the ways that this trait may affect a person's abilities when working with clients in health/social care.

Fast facts 1.1   A history lesson

Dignity has been a pertinent issue in relation to services for people with learning disabilities for many years. In the past most individuals with learning disabilities were placed in long-stay institutions which were often situated outside of towns and cities. These were generally char-acterised by a lack of dignity, and here are some examples of how they were treated.

Place

- Offered little or no privacy.
- Barren environments, with little or nothing to do.
- Institutions/hospitals often situated miles away from the person's community, family and friends.
- Little or no access to the outside world; everything that was considered to be necessary was within the institution.

People

- Personal identity was not promoted (wards had shared clothing and toiletries for all residents).
- Little in terms of personal possessions.
- Language was often stigmatising and undignified.

(continued)

(continued)

Process

- Inflexible regimes (for example, meals at set times).
- Lack of choice in meals.
- Family had to apply in writing to see their relative outwith the grounds.

(Royal College of Nursing, 2009)

Dignity

Dignity, from the Latin *dignitas*, meaning 'intrinsic worth', is the basis for both national and international procedures, both as a concept and as a legal precedent. Dignity as a guiding principle for the rights of human beings to be treated in certain ways and to certain standards by other human beings has been theorised on many levels (see Dworkin, 1995; Shotton and Seedhouse, 1998). However, on a practical level, it is a prerequisite (or in other words, an expectation) for all those working in healthcare, but we now understand that enhancing the dignity of others, especially those who are vulnerable, has been a difficult task in health and social care practice for many years.

Dignity as a concept

The concept of dignity is easy to discuss but difficult to define and is often used in the context of healthcare as a benchmark for quality. However, many recorded cases of bad practice in healthcare towards vulnerable groups have stated that practitioners 'failed to ensure the dignity of those they cared for' (Mencap, 2007; DH, 2012).

Reader activity 1.4   Dignity

- Define something which you consider dignified.
- What emotions does it provoke in you?
- Why?
- Now define something you consider undignified.
- What emotions does this provoke and why?
- Look at this web site which is a useful resource for care services looking to inspire dignity champions:
  http://www.dignityincare.org.uk/.

The term dignity appears in many ways but is most predominant in the Charter of United Nations, set up in 1945, which is intended to be the basis for universal behaviour across the world. Dignity is enshrined in the first governing principle of Article 1 of the Universal Declaration on Human Rights.

Fast facts 1.2   United Nations Declaration on Human Rights

The United Nations set a target for all nations in the form of a declaration on human rights in 1945 and to date approximately 192 member states have signed up to the Declaration and have incorporated it into their own laws and precedents. The Declaration has 30 separate statements or articles.

The promotion of dignity is enshrined in the first governing principle of Article 1 of the Universal Declaration on Human Rights: 'All human beings are born free and equal in dignity and rights. They are endowed with reason and conscience and should act towards each other in the spirit of brotherhood.'

Dignity as enforced through law

In the United Kingdom the right to dignity is enforced through law via the Human Rights Act 1998. It appears in the codes of conduct of most health professionals and there is a statutory requirement for all those working in healthcare to ensure the right to dignity for those in care. There is an obligation to enhance and ensure the dignity of all persons receiving healthcare and this is also regulated by the quality standard checks carried out by the Care Quality Commission (CQC) who are commissioned to regularly assess all healthcare services abilities in this area via planned and unplanned checks and investigations.

Fast facts 1.3   The Care Quality Commission

The Care Quality Commission has the responsibility to check and inspect all services that provide care based upon a set of government standards. The inspections can be as a result of a complaint or as a planned visit. Visits normally occur periodically. See www.cqc.org.uk/public.

Examples of reports detailing issues with enhancing dignity for people using care services include:

- www.cqc.org.uk/public/news/our-role-winterbourne-view-and-changes-we-will-make-protect-people-abuse
- www.cqc.org.uk/public/what-are-standards/your-rights-under-mental-health-act.

Respect

Respect is a term often used to imply placing a value upon someone or something. We use the terms interchangeably with our values and as a sign that we are placing ourselves and other things or people in a hierarchy. We are often encouraged to place ourselves lower down the hierarchy as a mark of respect:

- for others
- for your elders
- for your parents
- for authority or the law.

Self-respect is a separate concept, which, though connected closely with respect for others/things, holds a closer, more psychological and emotional relationship with our inner selves and the outer world. It is felt most keenly when our self-respect is threatened or indeed shattered by a lack or removal of respect by others. Many people talk of finding their self-respect again when they have regained control of their lives after being devalued or marginalised.

Reader activity 1.5   Socialised respect

Where did you learn to respect other people?

- At school?
- In your family?
- At work?
- From friends?

How do we change over our lifetime?

Respect for persons

Having and showing respect for those we care for is a function of health and social care, but how do we know that we share a commonality?

Respect towards other people can be illustrated in a number of ways:

- We can respect a person's legal rights through being *directive* (following certain practices).
- We can show respect *institutionally* to someone by calling them by a title (like Sir or Lord or Dr).
- We can have a healthy respect for a person as an *obstacle* who is easily provoked.
- We can show respect to someone (alive or dead) because they have done *worthy* things which you think are valuable (doing high quality work or giving time to a worthy cause).

Reader activity 1.6   Showing respect

How do healthcare workers react to those they care for in the following ways?

- Do they show respect by directing practice?
- Do they demonstrate institutional respect?
- Do they demonstrate respect for a person as an obstacle/object?
- Do they respect someone's worth?

Morally, however, we are encouraged to think about the respect for *all* persons as human beings and this provokes many philosophical debates. One philosopher called Immanuel Kant is often considered the founder of the concept called the 'categorical imperative' regarding respect and dignity, which has led to both the United Nations Declaration on Human Rights and also to modern healthcare practice (Henry, 1990). The challenge for health and social care workers is to demonstrate the same respect to all people regardless of their status, disability, age, etc.

Reader activity 1.7   Making a respect cake

- Create a virtual recipe for a respect cake.
- What ingredients would it include?
- What are the instructions?

Case study 1.1   Colin's story

Colin was a 58-year-old gentleman who died ten months after a diagnosis of oesophageal cancer, and this is the story of the last few months of his life which the people around him were able to make as comfortable as possible for him taking into account his preferences and wishes.

Colin was labelled as having a learning disability. He had been receiving care and assistance from health and social care professionals to some degree for the whole of his life. Colin had lived in a variety of different places including with his parents, in a learning disability hospital, and in various group living arrangements for people with learning disabilities run by health and social services. When he was diagnosed with cancer, plans were under way for Colin to move into his own home with 24-hour care from a dedicated team, and despite Colin's cancer diagnosis this move was still considered to be in Colin's best interest and something which he himself wanted to go ahead with.

Colin was not always an easy man to assist and would often refuse help and responded with difficult behaviour when anyone tried to insist that he complied. He often struggled to communicate his wishes verbally which often had led to confusion and misunderstandings on his side and also for those caring for him. This led to Colin's behaviour towards other people being labelled 'challenging'. Colin was also in receipt of specialist support from challenging behaviour services to help him and others around him communicate and behave in a mutually agreed way in an attempt to minimise the confusion and misunderstanding which could lead to Colin becoming distressed and challenging.

Colin had been supported by an array of different healthcare and social care professionals before his diagnosis of cancer, but other specialist healthcare professionals became involved in his care when he was diagnosed with oesophageal cancer, which, following investigation, was, at the point of diagnosis, deemed to be incurable. As soon as Colin received a diagnosis, the issue of relocation to a home of his own was discussed with him. Communication with Colin about his diagnosis and his future was handled very carefully. As Colin struggled to understand everyday issues in life, those who knew him well (his family and his carers) thought that he

(continued)

(continued)

would also struggle to understand his situation and his future life. Various ways to tell Colin were discussed and he was told simply and clearly that he was going to die soon and that he might be more comfortable in a place of his own with the support of other people.

Following several psychological support sessions with the Macmillan Nurse for people with learning disabilities, Colin was given the news in clear simple language that his diagnosis would shorten his life and he would die from his cancer. The Macmillan Nurse used both verbal words and accessible information pictures and DVDs to show Colin how his illness might progress. Colin responded initially by becoming withdrawn and spent more time in his room, he also appeared agitated and angry. This was taken as a sign that he understood elements of his situation (as this is a natural human reaction to bad news and to also to fear and frustration). Further discussion with Colin revealed that he thought he would not be able to stay in his new home because of his illness; however, when he was subsequently told he could remain in his new home with extra support until the end of his life, Colin's anxiety and agitation notably lessened.

It was agreed with Colin and his care workers that he would live in a small home of his own in his local community. Colin preferred the male care staff within his direct care team and he made this quite obvious in his responses to both male and female care staff. He appeared to have more respect for his male carers and was notably more verbally aggressive to the females in the team. Again Colin's preferences were considered and staff cover from females was kept to a minimum with the majority of his direct care team being males.

Colin's new home was close to the town and local community amenities that Colin knew well, including the health centre, the local pub and also a park and river. Colin enjoyed going to the pub and again the pub staff respected Colin and always asked when he came into the pub, 'Is it hot milk or beer today, Colin?' (as these were the drinks he usually requested). In reply, Colin always answered politely and there were never any confusion issues during Colin's visits to the pub as he enjoyed chatting and engaging with the locals in the pub.

The change in Colin's health state was assessed and his care planned by the local nurse who specialised in learning disability nursing and also palliative care. This was very important for Colin as she fully understood his needs as a person with a learning disability and also could coordinate the services, including Macmillan nursing. This nurse had the experience and skills to help provide appropriate symptom management for Colin, and through liaison with the district nurses and the GP could ensure the care Colin needed was facilitated. Throughout Colin's illness communication between health and social care professionals was an integral part of facilitating good care for Colin. Appropriate timely communication was also an important part of Colin's care and the use of accessible or adapted information helped Colin to understand the information being given to him, while also helping to alleviate any anxieties on receiving the information. Hence this minimised the episodes of challenging behaviour which often followed discussions with professionals.

The important aspects of the remainder of Colin's life were his ability to have some control and for other people to facilitate this to happen, without taking away his independence and preferences in his daily life, hence allowing him to maintain some control over what was happening. Colin had a brother with whom he had had a turbulent relationship over the years preceding his illness, Colin's brother attempted to support him following his diagnosis by visiting more often and encouraging Colin to talk about his illness and the future. Colin, however, resented his brother's input and their relationship broke down in the last months of Colin's illness when at Colin's request he asked his brother not to visit him again. Colin's brother was naturally upset by this but respected his wishes though he did attend Colin's funeral.

The way Colin was cared for by a variety of professionals including district nurses, day-to-day care staff, the physiotherapist and the occupational therapist, the challenging behaviour team, the specialist hospital oesophageal acute team, and also his brother and an independent advocate was considered important. The attention to his dignity as a human being and to the respect both by him for others and also by the team for him demonstrated good communication between the professionals involved and the facilitation of good end-of-life care for Colin. Colin was more receptive to healthcare professionals following his cancer diagnosis than he had ever been in his life, and this may have been because Colin realised he now needed the support of these people and he appeared to understand that these people were trying to help him and facilitate good care and symptom management to ensure Colin's needs were appropriately met from the point of his diagnosis until his death ten months later.

Key points arising from Colin's story

Compassion

The successes for Colin in the later stages of his life were related to the abilities of other people around him to anticipate his needs and also to respond to his needs. The ethical motivations to act for the benefit of another and to do no harm are referred to as:

- *beneficence*: this is the taking of action 'to positively benefit others';
- *non-maleficence*: this is deliberately behaving in a way 'which will do no harm'.

Both of these moral principles are a regular feature of care for people with life-threatening conditions or who are at the end of their lives. Examples include the decisions made by medical/nursing teams and families about rights to die or the treatment of a person with an eating disorder who refuses food. The topics are strongly debated in health and social care and often draw upon ethical principles and moral and personal beliefs.

The principle of compassion in care is also seriously debated (Tuckett, 2005). It is easy to assume that all professionally delivered care (the act of caring) is based upon exact and intense forms of beneficence and non-maleficence, which govern the behaviour of care-givers towards those clients/ patients in their care and indeed power. But how the power and control balance is decided or negotiated can be key to the relationship between the two parties. Showing compassion and the ability to go beyond the professional guidelines and history is often seen as an intrinsic and obvious sign of good care, but how is it negotiated and from whose point of view?

What is considered by a professional to be good care based upon guidelines, benchmarks and standards may not be seen in exactly the same way by the person receiving that care. The dilemma between the different views (or constructions) of care delivery is a real challenge for health and social care. Technically correct procedures based upon sound and evidence-based research which have looked at normative results (from a group of studies) may or may not be applicable to all patients/

clients who are learning disabled and construct the world from a different viewpoint and life history. Compassion may then be about modifying the care to meet the requirements of the individuals within the boundaries of evidence-based research and guidelines.

Reader activity 1.8   Compassion for Colin

Read Colin's story again and look for signs of compassion towards him:

- By whom and what did the individuals do?
- Was there a motivation (personal or otherwise)?

Understanding

The ability to understand another person's wishes, thoughts and feelings is often termed empathy. However, the ability to base one's own attitudes (and ultimately your actions) towards a person in your care, regarding their individual needs can be governed by your internal drives but also the external pressures you face.

Reader activity 1.9   Understanding Colin

- What facts do you think the care team used as a basis for their understanding about Colin?
- What information would be useful for a new member of the team?

Confusion and misunderstanding arising from working with people with learning disabilities

Mutually agreed

To mutually agree with someone involves a degree of flexibility, time and patience. This can be best seen as when two or more people make a decision and agree an identified goal/task. People with learning disabilities can often be involved in decision-making processes, however, they may require information in accessible formats to assist them in decision-making to achieve mutually agreed goals.

Reader activity 1.10   Agreeing with Colin

- What type of agreements would you imagine benefited Colin?
- Was there ever a case for overruling his wishes in his best interests?
- If so, why?

Compliance

Compliance relates to how agreeable and amenable individuals are in response to requests to comply with an intervention. This may be seen as a measure of how compliant they are. Many factors can affect an individual's ability to comply such as:

- level of cognitive function;
- sensory impairments;
- understanding of messages being given to them.

Many professionals may not fully understand how the individual with a learning disability uses alternative means of communication. Non-compliance can be mistaken for non-communication of wishes.

> **Reader activity 1.11   Communicating compliance**

Find types of alternative communication methods that can be used by people with learning disabilities:

- MAKATON
- picture book and symbols
- total communication
- objects of reference.

Communication

Communication is the way in which we send and receive information to each other. Communication can be giving or receiving messages with or without words. There are many forms of communication, e.g. written, verbal and non-verbal, gestures, facial expressions and body language. People with learning disabilities often require accessible information in various formats to help them to communicate with others to the best of their abilities. Some individuals may use only non-verbal communication which can often be very subtle, these individuals are therefore reliant on those who know them well and can interpret the individual's non-verbal communication so that their needs can be fully understood and appropriately met.

Confusion and misunderstanding

For people with learning disabilities, confusion and misunderstanding are all too often a problem. The behaviour of many people with learning disabilities can be misunderstood and their behaviour can be seen as disruptive and non-compliant when in fact the problem lies with the person's learning disabilities or, in some instances, other people's failure to understand the person's learning disability and usual methods of communication. This is why it is important that the person with learning disabilities is well supported by someone who can advocate on their behalf in situations where issues may arise, e.g. appointments within mainstream services where the individual is in a strange place with staff they do not know.

Labelling

Labelling theory tells us that social groups have a tendency to focus upon a person's difference and to attribute a label to this difference, which means the person is viewed as an outsider (Goffman, 1968). Very often a person with a learning disability may behave in ways that make him or her appear non-compliant when they are confused and unable to communicate their wishes. This can lead to the label of having challenging behaviour. This type of label has connotations of violence and aggression. Once a person is given this label, they are treated as requiring extra care and special resources.

Reader activity 1.12 Being labelled 'challenging'

What do you consider to be the advantages and disadvantages of being labelled 'challenging' like Colin?

Conclusion

This chapter 'Ensuring dignity and respect' is the first Guiding Principle. Many of the concepts will be re-visited throughout the book as more complex situations are discussed. The case study on Colin offers some interesting opportunities to consider the concepts of human drives, motivations, dignity, respect and the confusion and misunderstandings that can occur in the practice of caring for people with complex needs. This chapter has outlined the theories and facts that will underpin all good health and social care. The personal considerations undertaken in the reader activities may have proved surprising to some and be a revision for others, but are useful reminders of the personal and professional obligations to all of those in our care and especially those people (with learning disabilities and in other vulnerable states) who find understanding and comprehension more difficult.

Points to remember

- Human drives and motivation are important considerations for all health and social care providers.
- Legal and moral explanations of dignity and respect form the basis of professional codes of conduct and also the obligations of services to provide appropriate care for all clients and service users.

- Basic principles of ethical behaviour are applied to all encounters in health and social care.
- Moral codes of beneficence and non-maleficence form the basis for action in health interventions and provide the underpinning guidelines for planning care.
- Care and compassion agendas are important and are benchmarks for good quality care.
- The personal consequences of one's actions should be considered by everyone.
- Labelling theory can help us avoid discriminatory practice and become aware of the principles of individualised care packages.

Resources and online support

The following resources are useful:
The British Association of Occupational Therapists and College Occupational Therapists has a code for all those registered with it.
http://www.cot.co.uk/standards-ethics/standards-ethics

CSP (the Chartered Society of Physiotherapy) provides a code of conduct for all registered practising physiotherapists working in the UK.
http://www.csp.org.uk/tagged/code-conduct

GMC (the General Medical Council) registers doctors to practise medicine in the UK. Its purpose is to protect, promote and maintain the health and safety of the public by ensuring proper standards in the practice of medicine.
http://www.gmc-uk.org/about/register_code_of_conduct.asp.

HCPC (the Health Care and Professionals Council) regulates healthcare, psychology and social work professionals in the UK. The HCPC provides a set of standards for the conduct and ethics of those registered with the Council.
www.hpcuk.org/aboutregistration/standards/standardsofconductperformanceandethics.

NMC (the Nursing and Midwifery Council) is the regulatory body for all registered nursing and midwifes working in the UK. The Code of Professional Conduct outlines the statutory duties of nurses and midwives. The NMC was established under the Nursing and Midwifery Order 2001 and came into being on 1 April 2002.
http://www.nmc-uk.org/Publications/Standards/The-code/Introduction/.

There are additional guidelines for the conduct of health and social care support workers working in England, Scotland and Wales:

http://www.wales.nhs.uk/sitesplus/829/page/49729.
http://www.cot.co.uk/regional-local-groups/healthcare-support-workers-code-conduct-and-employer-code-practice.

http://www.skillsforcare.org.uk/qualifications_and_training/Minimumtrainingstandardsandcode
ofconduct/Minimum_training_standards_and_code_of_conduct.aspx.
http://www.hcswtoolkit.nes.scot.nhs.uk/induction-standards--codes/standards--codes
http://www.niscc.info/Conduct-120.aspx.

References

Beck, R.C. (2003) *Motivation Theory and Principles*. Englewood Cliffs, NJ: Prentice Hall.

Bragg, R. (1998) *All over but the shoutin*. England: Vintage.

DH (Department of Health) (2010) *Essence of Care*. London: HMSO.

DH (Department of Health) (2012) *Transforming Care: A National Response to Winterbourne View Hospital*. London: Department of Health.

Dworkin, R. (1995) *Life's Domination*. London: HarperCollins.

Goffman, E. (1968) *Stigma: Notes on the Management of Spoiled Identity*. Englewood Cliffs, NJ: Prentice Hall.

Goldberg, L.R. (1991) Language and individual difference: the search for personality lexicons, in L. Wheeler (ed.) *Review of Personality and Social Psychology*, vol. 2. Thousand Oaks, CA: Sage.

Henry, A. (1990) *Kant's Theory of Freedom*. New York: Cambridge University Press.

Herzberg, F. (1968) One more time: how do you motivate employees? *Harvard Business Review*, 46: 53–62.

Locke, E.A. (1997) The motivation to work: what we know, in M.L. Maehr and P.R. Pintrich (eds) *Advances in Motivation and Achievement*. Greenwich, CT: JAI Press Inc, pp. 375–412.

Maslow, A. (1943) A theory of human motivation, *Psychological Review*, 50: 370–396.

Mencap (2007) *Death by Indifference: Following Up the Treat Me Right! Report*. Available at: www.mencap.org.uk.

Royal College of Nursing (2009) *Dignity in Healthcare for People with Learning Disabilities*, RCN Guidance. London: RCN.

Shotton, L. and Seedhouse, D. (1998) Practical dignity in caring, *Nursing Ethics*, 5(3): 246–255.

Tuckett, A.G. (2005) The Care Encounter: pondering caring, honest communications and control, *International Journal of Nursing Practice*, 11: 77–84.

Wilson, J.Q. (1989) *Bureaucracy: What Government Agencies Do and Why Do They Do It?* New York: Basic Books.

Guiding principle 2: The importance of providing accessible information for people with learning disabilities

Pamela Inglis and Su McAnelly

Learning outcomes

After reading this chapter you will be able to:

- develop an understanding of the legal and moral obligations of all services to provide accessible information
- consider ways information is currently delivered and assess the accessibility for users with communication problems
- identify strategies for communicating information.

Introduction

He appreciated my contribution, but he thought the way they all learn best was when they discussed it amongst themselves....

One of the major difficulties for people with a learning disability is not having access to information which is essential to us all. People with a learning disability require the same access to information as you and I, as part of our society and of local communities. This is not merely a moral obligation, but because of the Equality Act (2010), it is now unlawful to discriminate against learning disabled people. As a requirement of the Equality Act (2010) the need not to discriminate applies to nearly all organisations and services, for example:

- hotels
- shops
- restaurants
- government organisations such as local councils
- hospitals
- doctors surgeries
- the courts.

This list is not exhaustive, but shows that we have a responsibility to make ourselves clear in the way that we communicate with people with a learning disability.

Reader activity 2.1   Making ourselves clear

Think of how many ways we can communicate a welcome to someone. For example, through saying it, throwing a welcome home party, a banner, a smile . . .

Now consider how you might give directions to someone who is unfamiliar with a large building, and who does not understand English. You will use gestures, your eyes, you might draw a simple map.

We all use different types of communicating, all of the time, it is not just in the spoken or written word; there are many ways to communicate.

Overcoming difficulties accessing information

Mencap (2002) have guidelines on how we can make information more accessible to people with a learning disability. This is not that difficult and can be used for other groups of people for whom English is not their first language, and who have only a basic understanding of English.

Importantly, accessible written information should not be child-like. It is about making it clear, therefore Mencap (ibid.) recommend that to make written information accessible it should:

- be in simple, clear and jargon free language;
- contain short sentences;
- have additional supporting images.

Reader activity 2.2   The importance of information

- Make a list of all of the types of information that are essential to you in a day. Think about this from when you wake in the morning (for example, what time is it?) until you go to bed in the evening.
- If you did not have access to this information, how much more difficult would your day be? How many other ways could you find out this information?

Types of information that are essential

Similarly, people with a learning disability have to know the same kind of information as you do. They have to know the time to get up, they have to use public transport, they have to understand choices for lunch, etc. However, this information is not always available to a person with a learning disability who may have a poor understanding of English, either written or verbal.

Reader activity 2.3   Becoming clear

Take the list below and consider what you believe the important points might be to communicate to the person with a learning disability. For example, in medicines, you may think that it is not that important that the person knows why/how the medicine works, but that s/he knows how many tablets to take at what time every day.

Rights
Housing
Police
The law
Health promotion
Health records
In-patient rights.

Part of making ourselves understood is not giving information overload to people. This is true of anyone in our society. Therefore, we need to consider what the most important things to know are and then try to communicate this first. As in the example above, often it is very difficult to understand how medicines work; our doctor usually does not go into detail, but s/he might tell us what they are for, how often and how many to take and what the possible side-effects are. The most important information is then written in an information sheet inside the box, and the instructions for use and any cautions (such as 'while taking this medicine avoid alcohol') are printed on the front of the box. However, if it is difficult to understand complex English, then it might as well be printed in an alien language.

Using plain English

A good place to start to consider alternative written words, to make ourselves clearer is a document by the Plain English Campaign (2001), called *The A to Z of Alternative Words*.

Reader activity 2.4   Plain English

Find other clear and plain English words for the following:

acquiescence	appropriate	approximately	beneficial
competent	compulsory	deficiency	detrimental

eligible	exclude	facilitate	generate
hereby	implement	jeopardise	locality
mandatory	neglect	obligatory	prescribe
prohibit	reduction	regulation	scrutinise
subsequently	terminate	ultimately	virtually

It is important when making information accessible that we avoid commonly used 'official phrases' such as 'age-appropriate' and explain what we mean without using jargon.

Using clearer words is only one way in which we may make ourselves understood, we should also pay attention to how the information looks and reads. It is considered more engaging if the reader is spoken to directly in the text – using personal language such as 'we', 'yours', and 'our' is more comfortable for the reader and can aid understanding.

Make sure that you explain the meaning of any difficult words that you may have to use. It is also helpful to ask your target audience how to explain difficult words.

Case study 2.1 The Dictionary of Difficult Words

In a study for the Department of Health in 2008, researchers Dr Tina Cook and Dr Pamela Inglis worked with men with a learning disability to discover how research might be understood. It is difficult to discuss research without using the word 'research', and other difficult words. They all worked together on a 'dictionary of difficult words' associated with research. The men in the study were also researchers and they designed the dictionary throughout using pictures which they thought helped explain the word and also through clear explanations of what the word meant. Here is an example:

Deciding whether to take part

> Consent means agreeing to take part in research.
> Part of consent is deciding whether or not you want to agree to take part.

The explanation worked well because it was not merely Dr Cook and Dr Inglis explaining it, but the men themselves who advised on how to explain it. So well are the difficult terms explained, that this dictionary now forms part of the materials available to healthcare students when they are learning about research at Northumbria University.

It is also important that you are consistent with the words that you use throughout. Do not change words that mean the same thing. For example: if using the word 'prohibit', do not change to 'ban' or 'forbid'.

Finally, the use of numbers, graphs and percentages can be overwhelming in any text. When writing for people with a learning disability, it may be best not to use the word for the number but write it as '7'.

Additionally, if using percentages, instead of saying 54.3%, a clearer way of saying this is to write 'just over half'. And while diagrams do help to make clear what is being said, graphs may not be easily

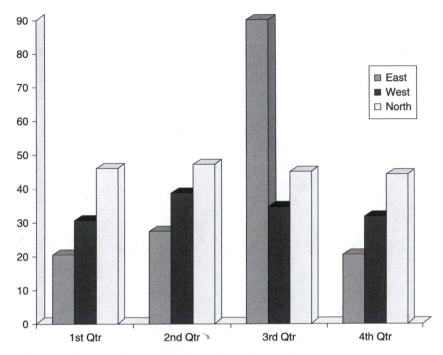

Figure 2.1 Example of information given in a graph

understood and may need to be explained (Figure 2.1). Instead of showing complicated graphs, you could say something like 'the east had the most'.

It is also important to ensure that you are writing, as you would speak, using sentences that are as short as possible. Additionally, do not use complex punctuation, such as semi–colons [;], as most people may not understand their usage. If your sentences are short and uncomplicated, then complex punctuation is not necessary.

Fast facts 2.1 A good practice guide

- Don't use jargon.
- Use plain English words and be consistent.
- If you must use jargon/difficult words, then provide an explanation of what those words mean.
- Don't include information that is not important, such as detail.
- Make the information flow, in a logical order.
- Use short sentences.
- Do not use complex punctuation.
- Use numbers not words.
- Avoid percentages and complex graphs, but explain the important bits.

Designing clear information

Consider how difficult and off-putting it is to receive lots of information, without breaks, pictures, tables, diagrams, etc. How many of us, for example, read all of the instruction leaflets that come with our mobile phones? Or the conditions and terms that we agree to when purchasing anything over the internet?

This information could easily be made clearer for us through how it is laid out and designed. Consider the 'quick start' booklets that many suppliers of electronic equipment provide, as they know that the average person will not use most of the information, or perhaps the technology that is possible – this is because this information is not accessible to us. It may be considered to be:

- too technical;
- too much to read;
- too long to read;
- boring.

To avoid this you should:

- Make sure that the text is broken into small important chunks.
- Use boxes, different colours, lists and bullet points to make the important information clear.
- Use titles and section headings to break up information and guide the reader through your work.
- Not hyphenate words or make points or sentences go over two pages, this can be confusing.
- Be consistent throughout.
- Use appropriate photographs, symbols or pictures to illustrate the text. Please see next section for further advice on this.

Reader activity 2.5   Quick starts

Find some instructions in your home (you have probably left them unopened in the box that your mobile phone or iPod/MP3 came with), and compare these to the 'quick start' booklet that they provide.

- How is this information different?
- List how the manufacturers make the 'quick start' booklet easier and more pleasurable to read.

There are certain rules that make information, no matter how technical, easier to understand. You will have listed them in the Reader activity 2.5.

Practice alert 2.1

- Do not write whole pages of dense text. Break it up with bullet lists or illustrations or boxes.
- Use large print to make things easier to see, and changing the size shows emphasis (Mencap recommend at least 12 point and 14 point for very important information). The font is important too – some fonts are much clearer than others to read, no matter what size the font is.
- Make sure that there is a good contrast between the colour of the print and the paper. Certain colours are better for individuals with poor sight and with some specific difficulties such as autism and dyslexia, and matt paper which is thick and does not show through the other side is essential for making text clear.
- Highlight what is important in the text through the font or bold, lists or bullet points. Underlining and block capitals are not advised.

Illustrating meaning

When using symbols, drawings and photographs, there are certain rules that you might apply. First, the images should go on the left and the text on the right; because in English, this is how the page is read. But more importantly the illustrations should be representative of whatever you are explaining. This should represent it in a clear way. The best way to help you choose clear and representative pictures is to ask the people who will be using the pictures. Asking the target audience is something marketing companies in our society do all the time, as when advertisements are aimed at women, they contain messages that are understood by women and include things that women relate to. Therefore, to ensure that the pictures or photographs are representative of the text and useful for wide access, then one should employ the help of the target audience.

Case study 2.2   Using pictures

The researchers with a learning disability working with Cook and Inglis (2008) helped to choose pictures that they thought would help people to understand the text, especially when they were describing difficult concepts such as research. Remember this study designed a pack to help people with a learning disability understand research and what questions to ask, etc. before they consented to, or took part in any research as participants or researchers.

They chose these pictures from clip-art to help to describe what research was – it used pictures and text and difficult words were in red so that the reader knew that those words were in the Dictionary of Difficult Terms that came with the pack:

It is a bit like being a detective.
You investigate the answers to questions.

(continued)

(continued)

Looking for clues

 Research helps you to answer questions and gather information.

Case study 2.3 is an extract from Cook and Inglis (2008, p. 53): these guidelines could help you consider the types of jargon you use in your communications with people with learning disabilities.

Case study 2.3   Jargon busting and difficult words

Jargon used in research may be discouraging for people who have had little opportunity to engage in research before.

> Do not use jargon, this is only a word that [the] university understands.
>
> (Peter, diary)

To understand more about research the men had to learn what certain terms meant and how certain words were used in the research context. Each time a word was not understood, it was discussed and 'translated'. For instance, the word 'consent' had not initially been understood, but after the men had watched the DVD, discussed different scenarios and talked together about it, they decided on a word that they would understand that meant the same thing.

> [On consent] Then we worked out that really, a shorter way of saying was that it was basically just to agree [to take part].
>
> (Alf)

Interviewer: And you keep saying you've got to document it. You've got to document it. What does document mean?
Respondent: Taking notes, Keith.

> Using pictures to represent a word or phrase did help understanding, as long as the same process in relation to recognising the meaning of the picture was undertaken as would be undertaken for the word. The picture used was agreed by the men on a consensus basis, but usually through checking that the man least able to understand the concept behind a word had understood what the picture represented.
>
> (Cook and Inglis, cited in DH, 2008, p. 53)

This showed how important it was to discuss, translate and represent words in order for people to fully understand. But difficult concepts may not be fully understood, or made understandable in a written or symbolic form. Sometimes it is necessary to enable people with a learning disability to learn in a constructive and 'recursive' way. The next section will discuss how this may be done successfully.

Using the principles of accessible information to help people with learning disabilities

The examples demonstrated in the study by Cook and Inglis (2008) show the ways in which you can help people with a learning disability to understand complex information.

> ### Reader activity 2.6   Understanding how people learn

Consider the example given in the Case study 2.4.

- Make notes.
- What surprised you?
- What methods were used to decide on the types of communication used?

Case study 2.4   Methodology

The men with learning disability in the study explained what had helped them learn best, about research, which is commonly described as a complex and often abstract concept to understand.

This study ensured that the men were co-researchers with Dr Inglis and Dr Cook, which meant that they had access to all of the information. They interviewed and worked hard at discovering and developing ways in which other people with a learning disability can understand research. Therefore, their understanding and informed consent were of huge importance to the study.

A CD was used, with all of the information read to them, as well as accessible text and illustrations in hard copy for information and consent forms. This enabled the men to listen to it at their own pace and to have the information in three different ways: written, pictorial and verbal, and this was reported as important to enabling their understanding and consent.

The men worked hard at explaining what in particular helped them to understand difficult concepts. They thought that what helped them most was the ways in which we all collaborated together. This included feeling that their opinion was important and also the ways in which we discussed complex concepts such as ethics. We did this in several ways and helped them to come to their own conclusions.

As they heard other opinions, this helped them to question their own understanding, enabling them to critique and assimilate understanding. One of the men stated:

> When we were discussing and debating stuff, during some of the discussion that we had, your mind slipped a few times before it settled. It's like you started it off and someone would say something. And it would be like, 'Erm, I'm not quite sure of . . .' And also then it started a bit of a debate up. And then by the time you finished the debate, you had most of the answers and then it was like, 'Eh, you know, we've just answered it.'

(David)

(continued)

(continued)

As the men's skills and knowledge developed, the men took over the facilitation of such discussions. So much so, that eventually:

> Keith has always been very positive about the benefits of working in a group. Today he said that although he appreciated my contribution, he thought the way they all learnt best was when they discussed it amongst themselves. The reason he gave for this, that he said quite proudly, was that they had learning disabilities and I hadn't. I wasn't in the club!
>
> (Researcher, field notes)

Another way of giving information was via a DVD, that was developed by the research team and a theatre company run by and for people with a learning disability. It showed six scenes about research, this was used to prompt discussion in a fun and interesting way. This also meant that we could repeat the DVD whenever we wanted to think about or talk about, for example, consent. The DVD was played at the beginning of each session, then a further scene was played cumulatively throughout the six sessions. This enabled the men to learn and to consolidate their learning, but was requested by the men, as we had originally intended to show one scene per week:

> In week three I noticed that there was a ripple of laughter about the joke in scene one [of the DVD]. They did not laugh when they saw it on week one. It has taken seeing it three times before they got the joke – before they understood. Glad the men asked to see all the scenes each week. If we had done it our way [each week only showing the scene relevant to the workshop materials], they would not have got it.
>
> (Researcher, field notes)

However, even though repetition was important to the men's understanding, it was not sufficient in itself, we also revisited complex concepts such as ethics in fun and interesting ways, enabling them to return to subjects and re-frame them and explore in more depth. We used role play, discussion, listening, sharing examples. We used pictorial representations and photographs to induce further discussion and understanding. One of the men commented:

> Because there was so much information to go through and so many angles and so much to discuss and talk about and come up with ideas for and think about. And you came to points where you were having to go away one week, come back next week and get just a bit more information and then go away again. And by the time you had finished it, you had, like, a mile-long list. And it was just incredible. And I did it and enjoyed it so much . . .
>
> (David)

In Figure 2.2 you can see that the men were given information in fun and interesting ways – hearing many views, using multiple ways to engage with materials, in a fun and collaborative way.

Then they had time in-between sessions (which were weekly) to think about what had been said, to discuss with the staff and each other, critiquing and assimilating what they had learned and to explore further through reading.

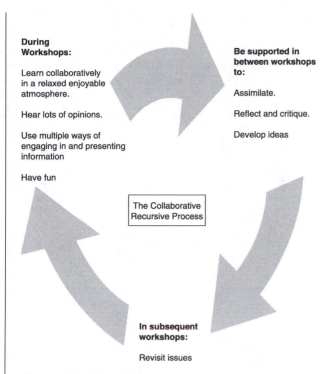

During
Workshops:

Learn collaboratively
in a relaxed enjoyable
atmosphere.

Hear lots of opinions.

Use multiple ways of
engaging in and presenting
information

Have fun

Be supported in
between workshops
to:

Assimilate.

Reflect and critique.

Develop ideas

The Collaborative
Recursive Process

In subsequent
workshops:

Revisit issues

Figure 2.2 The collaborative recursive process

The next week the men returned to the information, in other ways and the men particularly found the recursive nature important, and we built upon their previous knowledge and the recursive cycle began again. The following is a sample of the things they said:

That it was over six weeks and then had time to think about it after the six sessions.

Liked repetition.

Being in a group . . .

Jotting it down at the time and reading about it later helped me to go over it . . . I can look at it and think about it every day.

(Alf, diary)

Reader activity 2.7   Consider the key points

You have now read the quotations about the processes from a group of men who engaged in an exercise to provide them with assessable information. What do you consider are the key messages that we can take from this?

More information about accessible writing and images

Gilliford (2001), in his examination of access to healthcare, made a distinction between *having* access and *gaining* access. The former was taken to mean that a suitable service was available and physically accessible, whereas *gaining* access is when the user successfully gains entry into and uses a service appropriate to their needs. This distinction can equally be applied to accessing healthcare information, which, though it might be available, does not necessarily mean that the people can easily gain access to it.

The four major dimensions of access were defined as:

- wider determinants of health (pre-existing factors determining health and social policies affecting the health and well-being of the population);
- identification of need (personal recognition);
- organisation of healthcare (physical access dimensions);
- entry access (first contact health services, e.g. GPs) and continuing access (second or further contact health services).

Conclusion

The importance of considering all aspects of communication and the likelihood of it becoming inaccessible cannot be understated. In addition, the consequence of providing information which can mislead or cause confusion is both a moral and a legal issue for organisations and also individuals working with people with learning disabilities/difficulties. As people with learning disabilities are likely to access a number of social and healthcare environments containing a variety of services, the obligation is for all services to work hard to make their information written or otherwise as accessible as possible. You will learn in the next chapters of the book about various ways in which services can make adjustments in large and small ways which make a difference to the health and the social lives of people with learning disabilities, these often begin with accessible information.

You have seen from the study reported in this chapter that engaging and collaborating with groups of people with learning disabilities can provide useful ways to make services more accessible and also help the development of new services which meet the needs of service users more effectively.

Points to remember

- We have a moral and legal duty to make important information accessible for people with a learning disability.
- Do not make the message child-like, this is not necessary or helpful to adults with a learning disability.
- One way of communicating, such as using text, is usually not enough especially if the information is complex.
- We have to be creative and clear when communicating important information.
- Only use important information, detail is not always necessary.

- Make sure that the text is broken into small important chunks.

  - Use plain English, no jargon.
  - Use short sentences.
  - Do not use complex punctuation.
  - Use numbers not words.
  - Avoid percentages and complex graphs, but explain the important bits.
  - You can use boxes, different colours, lists and bullet points to make the important information clear.

- When using symbols, drawings and photographs, the images should go on the left and text on the right; this is because in English, this is how the page is read.
- Make sure that the target audience is involved in the design.
- Discuss, translate and represent words in order for people with learning disabilities to fully understand.

Reader activity 2.8   Test yourself quiz

- Which organisations does the Equality Act (2010) apply to?
- Which types of information need to be made accessible?
- What simple rules can you apply to written information to make it accessible to everyone?
- What are the implications of types of information being inaccessible?
- What sort of 'official type' words can be misunderstood?
- Which techniques for designing clear information would be the most successful for people with learning disabilities?
- Why is it important to collaborate with target groups such as people with learning disabilities?

Resources

BILD (British Institute of Learning Disabilities) is an organisation that promotes and develops learning resources, training and research, aimed at those working with people with learning disabilities. BILD's guidelines to health issues in accessible formats and EASY-TO-READ formats are found at: http://www.bild.org.uk/easy-read/.

The Equality Act (2010). This Act is the guiding force behind the statutory obligations of organisations to provide information which can be accessed by service users.
http://www.legislation.gov.uk/ukpga/2010/15/contents.

A simple guide to the Equality Act is found at:
http://www.equalityhumanrights.com/uploaded_files/EqualityAct/equality_act_employment_easyread.pdf.

Mencap (2002) *Am I Making Myself Clear? MENCAP's Guidelines for Accessible Writing*. London: Mencap. Mencap Accessibility Unit. This is an invaluable and essential resource which collates up-to-date guidelines and resources.
www.accessibility@mencap.org.uk.

Plain English Campaign. This organisation aims to make information accessible and understandable. http://www.plainenglish.co.uk/.

Cook, T. and Inglis, P. (2008). This research-driven report provides health and social services with guidelines about how to engage service users in the development of accessible information.

References

Cook, T. and Inglis, P. (2008) Participatory research with men with a learning disability, *Tizard Learning Disability Review*, 17(2).

Gilliford, M. (2002) What does 'access to health care' mean? *Journal of Health Service Research and Policy*, 7(3): 186–188.

Mencap (2002) *Am I Making Myself Clear? MENCAP's Guidelines for Accessible Writing*. London: Mencap.

3

Guiding principle 3: Providing equal access to services for people with learning disabilities

Pamela Inglis, Andrew Stafford and Kaydii Inglis

Learning outcomes

After reading this chapter you will be able to:

- appreciate the complex politics surrounding people with a learning disability and their care
- understand the effects of social attitude upon the care of people who are vulnerable in our society
- develop an understanding of the different barriers experienced by people with learning disabilities.

Introduction

A closed door may as well be a locked door if someone cannot physically open it.

Very often people with a learning disability do not have access to important aspects of life such as friendships, relationships, housing, medical treatment and information. Society treats these people in a certain way. There are certain models that society uses to deal with people with a learning disability and these are discussed in this chapter.

Case study 3.1   The Health Facilitation Team

A gentleman with a (moderate) learning disability and some behaviour which might present a challenge to healthcare access, as well as a mental health issue, was introduced to the Health

(continued)

(continued)

Facilitation Team (HFT). This gentleman was to be placed on a medication for his mental health issue which required monthly blood tests to monitor the levels of the drug in his bloodstream. Unfortunately, he was so anxious about having blood taken that he was unable to have his bloods taken by the clinic or by his practice nurse. This proved a huge obstacle to his good health.

The HFT then were asked to become involved as it was dangerous for him to continue with the medication if he could not have his blood monitored. Therefore, his mental health issue worsened. A member of the HF team visited the gentleman in his own home where he was comfortable and began a desensitisation programme.

This meant that she worked with the gentleman and the staff who cared for him and she chose a quiet time of day, a time when he was least anxious and with the staff he liked the best, and she gradually introduced the equipment for taking bloods, without him becoming anxious about it. This built up after careful planning to an ability to take bloods in his own home.

The HFT then trained and educated the local district nursing teams in the techniques, and in the ways in which the gentleman's bloods could be taken without inducing anxiety. The district nurse was also introduced to the gentleman who now successfully takes his blood monthly, so that his mental health may be safely treated by drugs.

Reader activity 3.1 Understanding other world views

Imagine having all of the information you hear and read every day to be written in a different language – one that you do not understand.

Now begin on a typical morning and imagine going throughout the day without understanding what is being said. For example, would you understand the morning news? Would you know which bus to get? Or understand the time to know when to leave?

Write down all of the problems that this would cause you until you go to bed that night. This will give you a snapshot of the difficulties experienced by people with a learning disability every day.

The important thing to remember is that most of the problems regarding access to the important things in our lives are not because of the person's learning disability, but because we as a society do not enable equal access to services, etc. for people who have particular difficulties. Please bear this in mind when reading the following section on the politics of learning disability. The later sections will use accessibility to good quality healthcare as an example of barriers and how to overcome them, for people with a learning disability.

The personal tragedy model

One of the ways in which we may set people apart is through a notion called the personal tragedy model. Personal tragedy is a discourse that views disability as an individual tragedy, not a social or political issue (Shakespeare, 1999; French and Swain, 2008), and enables us to treat people with a learning disability with pity and to control important aspects of their lives (Oliver, 1990). The centre of this difference is viewed as being within the person. In the treatment of people with a learning disability this has historically meant differentiation between people on the basis of different types of impairment. People with learning disability were separated from society and lived in huge institutions, and then separated from others with learning disability because they were 'cared for' in large houses that specialised in a particular impairment, such as epilepsy or profound disability. Such oppressive ways of viewing people encourage paternalistic and charitable interventions in people's lives by virtue of the fact of their impairment and the idea that they cannot care for themselves, or make decisions. This can sometimes be seen as positive for the staff caring for people with a learning disability as it may increase professional feelings of competence, caring and control, but does little for the quality of life of people treated in this way (Goodley, 1998).

Reader activity 3.2   You decide

In your adult life you will make many decisions alone and some that you will discuss with your friends and family. However, imagine that you could not make any decisions for yourself and those friends and family had to make all your decisions for you.

Taking a typical day, list some of the decisions that they will have to make. For example, when you got up, what you had for breakfast, what clothes you will wear, who you could see, where you could go, what time you go to bed, etc.

- Which decisions would you gladly hand over?
- Which ones might you share with someone?
- Which decisions would mean a great deal of difficulty for you if the decision was not to your liking?

Of course we all make decisions that our friends and family are involved in. If you choose to ask people to help you with a decision because you trust them, or they may know more about the issue, that's great. Few of us make all our decisions independently. The vital difference here is choice – people with a learning disability may not choose that such decisions be made on their behalf, but often have little say in this.

Normality, in this model, is defined by the non-disabled – and impairment is judged as a personal loss and a tragedy (Shakespeare, 1999). If you accept this view of learning disability, then this means that people who are judged as not being normal can be pitied and treated differently to others.

The medical model

The medical model classifies people according to the type and severity of their impairment; they do not have epilepsy, but become epileptic; they do not have impaired leg movement but become cripples. One characteristic that they have, their impairment, becomes the whole of what that person is defined as; just as in the personal tragedy model it sees difference as being within the person, and as something that is likened to a sickness or disease.

Erving Goffman (1961) studied the treatment of people in long-stay institutions and found that people were treated badly there. The institutions had many rules which were needed, it was argued, as medical therapy. Goffman thought that this was not true, and that the rules and regulations were the exercising of power by the medical staff there. He described the insular world experienced by the patients which meant that people living in long-stay hospitals became a number, rather than the separate personality they once were. These conditions were created, not always because of nurses and carers who were uncaring, but by overcrowding in under-stimulating environments, by lack of privacy and individual care, by lack of communication skills, by segregation of the sexes, by poor staff attitudes, by the labelling of people and by a consistent denial of individual needs.

Things slowly began to change in the mid-twentieth century when new ideas and disciplines were emerging, together with adverse reports from the long-stay hospitals and pluralist groups (Globe, 2008). In 1958, Jacques Tizard, a psychologist, placed children previously living in institutions in Brooklands House. The results of the experiment showed improvements in the cognitive ability and behaviour of the children, demonstrating that children raised in a more ordinary environment with more staff and a stimulating lifestyle would learn and develop; evidence of the harm of living in institutions was beginning to emerge. Later the United Nations Declaration of Rights of the Disabled (1971 and 1975), and *Better Services for the Mentally Handicapped* (DHSS, 1971), stated automatic hospitalisation should cease. This set out the framework for the relocation of people back into their local communities through maintaining that their local authorities had the duty to provide them with suitable accommodation. Following this, the National Development Group (1977) *Helping Mentally Handicapped People in Hospital* commented:

> [There are] 50,000 people living in hospitals, 20,000 of them have been there for more than 20 years . . . Anyone who looks at mentally handicapped hospitals today, cannot help but be struck by the discrepancy between the quality of life of the general population and that of the mentally handicapped hospital residents . . . The physical conditions under which mentally handicapped people are expected to live and work for year after year, have long been regarded as unacceptable for the rest of society . . . This comment has been reinforced many times by the media.

These were strong words and some believed that the hospitals would have to close immediately. However, 30 years later there were still people living in long-stay hospitals.

To an extent, such medical practices still occur today within some treatment and residential services, where people with behavioural or mental health needs, or people who have an autistic spectrum disorder, live together because of this diagnosis, rather than because they choose to live together. Currently, only 6 per cent of people with a learning disability have a choice of who they live with (DH, 2001).

Whether 'learning disability' is an absolute at all has long been debated (Brechin and Walmsley, 1989) and, in fact, in 1969 the American Association on Mental Deficiency (AAMD) placed the threshold for learning disability at an IQ of 85, 1 standard deviation away from the normal score (set at 100). This meant that 16 per cent of the population was considered to have a learning disability (Smith, 1976). This was subsequently re-thought in 1973, moving the threshold to two standard deviations from normal and learning disability was then defined as occurring at an IQ score of 70 or below (the threshold for learning disability today), and 2.25 per cent of the population was now categorised as having a learning disability (ibid.). Overnight nearly 14 per cent of Americans no longer had a learning disability – this constitutes an enticing argument for the social construction of learning disability.

During the 1970s, Wolf Wolfensberger was developing and refining his ideas on normalisation. He and others proposed that services should change so that people living in the institutions would be enabled to live a life close to the 'normal' enjoyed by the rest of society as possible (Globe, 2008). These ideas were based upon human rights and role theory.

Reader activity 3.3　How normal are we?

In Table 3.1 list what is normal and what is not normal – we have started you off.

Table 3.1 Definitions of normal and not normal

Normal	Not normal
2 arms and legs	4 legs
Being employed	Being unemployed
Abiding by the law	Criminal behaviour

There are lots of things you can comment on: weight, size, sexuality, religion, even age.

Now, take another look at your list, are there any cultures or times in history when the normal was not normal today?

Do the same, looking at when or where the not normal items may now be considered normal.

An example would include the normal notion of women working outside of the home, in other cultures, and not so long ago in our western culture, women working outside of the home was not considered normal.

Social role valorisation

Historically, social role valorisation (SRV) has impacted positively upon the lives of some people with a learning disability, who had previously lived in appalling conditions in institutions, but it has been criticised heavily almost since its conception (Gates and Beacock, 1997; Wolfensberger, 1998; Atherton, 2003). SRV is an ideology which is based upon the premise that people are devalued because they have more negative social roles than positive roles in society (Wolfensberger, 1998).

Reader activity 3.4　Role play

- List the positive and negative roles that you play in society. For example, my list may read something like Table 3.2, depending on who was writing it.
- Which of your roles do you think may be possible for people with a learning disability?

- Write a list for someone you know with a learning disability.
- How does this list differ from yours?

Table 3.2 Positive and negative role models

Positive		Negative
Mother	Nurse	Disciplinarian
Daughter	Wife	Unapproachable
Doctor	Lecturer	Academic supervisor

SRV suggests that changes in the behaviour of disabled people will lead to more positive social acceptance. Importantly, this message is about changing the behaviour of people with learning disability in order to be accepted by society, not about changing society. It proposes that certain groups of people in our society are devalued by the society because they do not fit in. Central to this belief is the proposal that these devalued groups can be elevated in the eyes of society, through increasing their valued roles and decreasing their devalued roles, by normalising themselves through skill acquisition and thus demonstrating to society that they are not that different from them – hence, this belief is often referred to as normalisation.

However, this presumes that people with a learning disability understand that they are not accepted by society and that they wish to be accepted and, further, that society will indeed include people with a learning disability if they appear to have more positive roles. Importantly, this model did not emerge from disabled people, but from academics and professionals. This is apparent in the views expressed within SRV. For example, it is society's values of independence, not disabled people's views, that SRV promotes; disabled people may have a completely different view of independence. For example, many people rely on others to live day to day; celebrities have entourages of people who care for their nutrition, their hair, who dress them, make their appointments, answer their mail, etc. – meaning they are not independent, but they are clearly still valued by society. As Martin Levine states:

> I may need help with some things but I'm not retarded. I can take care of myself . . . Everyone needs help. Some people need more. Even the ones on the outside – the normal people, have marriage counsellors and other people to help them.
>
> (Martin Levine, in Friedman-Lambert, 1987, cited in Goodley, 2001, p. 124)

In fact, disabled people may believe other values to be more important than independence. For example, having friends and family around them or being able to enjoy playing their own type of music in peace may be more important to people with learning disability than independence.

Wolfenberger's work appears to be based heavily in theory and its claims to be scientific are questionable (Robinson, 1989). Despite this, it impacts greatly upon some people with disability (PWD) whereby the carers for PWD spend a great deal of their time helping people to acquire skills that they may, or may not, wish to acquire in order to increase the likelihood of acceptance of people with learning disabilities into society. In doing so, they can generate immense pressures to achieve upon learning disabled people.

Current literature argues that using SRV as a model for all learning disabled people may not be ideal, but is still imposed by carers, integrated into current professional education, and its concepts and principles are still expressed in policies and legislation (Gates and Beacock, 1997; Atherton, 2003).

Therefore, one can imagine that it is the dominant beliefs of the time, that affect the way in which society acts upon PWD. What is important is that throughout the literature people with a learning disability have historically had little say about the beliefs and models affecting them, as these models originate from and are developed by academics and professionals, which is clearly unacceptable:

> The problem with that lot was that they'd never had a Down's Syndrome baby. 'Normal people' were in the association, I was the only one with Down's Syndrome working in that office for ten years.
>
> (Anya Sousa, cited in Goodley, 2001, p. 129)

The social model

Challenges to academic beliefs essentially began with the Union of the Physically Impaired Against Segregation (UPIAS, 1976) which was a group of disabled people in the 1970s who produced 'Fundamental Principles' that showed the way for the emancipation of people with impairments. This document was very influential in defining the social model of disability and the social oppression discourse.

The social oppression discourse is an alternative to the presentation of disability as an individualised problem, it proposes the idea that disability itself has been constructed as a form of social problem; much as how learning disability was reconstructed in America in 1973. Society, they argue, makes them disabled, not their impairment. It is through issues ranging from attitudes through to more practical things such as access to public transport and segregated schooling that disables them, not the impairment. It is living in a society constructed by and for non-disabled people that disables people with impairments (Oliver, 1991).

Reader activity 3.5   Beginning to create a new world view

Think about your favourite shop. Imagine you were in a wheelchair and had to access that shop alone, it may help to consider the following:

- How might you enter?
- Can you see and read/appreciate information or art on the walls of the shop?
- Can you see over counters?
- Can you see all of the goods for sale?
- How easy is it to get around that shop?
- How might people treat you differently?

These are all issues with the way that the shop and our society are constructed. If everything was developed only for people using wheelchairs, the world would look really different – the doors and ceilings might be lower, there would be ramps instead of steps and anyone without a wheelchair would look out of place, they would bang their heads on the ceiling and be viewed as different and a problem when accessing shops.

The negative ideas surrounding people with disabilities are challenged by the social model. Theorists, like Oliver (1990), draw our attention to the perceptions that society has about disabled people, commonly seen in terms of problems, and an inability to function normally. Disabled writers point out that even though they are classed as disabled they lead perfectly happy, useful and fulfilled lives (Swain and French, 2000). A disabled person may need 24-hour help in their everyday tasks, but this does not mean that their lives are not fulfilled. This is a judgement placed upon them by society; a value judgement based on someone else's experience. Their experiences may be different from most in our society, yet can still be fulfilling and valuable.

Throughout the 1980s and into the 1990s, changes through the Mental Health Act (1983) (MHA) developed new definitions and terminology and produced a code of conduct and guidelines for people using the MHA. But people with learning disabilities continued to be seen as a subset of those people termed 'mental' (Beacock, 2005). The Community Care Act (1990) set out the ways in which people should be better cared for within the community, rather than within specialist institutions. In 2001, the government released the first White Paper for 30 years on mental health: *Valuing People: A New Strategy for Learning Disability for the 21st Century* (DH, 2001). It was developed in consultation with some people with a learning disability and looked at the current problems and challenges: ageing, housing, employment services, quality, supporting carers and delivering change for the better. Implicit within *Valuing People* are the principles of SRV and the social model of health and disability. It added some value to *Better Services* (1971), but unfortunately called for similar actions to those expressed 30 years earlier, suggesting a lack of progress in the care and treatment of people with a learning disability in our society.

The affirmation model

The affirmation model (Swain and French, 2000) is a model that emerged from the disability literature and movement and has a positive view of disability and a proud group identity. Here, the differentness of people with a learning disability is celebrated, and sameness is not necessary. Importantly, this model emerged from the views of disabled people and here the beliefs and ideas reflect the view that people who are disabled do not have to change; and accordingly its implications for nursing practice differ from SRV. The affirmation model proposes that the solution for disabled people being devalued does not lie merely with a change of behaviour on the part of disabled people (as SRV suggests), but with the re-framing of their experience, for the eyes of everyone in society, in a more positive light.

The affirmative model of disability directly opposes the personal tragedy view of disability, and argues that having impairments can have benefits. The literature discusses cases of disabled people who have received a better education and escaped poor backgrounds because of their disability.[1] They take a different view in many respects from Wolfensberger (1988) in that, instead of attempting to impose social values to make people fit in, Swain and French (2000) argue that disability should include positive social identities of differentness. Disabled people do not need to change; but their experiences need to be re-evaluated by society in positive terms (ibid.).

Reader activity 3.6   Being positive

- List the reasons why you want to work with or care for someone who has a learning disability.
- List the positive aspects of having a learning disability.
- List the benefits our society might gain in changing to enable equal access for people with a learning disability.

Work by self-advocates (self-advocates are people with a learning disability who speak up on their own behalf, and sometimes on behalf of other disabled people) shows how people with learning disability can build strong, positive identities. The standards of this group do not necessarily have to reflect those of society, which include valuing youth, intellect, beauty and wealth. Such a positive and proud group identity, which has enabled the disabled movement to create positive images of and for themselves, enabled them to be equal *and* different. In line with affirmative models, carers should not only acknowledge value in difference, but champion it; relinquishing their power and responsibility to the independent choices of people with a learning disability (Inglis *et al.*, 2004).

Practice alert 3.1

- Always remember that how we describe people is very important, as it can lead to differential and often negative treatment.
- Always remember that learning disability is not a fixed condition, and is a constructed concept, developed by a world designed for people without a learning disability.
- Always remember that people with a learning disability may not be unhappy about having a learning disability, but may dislike the way that they are treated because they have a learning disability.
- While not ignoring the disadvantages people suffer because of having a learning disability, always be aware of the positive aspects of learning disability.

The next section will use health as an example of how we can bring about equal access to the important things in life, for people with a learning disability.

Health

It is widely acknowledged that people with a learning disability have greater health needs than the rest of the population, yet receive poor treatment from healthcare services. Hospital staff have a scant understanding of the needs of people who have a learning disability and can fail to provide necessary care:

- Nearly two out of every three carers are required to stay in hospital to support patients. Sometimes they are treated poorly, i.e. denied food and drink.

- Women with learning disabilities are commonly left out of health screening programmes such as breast and cervical cancers. The national uptake in the UK for the general population is 76 per cent and 85 per cent respectively. For women who have a learning disability, it is 50 per cent and 8 per cent.
- Uptake in services such as audiology is poor (8 per cent compared to 82 per cent in the general population).

People with a learning disability have the same rights as everyone else under the Human Rights Act 1998, and this means that services will have to change as commonly people with a learning disability may have communication difficulties and difficulty in recognising or expressing emotions, such as pain and discomfort.

Fast facts 3.1   Common co-existing conditions

PWD also have complex needs associated with common co-existing conditions (Table 3.3).

Table 3.3 Common co-existing conditions

Disability	Having a co-existing condition (%)
Physical disability	20–30
Epilepsy	15–30 (with 10% borderline)
Sensory impairment	30–40
Mental health disorder	6–10
Severe challenging behaviour	6

Source: Sign and Mental Health Foundation (2006); DH (1996, 2002).

In fact, while the life span in the general population is getting longer, the learning disabled population are more likely to die before the age of 50 and causes differ from the rest of the population.

Fast facts 3.2   The common health needs for people with a learning disability

People with a learning disability are:

- Three times more likely to die from respiratory disease.
- At higher risk of coronary heart disease (second most common cause of death).
- At risk of cardiac anomalies in specific syndromes (such as Down's Syndrome).
- At higher risk of gastrointestinal cancer and stomach disorders (gastric, oesophageal and gall bladder cancer are the most common).
- At higher risks of respiratory disorders – higher death rates associated with pneumonia, swallowing problems and asthma (early age) – the highest cause of death.

- At higher risks of dementia (22 per cent of people with a learning disability compared to 6 per cent of the general population).
- At higher risks of thyroid disorders (in fact, this is 55 per cent in people with Down's Syndrome).
- Younger when diagnosed with osteoporosis.
- At higher risks of sensory deficits (40 per cent have hearing problems); 4 per cent compared with 2–7 per cent of the general population.
- At higher risks of poor dental care – 36.5 per cent of adults with a condition and 80 per cent of adults with Down's Syndrome have unhealthy teeth and gums.
- At higher risks of weight anomalies – more likely to be under- or over-weight.
- At higher risks of behaviour which challenges service provision – 12–17 per cent.
- At higher risk of self-injury (highest rates of self-injury – 17.4 per cent with 1.7 per cent being severe and frequent).
- At higher risks of poor sexual health – low uptake in screening by women with learning disability. There are also higher rates of sexual abuse.
- At least 1 in 3 have problems with their mental health including:

  - Schizophrenia (3 per cent compared to 1 per cent of the general population).
  - Anxiety is more common among this group.
  - Depression (22 per cent compared to 5.5 per cent of the general population).
    (Barr *et al.*, 1999; DH, 2001; MENCAP, 2004, 2007; UKLDCNN, 2005; Commissioning Services DH, 2007; Michael, 2008).

There is an assumption that people with a learning disability have greater health needs because of their learning impairment. However, there is evidence to suggest that on the contrary, it is more to do with the social aspects affecting people with a learning disability, rather than physical aspects of some syndromes, for example, that are related to learning.

Fast facts 3.3   The social issues

The social issues include:

- Lack of choice and a reliance on others to create healthy opportunities.
- Little access to relevant health promotion information, which is not always in an easy-to-read format.
- Discrimination.
- Others' assumptions and attitudes.
- Poor access to healthcare.
- Environmental pressure.
- Traumatic life events.
- Psychological distress.

(continued)

(continued)

- Social restrictions.
- Social isolation.
- Stress.
- Poverty.
- Being part of a disadvantaged group.
- Barriers to good health such as poor diet or lack of accessible health information.
- Having few resources (such as friends and colleagues) to call upon in times of need.
- Having poor experiences of health services which may dissuade them from accessing services in the future.
- Having poor support networks, and few relationships, which lead to isolation and can be precursors for mental health issues.
- Additionally, they also tend to live in poverty (as they may not have access to employment), which includes poor housing.
- They may be put off visiting health professionals because of difficulty in accessing services, such as screening, nutrition, immunisation, contraception, exercise and life-style factors, such as smoking cessation.

Health information surrounds the general population, everywhere we turn; written, verbal, TV ads – but this may not be accessible for people with a learning disability to understand.

Other important barriers to accessing good healthcare are related to the healthcare they receive, and healthcare practitioners, rather than their learning impairment. Here issues are mainly something called diagnostic overshadowing. This is where healthcare practitioners believe that the presenting problems or symptoms are a feature of the learning disability, rather than ill health, therefore, the diagnosis of learning disability overshadows the diagnosis of ill health.

Case study 3.2   Overshadowing

A gentleman with severe learning disability had begun vomiting, had become very lethargic, and was unable to express any other symptoms, such as pain, that he may have been feeling. He was taken to his GP who suggested that it was a behavioural issue, and the man was inducing his vomiting, and that he was 'acting himself' by not doing what he was asked to do by his carers. This eventually got worse until he was still vomiting and not able to eat food.

Eventually he was so poorly that he was taken to the local Accident and Emergency hospital. He was given antibiotics for a week and recovered. This story could have ended very differently – by making an assumption that it was a behavioural issue because of his learning disability, rather than ill health. The GP blamed his symptoms on his behaviour, and therefore allowed the gentleman's' learning impairment diagnosis to overshadow other symptoms, and did not carry out any physical tests, but suggested that he should see a psychologist!

Thankfully, this particular episode ended well, but still meant that the gentleman was dehydrated, malnourished and in pain, for much longer than he should have been, had he not had a GP who considered his learning disability to be the main issue in his life.

- How do you think you might know that a person with a learning disability, who did not have verbal communication skills, was unwell?
- Find out if there are tools that might help you.
- Look up the Dis Dat tool on the web at: http://www.stoswaldsuk.org/adults/professionals/ disdat/Background%20to%20DisDAT/. This is a tool to aid in observing and identifying distress cues in people who have a learning disability.

A report was published in 2008 after a public inquiry into the early and unnecessary deaths of six people with a learning disability in England (Mencap, 2007). The authors of the report talked to many people: professionals, families, carers and of course people with a learning disability, and showed that there were many faults with the healthcare system in our country. This report is often referred to as the Michael Report (as Sir Jonathan Michael headed the Inquiry) but it was actually called: *Healthcare for All: Report of the Independent Inquiry into Access to Healthcare for People with Learning Disabilities*, July 2008, available at: www.iahpld.org.uk.

It made ten recommendations which the government agreed with. The first was about the education of staff to work with people with a learning disability. All healthcare staff should be appropriately educated and supported in practising in a non-discriminatory way, and this education should include the authentic involvement of people with a learning disability (Michael, 2008).

The law also tells us that we have to adjust services and organisations to fulfil their requirements under the Equality Act 2010 (formerly the Disability Discrimination Act, 1995) and offer people with a learning disability the following:

- accessible information;
- longer and accessible appointments;
- identification of learning disability;
- appropriate treatment when accessing generic services.

The services should provide proactive identifications of health problems through the inclusion of people with learning disability in their screening programmes.

- They should address health inequalities.
- They should reduce the gap in life expectancy.

Unfortunately, the latest report on unnecessary deaths of people with a learning disability states that there are currently 75 avoidable deaths identified. This number is expected to grow (Mencap, 2012).

What is really helpful for people with a learning disability and their health is if they have or someone who cares for them has a record of their baseline clinical vital observations, such as blood pressure, temperature and pulse. These may be taken by a practice nurse, at the GP or by electronic machines which can be purchased in any chemist. This is especially pertinent to people with a profound or severe learning disability and may give the first clue to their impending ill health. Further, it greatly helps any physician attempting to diagnose ill health, when they have an accurate record of their normal vital signs.

> ## Practice alert 3.2
>
> - Always remember that people with a learning disability have a legal and moral right to good quality healthcare.
> - Remember that people with a learning disability are not always able to describe and communicate symptoms of illness.
> - Remember that not all professionals understand what having a learning disability means for the person and the carers/family and should see the person and not the disability.
> - Do not confuse having a learning disability with physical ill health, or disease.
> - Use different forms of communication, and ensure that the information is without jargon, clear and brief.
> - Ensure that people with a learning disability have their vital signs checked at least twice a year – monthly is even better. This enables physicians to know what their normal state of health is. And as they give vital clues to one's general health – if taken regularly, such as monthly – can also help to identify any physical health problems sooner rather than later.

Getting it right

There are lots of ways in which people with a learning disability can gain access to quality health services, and this can be successful across many levels. Such as at a governmental level (for example, the Equality Act 2010) through offering incentives to GPs to deliver annual health checks, and through taking part in local health boards and committees with influence. People with a learning disability should be included in all health improvement initiatives.

But what is most important for this chapter is what can be achieved on an individual level for a person who has a learning disability. First, and what may be very beneficial to the individual and their carers/family, is ensuring that the person with a learning disability has access to specialist services when required, this can be done through contacting your local learning disability community nursing team.

This team is able to help with aspects of physical and mental health through actions, such as assessments, monitoring, clinical interventions and referral to specialist teams.

Additionally, there are health facilitation nurses who offer important access to acute and primary healthcare. They also help with health action planning and provide annual health checks for people with a learning disability.

Health action plans offer the individual an opportunity to access comprehensive assessment and planning for their physical health need – this can be anything from dental to podiatry needs. Health action plans are reviewed annually and offer guidance for healthcare practitioners in primary care working with the individual, but also supply information for the individual, their carers and family. And this aids good access to healthcare (note that is not always a nurse who develops a health action plan).

These examples and suggestions show that there are specialists who may help to ensure that people with a learning disability have good access to quality healthcare. And as individuals we can access such experts.

However, it is important that the individual has access to health information and health promotion too. The specialists may also help with this, but on an individual level there is much that can be done, such as developing interesting and fun ways of enabling people with a learning disability to access health promotion materials.

Reader activity 3.8 Dental care

- Think of ways in which you might encourage someone with a learning disability to brush their teeth twice a day.
- Consider how you may show the importance of teeth cleaning.
- What type of information might you use?
- What might you use to present the information in a clear and understandable way?
- What could you use as encouragement?

Conclusion

This chapter has taken the reader through a historical journey of the ways in which people with a learning disability have been treated in our society, and the negative effects that this has had upon them. Such effects include poor health and barriers to good quality and timely healthcare.

It is important that we treat people as individuals, with specific wants and needs, that we help them to access the same benefits as others in society and that we know when we might have to ask for help from specialists such as learning disability nurses. However, the real message of the chapter is one of how we might positively affect the lives of people with a learning disability whom we know and care for. These changes are often simple and practical, but are also our legal and moral duty.

Points to remember

- People with a learning disability have the same legal and moral rights as everybody else.
- Most of the issues about accessing good services, relationships and employment, etc. are not because people have a learning disability, but because our society is designed in such a way as to develop barriers for them to access things like information, choices, good quality services and even something as basic as healthcare.
- People with a learning disability are more likely to have mental and physical healthcare issues than the general population, yet are less likely to have appropriate and timely access to good quality services.
- People with a learning disability and health staff themselves often feel that health service staff are inadequately trained and lack the knowledge and skills to deal with the needs of people with a learning disability appropriately, and that staff require education in this area.
- People responsible for ensuring that people with a learning disability have access to good quality services, treatment, etc. do not understand what it means to have a learning disability.
- 'Diagnostic overshadowing' may lead to poor healthcare and pain and suffering, even death, for people with a learning disability.

(continued)

(continued)

- There are specialist nurses called Registered Nurses for Learning Disability (RNLD) who have specialist training in the health problems of those with a learning disability.
- There are specialist services available for people with a learning disability
- This chapter has explained the ways in which people with a learning disability may be viewed by society and what effects this may have upon their quality of life.
- If a learning disability is thought of as being within the individual, their issues, and a problem for the rest of society, then these people are treated with pity, control or isolation.
- On the other hand, if a learning disability is viewed as something that is developed because of a society that caters for people without a learning disability, therefore disadvantaging them, then we may find it fairer to help to change society so that it is more accessible and inclusive.
- Ensuring that PWD have equal access to the important things in life has benefits for the whole of society.

Note

1   This does not mean that people with a disability may not be more vulnerable to neglect and abuse because they are disabled or that aspects of disability are always seen as positive (Crow, 1996, cited in Shakespeare, 1999).

References

Atherton, H. (2003) A history of learning disabilities, in B. Gates (ed.) *Learning Disabilities Toward Inclusion*. London: Churchill Livingston.

Barr, O., Gilgunn, J., Kane, T. and Moore, G. (1999) Health screening for people with learning disabilities by a community learning disability nursing service in Northern Ireland, *Journal of Advanced Nursing*, 29(10): 1482–1491.

Beacock, C. (2005) The policy context, in T. Riding, C. Swan, and B. Swan (eds) *The Handbook of Forensic Learning Disabilities*. Oxford: Radcliffe Publishing.

Brechin, A. and Walmsley, J. (1989) *Making Connections*. London: Hodder and Stoughton.

Corbett, J. (1997) Chapter 6 in L. Barton and M. Oliver (eds) *Disability Studies: Past, Present and Future*. Leeds: The Disability Press.

DH (Department of Health) (2001) *Valuing People: A New Strategy for Learning Disability for the 21st Century*. London: The Stationery Office.

DH (Department of Health/Home Office) (2002) *Draft Mental Health Bill*. London: Department of Health.

DHSS (Department of Health and Social Security) (1971) *Better Services for the Mentally Handicapped*. London: Department of Health.

Equality Act 2010. London: The Stationery Office.

French, S. and Swain, J. (2008) *Understanding Disability: A Guide for Health Professionals*. Oxford: Churchill Livingstone Elsevier.

Gates, B. and Beacock, C. (eds) (1997) *Dimensions of Learning Disability*. London: Ballière Tindall.

Globe, C. (2008) Institutional abuse, in J. Swain and S. French (eds) *Disability on Equal Terms*. London: Sage.

Goffman E. (1961) *Asylums: Essays on the Social Situation of Mental Patients and Other Inmates*. Harmondsworth: Penguin.

Goodley, D. (1998) Supporting people with learning difficulties in self-advocacy groups and models of disability, *Health and Social Care in the Community*, 6(6): 483–446.

Goodley, D. (2001) *Self Advocacy in the Lives of People with Learning Difficulties*. Buckingham: Open University Press.

Inglis, P. A., Cooper, C., Oxbery, L. and Robinson, M. A. (2004) Square pegs in round holes? Nursing models and high secure settings. Paper presented at the 3rd International Conference for the Care and Treatment of Offenders with a Learning Disability. University of Central Lancashire, April 2004.

Mencap (1998) *The NHS – Health for All? People with Learning Disabilities and Health Care*. London: Mencap.

Mencap (2004) *Treat Me Right: Better Health Care for People with a Learning Disability*. London: Mencap.

Mencap (2007) *Death by Indifference*. Available at: www.mencap.org.uk.

Mencap (2012) *74 Deaths and Counting*. Available at: http://www.mencap.org.uk/sites/default/files/documents/Death%20by%20Indifference%20-%2074%20Deaths%20and%20counting.pdf (accessed 22 Feb. 2013).

Mental Health Act 2007 *Amendments of 2003 Act*. London: The Stationery Office.

Michael, J. (2008) *Healthcare for All: Report of the Independent Inquiry into Access to Healthcare for People with Learning Disabilities*. London: Department of Health.

Oliver, M. (1990) *The Politics of Disablement*. London: Macmillan Education Ltd.

Robinson, T. (1989) Normalisation: the whole answer? in A. Brechin and J. Walmsley (eds) *Making Connections*. London: Hodder and Stoughton.

Shakespeare, T. (1999) 'Losing the plot?' Medical and activist discourses of contemporary genetics and disability, *Sociology of Health and Illness*, 21(5): 669–688.

Shakespeare, T. (2008) Disability, genetics and eugenics, in J. Swain and S. French (eds) *Disability on Equal Terms*. London: Sage.

Smith, D.J. (1976) Twentieth-century definitions of mental retardation, in *Social Constructions of Mental Retardation*. Available at: www.mnddc.org/parallels2/pdf/99-MRI-MLW.pdf (accessed 12 Jan. 2008).

Swain, J. and French, S. (2000) Towards an affirmation model of disability, *Disability and Society,* 15(4): 569–582.

UKLDCNN (2005) *A Vision for Learning Disability Nursing: A Discussion Document.* London: United Kingdom Learning Disability Consultant Nurse Network.

UPIAS (1976) *Fundamental Principles of Disability*. London: Union of the Physically Impaired Against Segregation.

Wolfensberger, W. (1988) Common assets of mentally retarded people that are commonly not acknowledged, *Mental Retardation*, 26(2): 63–70.

4 Guiding principle 4: Personal and professional development through education and training

Su McAnelly

Learning outcomes

After reading this chapter you will be able to:

- identify your own learning needs in relation to adapting your skills and knowledge to meet the needs of people with learning disabilities
- explore the use of reflection and self-development tools in your professional role
- identify and analyse the role of leadership in adapting services to meet the needs of people with learning disabilities.

Introduction

> Education is the most powerful weapon which you can use to change the world.
>
> (Nelson Mandela Date unknown).

Personal and professional education and training

The health and social care of people with learning disability are often dependent upon a range of individuals; some paid, some unpaid and some professionally qualified and some unqualified and relatively unskilled. The ability of many of these individuals to assist people with range of learning disabilities to access good quality services is varied (see Michael, 2008 and Mencap, 2007).

It has long been argued that people with severe and complex learning disabilities who need even basic health or social care support experience barriers not always anticipated by non–disabled people (Swain *et al.*, 2004). One of the barriers can be the inability of service providers to apply adapted skills which can more successfully meet their needs. The chapter discusses the following personal issues that can affect your professional life:

- reflection;
- being flexible;
- accepting your abilities;
- learning new skills;
- management and leadership.

As shown in Chapters 2 and 3 which discuss the Guiding Principles of ensuring dignity and respect and providing accessible information, the law in the UK states that all public services are obliged to adjust their services to make it possible for people with disabilities to access them. For many service providers, mainstream health and social care workers and support staff, these adapted skills need to be acquired via some sort of specialist education and training and by refocusing the service delivery in a more accessible way. This may involve professional and personal development, leadership and management.

Reader activity 4.1   What would you do?

A new young female visitor to your service has only the ability to communicate via a picture book she carries around with her. She urgently needs to discuss her situation as she is suffering from domestic violence.

- What first steps would you take?
- What would be your learning needs?
- How would you adjust your own abilities and skills?

Personal development issues: reflection

The consultant and the receptionist in Case study 4.1 were faced with a dilemma and felt ill–equipped to deal with the situation presented to them. They would probably deal with the situation on this occasion and then have time to think about how this could have been more appropriately worked through. Reflecting upon events to review actions with the aim of improving skills and abilities is a positive method for both professionals and other health and social care workers.

Reflection and the process of examining one's own abilities and needs can be a useful starting point for practitioners in health and social care. The processes and models of reflection are often familiar reminders of our obligations towards our clients to remain forever vigilant about the extent of our personal and professional abilities and how these affect the care services we deliver and offer.

Case study 4.1   Mr Cadiz

A middle–aged man called Mr Cadiz has learning disabilities and a speech and language impairment. He cannot be easily understood verbally and he cannot hear sufficiently well to understand normal speech. He arrives in a consultant's waiting room after having been referred by his GP with a history of severe and lingering abdominal pain. He is holding his stomach and is complaining by moaning and pointing to his side. His mother is waiting outside as he does not want her to be present.

Mr Cadiz has already presented in a similar way to the local Accident and Emergency department in the previous months but he wouldn't allow anyone to touch his stomach or his affected side, and as a result he was sent home with some painkillers. He allowed his lady GP to examine him and she is now concerned that he needs further investigations.

His mother is quite elderly and frail and prefers not get involved in his examinations as she is afraid of him pushing her over. There is no other service which regularly supports the gentleman and his mother.

Both the receptionist in the waiting room and the consultant in his consulting room feel unable to communicate with Mr Cadiz effectively and feel ill-equipped to deal with the situation.

Using a reflective model can be a useful way of quickly checking out:

- What do we know?
- What do we need to know?
- How can we plan to change/improve?

The next section discusses three examples of reflective models which may be useful frameworks for the type of professional and personal reflection which could assist you in the challenges experienced, by amending and appraising your practice delivery for people with learning disabilities.

Schön's model of reflection

This model was developed by Donald Schön in the 1980s. This model is useful for helping us think about both *reflection in action* and *reflection on action.* This approach can be a useful way of learning from a particular event and encourages the immediate consideration of:

- what is happening now;
- reflection after the event of what did happen;
- identification of any possible learning.

This type of reflection is useful for people who prefer to learn from their experience and who are curious about their own actions and responses (Schön, 1983). Schön's theories regularly appear in nurse and health professional education, as they offer opportunities for students to think about the practice they engage in with clients and service users and to take time to reflect upon events and benefit from feedback from their assessors and mentors. This approach is less common among busy professionals who tend to have less time to spare for reflection and prefer tools and models which offer more structured reflection of overall practice and performance.

Kolb's cycle of experiential learning

David Kolb developed a cyclical model of learning and believed that learning is most successful when both knowledge and action come together. This familiar cycle is successfully used in professional learning portfolios and incorporates active participation and experimentation in the learning process. To be a successful experiential learner, a person should engage with the full cycle and develop this way of thinking as a habitual way of working reflectively. Kolb believed that we experience situations via feeling, watching, thinking and doing. He described the four phases of experiential learning (Figure 4.1):

- *Concrete experience phase*: This is the phase when the learner feels and learns.
- *Reflective observation phase*: This is the phase when the learner watches and learns.
- *Abstract conceptualisation phase*: In this phase the learner thinks and learns.
- *Active experimentation phase*: This is the phase when the learner actively engages and learns.

This approach to reflection is also commonly used in professional development and education and the busy professional studying may be engaged in the process of a reflective portfolio as part of their learning and development of skills and analysis.

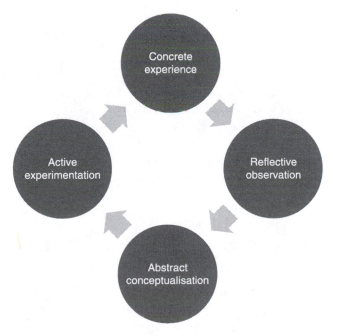

Figure 4.1 Kolb's cycle of experiential learning

Source: Kolb (1984).

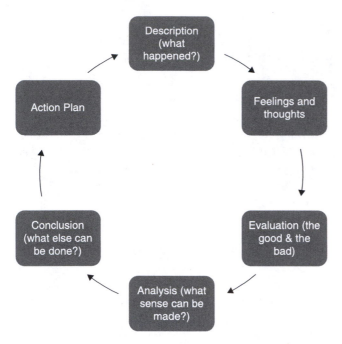

Figure 4.2 Gibbs' model of reflection

Source: Gibbs (1988).

Gibb's model of reflection

This model of reflection (Figure 4.2) helps you to think systematically about your experience and to make a plan of what you wish to achieve as a result of learning a new skill or a different way to look at a situation. This type of model is similar to the approaches advocated by Kolb and Schön but incorporates an action plan element and also asks you to be *honest* about the evaluation at the time of the experience. This type of honesty is key to the reflective process and becoming a responsive practitioner. This model of reflection is most notably used in practice situations and can assist individuals and teams to investigate new ways of working, but also forms the basis for many clinical supervision systems and appraisals.

Fast facts 4.1   Frameworks for reflection

Other reflective models are:

- John's (1995) framework for reflection;
- Borton's (1970) framework guiding reflective activities;
- Smyth's (1989) framework for reflection in action.

- Think about a recent event in which you did not perform very well.
- Choose a reflective model from the three examples and try to work through a reflective process for this event.
- Interpret the categories of the model according to your experience.
- Which one worked and why?

Personal development issues: being flexible

Becoming a flexible thinker with the ability to solve problems and try out new strategies is an acquired skill. Flexible thinking means finding more than one way to do something, it means stretching what you know enough make an educated guess that could be right (and if it is not right, that's still OK). Flexible thinking can be about finding out what you need to know and problem solving.

Fast facts 4.2 Useful resources

Here are some useful resources issued by the General Medical Council (GMC) to help practitioners reflect upon and learn new skills needed to make their own services more accessible:

http://www.gmc-uk.org/learningdisabilities/31.aspx
http://www.gmc-uk.org/learningdisabilities/302.aspx.

Critical thinking is one aspect of being a flexible practitioner which demands both the application of theory and professional judgement. You can become a flexible and critical thinking in five stages, according to the Insight technique by Kimberley Cohen:

- *Step 1 – Question.* Am I being flexible about this situation? How do I react to situations? This may involve aspects of your reflective journey outlined earlier in this section.
- *Step 2 – Recognise.* Begin to see where you are inflexible. View the change in yourself as a personal challenge not a hurdle.
- *Step 3 – Clarity.* Sometimes emotions and feelings can cloud judgements and this may lead to panic and over-reaction. Looking for a clear focus through both reflections and feedback from others can be a way of achieving some clarity on your skills.
- *Step 4 – Listen.* Taking deep breaths and listening to what you are saying to yourself can be a quiet way of taking stock and also giving you space to think more clearly.
- *Step 5 – Imagination.* Allow creative thoughts and expressions to envisage the ideal answer to your questions and problems. Allow yourself to be stretched.

Other approaches which can help with the development of a more flexible approach are:

- mindfulness training;
- meditation;
- life and career coaching (Kabat-Zin, 1990).

Applying a flexible approach

The case study of Mr Cadiz's visit to see the consultant demonstrates the complexities and barriers faced by people with disabilities when attempting to access services (French and Swain, 2012). The organisational contexts of the NHS, social services and other public bodies can be shrouded in mystery and fear for people with learning disabilities. But how can individuals make a difference?

Reader activity 4.3   How flexible can you be?

- Consider Mr Cadiz's story
- What amendments/adjustments, if any, could you make to the consulting experience?
- What difference would the amendments/adjustments make to Mr Cadiz? The consultant? The receptionist?

Fast facts 4.3   The Improving Health and Lives Project: the learning disabilities observatory (IHaL)

IHaL is a resource for healthcare professionals and others and gives advice and information (to organisations and individuals) about making reasonable adjustments to services and individual practice. A register is held of reasonable adjustment made by health services across England, Scotland and Wales. It is possible to find these examples at: www.improvinghealthandlives.org. uk/adjustments/.

Personal development issues: accepting your abilities

One aspect shared by most people working in caring professions and roles is work-based stress. The ability to deal with stress and the manifestations of stress can vary from one person to the next and also the individual agility to deal with stressful situations is important (Leka and Houdmont, 2010).

What is stress?

Stress is a feeling of threat; it is the reaction we instinctively feel to either run away (flight) or fight. The reaction to situations tells us that the external demands are exceeding our abilities to cope. This is stress. Our bodies react similarly whether the threat is a fierce dog (which we want to run away from) or an overwhelming day at work (which we need to complete, and it is a struggle).

Reader activity 4.4   Indicators of stress

Tick which indicators of stress you have experienced in the past few months:

- difficulty sleeping;
- loss of appetite;
- poor concentration or poor memory retention;
- performance dip;
- uncharacteristic errors or missed deadlines;
- anger or tantrums;
- violent or anti-social behaviour;
- emotional outbursts;
- alcohol or drug abuse;
- nervous habits.

Number of answers: _____. Now check your score:

1. You could be stressed.
2. You are probably stressed.
3. You are almost certainly stressed.
4. or more You are definitely stressed.

The solutions are either:

- reduce the external demand (remove the stresses)

or

- increase your ability to deal with the issues.

Managing stress by reducing the external demand

In our working lives as health and social care workers/professionals it is easy to see how demands placed upon our time and expertise increase. However, accepting our limits and becoming assertive about our own well-being and work-based management are often the tips to becoming a less stressed and more productive practitioner/worker.

> ## Fast facts 4.4   Becoming real
>
> * Covey's (2004) book, *The 7 Habits of Highly Successful People* offers good advice on how to prioritise your work and become more assertive and how to set achievable work-based and personal goals.
> * David Allen's handy hints in his (2002) book, *Getting Things Done* offers helpful ideas about managing the demands of care work and how to successful schedule.

Managing stress by increasing the ability to deal with issues

As we have mentioned, the ability to manage your own environment and your abilities can be increased by self-help techniques and also the adaption of programmes of support. Some individuals may benefit from more specialised help via a therapist or mental health workers trained in techniques such as cognitive behavioural therapy (CBT), neuro-linguistic programming (NLP) or psychotherapy. In some cases help with a healthy lifestyle through a personal health trainer or coach, incorporating keep fit and healthy eating, can help individuals manage their stress levels.

In addition, many people faced with minor stresses at work can benefit from additional education and training to equip them with more skills and competence. Many short courses are now delivered via on-line learning methods which can be work-based or part-time and self-directed. This type of learning offers greater flexibility to the busy worker.

Personal development issues: learning new skills

The challenges of health and social care work and, in particular, work with people with learning disabilities who often have complex health issues can mean new skills and new knowledge have to be learnt. The way we learn as adults can be governed by our individual characteristics, our environment and the method and type of learning activity we engage in.

Ideas about adult learning tend to be centred upon the classical theories of human behaviour (Merriam and Caffarella, 1998):

* Behaviourism
* Cognitivism
* Humanism
* Constructivism.

Behaviourism

This set of theories derives many ideas from the original psychological research findings of Watson, B. Skinner, Pavlov, and A. Bandura. The beliefs are based upon the central idea that learning is caused by external stimuli (called operant conditioning, according to Skinner) and that the learner is passive in the learning process, but responds according to external forces such as reward (positive reinforcement) or punishment (negative reinforcement) The central theme in behaviourism is that learning is promoted by giving positive reinforcement to encourage a change in behaviour.

Reader activity 4.5   Behaviourism at work

- What type of learning activity do you associate with behaviourism?
- Write a few notes about:

  - operant conditioning
  - classical conditioning

- How effective is it and why?

Cognitivism

This set of theories maintains a set of beliefs that learning occurs as result of the brain's abilities to process information (like a computer) and therefore the quality of the information put into the brain determines the learning or outcome. This 'black box' type approach to learning relies upon a change in the learner's schemata. Key cognitivist theorists are Gagne, Briggs and Bruner.

Reader activity 4.6   Learning theories

- Research the theorist A. Bandura.
- What are the main components of the social learning theory?
- What are the main benefits for learners?

Humanism

The key components of the humanist theories of learning is that all humans have the potential to learn. Basically, humanistic learning acknowledges that learning should be centred or personalised around the learner (student-centred learning) and the educator's role is to act as a catalyst to the learner's desire for knowledge and skills. Key contributors to this theory are Abraham Maslow and Carl Rogers. The elements of learning how to learn have been widely discussed by Carl Rogers and many more recent theories about student-centred learning and education approaches cite his work (Rogers, 1969).

Reader activity 4.7 How do you learn?

- Think of the last time you engaged in a learning activity.
- What type of learning theory do you think you were exposed to?
- How easy was it to identify the learning approaches you have experienced?
- Which type suits you and why?

Constructivisim

Constructivism as a type of theory about learning offers the ideas that learning is an active and constructive process. The learner is said to be the creator of their own learning and they are building upon experiences and encounters they have had in life. This type of approach encourages discovery and inquiry as methods for learning. The many learning methods employed tend to encourage collaboration between groups of learners and active learning through problem solving/orientation scenarios and real-life situations and simulations. Key theorists are J. Piaget, J. Dewey, and J. Bruner.

Reader activity 4.8 Constructing learning

Building 'communities of practice' is an approach that encourages groups with common values, aims and contexts to come together to learn and share learning.

- How could this approach help you with your work with people with learning disabilities?
- Who would be the communities?
- Would it involve people with learning disabilities themselves in the community?

Personal development issues: management and leadership

Dealing with changes to practice and also leading change can be a key role to play when creating a service that caters fully for the needs of clients (especially those with learning disabilities and complex health issues).

Your role could be:

- As a manager who takes responsibility for the actions of others and the overall delivery of care for people with and without learning disabilities.
- As an individual who is part of a team and sees an opportunity to make positive changes to enable better service access for clients with learning disabilities.
- You may be an individual practising or working with others in an interdisciplinary way to meet the needs of people accessing your services.

All of these roles will demand some sort of leadership skills and the ability to influence the actions and attitudes of others.

Leadership

There are many theories about leadership models, leadership philosophies and also leadership styles. A leadership model tends to refer to a structure containing a framework or a process which can be applied or followed. A model of leadership often has a diagram or flow chart which helps the application and communication of the model and can contain measurable components and triggers or goals/ standards to be achieved. The leadership model can be described as 'tool box'.

Reader activity 4.9   Leadership styles

Here is a list of key leadership styles:

- trait–based;
- behavioural ideals;
- situational and contingency;
- functional;
- integrated psychological.

Look up the definitions and key theorists for each model. What are the key components?

A leadership philosophy is a way of thinking about an approach. The philosophy is a set of beliefs and values by which adaptors of the way of thinking measure their behaviour and decisions. A leadership philosophy will influence and connect the adaptors' beliefs around fundamental principles of morality, fairness, ethics and power. A leadership philosophy can be likened to a 'compass' or code by which the followers govern their behaviour:

- servant
- authentic
- ethical
- values–based
- sources of power.

Leadership styles are more specific descriptions about the application of leadership. A leadership style is often governed by the attributes of the leader (good or bad) and can also be determined by the goal or outcome of the activity. Philosophies and models may dictate or influence a leadership style. A leadership style can be a 'tool' in the leadership model (that is adopted) 'tool box'. Here is a selection of leadership styles.

Transformational leadership

A person who is a transformational leader is described as inspiring and engaging. This ideal type of leader shares their enthusiasm for the clear goals they set and generates motivated followers. A leader with this style communicates well and draws other people into their world to achieve mutually beneficial goals and aims. Many transformational leaders also need to work with other people with an eye for detail as they are more attracted to motivating others.

Transactional leadership

This style of leadership is quite simply one of management and transactions between the leader and subordinates/followers. The focus is upon controlling and delegating through a system of rewards and punishment. Those who follow the leader's instructions are rewarded, those who don't receive no reward or receive a punishment. It is easy to see the root of the leader's power in this style which tends to reside in their authority and organisational position. Power rests with the leader's ability to direct tasks and to reward follows. This leadership style is often called a 'telling style' (Weber, 1947).

Reader activity 4.10   Transactional leader

- Can you think of a leader you have worked with who used a transactional style?
- What were the benefits and the problems?

Charismatic leadership

This type of leader is highly motivated to achieve goals and communicates these with a flair to others. These communication skills engage and inspire followers who respond with energy and passion for the goals of the leader. This type of leadership style can be similar to the transformational style but charismatic leaders tend to have personally focused goals rather than the group/shared goals of the transformational leader. A charismatic leader tends to be singularly responsible for the actions of others and without their full presence, the effect is weakened.

Reader activity 4.11   Charismatic leaders

- Think of a charismatic leader.
- What did they achieve and how?

Autocratic leadership

The role of the autocratic leader is to lead and be followed. Leaders of this type have complete power over those they lead and they make all the decisions. Working with an autocratic leader can be comfortable (as all the control is with the one leader), but also dissatisfying as there may be little opportunity to make suggestions or affect change. This type of leadership is highly efficient (especially in a crisis) and can suit some routine tasks and high outcome focused projects.

Reader activity 4.12   Autocratic leadership

- What type of activity suits an autocratic style?
- What are the benefits and the problems?

Management

Although often used interchangeably, there are big differences between leadership and management. Leadership (as we have discovered) centres upon influencing and directing people. Very often the leader of a group sets directions or outlines a vision. Management centres on controlling or directing a pre-set vision with established vision and values and involves influencing people but also controlling resources.

It is possible to have a single person who is the leader *and* the manager, but on occasions a leader may be absent and the manager ensures that all goals and priorities are met but no new direction or vision is required. Alternatively, a leader may emerge in a group without a manager and this can leave roles for others who will need to pick up the delivery of the tasks which emerge as a result of leader-inspired new directions.

Management styles

Just as leadership involves different styles, traits and attributes, management also has many versions and approaches. A management style can be influenced by a leadership style and alternatively can be of a set of skills which can be adopted for a purpose or task.

Fast facts 4.5   Other leadership styles

In addition to the above leadership styles there are many other theories about styles of leadership (Northhouse, 2010):

- bureaucratic;
- democratic/participatory;
- *laissez-faire*;
- task-orientated;
- people-orientated;
- servant.

Table 4.1 A summary of management styles

	Description	Advantages	Disadvantages
Autocratic	Senior managers take all the important decisions with no involvement from workers	Quick decision-making Effective when employing many low-skilled workers	No two-way communication, so can be de-motivating Creates a 'them and us' attitude between managers and workers
Paternalistic	Managers make decisions in best interests of workers after consultation	More two-way communication, so motivating Workers feel their social needs are being met	Slows down decision-making Still quite a dictatorial or autocratic style of management
Democratic	Workers allowed to make own decisions Some businesses run on the basis of majority decisions	Authority is delegated to workers which is motivating Useful when complex decisions are required that need specialist skills	Mistakes or errors can be made if workers are not skilled or experienced enough

A summary of management styles

Table 4.1 presents a summary of management styles. Change management is an area of importance to all public services and in particular in the rapidly changing environments of care services. The ability to affect and influence change for the good of the clients and users of services has become one of the greatest challenges for staff. Kotter (1996) outlines an eight-stage process for leading and managing change (Figure 4.3).

Reader activity 4.13 Management or leadership?

Look back at the case study of Mr Cadiz. What is required to make his care by the consultant successful?

- management?
- leadership?
- learning new skills?

Explain your thoughts.

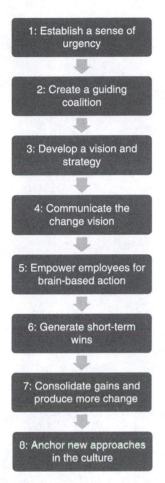

Figure 4.3 Kotter's eight-stage process for leading and managing change

Source: Kotter (1996).

Conclusion

This chapter has helped you consider your own development needs when working in health and social care, and also shown that acting upon your own needs is the basis for providing adaptable care for people with complex problems. Accommodating the needs of people with disabilities and various differences can often mean changing the way that a service is thought about, planned and delivered. This change may involve one or a number of the personal and professional development issues outlined in this chapter. The many frameworks and theories are guidelines for thinking and acting in an individualised way which ultimately can enable a more effective and equitable care service for clients with complex needs. These principles will be explored throughout the book as more complicated case studies are presented and the reader is encouraged to think deeply about the issues and resolutions required to assist people with learning disabilities successfully.

Points to remember

Personal and professional issues: Reflection

- Personal and professional development plays a key role in developing innovative ways to deliver and organise services to meet the complex needs of clients and service users.
- It is the responsibility of all personnel to consider their own development needs in relation to working with people with learning disability.
- Reflection and reflective models are useful ways of developing one's own skill and knowledge.

Personal and professional issues: Being flexible

- Professional and organisational boundaries can lead to inflexible working and can create barriers to access for people with learning disabilities.
- Becoming a flexible and innovative individual and team can be achieved by analysing the situation and using the tools of reflection, planning and effective communication.

Personal and professional issues: Accepting your abilities

- As professionals and as busy people we all need to accept our limitations.
- Commonly, stress and stress-related issues are cited as major reasons for work burn-out and poor performance in health and social services.
- Recognising the need for help and support is necessary and the availability of support is essential to providing effective and responsive professional services for people with complex problems.

Personal and professional issues: Learning new skills

- The ability to learn new skills and approaches is the key to developing one's practice.
- Learning can be individualised and focused.
- Knowing how we learn effectively can be a skill in itself.

Personal and professional issues: Management and leadership

- The correlations between leadership and management enable good services to develop.
- Woking with complex groups such as people with learning disabilities can demand good leadership and also sensitive management of communication and resources.

Resources

Books Beyond Words is a series of publications and resources which are designed to help people with communication problems and learning disability to access information. The service also delivers course and seminars.

www.booksbeyondwords.co.uk/

The Royal College of Nursing provides accessible resources to assist professional and personal learning and development. Here you will find online continuing professional development (CPD) resources relating to nursing care, career development and workplace issues. The resources are relevant to healthcare assistants, assistant practitioners, student and registered nurses across the range of care settings.
www.rcn.org.uk/development/learning/learningzone

References

Allen, D. (2002) *Getting Things Done: How to Achieve Stress-Free Productivity*. New York: Piatkus.

Borton, T. (1970) *Reach, Teach and Touch*. London: McGraw-Hill.

Covey, S.R. (2004) *The 7 Habits of Highly Successful People*. New York: Simon & Schuster.

French, S. and Swain, J. (2012) *Working with Disabled People in Policy and Practice: A Social Model*. Basingstoke: Palgrave Macmillan.

Gibbs, G. (1988) *Learning by Doing: A Guide to Teaching and Learning Methods*. Further Education Unit. Oxford: Oxford Polytechnic.

John, C. (1995) Framing learning through reflection within Carper's fundamental ways of knowing in nursing, *Journal of Advanced Nursing*, 22: 226–234.

Kabat-Zin, J. (1990) *Full Catastrophe Living: Using the Wisdom of Your Body and Mind to Face Stress, Pain, and Illness*. New York: Bantam Dell.

Kolb, D.A. (1984) *Experiential Learning as a Source of Learning and Development*. Englewood Cliffs, NJ: Prentice Hall.

Kotter, J. (1996) *Leading Change*. Boston: Harvard Business School Press.

Leka, S. and Houdmont, J. (2010) *Occupational Health Psychology*. Oxford: Wiley-Blackwell.

Mencap (2007) *Death by Indifference: Following up the Treat Me Right! Report*. London. Mencap.

Merriam, S.B. and Caffarella, R.S. (1998) *Learning in Adulthood: A Comprehensive Guide*. San Francisco: Jossey-Bass.

Northhouse, P.G. (2010) *Leadership Theory and Practice*. London: Sage.

Rogers, C. (1969) *Freedom to Learn*. New York. Merrill.

Schön, D.A. (1983) *The Reflective Practitioner*. New York: Basic Books.

Smyth, J. (1989) Developing and sustaining critical reflection in teacher education, *Journal of Teacher Education*, 40(2): 2.

Swain, J., French, S., Barnes, C. and Thomas, C. (2004) *Disabled Barriers – Enabling Environments*. London: Sage.

Weber, M. (1947) *The Theory of Social and Economic Organization*. New York: Free Press.

Guiding principle 5: Adapting your skills: thinking outside the box

Pamela Inglis and Angela Ridley

Learning outcomes

After reading this chapter you will be able to:

- consider definitions of learning disability; the issues, benefits and problems associated with defining others
- learn about the politics of disablement and understand broad categories of need
- consider the interface between learning disability and mental health issues
- discuss notions for people with a learning disability, including advocacy, employment, attributes, confidence, resilience and relationship
- list the positives of caring and the essential characteristics of a good practitioner and understand their importance
- have an awareness of standards of care and the legal framework.

Introduction

> People with learning disabilities don't know what self-advocacy means. Broken down it means speaking up for yourself . . . it means people must listen to me.
>
> (Downer, cited in Goodley, 2000; 80, 81)

Definitions of learning disability

Learning disability is difficult to define as it means many different things to different people. It is, however, defined in the literature and in legislation, for example (DH, 2001). The term is relatively new and replaced negative terminology such as 'mentally handicapped' which has links to charity as it literally states that they were 'cap in hand' (Gates, 2002). Learning disability is a term used in professional senses and as a political term, where it emphasises disability by society. The term has been rejected by the People First organisation, who prefer the term 'people with a learning difficulty'. Internationally, the terms change, but what appears to be emerging is the use of the term 'intellectual disability'.

Legally, the term has been replaced in the Mental Health Act (MHA) (1983) by 'mental impairment'. But impairment and disability mean different things:

- Impairment refers to the physical make-up of a person;
- Disability is a political term that refers to the disabling of people with impairments by a society built by and for people without impairments.

Throughout this chapter we will refer to 'people with a learning disability' – this suggests a group or category, and generally we argue voraciously for an individual more than a group approach. However, for the purposes of this book, we often have to use the group representation as a short-hand.

In saying that, terms used should always be associated with the person and not merely the impairment or the disablement. One accepted way is to refer to someone as a 'person/people with a learning disability', therefore, placing the person before the learning disability. The second way is more political and is a term preferred by self-advocacy groups such as The Lawnmowers (2005) and is 'learning disabled people'. Much like the general disability movement, this term is used to shift the emphasis from the person and place the disability back in the lap of society (Docherty et al., 2005, cited in Goodley and Geert Van Hove, 2005). See Chapter 3 for discussions regarding the social and affirmation models of disability.

Reader activity 5.1   Defining learning disability

- Imagine that an alien came down from outer-space and you had to explain to him what a learning disability was.
- Write down what you would say.
- What words would you use to describe the effects it has on someone's life?

Learning disability *is* difficult to define; it is not just an intellectual disability, it may have a global effect; it can mean people have social difficulties, it can affect our ability to communicate with people and affect people's behaviour. It is also associated with certain physical, behavioural or mental health needs which are not effectively met in our society (Mencap, 2004; UKLDCNN, 2005; Michael, 2008).

Not all the health issues affecting people with a learning disability are related to their learning impairment, but may be associated with the way that they are treated because of their impairment (for more information see Chapter 3, Equal Access). The main issue here is that one label attempts to cover all aspects of a person's life and needs, and the label changes depending upon who is defining it and for what purpose. Rarely are people with a learning disability asked what label they might prefer – and probably, like most of us, they would not like to be labelled as anything! Indeed, the label may affect the treatment of the person, but what is important is the way in which we treat individuals. One man in the study by Cook and Inglis (2008) described being labelled as having a banner over his head all of the time, proclaiming his learning disability!

Learning disability is a complex concept, there are many different wants and needs and sometimes it may be useful to think about broad definitions in assessing needs such as:

- *A mild learning disability* – people with a mild learning disability may not have been in touch with specialist services and may have been educated in mainstream schools, as most people live perfectly ordinary lives. Often they can read and write and are very good at disguising their disability. However, people with a mild learning disability may benefit from some support in coping with daily tasks such as budgeting, relationships, hygiene, housework, and finding and maintaining employment. Their disability may not be recognised, and they may not receive the support they need. Intelligence quotient (IQ) is not always a useful measure but often you might find those with a measurable IQ to be in the 60–80 range.
- *A moderate learning disability* – people with a moderate learning disability will have probably attended special education, will be able to make their needs and wishes known, but may struggle to live safely independently. They may be able to carry out everyday tasks such as making tea, or toast or warming things in the microwave oven. They will probably care for their own personal hygiene and have choices about what they like to wear and where they like to go. However, they will commonly benefit from 24-hour support for everyday tasks. The IQ range here will be around 50.
- *A severe/profound learning disability* – people with a severe or profound learning disability can commonly understand more than they can communicate and will need 24-hour support for most tasks. They may have a little verbal speech. Often we may need to attend to their personal care, feeding, hydration, dressing, etc. But we must always assure their dignity is maintained. We need to be more aware of non-verbal ways of communication such as facial expression and body posture, to understand if they are happy, in pain, or uncomfortable. Often their IQ is described as 0–35, or immeasurable. Commonly people with a learning disability have other physical and sensory impairments.

There are lots of ways in which people with a certain level of disability differ from each other, so caution should be used when thinking of learning disability in such broad terms. Of course we should treat people as individuals, not as a 'type'. It is not always useful to use such categories, as this may compound the problems associated with the categorisation of disabled people generally (Oliver, 1990).

Obviously, people with a learning disability have differing needs and wants, and different levels of ability. For example, people may have physical or sensory impairments, as well as a learning disability, and require 24-hour support. However, most people with a learning disability require little support to get on effectively with their everyday lives (MENCAP, 2004; UKLDCNN, 2005).

If we use such categories it may mean that particular views and opinions are applied to everyone in that group, despite their individual wants and needs. People with a learning disability are not only disabled; they are also men, or women, children, Christians, Buddhists, Muslims, tea drinkers, coffee drinkers, etc. They probably have more in common with others in their own peer group and families than they have with each other because they have a learning disability. Their disability may not be central to their identity, and this may be very sensible as common terms and views of people with learning disability are often negative (Wolfensberger, 1998; Swain and French, 2008).

| Reader activity 5.2   Negative definitions |

- How many of the terms that you used in the last exercise are negative and describe deficits? For example, IQ below normal, reduced ability to . . ., difficulty with . . .?
- Now, try describing what a learning disability is again, without using terms that are negative, or that describe deficits.

Practice alert 5.1

- Always remember that how we describe a person is very important, as it can lead to differential and often negative treatment.
- Always remember the positive aspects of people.
- You should put the person first, by saying 'a person/people with a learning disability'.
- Or if you are being political, you might say 'learning disabled people'.
- People with a learning disability may prefer the term 'people with a learning difficulty'.
- Often people do not like to be defined, or stereotyped at all.

Rarely is learning disability described in positive ways. There are, however, very positive parts of having a learning disability, and of being with people with a learning disability (Swain and French, 2000; Wolfensberger, 2001; Inglis *et al.*, 2003). For example, people with learning disability have been described as capable, loyal and enthusiastic employees who make other workers enjoy work more (Downs Syndrome Association, 2007; *Personnel Today*, 2007). They are also described as people who add something positive to society's diversity. Wouldn't it be boring if we were all the same (Brechin and Walmsley, 1989; Smith, 2000; Swain and French, 2000)? This positivity is very different to some terms used to describe people with a learning disability because we commonly concentrate on their needs, and the differences between them and the rest of society. Sometimes it is the legal and medical terms that promote the most negative attributes.

The importance of identity: what is wrong with legal and medical definitions?

Very often medical terms have been used to describe syndromes and enable people to understand the signs and symptoms of the learning impairment, difficulties and health issues that they may encounter. For example, people born with Down's Syndrome may have cardiac anomalies, frequent eye infections and upper respiratory tract infections and other possible health needs. This is important to know so that common health issues may be avoided, rigorous health surveillance is put in place and treatment may be offered.

But sometimes these terms instead are used as labels, and people with Down's Syndrome become referred to as 'Down's', and their individuality is lost in what people perceive that people with Down's Syndrome are like.

Reader activity 5.3   Medical misnomers

- List the medical terms that you know to describe a learning disability.
- How are these terms used in our society?
- Are there any which have poor or negative implications?

Reader activity 5.4   Defining Down's Syndrome

List the things that you know are associated with people with Down's Syndrome. This list will include physical and mental traits and perhaps personal attributes.

A fuller overview of Down's Syndrome is provided in Chapter 7 but for the purposes of this chapter it is important to note that everyone with Down's Syndrome does not have all of the traits that you listed, just because they have a similar genetic syndrome. Genes and chromosomes can be expressed in the individual in different ways. The syndrome may or may not be important to know, and we actually know little about the many causes of learning disability, few of which are genetic.

It may be important to know the genetic syndrome because of the extra help they may need, but Down's Syndrome babies are also born to different parents, socialised in different ways, have different wants, have varied IQ levels, i.e. they are as individual as you and I, they may look more like their siblings than other people with Down's Syndrome, in short, their Down's Syndrome does not affect every part of their being.

People with a learning disability may be treated differently in the legal system, and their legal status is not much different from people with a mental health issue (the Mental Health Act, 1983; 2007 amendments). Under this Act, people with a learning disability and people with a mental health issue who come within the Act are defined under one label: 'Mental Disorder'.

Of course, learning disability and mental health issues are two very different things, but they are linked in a way that people with a learning disability are more likely to have a mental health issue than others in society (see Chapter 20).

Reader activity 5.5   Similarities and differences

List the differences between mental health and learning disability. Now compare your list with what we have suggested.

Mental health and learning disability differences

- People with a learning disability are usually (but not always) born with a learning disability, and the learning disability is always acquired before the end of development (usually 18 years old).
- Usually (but not always) people with a mental health issue are diagnosed in adulthood.
- Learning disability cannot be cured, but we might help people to develop strategies and raise awareness in society (such as enabling equal access) so that they can live a good quality of life.
- Mental health issues may be helped through therapy, medication and counselling.

Mental health and learning disability similarities

- People with mental health and people with a learning disability may act in a way that other people think is bizarre.
- They may lack cognitive ability at times.
- Society often has low expectations about what these people can achieve.
- However, the way that they are most similar is the way in which they are treated negatively in society, viewed as different and treated with fear and pity.

Interestingly, Emerson (2003) found that children and adolescents with a learning disability were four times more likely to have a mental health problem, compared with their non-disabled peers. Similarly, it is more expected for an adult with a learning disability to develop anxiety disorders, adjustment disorder and post-traumatic stress disorder, compared to the rest of the population (Masi *et al.*, 2000; Turk *et al.*, 2005). What is interesting to note is that there were no gender differences in specific disorders reported, unlike the rest of the population.

> **Reader activity 5.6   Views of learning disability**

- How do you think most people in society view people with a learning disability?
- Why do you think that they are viewed this way?

What it really means; altering our perceptions

Great strides have been made through the disability movement to change the experiences of disabled people in our society and changing society's view of disablement. However, sometimes this does not positively affect the lives of people with a learning disability (Simone Aspis, cited in Chappell *et al.*, 2001; Goodley and Armstrong, 2001).

- In what ways are people with a learning disability discriminated against?
- What barriers exist for people with a learning disability in accessing paid employment?

This may be because people with a learning disability are seen as people for whom the social model of disability cannot apply, as the problem is viewed as one which occurs *within* people with learning disability and not just within the way society is structured (Goodley, 2001), thus viewing learning disability as different from other forms of disability.

'Can I speak now? You should see what I've got – I've got two arms and two legs, I'm not physically handicapped actually' (Anya Souza, cited in Goodley, 2001, p. 216). Docherty *et al.* (2005) state clearly that learning disabled people feel left out of the social model of disability. Yet they are disabled by society too; in the form of physical barriers, but also because of inaccessible information, jargon and offensive terminology which compound negative attitudes and justify people not listening to them and being patronising. For example, in an article entitled 'Disabled people's attitudes toward other impairment groups: a hierarchy of impairments', Deal (2003) describes the differing likes and dislikes of certain impairment groups that are held by disabled people and people without a disability. Unsurprisingly to most people who work within the field of learning disability, learning disability is reported to be one of the least desired disabilities. In fact, he states: 'When asking a person who uses a wheelchair what they find annoying, it is not uncommon for the response to be related to being thought of as someone with a learning disability' (ibid., p. 898).

Possibly because of this, some physically disabled people do not want to be associated with people with a learning disability. However, similar disabling barriers exist for people with a learning disability, and some of the disabling experience is shared. For example, there is still a general lack of awareness of disabled issues, and many disabled people still suffer bullying and harassment and general poor attitudes (Poole Partnership, 2006; Mencap, 2007; Quarmby, 2008). Reinders reminds us that even legislation may have little impact on people's lived experience: 'My son has all the rights the ADA [Americans with Disabilities Act] can secure, but he still has no friends' (Reinders, 2000, cited in Halstead, 2002, p. 36).

This book deliberately wishes to emphasise some of the positive aspects of learning disability and to throw out the common negative assumptions.

Stresses and resolutions

Often one may find it difficult to always be positive about the person with a learning disability when their life may be made so difficult by others' attitudes, lack of good access and lack of friends, etc.

Frequently we might find ourselves emphasising the person's need – just to enable them to have the services and adjustments that they need to live a fulfilled life. There should be a balance between not concentrating only on the person's needs, and also attending to those needs. Being positive about learning disability is not about ignoring the needs, but about ensuring that they are not the first and only part of the person that is attended to (Inglis, 2013).

Fast facts 5.1   Definitions

- It is difficult to define learning disability.
- Definitions are not always useful; medical and legal definitions are not always used in positive ways.
- Having a learning disability is different from experiencing mental health issues, but there are some similarities in their disablement.
- It is important to remember that even though people may have a learning disability, they are not always the same as others with a learning disability – they are first and foremost individuals.
- It is important not to use negative terms when describing someone.
- Even though we may want to emphasise the positives of someone with a learning disability, this does not mean that we do not pay attention to the ways in which they are discriminated against in society.

Challenging our professional and personal attitudes

As health and social care practitioners working with people with a learning disability we need to help them to develop a positive identity through rejection of the dominant view of normality. To do this we should challenge the dominant views that see the disabled experience as one of tragedy; instead we can assert the value and validity of the life experiences of disabled people as a liberating, positive, part of their identity. When we consider all of the disabling barriers to a positive life experience for people with a learning disability, this may seem difficult to do, but the next sections of this chapter offers some ways in which we may emphasise the positive and challenge views of tragedy.

Positive aspects of learning disability

In emphasising the positive, we may help to enable good access and life chances for people with a learning disability. Therefore we will attend to some of the ways in which people with a learning disability can and do positively contribute to our society.

Self-advocacy

People with learning difficulties sometimes don't know what self-advocacy means. Broken down it means 'speaking up for yourself' . . . it means people must listen to me, I can take a risk . . . Some parents won't want their kids to do things and they need to have their own support group.

(Downer, cited in Goodley, 2000; 80, 81)

Advocacy simply means speaking up on behalf of someone – either yourself or someone else. It is about using the beliefs of the person you are advocating for, and speaking out for their rights, wants and needs, despite your own personal view. Therefore, advocacy can be challenging.

Reader activity 5.8   Self-advocacy

- How do you think self-advocacy can help people with a learning disability?
- What might they speak out about?

Professor Dan Goodley worked with a self-advocacy group, made up of people with a learning disability, who were interested in ways in which this might help them and others with a learning disability. People with learning disability argue that self-advocacy offers important collective opportunities for the development of confidence and challenging oppression. Not everyone has to be a member of a group, or be particularly supportive to self–advocate. In fact, in labelling them as such, it may indicate other-ness, as we are called a self-advocate when we speak up for ourselves (Goodley, 2000).

One of the main ways to self-advocate is through challenging the negative views surrounding people with learning disability through '*accentuation of the positive*' (Goodley and Armstrong, 2001, p. 12), thereby overturning notions of dependency through emphasising abilities and attributes, that are important to self-advocates for their essential self-belief, interactions and risk-taking behaviour (Goodley, 1998).

The importance of self-advocacy is clear for Goodley (ibid.), where its actions were reported to enable the empowerment of people with learning disability more effectively than other methods. Docherty *et al.* (2005) are a group of self-advocates and researchers who strongly state that people with learning disability no longer want anyone else to speak on their behalf:

> Things have changed; the world has turned now. It's time to stop it always being professionals doing everything. We want people to listen to us and learn from us. We've seen tons of reports about learning disability . . . but most of the articles have been written by professionals who think they know about learning disability – people like Wolfensberger . . . but there's not a lot of writing from learning disabled people.
>
> (ibid., p. 31)

Self-advocates are now speaking out against:

- discrimination of them and their peers;
- barriers to good life chances;
- poor attitudes;
- inaccessible information (ibid.).

They argue that it is not their impairment, but low expectations and assumptions about what they can achieve that disable them in society, as many learning disabled people have jobs, relationships and children.

Practice alert 5.2

We must be open, ready and willing to listen to what learning disabled people want. Docherty *et al.* (2005) envisioned a world without the disabling barriers for people with learning disability – a world where:

- information is accessible;
- there are no more negative beliefs about learning disability;
- people with a learning disability are asked for their opinions, wants and needs;
- services are needs-led and not created for financial purposes;
- things are slowed down, so everyone does not have to rush;
- learning disabled people can complain and lose their temper (just as others do) without being labelled as displaying 'challenging behaviour';
- and where they can stand side by side with other disabled people to fight discrimination.

Docherty *et al.* (2005) work as self-advocates and are attempting to make their vision a reality through raising awareness in the following ways:

- writing articles;
- speaking to politicians (including the Prime Minister);
- being members of prominent boards;
- running workshops;
- making sure that their information is accessible for others with disabilities;
- generally attempting to show people that learning disabled people can do things and are not so different after all.

These show some of the ways in which we can ensure that people with a learning disability are consulted about important decisions. How can we make this happen?

Employment

In 1990 I heard about a job . . . I was desperate for the job. A teacher helped me fill in the application forms and I handed it in personally! I thought, 'I won't get scared.' Some of the questions they asked I didn't know, and I told them, 'I'm nervous.' They got back in touch with me two days later and told me I got the job. It brought tears to my eyes, it meant so much to get that job.

(Downer, cited in Goodley, 2001, p. 80)

Many people with a learning disability want to be employed and there is evidence that their employment may bring many benefits for the business and their non-disabled employees. This is evidenced from people with a learning disability and non-disabled people.

Fast facts 5.2   Employment

- *Community Care* magazine completed research in conjunction with *Personnel Today* suggesting that organisations are beginning to understand the potential of employing people with a learning disability.
- Nearly 60 per cent of the organisations employed people with a learning disability and 77 per cent reported this experience as positive.
- A separate poll of one thousand people with learning disabilities reported that employers needed to get better at opening up employment opportunities.
- Some 81 per cent of people with learning disabilities want to be employed but only 22 per cent actually are employed.

(Down's Syndrome Association, 2007; *Personnel Today*, 2007)

Reader activity 5.9   Employers

- Find out how employers are obliged by law to employ disabled people.
- What might make it easier for people with a learning disability to find a job?
- What do employers have to do?
- What do people with a learning disability have to do?

Disability discrimination legislation obliges employers to accommodate disabled people in the workplace. This can be done effectively through information and recruitment. Unfortunately, only 12 per cent of the organisations asked reported using special recruitment drives targeted for disabled people. This would obviously affect the amount of people with a learning disability entering employment. What is much more positive, though, is that 60 per cent of Human Resources professionals stated people with a learning disability are employed because of their contribution to the workplace and are being employed in more responsible positions than people realise. The positive outcomes gained from employing people with a learning disability are not limited to individuals' personal attributes, such employment demonstrates that employers who develop specialist approaches to recruitment mean that they attract talent from their competitors and benefit from 'ability hidden behind disability' (Griffiths, cited in *Personnel Today*, 2007, p. 3).

This shows that people with a learning disability really want to work, that they make positive contributions to the workplace and that the impairment is irrelevant. What is important, though, is the understanding of employers and the adjustments to work-based practices for disabled people.

A growing number of people with learning disability are self-employed and run their own businesses. The Lawnmowers, which is a theatrical group, is a particularly good example of this, and Anya Souza discusses her work designing and developing painted glass ornaments and decorations: 'I mean, here I am, living alone in my own flat and I do stained glass, which I sell' (cited in Goodley, 2000, p. 100).

Reader activity 5.10   Local searches

Find out about businesses designed to be run by and for people with a learning disability in your local area. These are likely to include the creative arts such as drama and information or training businesses.

Case study 5.1   Rosie's story: WorkFirst

Rosie is in her early twenties and has a mild learning disability. She is currently part of a government-funded scheme called 'WorkFirst' that offers support and work experience, through voluntary placements, with a view to securing paid employment.

Rosie's skills and knowledge included IT and administration skills and she is computer literate, working with databases, typing, and spreadsheets. Rosie needed some support to develop her skills in answering telephones and dealing with the public.

Rosie's dream job was working within an admin team and her allocated job experience placements reflected this. A position was then advertised for 16 hours paid at just above the minimum wage rate. She was supported to submit an application, with great care taken not to coach or prompt her – the work that she did on the application and interview was entirely her own. Of course, she developed this from her many work experience placements, and she did have the requisite skills and knowledge for the job.

Rosie secured an interview, but was unsuccessful for an appointment. Feedback was offered by the interview panel which was taken up by Rosie and her supporter. They were then informed that there had been 97 applicants for the post and the successful candidate was qualified to PhD level!

Since then, Rosie has secured a temporary part-time post within a team of administrators at a higher education institution, which had offered work experience placements for her.

Human factors – positive attributes

I feel that I've been more accepted into the community . . . That's not just because of the way I have got a place. My mum and I, we went for it, we said that people outside had to learn about people like me. That I wasn't daft, I wasn't a danger, I am a human being – I am just a normal person.

(Page, cited in Goodley, 2000, p. 85)

One of the ways to challenge negative views is to promote positive attributes which people possess. People with a learning disability, like other people, have many personal attributes.

List the positive attributes of the people you know who have a learning disability.

For example, it is reported that PWD make loyal and enthusiastic employees and make valuable contributions to the workplace, often out-performing people without disabilities (*Personnel Today*, 2007). People with Down's Syndrome are reported to bring the following advantages to the workplace:

- higher staff morale;
- good business practice;
- reductions in staff turnover;
- increase in staff attendance;
- development of previously untapped talent.

They are described as: 'Keen, reliable, flexible workers who are ready to start at short notice' (Down's Syndrome Association, 2007, p. 1).

'Would I say I have difficulties learning? No, I learnt well enough. I picked up things very quickly' (Anya Souza, cited in Goodley, 2000, p. 101).

Employing people with Down's Syndrome also demonstrates a positive corporate image as a business that adheres to regulations, equal opportunities and diversity in the workplace. People with Down's Syndrome are reported to be strong visual learners who learn through repetition, and their apparent partiality for routine can benefit the organisation as they are often reported as very meticulous in their work (Down's Syndrome Association, 2007).

People with a learning disability have also been reported to be encouraging to each other, especially through effectively using humour, as Goodley (1998, p. 445) reports in his study with four groups of self-advocates: 'In all four groups, there were particular members who were able to make people laugh and put themselves and others at ease.'

Recognising confidence and resilience

I've had an exciting life – I've enjoyed [working at] People First more than I did at the day centre because you do things all the time. I've done lots of things. I suppose there's not many self-advocates who could say they've been on the television twice!

(Page, cited in Goodley, 2001, p. 87)

Goodley (2000) describes the concept of resilience as closely linked to self-advocacy. He claims that resilience is contextualised in the time and the socialisation of the person and this is how self-advocacy groups may awaken a person to the potential of self-advocacy for their own confidence and resilience. It is an optimistic concept that questions the way that learning disability is viewed and how people's abilities are under-rated. Self-advocacy is one way that people with learning disability can grow in confidence and find opportunities to engage with positive support networks and gain employment in 'real' jobs.

Confidence and opportunity are good indicators of success in most people, and this is no different for disabled people. Raskind (2001) found that self-awareness, positive attitude and adapting to their learning disability was a better predictor of success than IQ in 41 former students in California. He found that children with learning disabilities were more likely to succeed if they possessed certain attributes he termed 'success attributes', which included self-awareness, proactivity, perseverance, goal setting, use of effective support networks and emotional coping strategies. As Page states: 'At first it's difficult, it took me a long time but you need to gain confidence for yourself. You also need to believe in yourself, what you're saying and what you need to do' (cited in Goodley, 2000, p. 85).

Similarly, Lemay (2005) suggests that people with a learning disability have great undiscovered potential. He believes that people's potential should be enabled as people are much more resilient than services believe: 'Resilience . . . should inspire our positive expectancies for individuals and push us to create the opportunities required to maximize developmental potential. Resilience should be the expected outcome and all our interventions should be animated by hope' (ibid., p. 6).

People with a learning disability have potential that may become apparent when society ends their oppression and when we discover how to unlock this potential. It is actually we as a society who have not yet discovered how to communicate properly with people with communication difficulties; or how to educate those who do not easily learn through our current methods.

Reader activity 5.12   Risks and opportunities

- How might we begin to offer more opportunities to people with a learning disability with whom we have contact?
- What risks may we take into account?
- How might we manage those risks successfully?

Interestingly, Raskind (2001) noted that successful people with a learning disability in his study compartmentalised their impairment, and saw this as only one part of themselves, not a defining feature. In fact, this is exactly the way in which we need to see the person's impairment – as just one aspect, ensuring that it does not consume their whole identity.

Case study 5.2   Giving opportunities

Cook and Inglis (2008) worked with men with a learning disability as co-researchers on a project that allowed the men to grow in confidence, self-awareness, ability and skills through adapting materials and by giving the men time to learn and question appropriately. The men gained a level 3 qualification (which is an 'A level' equivalent) from the university for their exceptional work. The men were always capable of this development, but reported lacking previous opportunities.

Therefore, it is important that people with a learning disability are not under-rated and are given opportunities to grow, develop, and make contributions to society.

Human factors and assets of love and relationships

Wolf Wolfensberger has written prolifically about people with learning disability and his work has had a most positive effect upon the services for many people with a learning disability (Atherton, 2003). In particular, he described people with learning disability as having certain assets. Lemay (2005) cites Wolfensberger (1988) as saying that people with a learning disability have 'common assets' that are repressed by their underprivileged lifestyle, which often includes poverty and poor life chances. He believes that it is because of their lack of life chances that people with learning disability have more ability to concentrate on being warm and means they are better equipped to recognise the needs of others, having a 'natural spontaneity' (Wolfensberger, 1988; Race, 2003, p. 213). Therefore, people with a learning disability tend to react well to human attention and kind-heartedness, making them fun to be around; where others have to engage their intellect, people with learning disability engage their 'emotions more than their intellect and challenge [others'] sentimentalities' (Race, 2003, p. 214). This may enhance friendships and help to create a positive self-image (Nunkoosing and John, 1997).

The level of impairment does not appear to alter this capacity for love. Smith (2000, p. 72) quotes DeVinck (1989, cited in Smith and Godfrey, 2002, p. 12), who describes the impact that his brother had on his life:

> Oliver could do absolutely nothing except breathe, sleep, eat and yet he was responsible for action, love, courage and insight . . . This explains to a great degree why I am the type of husband, father, writer and teacher I have become.

People with a learning disability may bring more than unconditional love, as is described above. They bring comfort to their families too, in diverse ways, just as the rest of the population do (Brechin and Walmsley, 1989):

> I went into hospital to have a cyst removed. When I came out, my Mam was very poorly. My brother brought my Mam a bed downstairs. She wouldn't go into hospital. So three nurses used to come every day, but she wouldn't let them touch her . . . after they had gone, I had to do it for her and make her bed. I used to sleep on a two-seater couch and I was up six or seven times a night. The nurses told me if I didn't stop and get some sleep I'd be gone before me mother. I used to weigh ten stones and I went right down to seven stones. After my Mam died, I could hear her shouting at me for a long time.
>
> (Kershaw, cited in Goodley, 2000, p. 90)

Positive effects on others

When Anya Souza was born with Down's Syndrome, the doctor described to her mother a gloomy view of Anya's future. A nurse then intervened; Anya states: 'Then a nurse came up to my mother and said, "Mrs Souza, your daughter will be fine. You'll get pleasure out of her." So I did, I gave her pleasure' (Anya Souza, cited in Goodley, 2000, p. 96).

People with learning disability have been reported to have positive effects on the lives of others which include enrichment such as teaching others to have qualities such as humility and fun, but also in practical ways, as carers and with financial help (Brechin and Walmsley, 1989).

Fast facts 5.3   Being an advocate

Wolfensberger (2001) explored the effects that becoming an advocate for people with a learning disability has on the advocates and their families (here advocates were professionals working with people with a learning disability as friends and supporters).

He uses his own experience and other literature to list the benefits of being an advocate for those he terms 'protégés' (here protégés are people with a learning disability):

- The capacity for love that people with learning disability have.
- Particularly, he notes a willingness to please and a genuine concern for others.
- Being with people with a learning disability who achieve despite their disability helps advocates to learn important things like determination.

Wolfensberger's advocates reported that through their work they learned that there are more important things than status, career and money and not to take the good things in their lives for granted; learning to be better people who were more accepting, patient and forgiving.

Similarly, Dune reports that when working in a specialist unit with people with a learning disability visitors unfamiliar with people with learning disability commonly have the same reactions:

Afterwards they talk primarily not about the programmes or staff, but about the great humanity of the experience of meeting the men and women who use the service. They are moved by the welcome and spontaneity, by the keen personal interest, and by the affectionate kindness and good humour. Clearly their hearts have been touched.

(2001, p. 2)

Fast facts 5.4   Positive assets

Through informal interviews with colleagues, Dune (ibid., p. 4) listed the positive assets of people with a learning disability:

- Openness
- Acceptance of others
- Presence, living in the now
- A calming influence through their slower pace of life
- Spontaneity and naturalness
- Enthusiasm
- Giving and generating loyalty and love
- Trust

(continued)

(continued)

- Helpfulness
- Capacity for forgiveness
- Builders of relationships and community.

Wolfensberger (1988) also suggested that people with a learning disability are:

- less likely to be impressed with status or money, but rather with what he terms 'heart qualities' (Race, 2003, p. 214);
- less likely to judge people, by whether they are good or bad, whether they keep promises or are honest or dishonest – not by their apparent important roles, etc.;
- more genuinely interested in their friends, and quick to help people in anguish, even if they are strangers;
- sometimes 'remarkably detached from worldly possessions' (ibid., p. 216), leading to a great aptitude for kindness and sharing, this sometimes means they may give away even their few possessions;
- 'remarkably trusting' (ibid., p. 215) even towards those who abuse them, and comments that when observed, this can be 'moving and consciousness raising' (ibid., p. 215);
- more likely to partake of, or come closer to, unconditional love.

Reader activity 5.13   Articulating attributes

Write down what you think of what Wolfensberger and others said about the attributes of people with a learning disability.

- What are the positives in what has been said?
- Which, if any, would you like people to think about you?
- What might be the negative side of describing people with a learning disability as loving, trusting and loyal?

Of course, this may mean that people with a learning disability may be more vulnerable, and this is something that we need to be aware of, because if someone is very trusting without discriminating, then they may be vulnerable to unscrupulous people and abuse.

What Wolfensberger and others describe may be part of the fun and enjoyment of being with someone with a learning disability. Unfortunately, this sounds uneasily like the idea of the 'super-cripple' described by disabled people and others, who 'bravely' overcomes difficulties (French and Swain, 2008, p. 27) and this is a commonly scorned portrayal of people with disabilities. Therefore, this may sound patronising to some people.

This is one of the difficulties of showing the positives of people with a learning disability, as it still shows them as 'other' and as a group or a 'type' rather than individuals.

- Which of the attributes you described above can be said of anyone you know without a learning disability?
- Which of the attributes could not be said of anyone you know without a learning disability?

Case study 5.3   Dr Pamela Inglis – my personal story. . . .

As a niece of Aunt Treesha who had Down Syndrome, it was by her physical features, as well as her idiosyncratic behaviours that I knew her; that fascinated and enchanted me, even as a child. It is difficult to find the words to describe how you feel, I suppose, as with any relationship of love; but more so here, where there may easily be accusations of patronage. I don't know why I loved spending time with Treesha, I just knew that I did. I knew that with her there was no pretence, no games; just genuineness – you could always be accepted as yourself. I think that this is a very attractive quality, and which we aspire to in the caring professions. There is some charm in the eccentric behaviours which sometimes single out people with learning disability and is the outward essence of their different-ness which should be celebrated (Robinson, 1989). This is also sometimes true of eccentric people who do not have a learning disability, for example, Quentin Crisp and more recently, Boris Johnson.

Reader activity 5.15   Definitions
and danger

What may be the dangers of highlighting the positive attributes of people with a learning disability?

After working with people with a learning disability for several years, an ex-member of the British Eugenics Society commented that: '[They] show such a variety of virtues – generosity, altruism, good will, sweet temper – that I began to think that a world peopled by mentally defectives might be an improvement on the present one' (cited in Goodley, 2001, p. 28).

Of course, by describing the positive aspects of people with a learning disability, one may fall into the same trap as negative discourses do; by generalising about people with learning disability, a group is created, and individuality and difference are lost.

The romanticisation of learning disability?

Robinson (1989) asks if describing people with a learning disability in romantic ways is twaddle, or is it that the rest of society that has been corrupted? This criticism is often thrown at sentimental stories of learning disability.

On one hand, there are sound arguments against the use of 'romantic' accounts of people with a learning disability. One good reason is the negative ways in which people with a learning disability are treated in our society – poverty, oppression and discrimination are hardly romantic. Also, by generalising about people with learning disability we use the same binary oppositions of good/bad, normal/abnormal judgements that are generally used against them; therefore, by saying that people with learning disability are essentially good, we are again stereotyping them, and individuality is lost.

Some people with a learning disability may have good attributes, but this does not make them all the same: good or bad. They are just attributes that exist in people – with or without a learning disability, and other less impressive qualities co-exist alongside these too.

We should not really be speaking about people with a learning disability; they should be speaking for themselves and such romantic qualities are not those which tend to be reported by academics in the literature as things that self-advocates say about themselves.

However, there are also sound arguments for 'romantic' stories. We cannot assume that people who cannot speak up for themselves would dislike the idea of being seen as a romantic figure with a huge aptitude for love and an ability to touch others and positively change them, like famous figures such as Mother Teresa, John Lennon, Gandhi, the Dalai Lama and Pope John Paul II.

It is important that positive stories about people with a learning disability are articulated and often they are steeped in feelings of admiration and love. They do not only have to be qualities judged by society as generally important or powerful.

Practice alert 5.3

- People with a learning disability have many attributes such as being good employees, loving and caring for others and making it enjoyable for others to spend time with them.
- Sometimes others find it difficult to understand that people with a learning disability have such useful attributes.
- This may be because often their disadvantages are commonly highlighted to enable them to get the help they need.
- However, it is important for us to work with people with a learning disability to highlight their needs and still recognise positive aspects of their lives.
- Some attributes termed 'romantic' may make people more vulnerable.
- It is very important to *treat people as individuals*, therefore, it may not be advantageous to discuss common attributes of people with a learning disability, as it can be viewed as indiscriminately treating them as faceless members of a group (Inglis, 2013).

Reader activity 5.16   Positives of caring

- Consider why you like working with people with a learning disability.
- Why did you choose this kind of work?
- What do you get out of it?

Human factors, professionalism and the positives of caring

Something that is not often discussed is the positives of caring for others. This is sometimes a very powerful motivator. The various issues highlighted above are familiar to the authors when working with people with a learning disability, and are some of the reasons why we enjoy it so much. Additionally, despite such opinions sometimes viewed as patronising, some are also highlighted in the results of studies (Inglis, 2010).

There are many accounts of the stressful nature of caring for people with complex needs but it also brings its own rewards (Grant *et al.*, 1998). Sometimes the rewards are:

* carers enjoying the achievements of the cared for;
* carers enjoying the intrapersonal aspects of the role (Grant *et al.*, 1998; see Preface).

Staff often describe the best part of their role as their interactions with service users. In addition, there are aspects of the caring professionals, some reported by service users, that may enable them to do their jobs well. In the literature, these are often referred to as 'good nurse characteristics' but can be just as valid in any profession where the caring role is involved.

Characteristics of a successful practitioner

The following is taken from the good nurse literature, but are just as valid when they include all caring professionals working with people with a learning disability. There are many opinions as to what characteristics enable good support but most commentators agree that the attributes should include:

* a knowledge base;
* a certain level of understanding and skill;
* a good education;
* a range of personal attitudes – moral or ethical traits (as described in Smith and Godfrey, 2002; Bjorkstrom *et al.*, 2006; Lofmark *et al.*, 2006; Scott, 2006).

> ### Reader activity 5.17   Personal characteristics
>
> * What personal characteristics do you think you need to provide good support for people with a learning disability?
> * How many are highlighted above?

Therefore, you should ensure that you know what you are doing, are responsible in your actions, and can develop skills which help you to do your job well. But importantly, you must remember that in order to use your knowledge and skill with competence, you need to use 'good' personal characteristics.

Smith and Godfrey (2002) carried out a qualitative study and found there was a link between not only knowledge and skill and the doing of the job, but also with the virtues and character of practitioners themselves.

Similarly, Bjorkstrom *et al.* (2006) found that the good characteristics were described in four main categories:

- doing good for others;
- being competent and skilled;
- having professional courage and pride;
- seeking professional development.

The category of doing good for others was the most frequently reported category and included characteristics like warmness and liking people, being tolerant, fair, interested, motivated and cheerful, and displaying a positive outlook on life. This is a topic discussed extensively in the caring professions where ethical practice includes seeing the people you care for as the same as you and therefore displaying empathy in interaction and in your practice (Scott, 2006).

Practice alert 5.4

Essential qualities of a supportive practitioner include:

- having integrity;
- being pleasant;
- being committed;
- showing understanding;
- being conscientious;
- being genuine and honest;
- showing common sense and kindness;
- having empathy;
- showing compassion;
- having a certain 'warmness';
- having a non-judgemental attitude;
- staff being mindful of the service user's (often) complex history to assess risks;
- managing risks in a humane and caring way.
  (Wilson and Startup, 1991; Smith and Godfrey, 2002; Scott, 2006; Reed *et al.*, 2007)

Using such personal characteristics to support those you care for enables your interactions with others to run smoothly, thus increasing the likelihood of a good working relationship/partnership and helps you to be a more effective practitioner.

Professionalism is often viewed as having a cold and distant feel to it. This should not be the case, as it is important that:

- We enjoy a good relationship with the people we care for.
- We view education, knowledge and skills as important to develop, through education, good honest supervision and reflecting on your own practice.

- You remember that you are responsible for ensuring that you have the correct education and training required to carry out your duties.
- You never do anything that you feel you are not adequately trained to do.
- You should ensure that you are practising in the correct way.
- You ask the opinions of those you care for, to ensure that your practice is effective.

Be aware that sometimes when we feel that we are being supportive, the people that we support might not feel the same way. French and Swain (2008, p. 86) state:

> [There are] two very strong and persistent themes [in disabled people's experiences of care]. The first is that disabled people do not necessarily believe that medical treatment and what it might achieve [are] the most important thing within their lives. A second theme relates to the lack of power disabled people have over their lives.

Therefore, we may believe that we are being professional and using good characteristics in our work with people with a learning disability, but we should be aware that our priorities are not always their priorities and we should always enable them to make their own choices. One of the main ways in which we can do this is by developing our knowledge and skill base. We can take courses, gain qualifications, and read about what is considered best practice.

Reader activity 5.18   On course for success

Make a list of courses you might attend, websites you might look at and books that you might read to ensure that you are developing professionally and using best practice.

Best practice is very important for carers because, even with the best of intentions, we may actually be harming the person we care for. Professionals refer to best practice as practice that has an evidence base: this means that someone has tried it out and it works well. Guidance from Mencap, the Down's Syndrome Association, Valuing People teams and the National Autistic Society often contain such best practice (see links below).

It is of utmost importance that we keep up to date with best practice and that we develop ourselves personally and professionally. We have the privilege to care for some of the most vulnerable people in our society and we have a responsibility (morally and legally) to ensure that care is of the highest quality and based on best practice.

Practice alert 5.5

- You are morally and legally responsible for carrying out high quality care for people with a learning disability.
- Knowledge and skill are very important, always be sure that what you are doing is the best practice.

(continued)

(continued)

- Good personal characteristics enable you to care more effectively.
- Never carry out duties that you feel you are not adequately trained to do, or that make you feel uncomfortable, or that you would not like to be done to you or your relatives.
- Always ensure that your practice is supportive of the person's wishes and that you offer choices.

A good rule of thumb might be that if you are asked to carry out duties that make you feel uncomfortable, or that you would not like to be done to you or your relatives, then do not carry out this duty (as you are responsible for your actions, despite who asked you to do it), and report your concerns to a supervisor or manager.

Standards of care

Standards of care in healthcare settings have been widely criticised by the media. The final report by Robert Francis QC (see link below to the report published by the NHS) concluded that patients were being routinely neglected. There is a growing litigious culture across industry, in healthcare this is no different, in fact, it appears to be heightened. The National Audit Office released figures in 2001 and again in 2007 which demonstrated that around £4 billion was needed for litigation costs. The National Patients Safety Association (NPSA) regularly publishes figures relating to accidents and deaths (see link below).

Where a standard of care is expected, a duty of care needs to be established, and will be assessed at the relevant time. Complications arise in this domain as it is not a universal obligation. The legal test was given in the legal precedent set out in *Donoghue v Stevenson* [1932], the famous ginger beer and snail case. Lord Atkin famously said in the case: 'You must take reasonable care to avoid acts or omissions which you can reasonably foresee would be likely to injure your neighbour.' There has subsequently been a variety of cases challenging whether a duty of care existed against police, fire services and ambulance services.

Practice alert 5.6

- For further reading on this, you may like to consider the judgment in the case of *Kent v Griffiths and Others* [2000].
- You may note the similarities with Lord Atkin's judgment and consider what the guidance is from your own or other professional regulatory bodies, particularly the General Medical Council.

The legal standard of care expected in healthcare was laid down in *Bolam v Friern* [1957]. The Bolam test tells us that in cases of medicine (for negligence), the standard is higher than that of a reasonable man. This is due to the professional identity and responsibility that healthcare practitioners hold. That they acted in accordance with the [practice] and did so as would any other responsible professional with same skill would do.

The Care Quality Commission is an independent regulator of hospitals, dentists, care homes and domiciliary support. All their reports are published and within the public domain, for further reading you can follow the link below to see how they highlight areas of good practice as well as gaps.

Person-centred agendas and approaches

Holism is a term referred to commonly within learning disabilities practice. According to the Nursing and Midwifery Council (2010):

> All nurses must practise in a holistic, non-judgmental, caring and sensitive manner that avoids assumptions, supports social inclusion; recognises and respects individual choice; and acknowledges diversity. Where necessary, they must challenge inequality, discrimination and exclusion from access to care.

See the link below in the resources. Person-centred care is a fundamental concept practised within learning disabilities. This is clear within the Valuing People agenda (see link below). The inclusion of people in decisions about care planning drives forward person-centred care. Furthermore, this allows carers and families to have a voice too. The robust processes of multi- and inter-professional working and the Care Programme Approach ensure checks and balances take place to afford an individual person-centredness.

Conclusion

This chapter has helped the reader to consider some of the difficulties associated with defining people with a learning disability and how it affects their relationships and practice. It listed some of the personal characteristics considered to be positive attribute of people with a learning disability, but warned of the difficulties this brings in terms of stereotyping, risk and individualised care and support.

The positive characteristics of successful practitioners were also discussed. It is important to have good knowledge and skill, but also to use positive personal and ethical characteristics in developing beneficial partnerships with the people that we support. Of utmost importance is that we ask people what they want, and what their priorities are in supporting them to do whatever it is they want to achieve, and we play a role in providing opportunities for them to develop and live a good quality life.

Points to remember

- People with learning disabilities should be listened to.
- Everyone with a learning disability is different with different wants, needs, likes, dislikes, positive and negative attributes.
- Health and social care practitioners have a duty to develop and adapt their skills so providing the best possible care.

Resources

Care Quality Commission www.cqc.org.uk/
Down's Syndrome Association, www.downs-syndrome.org.uk/?gclid=CLPa46DIybUCFcLHtAod
2TQAcA
General Medical Council www.gmc-uk.org/
Mencap www.mencap.org.uk/?gclid=COzO5ZHIybUCFYbHtAodGi8AOQ
National Audit Office www.nao.org.uk/
National Autistic Society www.autism.org.uk/
National Patient Safety Association www.npsa.nhs.uk/
Nursing and Midwifery Council www.nmc-uk.org/
The Francis Report www.midstaffsinquiry.com/pressrelease.html
Valuing People www.dh.gov.uk/health/category/policy-areas/social-care/learning-disabilities/

References

Atherton, H. (2003) A history of learning disabilities, in B. Gates (ed.) *Learning Disabilities: Toward Inclusion*. London: Churchill Livingston, pp. 41–60.

Bjorkstrom, M.E, Johansson, I.S. and Athlin, E.E. (2006) Is the humanistic view of the nurse role still alive – in spite of an academic education? *Journal of Advanced Nursing*, 54(4): 502–510.

Brechin, A. and Walmsley, J. (1989) *Making Connections*. London: Hodder and Stoughton.

Chappell, A.L., Goodley, D. and Lawthom, P. (2001) Making connections: the relevance of the social model of disability for people with learning difficulties, *British Journal of Learning Disabilities*, 29: 45–50.

Cook, T. and Inglis, P.A. (2008) *Understanding Research, Consent and Ethics: A Participatory Research Methodology in a Medium Secure Unit for Men with a Learning Disability*, Final Report. London: Department of Health.

Deal, M. (2003) Disabled people's attitudes toward other impairment groups: a hierarchy of impairments, *Disability and Society*, 18(7): 897–910.

DH (Department of Health) (2001) *Valuing People: A New Strategy for Learning Disability for the 21st Century*. London: The Stationery Office.

Docherty, D., Hughes, R., Phillips, P., Corbett, D., Regan, B., *et al.* (2005) This is what we think, in D. Goodley and G. Van Hove (eds) *Another Disability Studies Reader? People with Learning Difficulties and a Disabling World*. London: Garant, pp. 27–51.

Down's Syndrome Association (2007) *Information for Employers*. Middlesex: The Down's Syndrome Association.

Dune, J. (2001) *Image Matters*. Available at: http:/ www.frontline-ireland.com/Issue51_DUNNE.doc+assets+ learning+disability+wolfensberger&hl=en&ct=clnk&cd=13&gl=uk (accessed 12 Jan. 2008).

Emerson, E. (2003) The prevalence of psychiatric disorders in children and adolescents with and without intellectual disabilities, *Journal of Intellectual Disabilities Research*, 47: 51–58.

French, S. and Swain, J. (2008) There but for Fortune, in J. Swain and S. French (eds) *Disability on Equal Terms*. London: Sage, pp. 7–20.

Gates, B. (ed.) (2002) *Learning Disabilities: Towards Inclusion*, 4th edn. London: Churchill Livingston.

Goodley, D. (1998) Supporting people with learning difficulties in self-advocacy groups and models of disability, *Health and Social Care in the Community*, 6(6): 438–446.

Goodley, D. (2000) *Self Advocacy in the Lives of People with Learning Difficulties*. Buckingham: Open University Press.

Goodley, D. (2001) 'Learning difficulties', the social model of disability and impairment: challenging epistemologies', *Disability and Society*, 16(2): 201–231.

Goodley, D. and Armstrong, D. (2001) *Self-advocacy, Civil Rights and the Social Model of Disability. ESRC Research Grant. Final Research Report*. Available at: www.leeds.ac.uk/disability-studies/projects/selfadvocacy/final report.htm (accessed: 27 May 2008).

Goodley, D. and Van Hove, G. (eds) (2005) *Another Disability Studies Reader? People with Learning Difficulties and a Disabling World*. London: Garant, pp. 27–51.

Grant, G., Gowrad, P., Richardson, M. and Ramcharan, P. (2005) *Learning Disability: A Life Cycle Approach to Valuing People*. London: Open University Press.

Halstead, S. (2002) Service-user and professional issues, *Journal of Intellectual Disability Research*, 46(Suppl. 1): 31–46.

Inglis, P.A. (2010) Characteristics of nursing staff in medium secure settings, *Journal of Learning Disability and Offending Behaviour*, 2.

Inglis, P.A. (2013) Reinterpreting learning difficulty: a professional and personal challenge? *Disability and Society*, 28(3): 423–427.

Inglis, P.A., Robinson, M.A., Thornton, P. and English, G. (2003) Partnerships in nursing and education: enhancing the role of the specialist RNLD in forensic settings, paper presented at the 2nd International Conference for the Care and Treatment of Offenders with a Learning Disability, University of Central Lancashire, April. Available at: www.ldoffender.co.uk. (accessed 14 March 2005).

Lemay, R. (2005) Resilience, the developmental model and hope, *The Crucial Times*, 34: 5–6.

Lofmark, A, Smide, B. and Wikbald, K. (2006) Competence of newly-graduated nurses: a comparison of the perceptions of qualified nurses and students, *Journal of Advanced Nursing*, 53(6): 721–728.

Masi, G., Favilla, L. and Mucci, M. (2000) Generalised anxiety disorder in adolescents and young people with mild mental retardation, *Psychiatry*, 63(1): 54–64.

Mencap (2004) *Treat Me Right: Better Healthcare for People with a Learning Disability*. London: Mencap.

Mencap (2007) *Death by Indifference*. Available at: www.mencap.org.uk (accessed 10 June 2007).

Michael, J. (2008) *Healthcare for All: Report of the Independent Inquiry into Access to Healthcare for People with Learning Disabilities*. July 2008. Available at: www.iahpld.org.uk (accessed 10 August 2008).

Nunkoosing, K. and John, M. (1997) Friendships, relationships and the management of rejection and loneliness by people with learning disabilities, *Journal of Intellectual Disabilities*, 1(10): 10–18.

Oliver, M. (1990) *The Politics of Disablement*. London: Macmillan.

Page, L. (2000) Five life stories of 'top self-advocates', in D. Goodley (ed.) *Self-advocacy in the Lives of People with Learning Difficulties*. Buckingham: Open University Press, pp. 88–96.

Personnel Today Magazine (2007) Available at: www.personneltoday.com/Articles/2007/05/29/40782/learning- disabilities-are (accessed 9 Aug. 2007).

Poole Partnership (2006) *Positive About Disability Findings*. Available at: www.poolepartnership.info/uploads/reportFINAL.pdf (accessed 18 Aug. 2007).

Quarmby, K. (2008) *Getting Away with Murder: Disabled People's Experiences of Hate Crime in the UK*. London: Scope.

Race, D.G. (ed.) (2003) *Leadership and Change in Human Services: Selected Readings from Wolf Wolfensberger*. London: Routledge.

Raskind, M. (2001) Research trends: risk and resilience in people with learning disabilities. Available at: www.schwablearning.org/articles.aspx?r=622&f=relatedlink (accessed 12 Jan. 2008)

Reed, J., Inglis, P., Cook, G., Clark, C. and Cook, M. (2007) Specialist nurses for older people: implications from UK development sites, *Journal of Advanced Nursing*, 58(4): 368–376.

Reinders, H.S. (2000) *The Future of the Disabled in Liberal Society: An Ethical Analysis*. Notre Dame, IN: University of Notre Dame Press.

Robinson, T. (1989) Normalisation: the whole answer? In A. Brechin and J. Walmsley (eds) *Making Connections*. London. Hodder and Stoughton, pp. 247–252.

Scott, P.A. (2006) Perceiving the moral dimension of practice: insights from Murdoch, Vetlesen, and Aristotle, *Nursing Philosophy*, 7: 137–145.

Smith, D.J. (2000) The power of mental retardation: reflections on the value of people with disabilities, *Mental Retardation*, February, pp. 70–72.

Smith, K.V. and Godfrey, N.S. (2002) Being a good nurse and doing the right thing: a qualitative study, *Nursing Ethics*, 9(3): 301–312.

Swain, J. and French, S. (2000) Towards an affirmation model of disability, *Disability and Society*, 15(4): 569–582.

Swain, J. and French, S. (2008) *Disability on Equal Terms*. London: Sage.

Turk, J., Robbins, I. and Woodhead, M. (2005) Post traumatic stress disorder in young people with intellectual disability, *Journal of Intellectual Disabilities Research*, 49: 11.

UKLDCNN (2005) *A Vision for Learning Disability Nursing: A Discussion Document*. London: United Kingdom Learning Disability Consultant Nurse Network.

Wilson, A. and Startup, R. (1991) Nurse socialisation: issues and problems, *Journal of Advanced Nursing*, 16: 1478–1486.

Wolfensberger, W. (1988) Common assets of mentally retarded people that are commonly not acknowledged, *Mental Retardation*, 26(2): 63–70.

Wolfensberger, W. (1998) *A Brief Introduction to Social Role Valorization*, 3rd edn, rev., New York: Training Institute for Human Service Planning, Syracuse University.

Wolfensberger, W. (2001) What advocates have said, *Citizen Advocacy Forum*, 11(2). Edited version of a shorter keynote address given to the 2nd World Congress on Citizen Advocacy, Omaha, Nebraska, October 2000, pp. 4–27.

Cases cited

Bolam v Friern Hospital Management Committee [1957] WLR 582.

Donoghue v Stevenson [1932] AC 562.

Kent v Griffiths and Others, The Times Law Report, 23 December 1998; *The Times Law Report*, 10 February 2000; [200] 2 All ER 474.

6 Guiding principle 6: Delivering quality to people with learning disabilities

David Atkinson and Gwen Moulster

Learning outcomes

After reading this chapter you will be able to:

- identify what quality means and how it can be measured
- understand how quality monitoring has worked and how it has not
- select a number of frameworks which can be used to assess quality.

Introduction

> Providers have a duty of care to each individual they are responsible for, ensuring that services meet individual needs.
>
> Winterbourne View Report. DH (2012).

This chapter aims to explore what quality truly means in services that support people with learning disabilities. It will explore concepts of quality and look at what happens when quality fails. We will examine organisational approaches to assuring standards and perhaps most importantly explore what people with learning disabilities tell us that quality looks like. This chapter is the final guiding principles section and is intended to enable you to think and develop ideas about quality of care and the implications.

Case study 6.1   Jennifer's story

Jennifer, aged 35, presented many serious challenges to services. She had been homeless for several years because her placements regularly broke down. Historically, she had suffered from

(continued)

(*continued*)

significant loss throughout her life. She had no contact with her family, no friends and the staff she had built good relationships with had left, or she had been moved. Professionals and commissioners had consistently assessed Jennifer as needing robust, secure services. However, it was clear a person-centred approach might enable her to successfully move to her own home with a bespoke package of care designed to meet her needs and wishes.

An independent provider was found who then spent several months working with the in-patient service to get to know Jennifer. They learnt how to provide her with safe and effective care by working alongside her health support team. They built relationships and established what would make a good quality service for her. Jennifer had a number of requirements, but by far the most important one was her personal choice over who provided her care and support and how she spent her time. The effective continuation of her package of care and her increased personal satisfaction are evidence that the service she receives presents good quality both to her and to the commissioner who purchases the service on her behalf.

In the world of health and social care services the term quality is almost ubiquitous in mission statements and services' promotional materials. Politicians and leaders frequently talk about the need to deliver high quality services and many large organisations have quality strategies. The 1999 Health Act established a statutory duty of quality which was built upon by the Health and Social Care Act 2012, which laid out the duty of the Secretary of State for Health and the Healthcare Commissioners 'to improvement in quality of services' which requires that quality improvement outcomes should relate to the quality of user experience as well as the safety and effectiveness of services. In England, health and social care providers are monitored by an independent regulatory body called the Care Quality Commission (CQC) which was established in 2008. In the other three UK countries, health and social care providers are similarly regulated (Healthcare Improvement Scotland, Social Care and Social Work Improvement Scotland, the Regulation and Quality Improvement Authority in Northern Ireland and the Care and Social Services Inspectorate Wales and Healthcare Wales).

Reader activity 6.1   What do you understand by quality?

Think about the public services you use, these might include GP services, libraries, public transport, etc. Try to define what a high quality service looks like:

- to you personally;
- for your family;
- for other groups in your community.

In 2005, the Cabinet Office Strategy Unit proposed the use of service user held individual budgets as part of its paper, 'Improving the Life Chances of Disabled People'. This was presented as an attempt to give service users more choice and control over the social care services they use. Individual budgets are essentially cash payments to service users in lieu of community care services that they have been assessed as needing. These payments, rolled out in England from 2008 onwards, allow service users to choose for themselves the services they will access to meet their social care needs. This was followed by a government Green Paper on Community Care, promoting the importance of individualised support where power is held by the person and his or her family (DH, 2009). This provided the impetus for the continued growth of supported living services and the increased use of personal assistants and other homecare-type support. The use of personal budgets remains at the heart of the government's drive to increase the quality of social care and the 2012 Care and Support Bill includes plans for personal budgets to be introduced for all local authority-funded services users from April 2015. The quality, inspection and regulation of social care services are likely to become an important issue as more people opt for personalised supported living.

Personalisation

In 2007, the Department of Health published *Putting People First: The Transformation of Social Care*. *Putting People First* is a concordat that sets out a commitment to finding new ways to improve adult social care in England. The document set out plans to reform public services in order to create an increased focus on personalisation. Personalisation means that community care should be planned and delivered in a way that takes a more person-centred approach to what recognising what people want, building on their strengths and putting them at the heart of the decisions that are made about their care and support. It focuses on enabling people to make their own choices about how and when they are supported to live, rather than following a traditional service-driven model of provision where people access support of a nature dictated by the service provider. Personalisation aims to ensure that:

- People remain involved in their own communities.
- Effective advice and support are available to everyone.
- People can access services at an early stage in order to prevent crises from occurring.
- People receive support according to their individually assessed needs and preferences.

Fast facts 6.1   What people say about personalisation

I just want to control my own life . . . I like to socialise with other people and meet new friends. I just want to enjoy my freedom. I don't want people to control my life for me. I want to control it myself. That's what my Mum brought me up for, to control my own life.

Personalisation means, for me, that I want to be able to stay living in my own home. I want to be able to access every kind of public transport. I guess it's really about the ordinary, to be honest.

Public service reform has proceeded far more successfully where government has successfully articulated a story about reform . . . that has engaged the workforce.

(Social Care Institute for Excellence, n.d.)

Standards

In relation to driving quality standards across healthcare provision, the National Institute for Health and Clinical Excellence (NICE) has developed a set of quality standards using the best available evidence and based on the recommendations in the Health and Social Care Act (2012). These standards have been developed in collaboration with health and social care professionals and with input from people who use services, and take account of evidence from people's experience of using services, with regard to equality, safety, cost effectiveness and impact. NICE has recently assumed additional responsibility for creating similar guidance and quality standards for social care in England.

These NICE Standards should in future serve as a basis by which commissioners of services (including service users who hold their own individual budgets) can make informed judgements as to which service models to purchase.

Fast facts 6.2   What the NICE Standards will do

According to NICE (www.nice.org.uk/aboutnice/qualitystandards/qualitystandards.jsp), the NICE Standards will provide the following services:

- Health and social care professionals and public health professionals are to make decisions about care based on the latest evidence and best practice.
- People receiving health and social care services, their families and carers and the public will be able to find information about the quality of services and care they should expect from their health and social care provider.
- Service providers will be able to quickly and easily examine the performance of their organisation and assess improvement in standards of care they provide.
- Commissioners will be confident that the services they are purchasing are high quality and cost effective and focused on driving up quality.

As the independent regulator of health and adult social care, the Care Quality Commission is well placed to influence the quality of care in England. It is responsible for driving improvement and taking action if providers of care do not meet essential standards of quality and safety. It also supports the personalisation agenda by ensuring that service users have the power to make informed choices about the services they receive and have access to services that offer a seamless experience of care. The CQC has five priorities areas where they believe their role as regulator will enable them to significantly enhance the quality of outcomes for people who use services.

Reader activity 6.2   CQC priorities: how would you ensure this?

Make notes against the following five CQC priorities, to say how you feel you can personally support improved service quality.

1. Ensuring care is centred on people's needs and protects their rights.
2. Championing joined-up care so that health and social care are more coordinated.
3. Acting swiftly to help eliminate poor quality care.
4. Ensuring and promoting high quality care.
5. Regulating effectively in partnership.

In learning disability services English policy has been driven for over a decade first by *Valuing People* (DH, 2001) and latterly by *Valuing People Now* (DH, 2009). These policy initiatives have been mirrored by equivalent policies across Wales, Scotland and Northern Ireland (DHSSPS, 2004; Scottish Executive, 2000; and the National Assembly for Wales, 2002), establishing a common agenda founded on the promotion of rights, inclusion, choice and independence for all people with learning disabilities. There is broad consensus that all services should:

- *be individualised or person-centred* – ensuring that people and their preferences are central in determining the type of services they receive.
- *be provided locally* – effective services should be delivered in all areas rather than people having to move to distant areas to access the services they need.
- *be outcome-focused* – services should be able to demonstrate that they are effective in terms of meeting people's identified needs and equally in enabling service users to achieve their personal goals.
- *provide value for money* – care services can carry significant costs and therefore in justifying these costs, services must be able to deliver high quality outcomes.
- *be well coordinated and jointly commissioned* – health and social care providers should work closely together and where care and support are provided by multiple agencies, effective models of care coordination will be required in order that all providers are clear about their responsibilities.
- *not be institutionalised* – people's individuality should be respected and they should not be subjected to arbitrary rules and batch treatment in the services they use.
- *be community-based* – people should engage with all aspects of their local communities and not live their life separate from non-disabled members of society.
- *be open to scrutiny* – from regulators, commissioners, service users and their families.

Scandals

In spite of much fine rhetoric, quality can be difficult to recognise and monitor and a series of scandalous lapses of quality over the last decade have focused attention on what happens when quality systems fail for people with learning disabilities. These scandals include the following high profile examples:

- In Cornwall NHS Partnership Trust in 2006, reports revealed widespread abuses of people with learning disabilities in an NHS-run hospital and community-based services, including staff tying a service user down to prevent self-injurious behaviour, physical violence towards service users, excessive use of sedative medications and the punitive use of cold showers and withdrawal of food for discipline (Healthcare Commission, 2006). The Trust had previously been recognised as a top rated provider by the then regulator and predecessor of the CQC, the Healthcare Commission.

- In Sutton and Merton Primary Care Trust, in 2007, the Healthcare Commission reported on extensive institutional practices across hospital and community-based services with cramped environments, poor care practices and minimal opportunity to engage in constructive activities. Additionally, there was evidence that some service users had been physically and possibly sexually abused, mechanical forms of physical restraint had been employed, and there was minimal access to specialist support (Healthcare Commission, 2007). Just a couple of years earlier the PCT had been identified as a good service by the Healthcare Commission and yet performance would appear to have rapidly deteriorated unchecked.

- In 2004, Mencap published *Treat Me Right*, a report which highlighted the inequities of NHS healthcare provision to people with learning disabilities. In 2006, the Disability Rights Commission further emphasised concerns that people with learning disabilities were not afforded equitable access to healthcare services and treatment and as a consequence suffered more ill health and were more likely to die. In 2007, Mencap published *Death by Indifference*, a report which told the shocking stories of six people with learning disabilities who suffered potentially avoidable deaths while in various NHS healthcare services. A subsequent independent inquiry (Michael, 2008) and report by the Local Government Ombudsmen and Parliamentary and Health Service Ombudsmen (2009) both confirmed that people with learning disabilities were consistently being placed at risk within primary and secondary healthcare services due to institutional discrimination.

- In May 2011, a BBC *Panorama* television documentary showed undercover film footage of criminal aggression and degrading treatment of people with learning disabilities who were inpatients within the Winterbourne View, an independent hospital run by Castlebeck Care. Many of the perpetrators were subsequently gaoled and the hospital was promptly closed. The following reviews and investigations found there to have been a dysfunctional culture characterised by excessive use of physical restraint, inadequate access to advocacy services or engagement with families, poor recruitment practices and a failure to translate organisational policies into practice. External to the provider, it was noted that the safeguarding authorities had failed to respond to concerns which had earlier been raised with them, as did the CQC and local police services. It was also noted that commissioners of placements had failed to monitor quality within the service and effectively allowed service users to become permanently resident in a hospital setting (DH, 2012; Flynn, 2012).

- In 2012, Mencap published a further report, *Death by Indifference: 74 deaths and Counting*, this relayed details of more potentially avoidable deaths of people with learning disabilities within NHS services. At least 51 of these had occurred since the publication of Sir Jonathan Michael's Independent Inquiry in 2008.

So despite the myriad government strategies, guidance and 'tool kits' to support a process of change and quality improvement, supported by various regulatory frameworks and financial systems which aim to put people in control of their services, and systems for establishing clear standards by which service quality can be measured, there have been regular reports of poor quality care and support being experienced by people with learning disabilities and their family carers. It seems that while some essential underpinning principles of quality can be agreed, the differing perspectives of varying stakeholders gives rise to discrepant views as to how to objectively measure and monitor quality in operation. In this gap, poor quality services can continue to be delivered.

So, how, if these are examples of quality failings, how should it have been assured? The quality of care and services is fundamental in both health and social care. The *Darzi Report* (DH, 2008) suggested that in relation to NHS services, care should be safe and effective but should also focus on the users' experience of service receipt, noting that they should be 'treated with compassion, dignity and respect in a clean, safe and well managed environment' (ibid.).

Since 1992 UK healthcare services have been widely underpinned by clinical governance, this is the central strategy by which quality is assured. Clinical governance has been defined as: 'A framework through which organisations are accountable for continuously improving standards of care by creating an environment in which excellence in clinical care will flourish' (Scally and Donaldson, 1998).

Governance

Governance is an overarching concept which embraces a range of joined-up strategies by which to promote safe, high quality service. It applies across health and social care provision within both the state and independent sectors. The central underpinning themes of effective governance are:

- *User-focused* – the services should be user-focused and delivered in a fashion that is consistent with user-based perceptions of quality. Service user experiences should be sought and lessons learned from them.
- *Quality improvement* – services should strive to provide high quality care, tackle inequalities and update practice in line with emerging evidence. There should be clear policies aiming to ensure that risks are recognised and managed.
- *Leadership* – those who lead services need to be empowered to champion quality from the point of contact with users to strategic levels within their organisations. There should be clear lines of responsibility and accountability for care quality.
- *Staff focus* – staff need to have access to education and training in order to ensure the currency of their practice underpins high quality models of modern service delivery. Staff need to engage with effective supervision and appraisal structures in order to identify and rectify poor performance and ensure that their practice remains evidence-based.
- *Information* – service delivery needs to be underpinned by effective information. It is only by such arrangements that those responsible for service quality can be robustly assured that services are delivering against the quality agenda. User feedback data is essential as is a programme of audit whereby services continually measure their own services against benchmarked quality standards.

Organisationally, governance systems should connect service users and executive board members with a detailed information flow providing assurances to senior executive officers that care is safe, effective and user-focused. Governance requires an open service culture within which successes are celebrated and lessons are learned from mistakes.

Despite the introduction of these new systems, it is clear that no service exists in isolation; all are intrinsically linked to external organisations, including their commissioners, regulators, and other social and healthcare providers. The most dramatic failings of service quality have repeatedly been found when governance has been compromised across multiple agencies and where collaboration and coordination have been found to be dysfunctional. The Department of Health report on Winterbourne View (DH, 2012) highlighted the need for a shared, coordinated, cross-agency responsibility for quality of care, thereby ensuring the best of outcomes for people who use services.

Fast facts 6.3 The Winterbourne View Report

This report suggests 'Responsibility for safety and quality of care' depends on all parts of the system working together:

1. *Providers* have a duty of care to each individual they are responsible for, ensuring that services meet their individual needs and for putting systems and processes in place to provide effective, efficient and high quality care.
2. *Commissioners (NHS and local authorities)* are responsible for planning for local needs, purchasing care that meets people's needs and building into contracts clear requirements about the quality and effectiveness of that care.
3. *The workforce*, including health and care professionals and staff, have a duty of care to each individual they are responsible for.
4. *System and professional regulators* are responsible for assuring the quality of care through the discharge of their duties and functions.

When designing and delivering services it is important to acknowledge pressures from the external climate in which the services operate. In May 2011, Roe explored cost effectiveness issues relating to the provision of quality social care to people with learning disabilities against a background financial climate of financial recession, fiscal austerity and a consequent drive to achieve efficiencies across all public sector services. He felt that pressures on social care budgets posed a major challenge to services that deliver the highest standards of quality. He recognised that the Department of Health had earlier acknowledged these same tensions in a consultation document, *Transparency in Outcomes: A Framework for Adult Social Care* (DH, 2010), which stated: 'In previous times of financial difficulty, squeezing prices on care providers has led to a decline in the quality of the market, as higher quality provision has often suffered most – quality of commissioning makes a difference.' Roe asserted that the challenge of delivering high quality, cost-effective services is dependent on an ability to measure and compare quality. He cautioned that in the current financial climate:

> There is an urgent need for a 'stick in the ground' to establish the point below which service user entitlements, related budgets and the fees for providers should not go, if the downward spiral of quality care provision is not to commence.

Values

In its simplest form, quality might be perceived as that which is valued, however, valued by whom? Few values are universal and the aspirations of people with learning disabilities may be influenced by the values of differing professionals as well as their own personal values, those of their families and communities and of society more broadly.

- Having looked at some absolute failings of quality, in view of the current pressures on services, what does quality look like?
- How do we recognise it and how do we achieve it?
- Make notes on these questions.
- So in recognising what quality looks likes, which values should provide the yardstick to recognise and discriminate between differing degrees of quality?

Classically, Garvin, in 1988, suggested that there are five distinct approaches to understanding what quality means:

1. *Transcendent quality* – this perspective suggests that quality is not amenable to precise definition but rather that subjectively we each 'recognise it when we see it'. Transcendent quality is not a particularly helpful concept in understanding how we can ensure that we deliver idealised high quality services. It suggests quality is a subjective value-based judgement and does not allow comparisons of high versus low quality.

2. *Attribute quality* – here a more empirical approach means that quality is defined in terms of the quantification of a desired and measurable attribute and the 'finished product'. A quality service is one which measures highly against a specific quality outcome indicator– often this will lead to a focus on outcome measures.

3. *Process quality* – here quality is seen as arising from conformity to essential standards through processes. Here, it is not simply the outcome of a service which is focal to judgements of quality but also consideration of every step within the underlying processes, with quality being assured at every stage. Therefore, this implies a focus not just on what is done but also how it is done.

4. *Value-based quality* – quality is understood as a process which delivers an agreed and desirable level of performance for an acceptable cost. In essence, the highest quality services would be deemed to be those that perform to defined standards for the lowest cost. Commissioners of services have a keen interest in value-based concepts of quality, particularly given the current financial climate and in commissioning on the basis of evidence as to what does and does not work. This has led to a drive to understand and demonstrate the relative cost effectiveness of quality outcomes associated with varying models of care.

5. *User-based quality* – quality is understood as the capacity to meet the needs, desires and wishes of users. User-based quality is informed not by clinical evidence or the universal application of standards but rather by individualised users' expectations and aspirations, which are in turn established against a background context of societal and cultural norms. Users of services measure their subjective experiences of receiving services against their own expectations and on that basis come to a judgement as to the worth or quality of a service. Personalised approaches to service delivery have long been at the heart of national policy and so perhaps it is this concept of quality, more than any other, that should be the focus of our efforts to recognise, define and measure quality.

Attribute, process and value-based quality judgements are all made in light of a body of evidence regarding what is and is not effective, however, where the evidence base is limited, the search for quality assurance is difficult. Attribute and process quality are both standards-focused, and a range of standards frameworks has been developed (e.g. those developed by the CQC and NICE). However, a major challenge is in demonstrating that these quality standards are valid, i.e. that they are genuinely representative of what is universally considered to be indicative of quality. Even if appropriate and valid standards can be agreed upon, the next task is not much easier – how to measure performance against these standards. In some of those services described earlier where quality spectacularly and publicly failed, a number had previously been accredited as high quality services. Were the standards lacking validity or did inspection procedures fail to sensitively measure performance against them?

Fast facts 6.4   Dimensions of patient-centred care

The Picker Institute (2005) identified eight dimensions of 'patient-centred care' in a health context:

1. Swift access to health advice of consistent quality.
2. Effective treatment.
3. Information, advice and support for self-care.
4. Involvement in decision-making and respect for choice.
5. Attention to physical and environmental needs.
6. Emotional support.
7. Involvement of families/carers.
8. Continuity of care and smooth transitions.

The reviews that followed the scandalous lapses of quality described above provide clear evidence that things can go badly wrong for people with learning disabilities where person-centred care is absent. The Picker Institute's eight dimensions may form an appropriate framework for quality recognition and improvement initiative from a user-based perspective. It seems likely that the institutional abuses played out at Winterbourne View (DH, 2012) could not have happened if quality standards, based on a person-centred approach to care and service delivery, had been followed.

People with learning disabilities have much to say about what comprises quality. At the beginning of the last decade Paradigm UK, in partnership with Skills for People, the Valuing People Support Team and the Association for Supported Living, developed the 'REACH' Standards for supported living (Gitsham et al., 2002). These were developed to empower people with learning disabilities to check the quality of their own support and housing, and compliance with these standards has become a benchmark of quality within supported accommodation services. They provide a clear user-focused, standard-based quality framework that provides assurance of quality to service users, their families and those who commission services.

Fast facts 6.5   The REACH Standards

The REACH Standards comprise 11 person–centred statements which in combination describe user focused outcomes of high quality services. The REACH Standards (Wood and Kinsella, 2006) are:

- I choose who I live with.
- I choose where I live.
- I have my own home.
- I choose how I am supported.
- I choose who supports me.
- I get good support.
- I choose my friends and relationships.
- I choose how to be healthy and safe.
- I choose how I take part in my community.
- I have the same rights and responsibilities as other citizens.
- I get help to make changes in my life.

In developing the REACH Standards, Paradigm UK worked closely with people with learning disabilities who were recognised as 'experts by experience'. This has led to the development of numerous 'Quality Checker' services whereby people with learning disabilities, in some instances supported by advocacy organisations, will visit and audit the quality of services and report on the quality of user experience as well as making recomendations for quality improvement. Minney (2011) undertook a financial analysis of the benefits of using Quality Checker services over a two–year period. He reported that acting on Quality Checker recommendations improved the quality of user experience but also, in many instances, reduced the need for higher cost services in future. Financial returns suggested an average 11:1 return on investment within a five-year period (so for every £1000 spent on Quality Checker services, an organisation could expect to save £11,000). It is notable then that services of this nature offer returns, not just in terms of service quality but also in terms of efficiency savings. Such services effectively complement the activities of the CQC which are more concerned with ensuring services comply with essential standards relating to safety and the delivery of effective care.

Although not strictly applicable due to its status as a hospital, it is interesting to reflect on the fact that at Winterbourne View, none of the REACH standards would have been achieved. Most services users had been placed there using powers of compulsion conferred by the Mental Health Act and therefore had not chosen voluntarily to be there, nor could they choose with whom they lived. Service users had little or no say in how they were supported or by whom; they had minimal community contact and struggled to maintain contact with friends and to sustain relationships.

The Department of Health report on Winterbourne View put forward a series of 'I statements' which represent users' expectations and standards which should be met in high quality services delivered to people with learning disabilities or autism, who present with behaviours that challenge service. These potentially offer a similar framework to the REACH Standards, however, one that is applicable within hospital settings. These standards should not be viewed as aspirational and both organisations and services should be able to demonstrate objective evidence that they meet these standards.

Fast facts 6.6   Transforming care

According to DH (2012), high quality service means that people with learning disabilities or autism and behaviour which challenges will be able to say:

1. I am safe.
2. I am treated with compassion, dignity and respect.
3. I am involved in decisions about my care.
4. I am protected from avoidable harm, but also have my own freedom to take risks.
5. I am helped to keep in touch with my family and friends.
6. Those around me and looking after me are well supported.
7. I am supported to make choices in my daily life.
8. I get the right treatment and medication for my condition.
9. I get good quality general healthcare.
10. I am supported to live safely in the community.
11. Where I have additional care needs, I get the support I need in the most appropriate setting.
12. My care is regularly reviewed to see if I should be moving on.

Organisations and quality

The unique needs of people who have learning disabilities and their families require a focus on quality that is person-centred, taking on board all the things that may prevent them from accessing good quality care and services. This means that those who provide care or services may need to make continuous adjustments to their usual processes in order to accommodate individual needs and preferences, regardless of disability. This will ensure equity of quality outcome in terms of safe and effective services and user experience. While this can be a challenge, often equitable outcomes are easily achievable if the service provider thinks and acts in a different way. Getting it right for people with learning disabilities often means you discover strategies which lead to better outcomes for other users of services who have historically received poor quality services, and so the benefits of a more personalised approach can be translated into a demonstration of good quality for all. An example of such an approach is shown in Case study 6.2.

Case study 6.2   Our Hospital's Charter

The North London Acute Trust Summit has developed 'Our Hospital's Charter'. This is a statement of intent to provide good quality healthcare and experiences to people who have learning disabilities and their families and to improve health outcomes. It includes the principles of the Mencap 'Getting it Right' Charter (Mencap, 2008).

Whittington Health, an integrated acute and community Trust, is encouraging sign-up at all levels of the organisation. The Charter has been signed by the chief executive and Trust Board. A copy is on the Trust website and on the intranet and it is being used as a focus for assessing quality of care for people who have learning disabilities.

Several approaches have been adopted to check the quality of care. These include: patient experience electronic feedback machines in all wards and departments and at community clinics, focus groups for people who have learning disabilities and family carers, and a family and friends project. Secret shoppers also give feedback on quality.

Sometimes standards set within organisations can be a beneficial approach to improving quality. Agreed standards can help people who work in the organisation identify how well they are doing by measuring what they do against the standards. The standards are a statement of intent provided by the organisation for people who use the services. They can enable people to challenge if the quality of the service they receive is not consistent with the standards.

Quality in care is a broad concept that can be interpreted differently by different stakeholders. As a consumer, if I buy something, I want it to do what it says it will do, I want it to do it well without problems, and I want it to be priced accordingly. Experience tells us that if something is expensive does not always guarantee value for money or even good quality. As people with learning disabilities increasingly have their own budgets to buy care and services, expectations for quality will be very much based on cost and experience. Both aspects will be important and will need equal attention, so if a service is good but if it costs too much, people will not be able to afford to buy it. However, if a service is affordable but does not deliver what the person wants, they will not want to buy it.

Conclusion

In conclusion, then, we have seen evidence of an ongoing government commitment to giving people control of the care and services they receive. This includes increasing the financial power of those who use services as well as driving a clear agenda of personalisation. Learning disability services across the four UK countries have a clear and universal agenda which is about high quality, person-centred, local services that deliver demonstrable outcomes in terms of safe and effective care, as well as a quality user experience.

In spite of this background context, there have been a number of high profile examples of scandalous lapses of quality, and reflecting on these is essential if lessons are to be learned in order that quality can truly be achieved. We have considered approaches by which service providers and commissioners should be able to assure themselves of the quality of services, and we have reflected on the further threat of financial austerity on delivering quality. We have seen that quality can be conceptualised in many ways but that quality assurance is far from straightforward. In particular, we have seen that user-based approaches to understanding and delivering quality are achievable and can prove to be a cost-effective option.

This can only lead us to conclude that quality cannot be assured by politicians or strategists alone but has to be delivered at the interface between those who deliver services and those who receive them. The biggest single determinant of quality must therefore be the nature of human interactions between those providing care and support and those receiving it. The Quality Checkers have shown that this not only delivers quality but also a more cost effective way of delivering care and support. The quality challenge then is for all of us; we need to individually find effective ways to promote choice and maxmise independence. If we can do no more than pay lip service to this philosophy, care will continue to be compromised and further scandals will be reported.

Points to remember

- Lots of people talk about quality in relation to services, i.e. the government, the Department of Health, service providers, service users and their families and carers.
- Many organisations with an interest in quality have tried to identify essential standards by which quality can be recognised. However, quality remains difficult to define – everyone has a different take on what it looks like.
- Even if we can describe quality, it is difficult to recognise it in operation and to measure it. Governments are trying to drive quality by putting people with learning disabilities in charge of the money that is used to buy their services. The quality of services can be challenged by tight finances.
- Despite the existence of quality standards and systems to check services, some organisations have still delivered terrible services.
- Services need systems to monitor and check their own standards for quality and safety – this is known as governance.
- External organisations need to work together effectively to ensure that poor performance is recognised and dealt with.
- A combination of user-based and outcome-focused quality measures can lead to genuine improvements in terms of both quality and efficiency of services.
- For people with learning disabilities, day-to-day interactions with those who provide care and support are key to ensuring quality.

Resources

Care Quality Commission (CQC). The English care quality regulator.
www.cqc.org.uk/public

Foundation for people with learning disabilities. Provides access to forums where quality innovations can be shared.
www.learningdisabilities.org.uk.

Healthcare Improvement Scotland. The Scottish healthcare regulators' quality indicators.
www.healthcareimprovementscotland.org/previous_resources/indicators/ld_quality_indicators.aspx.

NHS Education for Scotland. Learning disability standards and guidelines.
www.knowledge.scot.nhs.uk/home/portals-and-topics/learning-disabilities-portal/resources/standards-and-guidelines.

NICE: The National Institute for Health and Care Excellence
www.nice.org.uk.

Northern Ireland Department of Health, Social Services and Public Safety
www.dhsspsni.gov.uk/index/phealth/sqs/sqsd-standards-service-frameworks/sqsd_service_frameworks_learning_disability.htm.

Skills for People. Quality Checkers in action.
www.skillsforpeople.org.uk/?q=what-we-do/quality-checkers.

Social Care Institute for Excellence. Source of high quality resources concerned with quality improvement.
www.scie.org.uk/topic/people/peoplewithlearningdisabilities.

References

DH (Department of Health) (2008) *High Quality Care for All: NHS Next Stage Review, Final Report*. London: Department of Health.

DH (Department of Health) (2009) *Shaping the Future of Care Together*, Green Paper. London: Department of Health.

DH (Department of Health) (2010) *Transparency in Outcomes: A Framework for Adult Social Care*. London: Department of Health.

DH (Department of Health) (2012) *Transforming Care: A National Response to Winterbourne View Hospital*. London: Department of Health.

DHSSPS (Department of Health, Social Services and Public Safety) (2004) *Equal Lives: Review of Policy and Services for People with Learning Disabilities in Northern Ireland*. Belfast: Stormont.

Flynn, M. (2012) *Winterbourne View Hospital: A Serious Case Review*. Gloucester: South Gloucestershire Safeguarding Adults Board.

Gitsham, N., Kinsella, P. and Hilson, N. (2002) *REACH: Standards in Supported Living*. Birkenhead: Paradigm.

Healthcare Commission (2006) *Joint Investigation into the Provision of Services for People with Learning Disabilities at Cornwall Partnership NHS Trust*. London: Healthcare Commission.

Healthcare Commission (2007) *Investigation into the Services for People with Learning Disabilities Provided by Sutton and Merton Primary Care Trust*. London: Healthcare Commission.

Local Government Ombudsmen and Parliamentary and Health Service Ombudsmen (2009) *Six Lives: The Provision of Public Services to People with Learning Disabilities*. London: TSO.

Mencap (2004) *Treat Me Right! Better Healthcare for People with a Learning Disability*. London: Mencap.

Mencap (2007) *Death by Indifference: Following Up the Treat Me Right! Report*. London: Mencap.

Mencap (2008) *Getting it Right*. Available at: www.mencap.org.uk.

Michael, J. (2008) *Healthcare for All: Report of the Independent Inquiry into Access to Healthcare for People with Learning Disabilities*. Available at: www.iahpld.org.uk.

Minney, H. (2011) *The Quality Checker: Why User experience*. Available at: www.minney-org/quality-checker-why-user-experience.

National Assembly for Wales (2002) *Fulfilling the Promises: Proposals for Services for People with Learning Disabilities: Consultation Documents*. Cardiff: National Assembly for Wales.

Picker Institute (2005) *Is the NHS Getting Better or Worse? An In-Depth Look at the Views of Nearly a Million Patients between 1998 and 2004*. Oxford: Picker Institute Europe.

Roe, D. (2011) *Cost and Cost Effectiveness Issues in Learning Disabilities Social Care Provision*. London: Languisson.

Scally, G. and Donaldson, L.J. (1998) Clinical governance and the drive for quality improvement in the new NHS in England, *British Medical Journal*, 317(7150): 61–65.

Scottish Executive (2000) *The Same As You? A Review of Services for People with Learning Disabilities*. Edinburgh: The Stationery Office.

Social Care Institute for Excellence (n.d.) *Personalisation: A Rough Guide*. Available at: http://www.scie.org.uk/publications/guides/guide47/.

Wood, A. and Kinsella, P. (2006) *REACH Standards in Supported Living: Service Review Pack*. London: Paradigm.

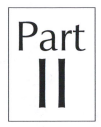

Part II

Assessment, screening and diagnosis

Emerson *et al.* (2005) highlighted the importance of involving people with a learning disability in health research as respondents had very different views of their health status and definitions of health compared to the professionals and organisations that provided the health service to them. In the main, respondents viewed health as something that allowed them to live a life they chose, e.g. going out independently, having friends, etc. While a move away from the medical model of health has led to more holistic definitions of health that recognise the bio-psycho-social impact on well-being, the professionals involved have not always recognised health in respect of these quality of life indicators. Emerson *et al.* identify that it is important that more research ascertains the views of people with a learning disability but suggest that responsibility for this should be led by healthcare professionals and their organisations. The Disability Rights Commission (2006) endorses this view and also provides clear guidelines on the legal obligations that organisations have to develop policy and practices that give people with disabilities a voice and the opportunity to be involved in their health services, including providing information that is accessible (available in a format that responds to their chosen method of communication, whether it is verbal or non-verbal).

The chapters in Part II are based on a case study. The case studies follow a lifecycle approach centred on one character 'Jem'. The scenarios given include discussion on a range of health and social care assessments conducted by professionals, families and carers.

The chapters that make up Part II are:

References

Disability Rights Commission (2006) *Equal Treatment: Closing the Gap. Health Formal Investigation Report: Summary for Practitioners.* London: Disability Rights Commission.

Emerson, E., Malam, S., Davies, I. and Spencer, K. (2005) *Adults with Learning Difficulties in England 2003/4.* London: HMSO.

7 Pre-/peri/-post-natal assessment, screening and diagnosis

Helen Atherton and Shaun Derry

Learning outcomes

After reading this chapter you will be able to:

- explore the range of assessments undertaken during pregnancy and childbirth
- identify pre-natal and post-natal screening tests
- consider the impact of diagnosis of a learning disability on the family.

Introduction

> The doctor said something about low intelligence, cardiac defects and a lifetime of caring. He then patted Louise's hand and left the room.

Preparing for the birth of a child is a unique and exciting time. On being asked to revisit the experience, parents often recall a variety of thoughts and emotions ranging from joy through to worries and anxieties, among which are those concerned with the health of the unborn child (Modh *et al.*, 2011). In the UK, the availability of pre- and post-natal screening and diagnosis offers parents the opportunity to establish the health of their child through the early detection of some physical and genetic-based conditions. While for some parents, such testing can offer the welcome reassurance that all is well, for others it can lead to a series of very difficult and ultimately life-changing decisions. This chapter explores assessment in pregnancy and childbirth in terms of the range of pre-natal and post-natal screening and diagnostic tests offered to parents across what has been termed the screening and testing pathway (NHS FASP Consent Standards Review Group and NHS Fetal Anomaly Screening Programme, 2011) (see Figure 7.1). The focus will be on the testing for Down syndrome or Down's syndrome, though it is acknowledged that a range of different conditions can currently be detected. This will undoubtedly rise with the development of more sophisticated methods of testing.

- Eyes that slant upwards
- Small ears
- Flat back of head
- Small mouth
- Protruding tongue
- Flattened nose bridge
- White spots on the iris (the coloured part of the eye), known as Brushfield spots
- Short fingers
- Broad hands with a single crease across the palm
- Loose skin on the back of the neck
- Loose joints (babies in particular may seem 'floppy')
- Poor muscle tone (hypotonia)
- Low birth weight
- Vertical skin folds (epicanthic folds) between the upper eyelids and inner corner of the eye

Figure 7.1 Physical characteristics of Down's Syndrome
Source: NHS Choices (2012).

In 2011, 2,307 abortions under category E (substantial risk that the child will be born with physical or mental abnormality resulting in severe handicap) were undertaken in England and Wales, 22 per cent (511) of which were specifically for Down's Syndrome (DH, 2011). Obviously, the offer, uptake and range of potential outcomes of such prenatal testing give rise to questions of a serious ethical and moral nature that includes human rights and the acceptance of disability in everyday society.

Case study 7.1   A Down's Syndrome baby

Louise Rogers was born into a middle-class family in the North-East of England. Her father, Jim, was the headmaster of the local secondary school and her mother, Anne, was a housewife. Louise, and her two siblings, Corin and Lauren, attended the local private school. All three left school and went on to university where Louise excelled in English Literature. During her time at university, Louise met Mark, a chemist. After finishing their higher education they moved back to the same city where Louise had been born. Mark began working for a local pharmaceutical company which required him to work abroad every few weeks. Louise returned to university to complete teacher training. Two months into the course she found that she was pregnant and gave birth to a daughter, JoJo. Unfortunately, Mark's work schedule, coupled with a new baby, took its toll on their relationship and they separated when JoJo was a year old.

When JoJo was 9, Louise met Luke, a labourer, in a local pub. They married 6 months into their relationship. Louise, now 28, fell pregnant again. JoJo was very excited at the possibility of having a new brother or sister. It was Luke's first child. Both Louise and Luke attended the preliminary antenatal check and dating scan, eager to see the first images of their baby. They met the midwife who asked questions about Louise's overall health and well-being. Among them was a question about pre-natal testing and the midwife asked Louise whether or not she wanted to have the 'foetus' screened for Down's Syndrome. This surprised Louise as she had not been offered this test in her first pregnancy and thought it was only for older mothers. The midwife explained that all women were now offered the test as a matter of course and it just meant having a 'bit more blood taken and another ultrasound'. Louise agreed to have the combined test as she viewed it as just being 'part of the process', and anyway she was still quite young, so she was sure everything would be fine. She was also pleased that this meant that she got to see more images of the baby.

The results of the combined test were a confusing mass of numbers but the midwife said that they essentially showed that Louise was at low risk of carrying a child with Down's Syndrome. The midwife gave them a copy of the results and told them to go away and enjoy the rest of the pregnancy. At 20 weeks, they found out that they were having a boy. They decided to call him Jem (Jeremy) after Luke's father.

Louise went into labour at 38 weeks. A baby boy was born after 14 hours in the presence of two midwives. After the birth, Louise was quickly shown Jem, then one of the midwives took him to be weighed and cleaned up while the other assisted Louise. After five minutes, the midwife caring for Jem called the other midwife over and they began to talk in hushed tones. One then disappeared and re-appeared with a doctor who very briefly examined the baby. After talking to the midwives, he came over to Louise and Luke and, without sitting down, said that he was very sorry, but he thought the baby had Down's Syndrome and that they would have to take a blood sample to be sure. He quickly said something about low intelligence, cardiac defects, and a lifetime of caring. He then patted Louise's hand and left the room. One of the midwives hurriedly dressed Jem and handed him to his father. She then also left the room saying that she thought they might have a leaflet somewhere about Down's Syndrome. The other midwife busied herself clearing up.

Both Louise and Luke were left in a state of shock, not fully understanding what this meant. Luke put the baby in the cot next to the bed and said that he couldn't cope and needed space and left the room. When he came back, he was visibly upset. He started shouting saying that it was obviously all his fault, as JoJo had been perfectly normal and that it was because he wasn't as intelligent as her father had been. He said that Louise's mother had been outside the ward waiting with JoJo but that he had told them to go because there was something wrong with the baby. He hasn't said what, except that it was serious. In truth, he had been too embarrassed to say what it was. Louise tried to calm him down but couldn't find the right words. She looked at the baby lying in the cot and tried to take stock of the situation. She couldn't imagine life with a child with Down's Syndrome yet couldn't imagine a life without her new baby.

What is Down's Syndrome?

Down's Syndrome is the most common genetic cause of learning disabilities. Prevalence is reported to differ between populations ranging from 1 in 319 to 1 in 1000 live births (Wiseman et al., 2009). The Down's Syndrome Association (DSA) (2012) have estimated there to be 60,000 people currently living in the UK with the condition. It is caused by the presence of an extra chromosome 21 in affected individuals, hence it is alternatively known as 'Trisomy 21'. Around 94 per cent of cases of Down's Syndrome are believed to be caused by the non-disjunction of the chromosomes during cell division. The remaining 6 per cent is attributed to a balanced translocation or mosaicism (Hartway, 2009). Translocation Down's Syndrome is the only form of the condition that is known to be hereditary. While Down's Syndrome transcends all races and social classes, the highest prevalence is among individuals born to older mothers (Graves Allen *et al.*, 2009).

All people with Down's Syndrome will have some level of learning disability, ranging from mild to moderate. They are distinctive through a range of physical features (see Figure 7.1), however, they should not be seen as a homogeneous group; as with all people, their physical appearance, personality and abilities will widely differ. People with Down's Syndrome can live happy, fulfilling lives, with many going to mainstream schools and learning to read and write; it is recognised, however, that they will always require some level of support to do this (DSA, 2012). While current estimates suggest that 92 per cent of parents in England and Wales choose to terminate a pregnancy after a positive diagnosis of Down's Syndrome (Morris and Alberman, 2009), this should not detract from the positive experiences of those caring for family members with the condition.

Physical health is one area in which people with Down's Syndrome, particularly those at the younger end of the age spectrum, are especially vulnerable. From birth onwards, they are at an increased risk for a number of congenital and acquired health problems that will require continual monitoring and prompt intervention from a range of healthcare professionals to ensure a good quality of life is maintained. The range of health conditions is available in Table 7.1 but it should be realised that they will not affect all individuals in the same way. Current life expectancy in this group is estimated to be around 60 years. This is thought to have quadrupled over the last 50 years due to improved treatment of respiratory infections and better access to cardiac surgery One significant health issue compromising longevity of life is

Table 7.1 Range of typical health problems found among people with Down's Syndrome

Condition	(%)
Hearing problems	75
Vision problems	60
Cataracts	15
Refractive errors	50
Obstructive sleep apnea	50–75
Otitis media	50–70
Congenital heart disease	40–50
Hypodontia and delayed dental eruption	23
Gastrointestinal atresias	12
Thyroid disease	4–18
Seizures	1–13
Haematologic problems	
Anaemia	3
Iron Deficiency	10
Transient myeloproliferative disorder	10
Leukemia	1
Celiac disease	5
Atlantoaxial instability	1–2
Autism	1
Hirschsprung disease	<5

Source: Bull and the Committee on Genetics (2011).

Alzheimer's disease which is significantly more prevalent among people with Down's Syndrome than the general population and has a much earlier onset, commonly occurring in the 30–40 age bracket; the highest incidence can be found among those in their early fifties (British Psychological Society and Royal College of Psychiatrists, 2009). This will be discussed further in Chapters 11 and 12.

Screening and diagnosis

Screening and diagnostic testing for learning disabilities have become increasingly common before and during pregnancy, and shortly after birth. Standard tests begin in the first week of an infant's life. Similarly, an awareness of the risk profile associated with increased maternal age has led to the provision of antenatal screening and/or diagnostic testing for Down's Syndrome. In recent years, however, there has been a trend towards a broadening of routine screening provision to, and an increased uptake by, all women, irrespective of age and other known risk factors (Tringham *et al.*, 2011).

Screening is the process by which an individual's risk of a particular condition is ascertained, in this case, the foetus or neonate. Antenatal screening carries no risk to the foetus, and screening tests are often non-invasive. Following screening, a risk-factor is ascribed to the individual that expresses the likelihood of the presence of a condition. Risk is categorised simply as lower or higher. Conditions are not definitively ruled out by a lower risk rating, nor are they definitively diagnosed with a higher risk rating (UKNSC, 2012). Women who receive a result which places their foetus in the higher risk category are likely to be offered further screening and/or the option of undertaking diagnostic testing (National Collaborating Centre for Women's and Children's Health (NICE, 2008)).

The purpose of diagnostic testing is to confirm the presence or absence of a condition. Antenatal diagnostic testing is usually invasive, and carries an associated level of risk to the foetus. As a result, diagnostic testing is not routinely offered to the wider population. Women who fall into the higher risk category due to pre-existing conditions, or higher risk screening results, may be offered diagnostic testing (Harcombe and Armstrong, 2008). Diagnostic testing is more precise than screening, and can offer a clear diagnosis of the condition of the foetus. There remains, however, a small margin for error in antenatal diagnoses as identified in the case study.

The three stages at which screening and/or diagnostic testing are available are pre-conception, antenatal, and post-natal. These will each be considered below.

Pre-conception

At pre-conception, the aim is to identify and ameliorate risk through parental screening, diagnosis, and subsequent risk management. Pre-conception care has become widely available in UK primary healthcare services. Administering folic acid supplements has become an established practice to reduce the risk of anencephaly, encephalocele, and spina bifida (Crider *et al.*, 2011). Reducing alcohol, tobacco, and illicit drug consumption reduces the risk of foetal alcohol syndrome (FAS) and intrauterine hypoxia. Genetic testing provides information pertaining to the carrier status of the parents and the associated risk to the child. Particular attention is given to those with pre-existing medical conditions, complications during previous pregnancies, and a family history of genetic conditions. Autosomal recessive conditions may be inherited by children whose parents are both carriers yet remain unaffected. The child will be affected if both parents' recessive condition is transmitted;

examples include phenylketonuria and Tay-Sachs' disease (Burke *et al.*, 2011). X-linked conditions, such as fragile X syndrome and Hunter's syndrome, are inherited from the maternal lineage. At pre-conception there are no certainties regarding the eventual outcome for the child. Parents-to-be with an increased genetic risk may receive support and information from genetic counsellors regarding ongoing reproductive decision-making e.g. alternative methods of conception (Riedijk *et al.*, 2012).

Practice alert 7.1

'Fragile X is diagnosed by a simple blood test. It is not about a label, but getting a diagnosis will help you to get the information and support you need' (Mencap, 2013).

Antenatal

Down's Syndrome is currently the main focus of antenatal screening and diagnostic testing for learning disabilities. Antenatal screening and diagnostic testing occur during weeks 11–20 of the pregnancy. If accepted, initial screening should be completed between 11 weeks–13 weeks and 6 days (Harcombe and Armstrong, 2008). A nuchal translucency scan – a specific type of ultrasound – and blood tests may be performed; this is known as the combined test (NCCWCH, 2008). During nuchal translucency scanning, the thickness between the spine and the nape of the foetus' neck is measured. An increased build-up of fluid leading to an atypical thickening is indicative of an increased risk of Down's syndrome. Evidence suggests that considering these tests in combination increases the accuracy of the results (Aldred *et al.*, 2010).

There are two main antenatal diagnostic tests for Down's syndrome. Chorionic villus sampling, completed during weeks 11–14, involves sampling the chorionic villi region of the placenta. The placental sample has the same genetic material as the foetus and, therefore, can be tested for chromosomal abnormalities. The UKNSC (2012) explains that amniocentesis should be completed during weeks 15–18, and this involves taking a sample of amniotic fluid. The sample contains foetal skin and waste cells which are suitable for chromosomal analysis. As the respective risk of miscarriage associated with these procedures is 1–2 per cent and 1 per cent, serious consideration is required prior to their uptake (Aldred *et al.*, 2010). The same sampling techniques are also used in the detection of other chromosomal conditions such as Fragile X syndrome.

Ethical and moral considerations associated with antenatal screening and diagnostic testing tend to divide opinion.

Reader activity 7.1 Diagnostic testing

- Consider your understanding of a learning disability. Make a list of what you consider to be the benefits and threats of antenatal screening and diagnostic testing.
- If this has impacted on your life or someone you know well, further advice and support are available through GP services or organisations such as the National Childbirth Trust, available at: www.nct.org.uk/pregnancy/antenatal-screening-and-testing-0.

Those in favour of pre-birth testing argue that early detection allows the family time to prepare for the child's potentially atypical needs. Other favourable arguments include the belief that parents are afforded a greater freedom of choice. Parents' perceived ability to care for a child with a learning disability, and expectations of the child's quality of life are often cited as influential factors in the decision-making process (Reid *et al.*, 2009). The opposing side of the debate includes scepticism about the reality of informed consent, the reliability of testing and the consequences thereof and decisions pertaining to termination and subsequent links to eugenic ideology. There is a school of thought, for example, which suggests that pre-birth testing justifies a modern, socially acceptable form of genetic cleansing (Reynolds, 2009). The complex nature of the decisions faced by parents in this position is indicative of the need for clear, impartial information about any and all possible courses of action.

Post-natal

For many children with learning disabilities, their diagnosis comes only when they are observed to be missing developmental milestones. Infants who have Down's Syndrome, however, often have specific, identifiable, physical characteristics which indicate an increased likelihood of the condition (see Figure 7.1). In cases where parents have decided not to undergo pre-natal screening, or received a false negative result, an initial diagnosis of Down's Syndrome is highly likely shortly after birth, usually within 48–72 hours (Charleton *et al.*, 2010). Once the suspicion of an infant having Down's Syndrome has been raised, as in Jem's case, chromosomal karyotyping – an investigation into chromosomal constituents – can be performed in order to provide a definitive diagnosis (Davidson, 2008). This test will also be completed following positive antenatal diagnostic testing in order to confirm the diagnosis. The parents of infants diagnosed with translocation Down's Syndrome may also be offered karyotyping and/or genetic counselling. Shortly after birth, all babies are subjected to a physical examination to establish their health status. As Down's Syndrome is statistically linked to an increased prevalence of health deficits (see Table 7.1), a number of these tests are of particular significance in light of a positive diagnosis. An enhanced screening protocol gives infants with Down's Syndrome the best possible start to their life.

Blood spot screening (the 'heel prick') includes tests for congenital hypothyroidism, which has a higher prevalence rate in people with Down's Syndrome, and phenylketonuria (PKU) (UKNSC, 2012). Hypothyroidism – defined by an underactive thyroid gland leading to insufficient levels of thyroxine – can cause physical and intellectual disabilities. PKU is typified by an inability to process phenylalanine, an essential amino acid. Infants diagnosed with PKU are treated simply with a low phenylalanine diet which can decrease symptoms such as the development of severe intellectual disabilities (Blau *et al.*, 2010). Early detection and treatment for both of these conditions increase the prospect of better long-term health.

Around 75 per cent of people with Down's Syndrome have some degree of hearing problem, therefore, the routine hearing test is important. Tests are straightforward and are often completed while the infant is asleep. Sight problems, including cataracts, are also noted at a higher prevalence rate in people with Down's Syndrome and will be detected during routine screening of the eyes. Differentiating from the routine screening assessment, infants with Down's Syndrome should expect to receive a routine echocardiogram (ECG) due to the increased likelihood of a congenital heart defect. Of those, the most commonly observed heart conditions are atrioventricular septal defects, which are discussed further in Chapter 8.

In addition to the routine screening tests provided to all neonates, the infant with Down's Syndrome may also require further and more in-depth screening. The higher prevalence of gastrointestinal, pulmonary and orthopaedic complications, alongside potential breathing difficulties due to nasal, sinus, and tracheal atypia, each require careful screening and subsequent treatment.

Reader activity 7.2   Understanding terms

- A number of terms may have been used within this chapter so far which may be unfamiliar, e.g. chorionic villi; amniotic fluid; tracheal atypia.
- Take some time to explore these terms in a dictionary to support your understanding where necessary.

Impact of diagnosis on the family unit

The birth of a child is a momentous occasion which stays with parents for the rest of their lives. Parents often recall specific minutiae from the day of their child's birth many years after the fact. Despite the distress and pain, the birth of a typical child is usually one of the happiest days of a parent's life. Raising a child with a learning disability, while acknowledging the inherent challenges, is overwhelmingly reported as a positive experience for the whole family, as the child grows, learns, and bonds with their parents and siblings. Families state that their child has enriched their lives and given them a different perspective. Some acknowledge that their child's learning disability has precipitated a deeper relationship between parent and child (King *et al.*, 2009). Although these feelings of fulfilment, happiness, and acceptance exist in the long term, they often necessitate a shift from the pre-diagnosis perspective.

The news that a child has a learning disability can be devastating for the family. Skotko *et al.* (2009: 752) report that parents were left feeling 'shocked', 'angry', 'devastated', 'overwhelmed', 'depressed', 'stunned', or 'helpless'. Guilt is also common when a diagnosis is received as parents ruminate on what they could have done differently during the pregnancy .Others conclude that they must have an underlying genetic pathology which has been inherited by the child, or that they have an inferior level of intelligence. These assumptions may manifest as feelings of embarrassment, shame, or self-blame as in the case study.

In the 1960s, Elisabeth Kübler-Ross conducted pioneering research into the psychological responses to death and dying. The culmination of this research was the seminal work, *On Death and Dying* (Kübler-Ross, 1969), which introduced the five stages of death (later renamed the five stages of loss):

1. denial (and isolation)
2. anger
3. bargaining
4. depression
5. acceptance.

Recent research has included the explicit acknowledgement that family and friends may go through the same grief processes in response to an unfavourable diagnosis or death (Kübler-Ross and Kessler,

2005). Furthermore, the concept of death has been expanded from biological death to include both social and psychosocial forms. Social death refers to the inability to fit into, or the ostracism from, the society of one's peers (Larkin, 2011). Psychosocial death is defined as the loss of a psychological and/ or emotional connection to a familiar person, e.g. a family member with dementia (Harwood, 2007). The diagnosis of an infant with a learning disability may present a combination of these definitions.

Reader activity 7.3   Professional help

Consider the range of health and social care professionals who could be involved in Louise and Luke's life following the birth of Jem. What roles and support should they provide? You may find it useful to look at the web pages developed by NHS Careers www.nhscareers.nhs.uk/.

Around the time of Kübler-Ross's initial research, John Bowlby – best known for his work on attachment theory – was also researching grief reactions. He suggested a four-stage process which included: protective defence, pining, despair, and recovery (Bowlby, 1980). These stages are characterised by:

- shock
- anger
- incomprehension
- yearning
- disorganisation
- reorganisation.

It is clear that a considerable overlap exists between these two theories.

Most of the research into the initial impact of the diagnosis of a child with a learning disability concentrates on either the parents or family as a unit or on the mother. Little research directly investigates how other family members are affected. Relatively little is known about the impact on the father. It is reported that fathers play an important role in maintaining positivity and supporting their partner (Dyer *et al.*, 2009). A number of touching, personal accounts exist, which help to highlight the family-wide experience. Andy Merriman (1999) recalls moments following the birth of his daughter, Sarah, who has Down's Syndrome. He recounts a debate as to whether or not the scene in the hospital room should be filmed. Elsewhere, he describes breaking down in a shop after being unable to decide which colour clothing to buy for his daughter; the usual 'pink for a girl' not seeming right for a girl with Down's Syndrome. Victor and Ivy Smith (Extra 21, 2012) recall that, upon receiving the news that their grandson had Down's Syndrome, and after the initial shock, their immediate concern was for the well-being of their son and his partner as well as for their new grandson. Siblings, too, may feel the impact of the diagnosis of a brother or sister with a learning disability. Although they may not recognise, understand, or much mind that their sibling has a learning disability, the impact they experience will often be linked to that of their parents (Seligman and Darling, 2007). Confusion and incomprehension of the situation, people talking in earnest and sombre tones, and their parents' distress, may each play a part in the initial reaction to their new sibling. While some of these experiences may not be restricted to specific family members, they illustrate the wider impact and the concurrent need for sensitivity and support.

Promoting informed decision-making

At the heart of professional involvement in and around pregnancy and birth is the promotion of parental autonomy (NICE, 2008). Despite the widely accessible nature of pre- and post-natal screening and diagnostic tests, and the argument of some that they have become a routine and largely accepted part of pregnancy and care of the newborn, the decision to opt for or decline testing remains the fundamental right of individuals. Ideally, such decisions should be made privately and where possible in partnership between couples (Skirton and Barr, 2010). They should be undertaken without duress and be in no way influenced by the attitudes and beliefs of professionals (NHS FASP CSRG and NHS FSP, 2011).

Health professionals have a professional obligation to facilitate informed choice with respect to screening and diagnostic testing. Key to this process is the provision of relevant, accurate, up-to-date, individualised, and evidence-based information. The quality of information provision is known to influence both parental adaptation to a diagnosis and subsequent decision-making (Muggli *et al.*, 2009). Where it is effective, it can lead to positive outcomes such as less decisional conflict and increased levels of satisfaction between parents (van den Berg *et al.*, 2005). When ineffectual, it can result in increased levels of parental fear, anxiety and feelings of disempowerment (Skotko, 2005).

Practice alert 7.2

- Clear guidelines and education exist to support professionals in facilitating informed choice.
- Undertake a search of the up-to-date literature to access professional guidelines in this matter.

The remainder of this chapter seeks to make the reader aware of some of the inherent difficulties in facilitating informed choice about testing in the face of an actual or potential diagnosis of learning disabilities, and the role of professionals in response to these. The term 'professionals' is used to refer, not only to those who are typically involved in maternal healthcare in the UK (GPs; midwifes, geneticists, genetic counsellors, paediatricians) whom you may have included in your list, but also to those whose role may be less formally recognised but is nevertheless potentially useful in ensuring informed choice e.g. the learning disability nurse or parent support groups. In doing so, it is recognised that difficult decisions can arise during the pre- and post-natal periods, but can also occur pre-conceptually when parents are deciding whether or not to try for a baby. This is particularly the case for parents whose own or family history suggests they may be at risk of having a child with a specific genetic defect (Human Genetics Commission, 2011). Even after the decision has been taken to terminate a pregnancy following a diagnosis of a foetal abnormality, parents still require information in order to make very complex, highly emotive, and often painful decisions. Regardless of the stage, the content of information and the way it is communicated by healthcare professionals can profoundly influence parents' response to a diagnosis and the way they view their child; it is also an event that is likely to remain vividly imprinted on their memories (Muggli *et al.*, 2009).

Specific guidance exists to direct professional involvement during the pre-conceptual, pre-natal and post-natal periods (Human Genetics Commission, 2011). The intention is not to cover each period in detail but to provide an overview of a range of overlapping issues with respect to the role of professionals in the potential screening and diagnosis processes, particularly in relation to Down's Syndrome. This will be supported by research that has investigated the views of a range of stakeholders in the process, including parents, health professionals and, crucially, people with learning disabilities themselves.

Practice alert 7.3

In the UK, all pregnant women can expect to be provided with information about the range of tests and options available along the screening and testing pathway. Such information should contain important details regarding the nature, purpose, risks, benefits, timings, limitations and potential consequences of testing.

The nature of information

Parental need for information will differ on the basis of both the nature of the conditions for which are being tested and the background and personal experiences of individuals themselves (France *et al.*, 2011). Available evidence suggests a wide range of potential variables influencing decision–making, ranging from age, religious and cultural beliefs through to beliefs about the morality of genetic screening and abortion. Perceptions of the condition for which screening is being carried out and previous experience of the condition are also known to be contributory factors. Farrelly *et al.* (2012) argue that it is the role of professionals to help parents explore these issues, while France *et al.* (2011) advocate allowing parents to raise their own concerns, thereby ensuring that information is tailored to their own subjective requirements, i.e. the management of the individual uncertainties they face and the decisions they, themselves, will have to live with. Parental control can also be achieved through 'offering' rather than 'providing' information thus responding to their right to know and their right to not to know (Schoonen *et al.*, 2012). This is crucial, as evidence exists to suggest that some parents are unaware that screening and diagnostic tests are 'optional'. Some report feeling pressurised into conforming to something some professionals are representing as 'routine' (Sooben, 2010).

During the course of the decision-making process, research has identified that parents not only seek to use 'professional' or 'biochemical' information (e.g. risk ratios; nature of procedures, their availability, the risk of miscarriage) but equally draw upon what the authors term 'lay' or 'experiential' knowledge; essentially, the personal experiences of others (France *et al.*, 2011). The need to understand people's lived experiences of either terminating a pregnancy on the basis of a foetal abnormality, or living and caring for a person with a genetic abnormality such as Down's Syndrome, has been perceived as an important facet of informed decision-making in this context. Indeed, it has been concluded that such information allows parents to create a vision for the future by living it through the accounts of others, and it is known to be highly valued and strongly desired by actual and prospective parents of children with Down's Syndrome. Research into parental decision-making processes demonstrates, however, that a balance between professional/biomedical and lay/experiential is not reflected in the information typically provided by professionals (Van Riper *et al.*, 2011). Evidence has shown a distinct bias towards the provision of medical facts with discussion on the lives of people with disabilities largely neglected. It has been claimed that this situation may be derived from parents and professionals approaching the nature of testing from different perspectives and values, with the latter group possibly influenced by cost-benefit ratios. Others, however, have attributed it to a lack of relevant knowledge and understanding about the lives of people with disabilities, in particular, those with Down's syndrome, or a lack of training and experience in disability issues in general (Hodgson and Weil, 2012). Inherently negative attitudes towards this group of people are also thought to exist. This may be implicit in the tendency of professionals to suggest termination in the face of a foetal abnormality, rather than commending other alternatives such as continuing with the pregnancy or adoption; professionals implying that by continuing the pregnancy parents are making the wrong choice is not uncommon.

Parents value positive information about the potential abilities of their child and it has been demonstrated that positively framed information can improve the overall experience of receiving a diagnosis (Dent and Carey, 2006). Yet a lack of currency, and a distinct bias towards negative outcomes, have typified the information provided to parents. This is also evidenced in the negative language employed in describing the situation such as 'tragedy' and 'burden' (Lalvani, 2011). In reality, such descriptors fail to accurately describe the way both parents of children with Down's Syndrome and people with Down's Syndrome themselves predominantly view their own lives. Even in the face of a diagnosis of severely life-limiting condition such Trisomy 18 (Edwards's Syndrome) and Trisomy 13 (Patau's Syndrome), parents who have chosen to go ahead with their pregnancy describe how their child has enriched their lives.

The NHS FASP CSRG and NHS FSP (2011) have called for a balanced perspective of the conditions which are being tested for, yet it has been conceded that this notion of 'balance' is difficult to quantify. Using the experience of parents, and those involved in the provision of both pre- and post-natal genetic counseling, Sheets *et al.* (2011a) compiled a list of 34 items that reflect what is deemed essential information to be presented to parents in the initial discussion following a diagnosis of Down's Syndrome, whether that is pre-natally or post-natally, some of which are presented in Figure 7.2. This is useful for prompting professionals to cover key topic areas, however, the authors caution against its use as mere checklist. Furthermore, they corroborate the views of others that professionals must seek to establish the individual's personal requirement for information, taking into account parental values, coping strategies and support networks.

Reader activity 7.4   A balanced perspective

Reflect on your current ability to provide a balanced perspective on the lives of people with Down's Syndrome. Identify some areas for your personal and professional development. This may include looking for positive life stories and images.

While it may be the case that people are requesting more social information about people with Down's Syndrome, such as their ability to make friends, engage in meaningful relationships, and participate in family life (Skokto *et al.*, 2011), their right to know and their right not to know such information needs to be upheld. Although for some such information may be pertinent and helpful, for others it may make the ultimate decision more difficult to make (Skirton and Barr, 2010).

Communicating key information

It is not only the content of the information provided that is important in facilitating parents to make informed choices, but also the way that it is communicated. Poorly presented, incomprehensible and

1 DS is caused by extra genetic material from chromosome 21. DS may be suspected based on physical findings, but the diagnosis is confirmed by chromosome analysis.

2 Individuals with DS have a variable range of intellectual disability from mild to moderate.

3 Babies with DS have delays in achieving developmental milestones and benefit from early intervention including physical, occupational and speech therapy.

4 80% of babies with DS have hypotonia.

5 50% of babies with DS have one or more congenital abnormality: 40–60% of babies with DS have a heart defect and 12% have a gastrointestinal defect that may require surgery. Assistance with referrals to specialist is appropriate for identified complications.

6 Children with DS are more like other children than they are different.

7 Raising a child with DS may involve more time commitment than typical children.

8 Individuals with DS can

participate in community sports, activities, and leagues

learn in a special education class or may be included in regular classes, and most can complete high school

be employed competitively or in a workshop setting

live independently or in a group home

have friends and intimate relationships.

9 Life expectancy extends into the fifties or sixties.

10 Information on local support groups, advocacy organisations, early intervention centres, printed material, fact sheets, books, specialist referral(s) as needed, and the option to contact a family raising a child with DS should be offered.

11 A personalised recurrence risk for future pregnancies should be offered.

Figure 7.2 Essential information about Down's Syndrome
Source: Adapted from Sheets *et al.* (2011a).

ill-timed information can increase the anxiety levels of parents, leading some to lose control of the situation and acquiesce to what they perceive to be the demands of health professionals (Sooben, 2010). Both information overload and conversely a lack of information have been cited as problematic issues, as is the feeling of being rushed into making difficult decisions. Particular attention has also been given to the difficulty of understanding complex information such as risk ratios in screening while stressed and anxious (Durand *et al.*, 2010).

Parents need to be able to understand and assimilate key information if they are to make an informed choice. Key information should therefore be made available in a variety of formats, responding to the personal requirements of individuals.

Practice alert 7.4 Key information

Current research indicates that parents value books, leaflets, and professional recommended websites that incorporate graphs, videos and other visual material. The provision of these should allow parents to assimilate information away from the stress of the clinical environment, though special consideration needs to be given to those for whom written language may be a barrier to understanding English.

Muggli *et al.* (2009) advocate a family-centred approach to the provision of information and there is an increasing availability of resources to support parents in conveying the meaning of a diagnosis to other family members, including other children. A good example of this is a colouring book produced for young children about Down's Syndrome (Bell and Aguila, 1998) and the book *Fasten Your Seatbelt*, written for teenagers (Skotko *et al.*, 2009). During the course of consultations, professionals may either provide material or direct parents to websites of organisations that contain lists of relevant resources (see Resources section below).

Parents often comment on the failure of professionals to respond to their emotional needs and the highly clinical way that information is conveyed. Many parents have criticised health professionals for failing to see their children as having value, being unique and being foremost a child. Moreover, there is a reluctance of health professionals to be drawn on the child's potential abilities (Sooben, 2010). This negativity and insensitivity towards the feeling of the parents can serve to heighten levels of distress and anxiety and indeed feelings of being different. This can be amplified by the battery of routine and diagnosis-specific tests that the child will undergo in the first few days and, again, professionals are responsible for ensuring that parents receive key information about such procedures, including risks and potential outcomes.

Feelings of difference can be further exacerbated through the ill-timed sharing of a diagnosis, which in some cases is done before the parents have had chance to bond with their newborn as a child rather than a child with a disability. To counter this, professionals are urged to normalise the process as much as possible, beginning by congratulating the parents on the new arrival (Bull and the Committee on Genetics, 2011). The need to convey the diagnosis in private and, where possible, with both parents present is considered essential practice (Sheets *et al.*, 2011a). There is disagreement, however, over other interventions. Some suggest a supportive environment may be facilitated by the availability of a private room, while others indicate this may accentuate feelings of difference. This suggests that the way parents are told about a diagnosis should, where possible, be tailored to their needs. Further up-to-date guidance for professionals on communicating a pre- or post-natal diagnosis of Down's Syndrome can be found in the work of Sheets *et al.* (2011b).

Finding out about Down's Syndrome

Experiential knowledge and understanding have been shown to be important facets of informed decision-making surrounding screening and diagnostic testing. It is this type of information, as opposed to medical facts, however, that may be the hardest for many health professionals to draw upon. Van Riper and Choi (2011) argue that this lack of knowledge, or indeed knowledge that is biased towards the negative aspects of having a child with a learning disability, may be attributed to the limited opportunities health professionals have to experience the lives of families outside of the clinical environment. In order to address this deficit, health professionals need to be prepared to educate themselves about the day-to-day lives of this group, not only to educate parents, but to challenge existing professional negative assumptions (Brasington, 2007). Nowadays, the internet provides a ready and accessible source of such information and can be equally useful for parents wishing to find out more. The websites of both NHS Choices (2012) and the Healthtalkonline (2012) contain footage of individuals discussing their lives with Down's Syndrome and other conditions. Such accounts are similarly found on the websites of many national support organisations dedicated to improving the lives of those with specific forms of disability. These websites provide a rich source of key information, including the personal accounts of those living with the condition. One such organisation is the Down's Syndrome Association, who are currently running an interactive training programme called 'Tell it Right, Start it Right' to educate professionals working in maternity services (DSA, 2012). Many similar organisations exist and information about their activities can be found by doing a quick internet search, or through *Contact a Family* which provide a comprehensive database of different conditions and available services (CAF, 2012). Many such organisations will have telephone help-lines and often branches where access to local support groups can be attained (Sykes, 2010). Information about such groups can also be found through Children's Centres which are now located in many areas. Support groups also exist virtually on social networking sites such as Facebook and in the form of other online groups (see Janvier *et al.*, 2012).

Reader activity 7.5 Accessing information

Identify the range of individuals and organisations who could provide information and support regarding the lives of people with Down's Syndrome in your local area.

As the child grows older, it is likely that they will come into contact with specialist services at some time or other and it is the knowledge and understanding of those working in such services that represent an extremely useful resource for professionals in maternity services. Learning disability nurses, for example, work with both children and adults with learning disabilities across a range of settings and, therefore, have a detailed knowledge and understanding about their lives (DH, 2007). A significant part of their role is the provision of education and this extends to other healthcare professionals who may be involved in the care of this group. Most towns and cities will have a community learning disability team, the details of which can be obtained by accessing the internet sites of local NHS trusts. Additionally, some are fulfilling the specialist role of liaison nurses in general hospitals (Trueland, 2010). There is currently little evidence of learning disability nurses being involved at the point of birth of a child with learning disabilities but the knowledge and skills that they could bring to such a situation should not be underestimated.

Conclusion

In recent years, screening and diagnostic testing before and during pregnancy, and shortly after birth, has become accessible to a broader demographic. Aside from the serious and difficult decisions facing parents regarding conception, the continuation or termination of a pregnancy, and the moral and ethical debate that exists around the subject, an increase in the availability of such tests raises further questions for both parents and professionals. The diagnosis of a foetus or neonate with a learning disability can have a dramatic effect on the family unit, irrespective of the stage at which the news is delivered. Initial reactions to this news may have a long-lasting and pervasive effect on the parents' perspective of the future outcome for the child. Biased information, either implicitly or explicitly, may influence the parents' decisions pre-birth, or colour their judgement post-birth. Healthcare professionals need to have a good level of knowledge and understanding of conditions such as Down's Syndrome, acknowledging both medical implications and experiential accounts of each course of action. According to much research, the current general trend appears to indicate that healthcare professionals maintain a focus on negative aspects of conditions such as Down's Syndrome, or at least the implication is reflected in their approach to delivering the news. Rather than simply suggesting a reversal of this approach, the presentation of a balance of relevant, understandable information including both positives and negatives should be offered in a timely manner and within a supportive environment. Although it is acknowledged that this approach has inherent difficulties, there is a growing research base which professionals may use in order to facilitate the process. Furthermore, specialist professionals such as learning disability nurses may prove to be invaluable resources. It is crucial that this information is delivered dynamically, dependent on the parents' requirements, and equally that parents have the right not to know if they so choose. By adopting a balanced approach to information sharing, allowing the parents time and space to make decisions, and respecting their right to give or withhold informed consent free from pressure or coercion, the healthcare professional allows the parents the opportunity to make decisions which they believe are in their family's best interests, and, where necessary, to form renewed perspectives based on realistic expectations.

Points to remember

- Screening and diagnostic testing may be offered at the pre-conception, antenatal, or post-natal stages.
- Receiving a diagnosis is an extremely anxiety-provoking and life changing experience.
- Children with learning disabilities often have additional health needs. Early screening can also detect these.
- Parents and prospective parents have a right to know and a right not to know. Professional skill and insight is essential in ensuring parents are well supported in making informed decisions.

Resources

ARC
www.arc-uk.org

Contact a family
http://www.cafamily.org.uk/

Down's Heart Group
www.dhg.org.uk

Down's Syndrome Association
http://www.downs-syndrome.org.uk/

Down Syndrome Ireland
www.downsyndrome.ie

Down's Syndrome Scotland
www.dsscotland.org.uk

Genetic Alliance UK
www.geneticalliance.org.uk

Healthtalkonline
www.healthtalkonline.org

Mosaic Down Syndrome UK
www.mosaicdownsyndrome.org

SANDS
www.uk-sands.org

SHINE
www.shinecharity.org.uk

SOFT UK
www.soft.org.uk

References

Aldred, S.K., Deeks, J.J., Neilson, J.P. and Alfirevic, Z. (2010) Antenatal screening for Down's syndrome: generic protocol (protocol), *Cochrane Database of Systematic Reviews 2010*, issue 4. Art. No.: CD007384. DOI: 10.1002/14651858.CD007384.pub2.

Bell, A.L. and Aguila, D.D. (1998) *What You Should Know About Down Syndrome*. colouring book accessible.

Blau, N., van Spronsen, F.J. and Levy, H.L. (2010) Phenylketonuria, *The Lancet*, 376(9750), 1417–1427.

Bowlby, J. (1980) *Attachment and Loss: Loss: Sadness and Depression*. London: Hogarth Press with the Institute of Psycho-Analysis.

Brasington, C.K. (2007) What I wish I knew then . . . reflections from personal experiences in counselling about Down Syndrome, *Journal of Genetic Counselling*, 16(6): 731–734.

British Psychological Society and Royal College of Psychiatrists (2009) *Dementia and People with Learning Disabilities*. London: BPS.

Bull, M.J. and the Committee on Genetics (2011) Clinical report:health supervision for children with Down Syndrome, *Pediatrics*, 128(2): 393–406.

Burke, W., Tarini, B., Press, N.A. and Evans, J.P. (2011) Genetic screening, *Epidemiologic Reviews*, 33(1): 148–164.

Charleton, P.M., Dennis, J. and Marder, E. (2010) Medical management of children with Down syndrome, *Paediatrics and Child Health*, 20(7): 331–337.

Contact a Family (2012) *Down Syndrome*. Available at: www.cafamily.org.uk/medical-information/conditions/d/down-syndrome/ (accessed 6 Sept. 2012).

Crider, K.S., Bailey, L.B. and Berry, R.J. (2011) Folic acid food fortification: its history, effect, concerns, and future directions, *Nutrients*, 3(3): 370–384.

Davidson, M.A. (2008) Primary care for children and adolescents with Down syndrome, *Pediatric Clinics of North America*, 55(5): 1099–1111.

Dent, K.M. and Carey, J.C. (2006) Breaking difficult news in a newborn setting: Down Syndrome as a paradigm, *American Journal of Medical Genetics, Part C, Seminal Medical Genetics*, 142C(3): 173–179.

DH (Department of Health) (2007) *Good Practice in Learning Disability Nursing*. London: DH.

DH (Department of Health) (2011) *Abortion Statistics, England and Wales: 2011*. Available at: http://transparency.dh.gov.uk/category/statistics/abortion (accessed 28 Aug. 2012).

Down's Syndrome Association (2012) *Key Facts and FAQs*. Available at: www.downs-syndrome.org.uk/ (accessed 1 July 2012).

Durand, M.A., Stiel, M., Boivin, J. and Elwyn, G. (2010) Information and decision support needs of parents considering amniocentesis: interviews with pregnant women and health professionals, *Health Expectations*, 13(2): 125–138.

Dyer, W.J., McBride, B.A. and Jeans, L.M. (2009) A longitudinal examination of father involvement with children with developmental delays: does timing of diagnosis matter? *Journal of Early Intervention*, 31(3): 265–281.

Extra 21 (2012) *A Grandparent's View*. Available at: www.extra21.org.uk/ (accessed 4 Sept. 2012).

Farrelly, E., Cho, M.K., Erby, L., Roter, D., Stenzel, A. and Ormand, K. (2012) *Genetic Counseling for Prenatal Testing: Where Is the Discussion About Disability?* Available at: http://www.ncbi.nlm.nih.gov/pubmed/22297411 (accessed 28 Aug. 2012).

France, E.F., Wyke, S., Ziebland, S., Entwistle, V.A., and Hunt, K. (2011) How personal experiences feature in women's accounts of use of information for decisions about antenatal diagnostic testing for foetal abnormality, *Social Sciences and Medicine*, 72(5): 755–762.

Graves Allen, E., Freeman, S.B., Druschel, C., Hobbs, C.A., O'Leary, L.A., Romitti, P.A., Royle, M.H., Torfs, C.P. and Sherman, S.L. (2009) Maternal age and risk for Trisomy 21 assessed by the origin of chromosome nondisjunction: a report from the Atlanta and National Down Syndrome Projects, *Human Genetics*, 125(1): 41–52.

Harcombe, J. and Armstrong, V. (2008) Antenatal screening: the UK NHS antenatal screening programmes: policy and practice, *InnovAiT*, 1(8): 579–588.

Hartway, S. (2009) A parent's guide to the genetics of Down Syndrome, *Advances in Neonatal Care*, 9(1): 27–30.

Harwood, I. (2007) A family facing end of life issues of a person with learning disabilities: a personal reflection, *British Journal of Learning Disabilities*, 35(2): 102–106.

Healthtalkonline (2012) Antenatal screening. Available at: http://healthtalkonline.org/peoples-experiences/pregnancy-children/antenatal-screening/topics (accessed 10 April 2014).

Hodgson, J. and Weil, J. (2012) Talking about disability in prenatal genetic counseling: a report of two interactive workshops, *Journal of Genetic Counseling*, 21(1): 17–23.

Human Genetics Commission (2011) *Increasing Options, Informing Choice: A Report on Preconception Genetics Testing and Screening*. London: Human Genetics Commission.

Janvier, A., Farlow, B. and Wilfond, B.S. (2012) The experience of families with children with Trisomy 13 and 18 in social networks, *Pediatrics*, 130(2): 293–298.

King, G., Baxter, D., Rosenbaum, P., Zwaigenbaum, L. and Bates, A. (2009) Belief systems of families of children with autistic spectrum disorders or Down syndrome, *Focus on Autism and Other Developmental Disabilities*, 24(1): 50–64.

Kübler-Ross, E. (1969) *On Death and Dying*. New York: Macmillan.

Kübler-Ross, E. and Kessler, D. (2005) *On Grief and Grieving: Finding the Meaning of Grief Through the Five Stages of Loss*. New York: Macmillan.

Lalvani, P. (2011) Constructing the (m)other: dominant and contested narratives on mothering a child with Down syndrome, *Narrative Inquiry*, 21(2): 276–293.

Larkin, M. (2011) *Social Aspects of Health, Illness and Healthcare*. Maidenhead: McGraw-Hill Education.

Mencap (2013) *All About Learning Disability and Other Conditions*. Available at: www.mencap.org.uk/all-about-learning-disability/about-learning-disability/learning-disability-and-other-conditions/fragile-x-syn.

Merriman, A. (1999) *A Minor Adjustment: The Story of Sarah – A Remarkable Child*. London: Macmillan.

Modh, C., Lundgren, I. and Bergbom, I. (2011) First time pregnant women's experiences in early pregnancy, *International Journal of Qualitative Studies in Health and Wellbeing*, 6(2): 10. DOI. 3402/qhw.v6i2.5600.

Morris, J.K. and Alberman, E. (2009) Trends in Down's syndrome live births and antenatal diagnoses in England and Wales from 1989–2008: analysis of data from the National Down Syndrome Cytogenetic Register, *BMJ*, 339: 637–94

Muggli, E.E., Collins, V.R. and Marraffa, C. (2009) Going down a different road: first support and information needs of families with a baby with Down syndrome, *Medical Journalists Association*, 190(2): 58–61.

NHS Choices (2012) *Down's Syndrome*. Available at: http://www.nhs.uk/conditions/downs-syndrome/pages/introduction.aspx (accessed 3 Sept. 2012).

NHS FASP Consent Standards Review Group and NHS Fetal Anonmaly Screening Programme (2011) *NHS Fetal Anomaly Screening Programme Consent Standards and Guidance* London: NHS FASP.

NICE (2008) *Antenatal Care: Routine Care for the Healthy Pregnant Woman*. Available at: http://publications.nice.org.uk/antenatal-care-cg62 (accessed 7 Sept. 2011).

Reid, B., Sinclair, M., Barr, O., Dobbs, F. and Crealy, G. (2009) A meta-analysis of pregnant women's decision-making processes with regard to antenatal screening for Down syndrome, *Social Science and Medicine*, 69(11): 1561–1573.

Reynolds, T.M. (2009) The ethics of antenatal screening: lessons from Canute, *The Clinical Biochemist Reviews*, 30(4): 187–196.

Riedijk, S., Oudesluijs, G. and Tibben, A. (2012) Psychosocial aspects of preconception consultation in primary care: lessons from our experience in clinical genetics, *Journal of Community Genetics*. Available at: DOI: 10.1007/s12687-012-0095-z.

Schoonen, M., Wildschut, H., Essink-Bot, M.L., Peters, I., Steggers, E. and De Konig, H. (2012) The provision of information and informed decision-making on prenatal screening for Down syndrome: a questionnaire- and register-based survey in a non-selected population, *Patient Education and Counselling*, 87(3): 351–359.

Seligman, M. and Darling, R.B. (2007) *Ordinary Families, Special Children: A Systems Approach to Childhood Disability*, 3rd edn. New York: The Guilford Press.

Sheets, K., Best, R.G., Brasington, C.K. and Will, M.C. (2011a) Balanced information about Down syndrome: what is essential? *American Journal of Medical Genetics, Part A*, 155(6): 1246–1257.

Sheets, K.B., Crissman, B.G., Feist, C.D., Sell, S.L., Johnson, L.R., Donahue, K.C., Masser-Frye, D., Brookshire, G.S., Carre, A.M., LaGrave, D. and Brasington, C.K. (2011b) Practice guidelines for communicating a prenatal or postnatal diagnosis of Down Syndrome: recommendations of the National Society of Genetic Counselors, *Journal of Genetic Counseling*, 20(5): 432–441.

Skirton, H. and Barr, O. (2010) Antenatal screening and informed choice: a cross-sectional survey of parents and professionals, *Midwifery*, 26(6): 596–602.

Skotko, B.G. (2005) Prenatally diagnosed Down syndrome: mothers who continued their pregnancies evaluate their health care providers, *American Journal of Obstetrics and Gynecology*, 192(3): 670–677.

Skotko, B.G. and Levine, S.P. (2006) What the other children are thinking: brothers and sisters of persons with Down syndrome, *American Journal of Medical Genetics, Part C*, 142C(3): 180–186.

Skotko, B.G. and Levine, S.P. (2009) *Fasten Your Seatbelt*. Bethesda, MD: Woodbine House, Inc.

Skotko, B.G., Capone, G.T. and Kishnani, P.S. (2009) Postnatal diagnosis of Down syndrome: synthesis of the evidence on how best to deliver the news, *Paediatrics*, 124(4): 751–758.

Skotko, B.G., Levine, S.P. and Goldstein, R. (2011a) Having a son and daughter with Down syndrome: perspectives from mothers and fathers, *American Journal of Medical Genetics, Part A*, 155(10): 2335–2347.

Skotko, B.G., Levine, S.P. and Goldstein, R. (2011b) Having a brother or sister with Down syndrome: perspectives from siblings, *American Journal of Medical Genetics, Part A*, 155(10): 2348–2359.

Skotko, B.G., Levine, S.P. and Goldstein, R. (2011c) Self-perceptions from people with Down syndrome, *American Journal of Medical Genetics, Part A*, 155(10): 2360–2369.

Sooben, R.D. (2010) Antenatal testing and the subsequent birth of a child with Down syndrome: a phenomenological study of parents' experiences, *Journal of Intellectual Disabilities*, 14(2): 79–94.

Sykes, M. (2010) Delivering a support group for siblings of children with learning disabilities, *Nursing Times*, 106(4): 15–16.

Tringham, G.M., Nawaz, T.S., Holding, S., McFarlane, J. and Lindow, S.W. (2011) Introduction of first trimester combined test increases uptake of Down's syndrome screening. *European Journal of Obstetrics and Gynaecology and Reproductive Biology*, 159(1): 95–98.

Trueland, J. (2010) New evidence that liaison nurses make a difference, *Learning Disability Practice*, 13(1): 6–7.

UK National Screening Committee (2005) *Screening Choices: A Resource for Health Professionals Offering Antenatal and Newborn Care. Unit: Informed Choice in Antenatal and Newborn Screening.* Available at: http://cpd.screening.nhs.uk/choicestoolbox/units/informed-choice.pdf (accessed 28 Aug. 2012).

UK National Screening Committee (2012) *Screening Tests for Your Baby*. Available at: www.screening.nhs.uk/ (accessed 14 July 2012).

Van den Berg, M., Timmerman, D.R.M., ten Kate, L.P., van Vugt, J.M.G. and van der Wal, G. (2005) Are pregnant women making informed choices about prenatal screening? *Genetics in Medicine*, 7(5): 332–338.

Van Riper, M. and Choi, H. (2011) Family-provider interactions surrounding the diagnosis of Down syndrome, *Genetics in Medicine*, 13(8): 714–716.

Wiseman, F.K., Alford, K.A., Tybulewicz, V.L.J. and Fisher, E.M.C. (2009) Down syndrome: recent progress and future prospects, *Human Molecular Genetics*, 18(1): 75–83.

8 Developmental issues in early childhood

Helen Laverty

Learning outcomes

After reading this chapter you will be able to:

- explore early-day emotions of the family with a new baby who has Down's Syndrome
- consider the assessment of a common cardiac anomaly associated with Down's Syndrome
- appraise the attachment and disassociation processes different family members go through at the time of diagnosis and in the early years of a child's life
- identify strategies for supporting families and consider how to scaffold their development as a family with a member who has a disability vs. becoming a disabled family.

Introduction

> I think at first it shook our perfect world, but now in three years our world has broadened. We have watched something wonderful grow.

This chapter allows you to further explore the experiences of Louise, Luke, JoJo and Jem, and takes you through the early years and tribulations of their life as a family. The chapter relies on narratives from both parents and offers reflective exercises for the reader to engage with either independently or in study groups. There are both published text and internet resources for the reader to explore further.

Case study 8.1   Family history

This case study considers Jem's family history and is presented as personal reflections from his parents. Each narrative is numbered allowing the reader to cross-refer them during reflections.

(continued)

1. *Louise*: Looking back on those first few hours of Jem's life, it's hard to explain those intense emotions, the feelings of isolation, and desperation as it seemed like some big hand had come and taken our chance at family life away, and as if we hadn't had so much prejudice to contend with anyway. I had so loved being mummy, and loved him as soon as we knew he was on his way, I remember looking over to him and thinking he looked so cute. I wanted to know all those normal mummy things like weight and length, but can't honestly remember being told them; he'd got such a shock of hair, and was snuggled up tight in a blanket, so I just picked him up and sang to him 'You are my sunshine, my only sunshine . . .'

2. The leaflets the midwife brought back were horrid! They showed pictures of people wearing old-fashioned clothes, and obviously nappies, doing demeaning activities and had the audacity to talk about meaningful productive lives! I just dropped them on the side. The other midwife who had helped deliver Jem came back a bit later when it was a bit quieter. She sat and cooed at him, then said that she would take me upstairs to a special care baby unit, and settle us in. Why did I need to go to SCBU? Where was my husband? And why couldn't I go home that day? were all questions I wanted answering but I seemed to be wrapped in a cocoon of fog and simpering smiles.

3. *Luke*: Long story short, after kicking the wall, blowing off steam and rambling on the phone to my brother, I realised what I had done and came back to find Louise and Jem. It's a good job she's forgiving, and we just sat there in that little bedroom holding each other and not even daring to think about tomorrow, and all the time that pile of leaflets were sat accusingly on the bed.

4. Louise's mother turned up about an hour later with my brother in tow. He'd told her that Jem had got Down's Syndrome, and all she wanted was a cuddle, funny, I'd always thought up till then that she didn't like me! Anyway she's quite a forceful character, and when she picked him up she said to Louise, 'Your son is hungry', so that sort of switched that warrior mummy on in her and she asked if she should breastfeed him like she had done JoJo.

5. We spent those first couple of nights waiting for the next whammy, and that came on the Wednesday! JoJo had been brought to visit and that coincided with the doctor's visit. She was quite young, made a fuss of both the kids and then asked if any of us had any questions. JoJo asked why her brother was wearing lipstick! We just laughed, but the doctor said: 'That's probably because he's got a problem with his heart!'

6. *Louise*: We've come a long way since then: Jem was diagnosed with an Atrio Ventricular Septal defect and operated on when he was about 8 months. Up until he came out of surgery, we seemed to live each day holding our breath. He was so poorly, we didn't know if he'd live, and that bubble of fog and cotton wool seemed to hold us all back as a family, even JoJo, she seemed stuck too. Then one morning there was some rubbish on the telly about making lists of questions before you could make *a* change or even ask the questions at a meeting.

7. *Luke*: When I look out the window today, waiting for him to come home from school, it's hard to imagine all of those things we went through in the early days, you know, from not expecting him to live, or survive surgery, or even our marriage surviving. We've made some amazing friends on this trip, and have lost some whom we realise didn't matter in the first place. Louise, who is far more practical than me, decided we should put some information together that would help other parents in our 'foggy world' find some real answers and solutions that suit them and their family best.

To begin the learning process, reflect back on the case studies in Chapters 7 and 8 and complete the learning activity in Table 8.1. This guided reflection encourages you to consider your own thoughts, feelings and beliefs. It asks you to draw on your experiences and those you might have read about or witnessed in the media.

Table 8.1 'So what? Then what? Now what?'

So what has that made you...	Think?	Feel?	Want to do?	Remember?
Then what do you want to do about those feelings and thoughts	Feelings	Feelings	Thoughts	Thoughts
Now what would you do if	You were in that situation?	You were asked to take part in that scenario?	Wanted more knowledge to face the scenario?	Wanted to support that family?

Adapting to a diagnosis

All new families, regardless of any label that has been attached to their baby (boy, girl, poorly, Down's Syndrome, physical impairment – the list is endless), go through a period of adaption; this is often described in terms of surviving, searching, settling in and separating (Figure 8.1). It is how well an individual family is supported that will enable this process to be family-centred and empowering, rather than labelled and disempowering (Miller, 1994; Quinn, 1998).

↑Outer search

Surviving → Searching → Settling in → Separation

↓Inner search

Figure 8.1 The process of adaptation
Source: Miller (1994).

Surviving has been described by some families as the motions you go through and the actions you take as a family when something completely beyond your control has rocked your world and how you thought you would live in it. Even families who knew before birth their baby would have Down's Syndrome find the whole surviving process a minefield of 'What if's?', 'Why us?' and 'What's next?'

Families with a pre-natal diagnosis of Down's Syndrome frequently describe how there is no rite of passage out of surviving, just one day you find you are living and thriving again, but spend a long time waiting for the next whammy to knock that sense of 'today well lived' away. The support of a professional will enable more 'days well lived' to occur, and effective parent partnerships to be established.

In the second part of the case study, Louise describes being wrapped in a cocoon of fog and simpering smiles; many families when recounting their birth stories to you will have often 'forgotten' or 'over-looked' the positive aspects – such as feelings of love and elation as the label and negative health outcomes/prospective is paramount in that family's story. There is great benefit to be derived from supporting the family members to complete a more 'ordinary' baby day story, that includes the things everyone expects in such stories: time of birth, gender, weight, Apgar Score.

The Apgar test offers great reassurance to new parents. Most babies are judged to be in good health, but if the newborn does require medical help, health professionals have a baseline on which to build the success of their interventions know it right away. The procedure has been a routine part of new life since anaesthetist Virginia Apgar published it back in 1953 (Baby Centre, 2013) (www.babycentre.co.uk/a3074/apgar-scale#ixzz2JSJNbO4W).

Practice alert 8.1

Encourage parents with babies/young children who have a learning disability to document and record important developments in the child's life as they would a child without disabilities.

During the surviving period parents either just cope or can react to the news, situation, and diagnosis. Both strategies can be either healthy or cause a family to get 'stuck': often as professionals we meet families with adult sons and daughters who have learning disabilities who are still surviving because they haven't been supported to move on from just coping; by the same token the concept of reacting can cause huge rifts in the way the family see the support offered and approaches the professionals take. So what is the difference? Families who just cope are often the ones who become overlooked: descriptions in case notes of 'mum settled well, baby feeding and dad back at work' on the surface appear incredibly positive, but when you explore the application of a vicious circle (Figure 8.2) to the case study and consider how the belief that the family will just get on with 'it' impacts on the family's holistic health, then a balance of coping and reacting has got to be seen as healthier.

Marcia Van Riper has undertaken extensive research into the impact of a child with Down's Syndrome (DS) on family well-being and development (Van Riper, 1999a, 1999b, 2000, 2003, 2013, in press; Van Riper and Cohen, 2001; Van Riper et al. 1992a; Van Riper et al. 1992b; Van Riper and Selder, 1989). She identifies the flowing issues:

> While the birth of a child with DS may initially be viewed as a tragedy, this interpretation usually changes dramatically over time. For example, one mother said, 'All of us have learned to look beyond face value. Before our son was born, there were no disabilities in our very large family. I think it at first shook our perfect world, but now in three years our world has broadened. We have all watched something wonderful grow out of what was initially felt as a tragedy.'

Uncertainty is a major characteristic of the life transition experienced following the birth of a child with DS.

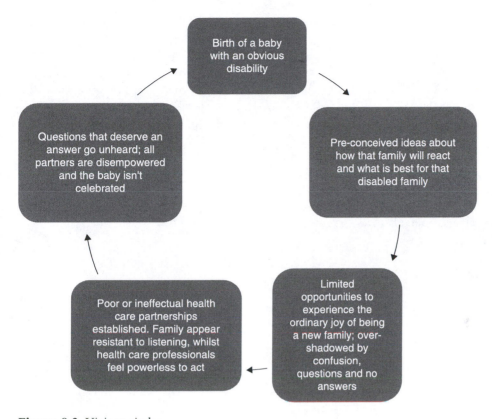

Figure 8.2 Vicious circles

Initial sources of uncertainty

- *The unexpected diagnosis of DS.* Despite increased use of pre-natal testing, many parents are unaware of their child's diagnosis of DS until after the child's birth. Most parents enter the birth experience expecting to have a healthy child, not one with health problems and developmental delays. One mother noted: 'When a child is conceived; a dream is born. The dream image [is of] a healthy, strong, and clever child who with confidence and success, fulfils a parent's desire to bear a child . . . when we received the news that she had DS, it was as if the child of our dreams had died.'

- *Parental concern about the child's future and the family's future.* For many new parents, becoming aware of their child's diagnosis of DS and associated health, development, and educational needs is like entering a whole new world – a world filled with healthcare providers from a wide variety of disciplines, support groups and early intervention programmes. It is a very different world than the one they imagined and for which they planned. Some parents report feeling the need to pin down or forecast the future.

- *Apprehensions regarding parenting abilities.* Initially, many new parents feel inadequate or unprepared to care for a child with DS. Early access to support and guidance from professionals with expertise in DS, as well as other parents of children with DS, can play an important role in decreasing apprehensions about raising a child with DS. Unfortunately, not all parents get this. Parents with inadequate support and guidance are more likely to have difficulty dealing with the ongoing challenges associated with raising a child with DS and may experience decreased individual and family well-being.

- *Initial responses of healthcare providers.* The initial responses of healthcare providers can have a profound impact on parental uncertainty. Parents who are informed of their child's diagnosis of DS in a caring, sensitive manner by healthcare providers, who have access to up-to-date information about children with DS and their families, experience less uncertainty and are in a better position to deal with the ongoing challenges associated with raising a child with DS. Parents who are given outdated information in a cold, uncaring manner may have difficulty moving forward. According to one father: 'The failure of others to inform us adequately from the start – that fostered a climate of uncertainty.' A mother noted: 'They generally ignored me and avoided talking about my daughter. They didn't realize that what I wanted and needed was someone to say, 'Now she's here, it is time to go on', they made time stand still. I couldn't move forward' (Van Riper, 2013).

Additional health needs

Latest research suggests that in every 700 births, one baby will be born with Down's Syndrome. Approximately 47 per cent of these babies will also have a congenital heart problem. The whole range of heart defects may be found in people with Down's Syndrome. Some are mild and cause few problems, but they are more commonly of a serious nature, though with modern techniques the majority are operable with excellent success rates. Although it is only rarely found in the non-Down's population, the most common defect in children or adults with Down's Syndrome is the atrioventricular septal defect (AVSD). This often has a common single valve in the middle of the heart and a large hole between the two sides of the heart. This serious defect affects the centre of the heart and there is often no heart murmur, thus adding to the possibility of late diagnosis.

The most common sort of heart defect which makes the child blue with Down's syndrome is Tetralogy of Fallot. This may be found in combination with AVSD. Most experts are now convinced that patients with Down's Syndrome are more prone to pulmonary hypertension/pulmonary vascular disease than their non-Down's peers. Successful surgery will usually prevent the continuation of pulmonary hypertension and the development of pulmonary vascular disease. Early diagnosis of a heart problem is essential so that surgery can be performed before 6 months of age. Many of the early symptoms of a major heart defect, e.g. poor weight gain, lack of energy, feeding problems, are often mistaken (both by professionals and parents) for characteristics of Down's syndrome itself. All babies with Down's Syndrome (symptomatic or otherwise) should be offered a heart scan as soon as possible to establish their cardiac status. Many parents express the need for guidance on how to recognise signs of heart failure; they are naturally anxious to recognise any changes in their child which may require medical treatment, but at the same time do not wish to be labelled as 'neurotic and over-anxious'. It can be a fine balance for already experienced parents and exceedingly difficult where this is the first child. Severe early feeding difficulties are often a major problem for these babies. However, with patience and perseverance breastfeeding can be successful and should not be discontinued due to poor weight gain without consideration and discussion. Whether breast- or bottle-fed, many DS babies will need calorie supplements and feeding via a naso-gastric tube to facilitate weight gain.

An AVSD is the most common congenital heart defect found in children with Down's syndrome, accounting for 50 per cent of the total. In its complete form, there is a hole in the wall between the top chambers (atria) and a hole in the wall between the bottom chambers (ventricles), and one common valve between the two atria and the two ventricles. In the partial forms there may not be a hole between the bottom chambers (ventricles) or the mitral and tricuspid valves may not be joined together, but either or both may leak, known as valve incompetence. Because of the high pressure in the left ventricle (needed to pump the blood around the body), blood is forced through the holes in the septum (central heart wall) when the ventricle contracts, thus increasing the pressure in the right ventricle. This increased pressure (pulmonary hypertension) results in excess blood flow to the lungs.

Clinical examination may show an enlarged heart and liver, and a diagnosis of 'heart failure' may be given. This is not as frightening as it sounds – it is in fact the medical term used to indicate that the heart is working inefficiently due to the demands the body is placing on it. Because of the flow of blood from one side to the other, the heart has to work harder than normal. Not all children will exhibit symptoms early in life, and those that do will not necessarily show all of the symptoms discussed. Early treatment may involve the use of diuretics such as Frusemide and Spironolactone to control the fluid retention around the body and to reduce the volume of blood in the circulation, thus making the heart's workload easier. These may be used in conjunction with other drugs such as Captopril, to make it easier for blood to pass to the body, rather than back through the hole to the lungs. Slow weight gain may lead to the addition of additives such as Calogen, Maxijul or Duocal to a baby's milk to increase calorie intake.

Practice alert 8.2

The majority of cases of AVSD are suitable for surgical intervention; this generally takes place within the first six months of life. If the condition is left unoperated, the increased blood pressure in the lungs causes damage which eventually makes surgery impossible, as the body adjusts to these pressures and could not cope with the surgery.

Often following surgery there remains a leaky valve which requires regular monitoring in case more surgery is needed, though in many cases the heart copes very well with the leakage and no further treatment is required. Sometimes bouts of illness may place an additional strain on the leaky valve, but this may be alleviated by treatment with diuretics for a short period. There may be times when all chest infections require quite energetic treatment. The repeated use of antibiotics, if used properly, is very helpful and does not reduce the child's resistance to infections.

Parents of people with Down's Syndrome face the same worries as all parents when their child is diagnosed with a congenital heart defect, but they may also worry about 'prejudice' in their treatment and question the motives of hospitals in recommending or advising against surgery. It is quite acceptable to ask for a second opinion at a different hospital if parents have any concerns, and this will not affect any future treatment at either hospital. As with all children, bouts of illness and hospitalisation can cause temporary delays, even setbacks, in development, but no direct link between mental ability and a heart condition is to be expected. Occasionally, parents disbelieve the severity of their child's heart condition, particularly as some show very few symptoms in their early years, i.e. the period when the pulmonary vascular resistance is rising and to a great extent compensating for the effects of the defect. This 'honeymoon period' is only temporary; therefore the optimum time for surgery is often when the child is very young before complications can occur. Many people with Down's Syndrome, even those with severe heart problems, attend mainstream schools and lead full and active lives. Programmes of stimulation, such as Portage or physiotherapy, are often recommended for people with Down's syndrome, and parents may worry about the strain that physical exercise may place on the heart. They must, of course, ask the opinion of their medical advisors, but a good level of exercise is beneficial to the child.

> It is easy to underestimate the effect which the news of a heart problem has on the parents of a child already diagnosed with a learning disability. Having already come to terms with one disability, which for some parents is extremely difficult, they have formed a very strong and protective bond with their child. Well-meaning, but sometimes insensitive words can be extremely painful for these parents, especially if surgery is not possible or not recommended. Waiting for an operation, or worse still living with the knowledge that their child cannot have surgery, can be a very stressful time.
>
> (Down's Heart Group, 2005)

Supporting families

It's a huge privilege to support parents during the birth of their happy, healthy baby. But what if the baby is still happy and healthy but you suspect an intellectual disability? Go back to Figure 8.2, reflect on how the vicious circles do little to support a developmental process of living, loving and/or learning for either family members or healthcare professionals. This vicious cycle can start when a baby has an obvious disability, and moves on to the preconceived ideas we as health and social care professionals have about that family and how they will react and what we believe is best for that *disabled family*. It limits opportunities for families to experience the ordinary joy of being a new family and is over-shadowed by confusion, questions and no answers. Because of pre-conceived views of both the disability and how a family will react, poor or ineffectual healthcare partnerships are established. To us, the family appear resistant to listening and we as healthcare professionals seem resistant to hearing too, all partners feel powerless to act. There are questions that deserve an answer and go unheard; these questions can come from any family member; all partners are disempowered and despite all of this, there is a new baby whose entry into the world needs celebrating!

Vicious circles can be changed into learning circle by a fundamental shift in thinking, feeling, developing and action. Learning circles promote the individuality of families and put baby first (Baby First, 2013). Figure 8.3 shows how this shift in thinking can have a more positive impact on subsequent assessment, screening and diagnosis for the child with Down's Syndrome.

Learning circles promote the individuality of families and put the child first. The birth of the baby is celebrated and new families are supported to behave the same as any other. The healthcare needs of the child are addressed in an empathetic, open and proactive way. Families are valued equally, and effective partnerships between the healthcare team and the family are established, nurtured and develop. The focus is on the child, not the disability.

Reader activity 8.2 Providing information

- Read narrative 3 in the case study and consider your thoughts and feelings in relation to materials you have seen.

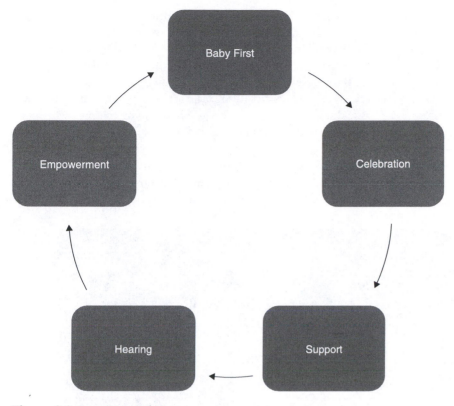

Figure 8.3 Learning circles

- Conduct an internet search and see what information you can find on understanding what Down's Syndrome is.
- Choose one leaflet, web page or article and consider the following questions:
  - What information was provided?
  - Was it aimed at a particular group, e.g. parents or healthcare professionals?
  - Was it easy to understand? Did it use jargon?
  - Did it portray people with Down's Syndrome in a positive light?

When we provide information to parents, we need to consider how accessible it is. We also need to think about how useful the information is which we can only do by evaluating it and talking to parents and carers who have used the services. Proactive support means that you will try to find more positive information for families and act as a signpost in those early days to answer seeking. Think about some of the information the general public can access via the web and consider how this would enhance their family life or over-shadow it.

There is merit in revisiting previous learning in communication and interpersonal skill, in particular, the work of Carl Rogers and his client–centred therapy model. He published his major work,

Client-Centred Therapy in 1951, in which he identified three special qualities: warmth, empathy and congruence. Think about how you would integrate these concepts into supporting Jem's family; and then more importantly as a healthcare professional listening later in this family's life when they want to tell their story. Seedhouse (2008) explores ethical decision-making in a framework and suggests it is a useful tool to consider learning through reflection (Figure 8.4).

Considering the different aspects of the grid enables us to challenge our own thinking and that of others. It questions our priorities and encourages a more balanced and involved approach to care decision-making. This is of particular importance in managing and supporting parents' reactions and often distress in supporting their child in the early years. As previously mentioned, the reactions we see from parents can often be a source of disharmony both in their relationships with each other, extended family members or with the health and social care team. Reactions range from confusion to fear to incompetence; and are based on grief, anger, guilt, the need to blame and helplessness.

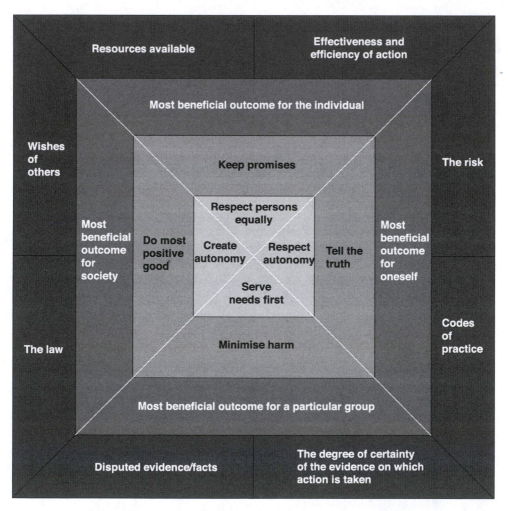

Figure 8.4 The Seedhouse Grid

Source: Adapted from Seedhouse (2008).

Louise's reaction when her mother tells her Jem is hungry demonstrates how positive action can be taken in the surviving stage of this family's journey, but also how the healthcare team could have facilitated something proactive in this 'baby day story'.

> Research studies around breastfeeding and breastfeeding patterns among mothers of infants born with Down Syndrome remain an underreported research phenomenon. About 700 infants are born with Down's Syndrome every year in the UK and for many the ability to breastfeed may present with a range of difficulties in the first few days of life often as a consequence of facial and other anatomical structural abnormalities associated with Down's Syndrome. Despite compelling evidence within the general population that breastfeeding can help with physiological and emotional wellbeing of both mother and child, there is a profound gap as to how new mothers of infants with Down Syndrome are supported with infant feeding decision-making and their personal experience of breastfeeding.
>
> (Sooben, 2012)

Feeding baby

Babies with Down's Syndrome have a tendency to early feeding problems possibly as a result of poor muscle tone, and babies with a heart problem also tend to have problems as they tire easily when feeding. So babies who have a heart defect and Down's syndrome have two things making it harder for them and poor feeding and slow weight gain. The Down's Heart Group offer the following advice on breastfeeding:

- Sucking is hard work so make it as easy as possible. If you are breastfeeding, try expressing a little milk to start with to get it flowing before you latch baby on, that way they get an immediate reward for their efforts and don't waste valuable energy stimulating milk production.
- If you are having problems breastfeeding and have to feed breast milk from a bottle for a while, do keep putting the baby to the breast and try stimulating the baby's mouth with your finger before feeds. Stroke gently around baby's mouth and cheek, put your clean finger in their mouth to help with sucking and gently stroke downwards on their throat to encourage swallowing. Be persistent, it may take a while but eventually your baby will get the hang of feeding.
- If you are expressing breast milk, a hand pump can become hard work, consider investing in an electric pump or enquire about borrowing one from your local special care unit, N.C.T. or La Leche League.
- If you are breastfeeding but not producing enough milk for your baby's needs, they can still benefit from however much breast milk is available and the remainder of their feeds can be made up with formula.
- Breast milk can be given with a bottle or even by naso-gastric tube (a tube that goes directly into the stomach via the nose and throat) if baby tires too easily to feed on their own.
- You may consider using a supplemental nurser, which is like a bottle of milk hung round mum's neck leading to a fine tube which is taped to the breast. The milk feeds by gravity so baby doesn't have to suck hard but is still latched on to the breast.
- If you decide to give up breastfeeding because your baby is not putting on enough weight and you have been advised to do so, it is worth continuing to express milk and freeze it for a few

weeks more. That way, if the change to formula doesn't give the desired weight gain, it is possible to revert back to breastfeeding if you want.

- Breast milk is recommended for babies as through it the mother passes on much of her own immunity to infection. This is of course even more important when the baby has a heart condition, particularly prior to surgery, but you should not feel bad if your baby is not breastfed or you are unable to breastfeed for very long.
- Expressed breast milk can be placed in sterile bottles and stored in the freezer to be used later. This can be particularly useful if your baby is in hospital for a few days and around admission for surgery.

Meeting milestones

Reader activity 8.3 Inner and outer searches

All parents, regardless of the label that has been attached to their child, compare, contrast and anticipate their child's next move and use others, and media sources as a guide or reference point. Families begin a search while they are still surviving; it's both an inner and outer search. The inner search is about asking questions of themselves in relation to how they will cope, how will they find the resources to deal with what is happening to their family? The outer search starts with questions to others that demand answers. Professionals need to consider the following needs of parents:

- Parents need a focus with goals that are achievable for their child. They need to be able to acknowledge that development is possible even if it may be at a slower rate than the child's peers.
- Parents need strategies for support especially when they feel fed up with just coping as opposed to receiving what they need to ensure the well-being of the whole family.
- Parents need timely and accurate information real answers to their questions, even if this means what they want and need being not readily available.

Table 8.2 Reflective table

What we think we know	What we want to know	What we don't know	What shall we do?	
The baby has have Down's Syndrome	What will that mean to us?	Anything about Down's Syndrome	Ask for real information	
Our baby has a serious heart complaint	What can be done about it?	How serious it is	Ask for real information	
What do we tell other people	How will they react	How much support we'll need	Stop meeting the devil half way!	
So what has that made you	Think	Feel	Want to do	Remember

Then what do you want to do about those feelings and thoughts	Feelings	Feelings	Thoughts	Thoughts
Now what would you do if	You were in that situation?	You were asked to take part in that scenario?	Wanted more knowledge to face the scenario?	Wanted to support that family?

Reader activity 8.4   Age line

Draw a line on a piece of paper to represent an age line from the birth of a child to the age of 10. Add on the following developmental points noting at what age you feel a child should have achieved them.

1. Holding head up independently
2. Walking independently
3. Using descriptive text in conversation
4. Writing their name
5. Reciting the alphabet
6. Able to catch a ball.

Parents will usually be very aware of when peers of their child have achieved milestones and will become very anxious when their own child doesn't. Think about some of the information about learning disabilities and their causes that is readily available in the public domain and how proactive and helpful it is to families. As professionals we are all too aware of the need for accurate scientific assessment that provides the baseline from which we can plan our interventions – but how important are these to parents? And perhaps more importantly, how far do they go to instil confidence in the service for parents and ensure that their son or daughter receives gold standard care? As has already been seen in Chapter 7, a host of different healthcare professionals will work alongside the family but in terms of development it is important to recognise the role, advice and support offered by a health visitor.

Practice alert 8.3   Health visitor

Health visitors support and educate families from pregnancy through to a child's fifth birthday (NHS Careers, 2013). Common tasks include:

- offering parenting support and advice on family health and minor illnesses;
- new birth visits which include advice on feeding, weaning and dental health;
- physical and developmental checks;
- providing families with specific support on subjects such as post-natal depression.

Developmental assessment is essential for the following reasons:

- It challenges the care-giver to describe the individual in developmental terms.
- From that follows an acknowledgement of developmental need.
- We need to acknowledge that the professionals' perceptions of what an individual cannot do has often been influenced by the design of the assessment schedule and translated into the jargon and myth of never will do.
- Parents predominantly have a more realistic view of their son and daughter, after all, they have been there 24 hours a day, 7 days a week (Laverty and Reet, 2001).

All parents want the best life chances for their child and early developmental chances are especially important for the child with any learning disability, as it is the foundation for holistic long-term functional outcomes for the child in areas of movement, play, social interaction, communication and independence. In the early days of their child's life, parents will often need to be encouraged to interact with their baby, just ordinary things like cuddling, cooing and communications.

Down Syndrome Ireland state:

> Parents will naturally have questions about the likely severity of their child's possible delay. As a result of such logical questions, parents may focus on the rate of their child's gross motor development because this is the first test of the child's developmental rate. The rate of gross motor development in children with Down Syndrome is influenced by three primary physical problems that affect their gross motor development: hypotonia (low muscle tone), decreased strength, and hypermobility of the joints (loose joints). In order to cope with these problems, they may develop compensatory movement patterns that can lead to problems later in life. For example, some children with Down Syndrome may lack stability, and will compensate by standing and walking with their feet wide apart, knees stiff, and their feet turned out. If this atypical pattern is allowed to persist, problems will develop in their knees and feet, walking will become painful, and their endurance will be diminished.
>
> (see Resources)

Physical needs

According to Winders (2007):

> The appropriate goal of physiotherapy is not to accelerate their rate of gross motor development, as is commonly assumed. Rather, the goal is to facilitate their development of gross motor skills, while minimizing the development of abnormal compensatory movement patterns that children with Down Syndrome are prone to develop. *The opportunity is for parents to use the arena of gross motor development to begin to understand how their child learns.* Ideally, physiotherapy services should be started at 1–2 months of age in this population. Children with Down Syndrome are seen weekly or every 2 weeks until they are able to walk, and then monthly for the first 4–6 months of walking to refine their walking pattern. Physiotherapy typically ends when the child is able to walk with an efficient pattern, run, walk up and down stairs, jump, and ride a tricycle.

Developmental assessments will progress from gross motor skills to language, fine motor skills and social skills. This will be alongside other physical assessments that measure growth in height, weight and sensory function.

Communication

While early professional intervention will help both the child and the family, in the search for resources parents are often best advised to concentrate on areas that will enhance social integration for their child; motor development, social understanding, self-help skills and behaviour, play, and speech and language skills, are obvious choices.

> Visual processing and visual memory skills are strengths in children with Down Syndrome and can be used by parents and therapists to support children's learning. By 5 years of age, many children with Down Syndrome can achieve some of the same developmental targets as their peers, if this is expected of them. Most will be walking, toilet trained and able to feed themselves and dress with minimal help. Most will be able to fit into the expectations of the mainstream classroom, regulate their own behaviour and behave in a socially acceptable way. Most children will have significantly delayed spoken language. They will understand more than they can say, and their spoken language will not be clear. Many will have some of the basic concepts and knowledge for learning number, maths and reading. These achievements are possible, provided that parents have high expectations for social development and good behaviour from the first year of life, and that services offer targeted support for motor develop-ment and speech and language development. Like all children, progress for children with Down Syndrome is influenced by family life and parents' child rearing skills, inclusion with peers at home and in preschool, and the quality of education available. It is also influenced by biological make-up, and some children with Down Syndrome are born with more biological disadvantages than others. The first priority for parents is to maintain normal family life. The most powerful influence on the progress of a baby with Down Syndrome is to be loved, wanted and absorbed into the everyday life of the family and of the community. Specific teaching and therapies will definitely help, but must be kept in perspective and not allowed to create stress and anxiety for families.
>
> (Buckley and Sacks, 2001)

There is merit in the reader finding out about early intervention schemes in their locality, in partic-ular the National Portage Association. Portage is a home-visiting educational service for pre-school children with additional support needs and their families (National Portage Association, 2013). Its broad aims are:

- to work with families to help them develop a quality of life and experience for themselves and their young children in which they can learn together,
- to play together, participate and be included in their community in their own right;
- to play a part in minimising the disabling barriers that confront the young children and families receiving Portage services;
- to support the national and local development of inclusive services for children.

Figure 8.5 highlights further findings from the work of Marcia Van Riper in relation to child development.

Conclusion

To conclude, no one can predict how a family will react or cope with the information they are given about their child's learning disability, and/or associated complex health needs; however, the support offered by members of the health and social care team will enable that 'grounding' as a family to happen more congruently. A vicious circle starts when a baby's obvious disability becomes the focus of the healthcare professional's attention. Care becomes dominated by preconceived ideas and what we believe is best for that *disabled family*. It limits opportunities for families to experience the ordinary joy of being a new family and is over-shadowed by confusion, questions and self-doubt.

The disabled family label often enforces stereotypic roles within healthcare. There are questions that deserve an answer and go unheard. Eventually all partners, both family and healthcare professionals are disempowered and this reinforces everyone's focus on the one tangible factor – *the disability*. Despite all this there is a new baby whose entry into the world needs celebrating! Learning circles

---

- Families of children with DS generally experience higher levels of stress than families with typically developing children because families of children with DS are subject to the challenges faced by families of typically developing children, plus the additional challenges associated with raising a child with DS (increased care-giving difficulties, changes in roles, and increased time demands).
- While some families find it difficult to adapt to the ongoing challenges associated with parenting a child with DS, other families are resilient and thrive. The availability of individual, family, and community resources plays an important role in how families adapt to the ongoing challenges associated with raising a child with a chronic condition. In communities with limited resources, families end up spending a great deal of their time looking for and/or creating their own resources. In addition to being time-consuming, this may lead to a decrease in individual and family well-being. So unfortunately, at present, geography or where you live does seem to matter. Currently there is a need to help more families gain access to available services and resources. There are some wonderful online resources concerning children with DS and their families, but these resources only can be helpful to families if they can access them.
- On measures of individual, marital, and family functioning, families of children with DS are more comparable to, than different from, families of typically developing children.
- Parents of children with DS who have positive, family-centered relationships with health care providers report greater satisfaction with care, as well as higher levels of psychological well-being and family functioning.
- Both parents and siblings of children with DS report that their lives have been profoundly influenced by the experience of living in a family that includes a child with DS. More importantly, they report that the positive consequences of this experience far outweigh the negative consequences. Positive consequences included: bringing the family closer together, learning the true meaning of unconditional love, putting things in proper perspective, and appreciating diversity.

Figure 8.5 More key findings

Source: Van Riper (2013).

promote the individuality of families and put baby first. The birth of the baby is celebrated and new families are supported to behave the same as any other. The healthcare needs of the baby are addressed in an empathetic, open and proactive way. Families are valued equally, and effective partnerships between the healthcare team and the family are established, nurtured and evolve. The focus is on the baby not the disability.

Sometimes you can have too much of a good thing. Families often feel overwhelmed with information and this can often go unused. We need to target information and present it in a way that is appropriate. Otherwise, information can paradoxically have a disempowering effect. And sometimes we need to leave well alone, give families space to work out for themselves how much help they want, when they want it and in what format, we cannot adopt a 'one size fits all' approach.

Points to remember

- Parents need sensitive, informed, patient, caring professionals throughout the child's early years.
- A listening ear is essential.

Resources

Down's Heart Group
www.dhg.org.uk/

Down's Syndrome Ireland
www.downSyndrome.ie/

National Portage Association
www.portage.org.uk/

NHS Choices: Down's Syndrome Diagnosis
www.nhs.uk/Conditions/Downs-Syndrome/Pages/Diagnosis.aspx

NHS National Genetics Education and Development Centre
www.geneticseducation.nhs.uk/

References

Baby Centre (2013) Baby Centre: Apgar Score. Available at www.babycentre.co.uk/a3074/apgar-scale# ixzz2JSJNbO4W (accessed 24 April 2013).
Baby First (2013) University of Nottingham. (RLO CETL, UCC and the University of Nottingham). *Baby First Baby Book*. Available at: www.nottingham.ac.uk/nmp/sonet/rlos/learndis/babyfirst/ (accessed 24 April 2013).

Buckley, S. and Sacks, B. (2001) *An Overview of the Development of Infants with Down Syndrome (0–5 Years): Overview Part_1 (Down Syndrome Issues and Information)*. Down Syndrome Educational Trust, 20 Sept.

DH (Department of Health) (2001) *Valuing People: A New Strategy for Learning Disability for The 21st Century*. London: The Department of Health.

Disability Rights Commission (2006) *Equal Treatment: Closing the Gap. Health Formal Investigation Report*. London: Disability Rights Commission.

Disability Rights Commission (2007) *Equal Treatment: Closing the Gap. One Year On*. London: Disability Rights Commission.

Down's Heart Group (2013) *Reference Sources*. Available at: www.dhg.org.uk/information/resources.aspx (accessed 24 April 2013).

Emerson, E. and Hatton, C. (2008) *People with Learning Disabilities in England*. Lancaster: Centre for Disability Research (CeDR), Lancaster University.

Miller, N. (1994) *Nobody's Perfect*. San Francisco: Brookes Publishing Co.

Morris, J.K. and Alberman, E. (2009) Trends in Down's Syndrome live births and antenatal diagnoses in England and Wales from 1989 to 2008: analysis of data from the National Down Syndrome Cytogenetic Register, *BMJ*, Oct 26; 339:b3794.

Laverty, H. and Reet, M. (2001) *Planning Care for Children in Respite Settings: Hello, This Is Me*. London: Jessica Kingsley.

National Portage Association (2013) National Portage Association: Welcome to Portage. Available at: http://www.portage.org.uk/ (accessed 24 April 2013).

NHS Careers (2013) *What Do Health Visitors Do?* Available at: http://www.nhscareers.nhs.uk/explore-by-career/nursing/careers-in-nursing/health-visiting/what-do-health-visitors-do/ (accessed 24 April 2013).

Quinn, P. (1998) *Understanding Disability: A Life Span Approach*. London, Sage Publications.

Rogers, C. ([1951] 2003) *Client Centred Therapy: Its Current Practice, Implications and Theory*. London: Constable.

Seedhouse, D. (1998) *Ethical Grid*. Available at: www.priory.com/images/ethicgrid.JPG (accessed 11 September 2012).

Seedhouse, D. (2008) *Ethics: The Heart of Health Care*. New York: Wiley.

Sooben, R.D. (2012) Breastfeeding patterns in infants with Down's Syndrome: A literature review, *BJM*, March 2012. 20(3).

Van Riper, M. (1999a) Maternal perceptions of family-provider relationships and well being in families of children with Down Syndrome, *Research in Nursing and Health*, 22: 357–368.

Van Riper, M. (1999b) Living with Down Syndrome: The family experience, *Down Syndrome Quarterly*, 4: 1–11. Available at: http://www.denison.edu/collaborations/dsq/vanriper.htrnl.

Van Riper, M. (2000) Family variables associated with sibling well being in families of children with Down Syndrome, *Journal of Family Nursing*, 6: 267–286.

Van Riper, M. (2003) A change of plans: the birth of a child, with Down Syndrome, *American Journal of Nursing*, 103: 71–74.

Van Riper, M. (2013) Down's Syndrom.com. *What Families Need to Thrive*. Available at: http://www.downsyn.com/thrive.php (accessed 24 April 2013).

Van Riper, M. (in press) Families of children with Down Syndrome: responding to a 'Change of Plans' with resilience, *Journal of Pediatric Nursing*.

Van Riper, M. and Cohen, W. (2001) Caring for children with Down Syndrome and their families, *Journal of Pediatric Health Care*, 15: 123–131.

Van Riper, M. and Selder, F. (1989) Parental responses to the birth of a child with Down Syndrome, *Loss, Grief and Care: A Journal of Professional Practice*, 3: 59–75.

Van Riper, M., Pridham, K., and Ryff, C. (1992a) Symbolic interactionism: a perspective for understanding parent–nurse interactions following the birth of a child with Down Syndrome, *Maternal Child Nursing Journal*, 20: 21–39.

Van Riper, M., Ryff, C., and Pridham, K (1992b) Parental and family well-being in families of children with Down Syndrome: a comparative study, *Research in Nursing and Health*, 15: 227–235.

Winder, P. (2007) *Gross Motors Skills in Children with Down Syndrome: A Guide for Parents and Professionals*. Bethesda, MD: Woodbine House.

9 The health needs of adolescence

Jo Lay

Learning outcomes

After reading this chapter you will be able to:

- identify adolescence as a major life transition from a holistic health perspective
- explore screening and assessment strategies that can be used to promote effective plans for young people in adolescence
- examine the impact of a learning disability on the experience of adolescence.

Introduction

Adolescents – young people between the ages of 10 and 19 years – are often thought of as a healthy group. Nevertheless, many adolescents do die prematurely due to accidents, suicide, violence, pregnancy-related complications and other illnesses that are either preventable or treatable. Many more suffer chronic ill-health and disability. In addition, many serious diseases in adulthood have their roots in adolescence. For example, tobacco use, sexually transmitted infections, including HIV, poor eating and exercise habits, lead to illness or premature death later in life.

(WHO, 2013)

Adolescence can be a difficult time for any young person and their families and friends. This chapter seeks to examine positive approaches to supporting young people with learning disabilities at this transition time in their life. It will explore what this transition is and how a learning disability can impact on these life changes.

The Royal College of Paediatrics and Child Health (RCPCH, 2003) believe that adolescence should be defined developmentally as opposed to by age as a young person's experience by age can differ greatly. Physical maturity in particular can differ greatly. The FPA (2013) remind us that having a learning disability will not in itself stop a person from reaching adulthood, going through puberty or having sexual feelings. We cannot and should not try to make assumptions about individuals based on their learning disability, but should be aware of the issues that impact on transition. Priestley

(2003) suggests a number of classifications used to identify the socially constructed term 'youth'. These include age categories: Social organisation – the points at which young people take on roles and responsibilities; Cultural – focusing on the development of identity; and physical maturation. Disability can impact on all these classifications. For this reason, no one definition will be adhered to in the chapter, rather, each classification will be discussed based on its significance to particular topics. The terms adolescent, youth, young people, and teenagers are used interchangeably in discussion.

Case study 9.1   Jem's 19th birthday

Jem has just celebrated his 19th birthday but it didn't feel like much of a celebration. He invited some of the people from college over to his house but no one came. He had been really looking forward to introducing them to his mum and Tom. Mum worries about him a lot and Jem thought she would feel better if she could see how cool his friends from college were. Jem started college two months ago. Some of his mum's friends seemed surprised that he was doing a computer course. They weren't mean about it but Jem could see on their faces they were surprised. It makes him angry when people think he's stupid because of the Down's Syndrome. Why do they have to make him different all the time? Some of the teachers at college are like it too, saying he doesn't have to finish work if it's too hard! He does better than Matt who sits next to him. Matt is cool though. He lets Jem hang around with him and his mates at lunch. Matt explained that Jem shouldn't have to put up with some of the teachers' attitude and is going to help him do something about it. They're meeting in the college car park with some other boys next Monday evening to do it but Jem doesn't know what 'it' is yet. Still it serves Mr Brownlee right. But why didn't Matt come round on Jem's birthday? He'd pulled a funny face when Jem gave him the party invitation but he did say he'd probably come. Tom's mum had called in the morning to say that Tom had a bad cold and couldn't make it. Tom had wanted to talk to Jem on the phone but Jem felt angry and let down by him and refused to talk. Tom had been Jem's best friend at school but he wasn't at college. Tom didn't do anything now. His mum wouldn't let him go to college and Jem was starting to think he was a bit of a baby.

Jem feels angry and fed up a lot of the time. Mum says he's turning into a 'right grumpy teenager' and needs to learn to grow up. Jem thinks he is growing up but mum doesn't seem to realise it. That is what makes him grumpy and angry.

Reader activity 9.1   Charter for working with young people

What do you perceive to be the most important tenets of working with young people? You may like to discuss this with family members, colleagues or friends. It can be useful to set this out as a charter or standard, e.g.

When working with young people I will

- listen to opinions before reacting
- prepare them for independence, etc.

Once you have your list, try and prioritise it. Are there some aspects that are more important than others?

Figure 9.1 shows a charter developed by young people using the Merseyside Connexions service. Thinking about this charter provides a positive introduction to working with young people by promoting their needs, wishes and aspirations. From the earlier chapters of this book we know that the needs of people with a learning disability are diverse, based on individuality but also the wider spectrum of disability and the impact this has on services required. Planners and commissioners need to consider screening measures if they are to ensure that appropriate services are in place. This is particularly important in the transition from child services to adult. The *Valuing People* White Paper (DH, 2001) introduced Local Partnership Boards to determine local needs and services for people with a learning disability through Joint Investment Plans (JIPs). Kerr (2001, p. 157) stated: 'Planning learning disability services at a population level requires information about current service gaps and estimates of future need.' Previous attempts at screening had focused on measurements that addressed level of disability as opposed to numbers of people requiring services such as the Social and Physical Incapacity Scale. Surveys and scales which measure severity of disability may identify data in terms of physical support requirements but lack the holistic health assessment that is needed to plan for the future. The impact of disability has many differentials which may include personal character; family support, etc. It is therefore not practical to have a 'one-size-fits-all' prediction on service need in this way.

Health promotion

Bartley (2008) identified that the focus on health needs assessment has been part of the NHS for some time but information has been sorted from secondary data as opposed to direct user involvement. Health Needs Assessment is a systematic way of measuring the health needs of a population (NICE, 2009) and setting objectives for further development. There remains a policy commitment to people with learning disabilities that health provision should be made within mainstream services

---

- We have the right to share our problems and receive support.
- We have the right to impartial advice and accessible information.
- We have the right to be treated with respect and taken seriously.
- Information remains confidential, unless we have been told otherwise.
- Young people must be free from the risk of harm when working with Connexions.
- We have the right to equal opportunities and will not be judged.
- We as young people have a right to be listened to and heard.
- We have the right to make comments or suggestions about the services provided for young people.

Figure 9.1 A Youth Charter

Source: www.connexionslive.com/AboutConnexions/YouthCharter/Default.aspx.

with specialist support as necessary. It is now more widely accepted that users of services should be consulted about their needs and the direction of policy and provision. Health promotion is considered as a wider topic in Chapter 26. The Common Assessment Framework (CAF) was introduced as a holistic, non statutory assessment in 2006 by the then Department for Education and Skills. It was part of a policy direction that recognised the importance of joint working arrangements in all children's services. According to the Department of Education (2012), the CAF should be used when:

- a practitioner is worried about how well a child or young person is progressing (e.g. concerns about their health, development, welfare, behaviour, progress in learning or any other aspect of their well-being);
- a child or young person, or their parent/carer, raises a concern with a practitioner;
- a child's or young person's needs are unclear, or broader than the practitioner's service can address.

The CAF process is voluntary and informed consent must be given. It is a request for services rather than a referral. There are four stages to the process (see Figure 9.2). Each stage is supported by specific assessment tools and checklists. Once needs have been met, the process finishes and the CAF is closed.

Health promotion is key in developing services that actively meet adolescent health need. RCPCH (2003) made some key recommendations in the development of this:

1. It must be recognised that, like other groups in the population, socio-economic circumstances and social inclusion have a profound impact on the holistic health status and well-being of young people.
2. Emphasis should be on health promotion rather than health education. Biological and psychological changes in adolescence develop thought processes that include development of identity, meaning and ideology. Health-promoting strategies that are utilised in adolescence can form the behaviour exhibited as an adult.
3. Relationship and parenting schemes should be available for vulnerable groups.
4. Support for adolescents from vulnerable or excluded groups such as those with long-term health conditions or disabilities needs to be developed.
5. Health needs must be considered in the context of other needs such as employment, housing, further education, etc.
6. Local health organisations must consider their screening tools in identifying the number and projected needs of adolescents in their community, making sure resources are allocated to reflect this.

WHO (2013) suggest that there are a number of small-scale health initiatives which support adolescents but the priority should be on advice and recommendations which develop existing generic health services to become 'adolescent-friendly'. In order to deliver this, services should be measured against the following criteria:

1. *accessible* – Are adolescents able to access the services provided? Accessibility can be measured in terms of environment, time, transport, etc.
2. *acceptable* – Are services provided in a way that appeals or meets the expectations of adolescents? This considers the motivation of adolescents in having their healthcare needs met.
3. *equitable* – Are all adolescents able to access this service? This is particularly relevant if considering the needs of a socially excluded group such as the learning disabled.

1. Early identification of needs.
2. Assess those needs.
3. Deliver an integrated service using a 'Team Around the Child' (TAC) approach.
4. Review progress.

Figure 9.2 The CAF Process

4. *appropriate* – Do services reflect adolescent need? How is need identified? To what extent has there been user involvement?
5. *effective* – Are the right health services provided in the right way and do these make a positive contribution to health?

Service user involvement should be prominent in this. The Department of Health (2011) published a self-assessment tool for health services to measure their own quality in providing health services to young people. The assessment tool criteria consider 10 themes, similar to the WHO guidance:

1. accessibility
2. publicity
3. confidentiality and consent
4. environment
5. staff training, skills, attitudes, values
6. joined-up working
7. involvement of young people in feedback, monitoring and evaluation
8. health issues for adolescents
9. sexual and reproductive health services
10. specialist and targeted child and adolescent mental health services (CAMHS).

The final two themes relate to specialist services but are important considerations in meeting the needs of adolescents or young adults with a learning disability. Indeed, sexual health is an area that can be still seen as taboo or avoided by health services and families. It is essential to address this issue to promote health, relationships and understand vulnerability.

Mental health

Figures vary on the incidence of poor mental health in children and adolescents but it is recognised that this is a very difficult and confusing time for young people. It is estimated that 10–20 per cent of this group experience mental health difficulties. Adolescents typically develop coping strategies to deal with life's stresses and disappointments. This development varies between individuals in terms of the emotional distress it causes and the length of time it takes to go through this process. It requires cognitive skills to identify and explore thoughts and feelings and consider how to manage these. It can be hard to understand and accept that the human condition is not perfect and that we all make mistakes, and yet as parents or carers we can often put pressure on young people to be that perfect person. Research has considered the desire for young people to conform and be part of a group that provides unity and shared focus, whether that is through fashion, music, sport or other cultural or societal perspective. Within this conformity, an adolescent may still feel they are challenging authority and making their own decisions, often because it feels anti-establishment or is against their own parent's wishes or belief systems. In the case study we can see a number of areas where Jem is questioning authority and his feelings about this. He shows a good level of cognitive skill, even recognising why his mum might be worried about him. The spectrum of learning disability suggests that many young people will not have these skills but what is important is that assumptions are not made on the basis of disability and that appropriate assessment and strategies are put in place.

Fast facts 9.1   Childhood mental health problems

'One in ten children aged 5–16 years has a clinically diagnosable mental health problem. At any one time, more than a million children will have a diagnosable mental health disorder and mental illness in childhood and adolescence costs up to £59,000 per child every year' (www. gov.uk/government/news/children-and-teenagers-to-benefit-from-successful-adult-mental-health-therapy).

The National Institute for Mental Health (NIMH, 2013) note that though adolescence is when we are usually at the peak of our physical and mental capacity, it is a hazardous time for our mental health. They suggest that mortality rates rise quickly between early and late adolescence. They also state that 'rates of death by injury between ages 15 to 19 are about six times that of the rate between ages 10 and 14. Crime rates are highest among young males and rates of alcohol abuse are high relative to other ages.'

Taggart *et al.* (2010) state that a large number of empirical, international studies are clear that young people with a learning disability are more likely to experience behavioural and emotional difficulties compared to their non-disabled peers. They undertook research which attempted to identify early signs of emotional distress which could then be incorporated into assessment tools. They compared individuals, life events and family and socio-economic risk factors. Individual and risk factors that impacted on emotional health and well-being for this group, in comparison to non-disabled peers were:

- poor physical health;
- poor mental health;
- self-injurious behaviour;
- challenging behaviour;
- hyperactivity;
- being bullied;
- a higher number of significant life events.

Reader activity 9.2   Significant life events

- Make a list of what you consider might be significant life events for an adolescent.
- Why do you think a 'learning disability' may make the adolescent more susceptible to emotional distress as a result of these events?

- Attention Deficit Hyperactivity Disorder (ADHD)
- Anxiety
- Autism
- Asperger's syndrome
- Behavioural problems
- Depression
- Eating disorders
- Obsessive Compulsive Disorder (OCD)

Figure 9.3 Common mental health issues among young people

'Morbidity mainly arises from chronic illness and mental health problems, with the likelihood of long-term adverse consequences, and a crucial relationship between physical, mental and social health' (RCPCH, 2003, p. 12). Taggart *et al.* (2010) found that family and socio-economic risk factors were living in one-parent families; living in rented accommodation; parental unemployment; substance abuse; residing in services and living in low socio-economic communities. Services need to acknowledge the exacerbated impact adolescence can have on the health and well-being of someone with a learning disability. As professionals, we need to be aware of the potential physical and emotional changes that occur during this transition.

Recent research into the developing brain has challenged previous thinking on brain maturity. It was previously thought that grey matter was at its peak in childhood. Grey matter forms the outer layer or 'cortex' of the brain responsible for thoughts and memory. Recent scans have suggested that the brain does not fully mature to its optimum level of grey matter until adolescence. Studies also showed that different parts of the cortex mature at different rates with those areas responsible for more basic functioning, developing first. The implication of this is that the areas of our brains that control responses to emotions and thoughts are the last to mature. NIMH (2013) suggests that this can help us to understand why teenagers may behave on impulse, often with disregard to risk. However, this research needs to be seen in the context of other stimuli such as family relationships, culture, peer pressure, environment, etc. Figure 9.3 shows some of the more common mental health illnesses experienced by teenagers and young people.

Many of the mental health issues identified in Figure 9.3 are discussed in Chapters 15, 17 and 20. The Developmental and Well Being Assessment (DAWBA) (Goodman *et al.*, 2000) was developed to generate ICD-10 and DSM-IV psychiatric diagnoses on 5–16-year-olds through a series of questionnaires, interviews and self-monitoring techniques. In the UK people with learning disabilities and identified mental health needs are diagnosed using these criteria.

Fast facts 9.2   Psychiatric diagnoses sources

- The *International Classification of Disorders*, ICD-10, categorises mental and behavioural disorders.
- The *Diagnostic and Statistical Manual of Mental Disorders*, DSM IV, is published by the American Psychiatric Association and covers all mental health disorders for both children and adults.

Chapter 3 introduced the reader to the concept of mental capacity. It is useful to recap and consider the implications of legislation in regard to consent and involvement in health. Mental capacity assessments are not always appropriate to use with adolescents under the age of 16 as they are still developing their competence and understanding. Under the Mental Capacity Act (2005) Code of Practice, 'children' are defined as being under the age of 16. 'Young People' are those aged 16–17 years. This is different to the Children's Act (2004) which refers to anyone under the age of 18 as a child. The Mental Capacity Act does not apply to children under the age of 16 with two exceptions:

1. The Court of Protection can make decisions about a child's property or finances (or appoint a deputy to make these decisions) if the child lacks capacity to make such decisions within Section 2(1)* of the Act and is likely to still lack capacity to make financial decisions when they reach the age of 18 (Section 18(3)).
2. Offences of ill treatment or wilful neglect of a person who lacks capacity within Section 2(1)* can also apply to victims younger than 16 (Section 44).

(www.cambridgeshire.gov.uk/NR/rdonlyres/262F794F-3C54-4541-
81BD-D87B135312D8/0/MCAandChildren.pdf)

Most of the Mental Capacity Act applies to young people between the ages of 16 and 17 with just three exceptions:

1. Only someone over the age of 18 years can make a lasting power of attorney.
2. You must be older than 18 years to make an advance decision to refuse medical treatment.
3. The Court of Protection can only make a statutory will for someone aged 18 and over.

Support strategies

Popular therapies for supporting the mental health of young people are 'talking therapies', i.e. those therapies that encourage self-reflection. The Mental Health Foundation (2013) defines talking therapies as those therapies which help you to understand negative thoughts and feelings and make positive changes. Talking therapies are also called talking treatments; counselling; psychological therapies or treatments and psychotherapies. Hernandez-Halton *et al.* (2000) developed a psychotherapy service for children, adolescents and adults with a learning disability in London. They noted that a number of the referrals they received stated that the individual had been abused. They were not surprised by this, considering other research which highlights higher levels of abuse in vulnerable people compared to the rest of the population, but they were keen to explore the efficacy of talking therapies as treatments. These therapies can too easily be dismissed for the learning disabled due to recognised communication deficits. Hernandez-Halton *et al.* identified the importance of the assessment process in differentiating between the learning disability and the emotional distress in order to support the patient to make sense of their emotions. The team recognised that for many people with a learning disability, verbal communication can be difficult. Patients, particularly children, were able to express feelings through other mediums such as art, drawings and play things. However, verbal communication was still an essential element and continues to be seen as a barrier to access. In the case study, Jem would appear to have the communication skills to explore talking therapies as a way of understanding the changes that are happening to him. In a 2011 press statement, MP Paul Burstow said: 'We know psychological therapies work. Our aim is to transform existing mental health services for children so our children get the best treatment possible, from services that are more responsive to their needs.' The government pledged to spend £32 million increasing children's access to psychological therapies. This was part of an overall mental health strategy 'No Health without Mental Health' (DH, 2011b) which has six objectives:

1. More people will have good mental health.
2. More people with mental health problems will recover.
3. More people with mental health problems will have good physical health.
4. More people will have a positive experience of care and support.
5. Fewer people will suffer avoidable harm.
6. Fewer people will experience stigma and discrimination.

These objectives can be viewed positively for the learning disabled in light of well-researched problems in inequalities in health (Parliamentary and Health Service Ombudsman, 2009). These objectives should inform the assessment processes which health services implement. In the last 20 years it has been recognised that a higher proportion of people with learning disabilities than the general population experience emotional disturbance and mental illness. Raghavan (2007) suggests that despite policy directives guiding people with a learning disability towards mainstream services, it is in specialist learning disability services where most assessment and care is received. For children and adolescents with a learning disability, this specialist support is likely to be found through child community learning disability teams; CAMHS teams and Specialist Inclusive Learning Centres (SILCS).

Practice alert 9.1

Children and Adolescent Mental Health Teams (CAMHS) were established as inter-professional teams of professionals who are experienced in assessing, understanding and meeting the needs of this group. Staff within the team may be:

- psychiatrists
- social workers
- nurses
- occupational therapists
- psychologists
- psychotherapists
- counsellors
- family therapists
- arts therapists
- primary mental health worker
- outreach workers.

Services can introduce a range of other therapies to young people and their families, such as behavioural assessment and family therapy. This support can be sought through GP referral or accessed directly through voluntary organisations. Weare (2010) identifies that voluntary sector organisations play an important role in offering support to adolescents in schools.

Reader activity 9.3 Support information

- Undertake an internet search to see which organisations you can find, locally and nationally, which offer healthcare support and advice to adolescents.
- What criteria might you use to consider the quality of the information provided?

Behaviour management

Jem is experiencing some difficulties with his behaviour, as noted in the case study. These feelings of anger are natural in adolescents but for Jem there is a risk that the behaviour can be misdiagnosed and attributed to his learning disability, this is known as 'dual diagnosis'. Wheal (2004) suggests that it can be hard to understand young people and that their behaviour can frequently be misinterpreted. She outlines this in Figure 9.4 where the points on the left fit with those on the right.

Figure 9.4 highlights the importance of assessment strategies which seek to support the young person in understanding and subsequently participating in their own behaviour management.

Functional Behavioural Analysis is part of the process of behavioural psychology which uses operant conditioning to consider the relationship between stimuli and responses. This asks the questions, are there triggers that make someone behave in a particular way? Can we introduce or can the young person use different stimuli to change the behaviour? The first phase is to assess the behaviour using an ABC chart.

A = *Antecedent*: What was happening before the behaviour occurred? Consider issues such as the environment or interventions from another person. It is important to consider antecedents thoroughly without jumping to conclusions as to causes of behaviour.

B = *Behaviour*: What actually happened? How was this communicated?

C = *Consequence*: What were the immediate consequences of the behaviour? Who did what? Who said what? How did the young person, and others around them, feel?

Wheal (2004) identifies a further two elements to this analysis as:

D = *Design*: Use the information gathered to plan how to avoid the behaviour in the future.

E = *Enter*: The focus is on positive interaction with the adolescent which values them and shares commitment.

Maloret (2006) compares behavioural interventions with psychotherapies, suggesting that behavioural assessment focuses on the behaviour rather than cause. Talking therapies are concerned with the root cause of behaviour and how the individual can be supported to manage or move on from this.

Refuses to do something	Can't do something
Says it's stupid	Doesn't understand
Won't speak	Doesn't know what/how to say
Rants and raves	I'm embarrassed
Acts the fool	Is unsure
Gets angry	Needs attention
Shows off	Is worried

Figure 9.4 Difficulties in understanding, two perspectives

Professionals need to consider individual behaviours in the light of other holistic healthcare needs. The Developmental Behavioural Checklist (DBC) is a 96-item checklist which assesses a broad range of emotional and physical disturbance in children aged between 4 and 18 years. It should be completed by someone who has known the young person for at least 6 months and should take no more than 15 minutes to complete (Tonge and Brereton, 2011). Each behavioural item is given a rating score (0 = not true; 1 = sometimes true; 2 = very/often true). This assessment can identify a total behaviour problem score. Analysis of this can aid professionals and families in identifying the best support strategy for the young person. It has been used effectively with young people on the autistic spectrum.

Adolescence and transition

Behavioural and emotional changes are symptomatic with the period of transition in adolescence. The term transition identifies the changes that are happening to the young person in preparation for adulthood. *Valuing People* (DH, 2001) extended Connexions services to meet the needs of young people with learning disabilities, aged 13–19. Connexions provide personal advisors to young people and have the following objectives:

- Raising aspirations – setting high expectations of every individual.
- Meeting individual need – and overcoming barriers to learning.
- Taking account of the views of young people – individually and collectively, as the new service develops and as it is operated locally.
- Inclusion – keeping young people in mainstream education and training and preventing them from moving to the margins of their community.
- Partnership – agencies collaborating to achieve more for young people, parents and communities than agencies working in isolation.
- Community involvement and neighbourhood renewal – through involvement of community mentors and through personal advisers brokering access to local welfare, health, arts, sport and guidance networks.
- Extending opportunity and equality of opportunity – raising participation and achievement levels for all young people, influencing the availability, suitability and quality of provision and awareness of opportunities.
- Evidence-based practice – ensuring that new interventions are based on rigorous research and evaluation of 'what works' (Department for Education and Employment, 2000).

These objectives recognise the impact of transition. Policy had identified the importance of this transition as a priority in funding and services for some time, but research suggests that there is much

1. To provide a smooth process between childhood and adulthood;
2. To create choices and opportunities that otherwise may be overlooked;
3. To promote empowerment and an enabling culture;
4. To encourage and develop inter-professional and inter-agency working;
5. To support young people to identify their needs and wants in a positive future;
6. To identify access to mainstream services;
7. To consider future opportunities whether that be employment, Further Education, Higher Education or other training.

Figure 9.5 Aims of transition
Source: Adapted from Kaehne and Beyer (2009, p. 141).

variation across the UK in how successful this is. Figure 9.5 shows the aims of transition. Kaehne and Beyer (2010) believe that past failures in transition were attributed to lack of service user involvement and general social exclusion, but they identify a less publicised reason for such failures. This problem is a difference in expectations and outcomes between care providers, such as schools and social workers, and the parents of the adolescent. Kaehne and Beyer undertook research with two cohorts of students between 2005 and 2007, and found that there was a marked difference between the views of carers and professionals. Carers focused on changes within the family during transition whereas teachers and support staff focused on growing independence and the development of social skills. As the parent of an adolescent, I recognise the importance of independence and skills but also acknowledge the huge impact that 'stroppy' behaviour can have on the day-to-day functioning of a family. This is no different in Jem's case in the case study. His needs and behaviour are that of a 'typical' young adult. It is perhaps ironic that this typicality meets the philosophy of normalisation and social role valorisation, long-held belief systems in learning disability services. However, to Jem, this is a confusing time where he feels 'different' and excluded.

It is important to recognise that transition planning is not just for those young people who can identify needs and articulate them. The nature of a learning disability makes communication and social interaction difficult for a large number of adolescents. Cognitive impairment can make this an even more confusing and challenging time. The challenge is to families and services to adapt and adjust to make transition a reality for the individual. 'Reality is difficult. There is no way around this fact. One of the difficulties is to acknowledge and live with one's limitations. We all have them, but having a learning disability makes these limitations more concrete' (Hernandez-Halton et al., 2000, p. 124). Young people need support which recognises their potential and ability to develop competence. This requires realistic goals based on clear assessment but this should be motivational.

Independence and skills teaching

All those involved in the care and support of adolescents need to consider their understanding of the word 'independent'. Dictionary definitions suggest it means being free from the control of others. In services for the learning disabled, independence was traditionally seen as the ability and skill to undertake tasks. This could be misinterpreted as undertaking these skills alone as opposed to needing help or assistance. Being free from the control of others implies that we are empowered to make choices and decisions. We all need information and support to be able to do this. The levels of support and guidance we require will differ, based on our individual needs, abilities and preferences. The key message here is one of choice and control. It is too easy within learning disability services to make assumptions about an individual's likes, dislikes and need based on communication deficits. This is disempowering and unacceptable from a human and civil rights perspective. This does not mean it is always easy to support individuals with complex disabilities to exercise their rights to decision-making, but it is our responsibility to try. Person-centred planning tools are an excellent way of promoting this perspective in meeting needs.

Person-centred approaches to supporting the learning disabled were made explicit in the government White Paper, *Valuing People* in 2001 (DH, 2001) and celebrated as a way for an individual to maximise choice and control in their lives, including access to health.

> A person–centred approach to planning means that planning should start with the individual (not with services), and take account of their wishes and aspirations. Person-centred planning is a mechanism for reflecting the needs and preferences of a person with a learning disability and covers such issues as housing, education, employment and leisure.
>
> (ibid., p. 45)

Patient- or person-centred approaches to health are increasingly seen as more efficient as they promote good communication between the clinician and patient but research to support this is lacking (Lewin *et al.*, 2009). The Mental Capacity Act (2005) is based on person-centred principles and gives legal backing to previous guidelines for good practice (Mencap, 2010). It gives responsibility to all healthcare professionals to follow person-centred guidance in addressing issues of choice and consent in healthcare with the learning disabled. The key principles of this include the person being at the centre of any planning and discussion. This does not mean decisions are simply taken in their best interests but ways are sought to actively involve them in decision-making using accessible communication systems when necessary. Family and friends should be full partners in this process (DH, 2001). Information, advice and guidance (IAG) services are essential in supporting young people and their families to plan.

Reader activity 9.4   Life planning

- Identify the areas of life planning that a typical older adolescent might be involved in.
- What might the potential difficulties be in these areas of planning for someone with a learning disability?

It is necessary for information and guidance services to recognise these difficulties, not to see barriers in terms of life planning but to be able to problem solve and seek appropriate assessments which enable the adolescent to see a positive future. Different health and social care professionals will have their own tool kit of assessment strategies based on the different roles they may play in guidance and support. One such strategy commonly used by learning disability nurses is the 'Human Needs Model' developed by Roper, Logan and Tierney (1996). Nursing models are frameworks which support nurses to meet individual's needs through a process of assessment, diagnosis, planning, implementation and evaluation. The Roper *et al.* (1996) model covers the five dimensions of psychological health; physiological health; socio-cultural health; political-economic health and environment. The assessment component of this

- Maintaining a safe environment
- Communication
- Breathing
- Eating and drinking
- Elimination
- Washing and dressing
- Controlling temperature
- Mobilisation
- Working and playing
- Expressing sexuality
- Sleeping
- Death and dying

Figure 9.6 Activities of living

model is called the 'Activities of Living' and considers 12 items in respect of an individual's independence and potential for independence (see Figure 9.6). Critics of this model suggest that it is too simplistic but supporters argue that this simplicity is one of its strengths.

These activities can provide a useful baseline assessment for young people wishing to be more in control of their support or thinking about moving on from the parental home. When considering each activity, those involved must be clear about their understanding and interpretation of each activity. For example, within the activity 'expressing sexuality' you might think about self-identity, developing relationships, etc.

Once assessments have identified areas for personal development in health, the young person may need support in developing their skills and competence in these areas. The health and social care professional should give consideration to the learning style of the individual (see Practice alert 9.2). This might involve some experiments with concentration and memory that involves the person and motivates them in exploring their own learning.

Practice alert 9.2

There are different types of learning:

- visual – watches or reads
- auditory – listens
- kinaesthetic – does (hands-on)
- multimodal – a mixture of learning styles.

Different learning theories explore the purpose, focus and belief systems of learning and influence how learning is developed. One example is behaviourism which we have already considered in relation to challenging behaviours. Task analysis is a process which breaks tasks down into component parts to work towards a target or goal. An example of this can be given in breaking down the task of buttoning a coat:

Aim: To button a coat independently. The steps are:

1. Supported to put coat on.
2. Encouraged to locate first (top) button hole with left hand.
3. Pushes index finger through this button hole.
4. Holds top button with right hand.
5. Moves the button towards the left hand.
6. Trace the button along the index finger into the hole.
7. Move the left hand to hold the button.
8. Pull it through the hole.

The Bereweeke Skills Teaching Assessment Checklist (Jenkins *et al*, 1983) uses the approach of task analysis in planning. It was developed for adults with a learning disability but can still be a useful tool in supporting older children. Other functional assessments are used within education services. Some examples of these are:

- Assessment of Basic Language and Learning Skills
- Vineland Adaptive Behaviour Scales.

Sexuality and relationships

Sexuality is addressed in detail in Chapter 18. These paragraphs take an adolescent perspective on the topic. The Family Planning Association (FPA, 2013), a sexual health charity, suggest that children between the ages of 9 and 13 need to know about:

- puberty changes and body parts;
- sex and reproduction;
- sexual orientation;
- contraception and sexually transmitted infections;
- pregnancy choices, including abortion;
- periods, wet dreams, masturbation;
- love and relationships.

There is no evidence to suggest that young people with a learning disability have different needs to this but we need to consider their level of understanding, maturity and ability to communicate to ensure we deal with this topic appropriately. In determining physical maturity consideration must be given to the stage of puberty that the young person has reached. Puberty is the time in a person's life when the body has reached sexual maturity and sexual organs become functional. It is caused by the release of the sex hormones testosterone and oestrodial (NHS Choices, 2012). Puberty causes physical changes which can include rapid growth spurts, growth of breasts in girls and the penis in boys. It also can cause psychological and behavioural changes, as have already been discussed. For girls, puberty usually occurs between the ages of 8 and 14, with the average age being 11 years. For boys, puberty usually occurs between 9 and 14 years, with an average age of 12. There can be complications in puberty with puberty delayed or happening early (precocious). Adolescents with a learning disability are more prone to difficulties due to connections between precocious puberty and brain damage/disease. NHS Choices (2012) identify the main causes of precocious puberty as:

- problem in the brain (such as a tumour);
- brain injury due to head trauma;
- an infection of the brain (such as meningitis);
- a problem in the ovaries or thyroid gland;
- an inherited tendency (it may run in your family).

If parents or carers have concerns about the onset or delay in puberty they should seek advice through a GP.

Puberty will usually see the start of personal and sexual relationships developing for a young person. It can be difficult for parents to recognise their child as having sexual feelings or needs, particularly if their cognitive impairment is severe. It is important that protection of a vulnerable person is key. This includes the young person having information. The Resources section at the end of this chapter identifies the web pages for FPA, who have experience in meeting the needs of the learning disabled. Their suggestions for what teenagers should know about sex is given in Practice Alert 9.3.

Practice alert 9.3

- They should not give in to pressure to have sex if they're not ready.
- They should not pressure their partner to have sex.
- They should use condoms to help prevent sexually transmitted infections and pregnancy.
- They should know about other types of contraception.
- That it's not just about sex and biology. It's about relationships, puberty and body changes, love and feelings, like self-esteem.
- They should know about sex in the media.

(FPA, http://www.fpa.org.uk/helpandadvice/
parentsandcarers/talking-with-teenagers)

Risk assessments

Risk assessment is an essential element of child protection but is also an important tool in encouraging choice and autonomy. Titterton (2005, p. 9) states that 'Risk provides an innovative and challenging way of bringing about genuine change in the way health and social services are conceived, planned and delivered.' This requires professionals to work with young people and families in balancing the potential for risk with supporting the young person to develop life skills and decision-making. This balancing act requires excellent communication skills from professionals to develop therapeutic relationships in supporting parents to see the holistic picture of the individual and providing them with reassurance. Assessing risk can be seen as a way of avoiding an unwanted outcome but it can also be seen as way of managing barriers to achieve a positive outcome. Titterton suggests that an approach which is overly focused on safety can ignore some of the needs of vulnerable people and potentially deny choice and autonomy which can reduce self-esteem and respect. Bates and Silberman (2007) support a widely held view that person-centred risk assessment provides a way forward and identify seven criteria which this type of assessment should fulfil:

- involvement of service users and relatives in risk assessment;
- positive and informed risk taking;
- proportionality;
- contextualising behaviour;
- defensible decision-making;
- a learning culture;
- tolerable risks.

Adoption of these criteria requires services to be clear about their commitment to the young person. This circles back to the start of the chapter when you were asked to consider the important tenets of working with young people.

Points to remember

- We need to listen and value the contribution that young people make.
- We must make sure that information is available and accessible on issues that affect the person.
- We must appreciate the difficulties associated with the transition of adolescence and the impact that disability can have on this.
- We should employ an inter-professional approach to assessment which acts on best practice and professional knowledge.
- We must ensure a learning culture which recognises individual learning needs and accepts that mistakes can be learnt from.
- We must remember that young people are individuals first.

Resources

Young Minds Professionals
These web pages provide links to Child Adolescent and Mental Health Services across the UK.
www.youngminds.org.uk/training_services/policy/camhs_in_the_uk

More information on the Development and Well-being Assessment, including interview and questionnaire sheets, is available at www.dawba.com/.

FPA (Family Planning Association). The FPA provides training for professional s supporting people with a learning disability in areas of sexual health: http://www.fpa.org.uk/.

The National Transition Support Team (2011) have written a paper on person-centred approaches for young people, available at: http://www.transitionsupportprogramme.org.uk/pdf/NTST_Person_Centred_Approaches.pdf.

References

Bartley, J. (2008) Assessing population health needs of children and young people, in V. Thurtle and J. Wright (eds) *Promoting the Health of School Age Children*. London: Quay Books.

Bates, P. and Silberman, W. (2007) *Modelling Risk Management in Inclusive Settings*. London: National Development Team. Available at: www.ndt.org.uk/docsN/ET_SIrisk.pdf.

Department for Education and Employment (2000) *Connexions: The Best Start for Every Young Person*. Sheffield: Department for Education and Employment.

Department of Education (2012) *The CAF Process* http://www.education.gov.uk/childrenand-youngpeople/strategy/integratedworking/caf/a0068957/the-caf-process (accessed 12 Jan. 2013).

DH (Department of Health) (2001) *Valuing People: A New Strategy for Learning Disability for the 21st Century*. Cm. 5086. London: Stationery Office.

DH (Department of Health) (2011) *Self Review Tool for Quality Criteria for Young People-Friendly Health Services*. Available at: https://www.gov.uk/government/publications/self-review-tool-for-quality-criteria-for-young-people-friendly-health-services (accessed 10 Feb. 2013).

DH (Department of Health) (2011b) *No Health without Mental Health: A Cross Government Outcomes Strategy for People of All Ages*. London: Department of Health.

Emerson, E., Malam, S., Davies, I. and Spencer, K. (2005) *Adults with Learning Difficulties in England 2003/4*. London: NHS Health and Social Care Information Centre.

FPA (Family Planning Association) (2013) *Talking to Children aged 9–13*. Available at: www.fpa.org.uk/helpandadvice/parentsandcarers/talking-to-children-aged-nine-to-thirteen (accessed 10 Feb. 2013).

Goodman, R., Ford, T., Richards, H., Gatward, R. and Meltzer, H. (2000) The development and well being assessment: description and initial validation of an integrated assessment of child and adolescent psychopathology, *Journal of Child Psychology and Psychiatry and Allied Disciplines*, 41: 645–656.

Hernandez-Halton, I., Hodges, S., Miller, L. and Simpson., D. (2000) A psychotherapy service for children, adolescents and adults with learning disabilities at the Tavistock Clinic, London, UK, *British Journal of Learning Disabilities*, 28: 120–124.

Lewin, S., Skea, Z., Entwhistle, V., Zwarenstein, M. and Dick, J. (2009) *Interventions For Providers to Promote a Patient-Centred Approach in Clinical Consultations*. Chichester: John Wiley & Sons Ltd. Available at: http://www.thecochranelibrary.com/view/0/index.html (accessed 23 June 2010).

Jenkins, J., Felce, D. and Mansell, J. (1983) *The Bereweeke Skills Teaching System: Assessment Checklist*. Windsor: NFER.

Keahne, A. and Beyer, S. (2009) Views of professionals on aims and outcomes of transition for young people with learning disabilities, *British Journal of Learning Disabilities*, 37: 138–144.

Keahne, A. and Beyer, S. (2010) Stroppy or confident? Do carers and professionals view the impact of transition support on young people differently? *British Journal of Learning Disabilities*, 39: 154–160.

Kerr, G. (2001) Assessing the needs of learning disabled young people with additional disabilities, *Journal of Learning Disabilities*, 5(2): 157–174.

Maloret, P. (2006) Mental health issues and adults with learning disabilities, in I. Peate and D. Fearns (eds) *Caring for People with Learning Disabilities*. Chichester: John Wiley & Sons Ltd.

Mencap (2010) *Involve Me: Practical Guide. How to Involve People with Profound and Multiple Learning Disabilities (PMLD) in Decision-Making and Consultation*. Available at: www.mencap.org.uk/sites/default/files/documents/Involve%20Me%20practical%20guide_full%20version.pdf.

Mental Health Foundation (2013) Available at: www.mentalhealth.org.uk/help-information/mental-health-a-z/T/talking-therapies/ (accessed 18 April 2013).

National Institute for Mental Health (2013) The teen brain still under construction. Available at: www.nimh.nih.gov/health/publications/the-teen-brain-still-under-construction/complete-index.shtml (accessed 13 April 2013).

NHS Choices (2012) Puberty. Available at: www.nhs.uk/Conditions/Puberty/Pages/Introduction.aspx (accessed 10 March 2013).

NICE (2009) *Health Needs Assessment Workbook*. Available at: www.nice.org.uk/aboutnice/whoweare/aboutthehda/hdapublications/health_needs_assessment_workbook.jsp (accessed 10 April 2014).

Parliamentary and Health Service Ombudsman (2009) *Six Lives: The Provision of Public Services to People with Learning Disabilities*. London: The Stationery Office.

Priestley, M. (2003) *Disability: A Life Course Approach*. Cambridge: Polity.

Raghavan, R. (2007) Mental health disorders in people with learning disabilities, in B. Gates (ed.) *Learning Disabilities: Toward Inclusion*. London: Churchill Livingstone.

RCPCH (Royal College of Paediatrics and Child Health) (2003) *Bridging the Gaps: Healthcare for Adolescents*. London: RCPCH:

Roper, N., Logan, W. and Tierney, A. (1996) *The Elements of Nursing: A Model for Nursing. Based on a Model of Living*, 4th edn. London: Churchill Livingstone.

Taggart, L., Taylor, D. and McCrum Gardner, E. (2010) Individual, life events, family and socio-economic factors associated with young people with intellectual disability and with and without behavioural/emotional problems, *Journal of Intellectual Disabilities*, 14(4): 267–288.

Titterton, M. (2005) *Risk and Risk Taking in Health and Social Welfare*. London: Jessica Kingsley Publishers.

Tonge, B. and Brereton, A. (2011) Overview of the Developmental Behaviour Checklist. Available at: www.med.monash.edu.au/spppm/research/devpsych/actnow/download/factsheet09.pdf (accessed 10 April 2013).

Weare, K. (2010) Promoting mental health through schools, in P. Aggleton, C. Dennison and I. Warwick (eds) *Promoting Health and Well-being through Schools*. London: Routledge.

Wheal, A. (2004) *Adolescence: Positive Approaches for Working with Young People*. Dorset: Russell House Publishing.

WHO (World Health Organisation) (2013) Adolescent health. Available at: www.who.int/topics/adolescent_health/en/ (accessed 22 April 2013).

10 Determining health and social care in adulthood

Mary Dearing and Debbie Crickmore

Learning outcomes

After reading this chapter you will be able to:

- identify some commonly used assessment tools in adult health and social care
- highlight the value of working with others to share information
- use assessment findings to plan and deliver care that places the individual at the centre
- encourage reflection on your experiences.

Introduction

> It's Jeremy now . . . thankyou very much!

This chapter will consider a range of health and social care assessments upon which care and support of adults with learning disabilities may be based. By continuing our journey with Jeremy, we'll consider how he came to the situation described above, what happened when he became acutely unwell and how he was supported to go forward to the next phase of his life.

Case study 10.1   Jeremy's life

As he approaches 30, Jem prefers to use his real first name of Jeremy as he feels it's more suited to his independent adult life. He holds a tenancy on a Local Authority one-bedroom ground floor flat in a housing estate on the outskirts of the city. It's a few miles from his mum who says 'It's not the best of areas' but he likes it. There's a parade of shops close by where young people meet up and they acknowledge him when he passes. His flat faces into a square of other properties and he's on nodding acquaintance with some of his neighbours.

(continued)

(continued)

Jeremy has two hours support twice a week from Anne, directed at budgeting and menu planning. She's a nice enough woman but sometimes Jeremy feels like she's his mum, after all, it's his money and it's up to him how he spends it. Once or twice lately when Anne calls, he's even pretended he's not in. He knows this isn't the right way to do things but wants to work out himself how to speak up about how he feels. When Anne was off recently, a younger guy, Chris, helped and that somehow felt different – better. It was good to be able to talk to a man about the stomach pains he'd been having. Chris thought Jeremy might be constipated and suggested increasing the amount of fruit and vegetables he eats and drinking more fluids.

Working three shifts a week at a large local supermarket, Jeremy's first paid job was collecting trolleys but when one of the supervisors noticed he was helping some of the women in the bakery with the computerised ordering system, he was moved into the warehouse to help with stock control. Jeremy enjoys his work and loves the banter that goes on in the warehouse. He looks forward to the Christmas party each year and is never without a dance partner.

While at work last Friday evening Jeremy experienced severe abdominal cramps and nausea. Stan, his co-worker in the warehouse, was really worried about him and gave him a lift to the local Walk-in Centre where he was seen by a nurse practitioner. When the nurse examined Jeremy's abdomen, it was so tender that she explained he should go to hospital. She would urgently refer him by letter to Accident and Emergency.

While waiting for a taxi, Jeremy begins to worry about what will happen at the hospital. The last time he went there was to see his granddad just before he died from bowel cancer. Jeremy is scared that he too will die.

Assessment

Assessment is an important function as it provides the basis for individualised support, avoiding blanket, 'one-size-fits-all' services and 'doing things the way we've always done them' mindset. If we can work with someone to find out what they need and want, then we're on the way to figuring out how to support them to achieve those goals. It helps us prioritise, solve problems, facilitate learning and identify areas where there could be an issue before it arises. So, it's not only an active process that should put the individual at the centre, but could be proactive and, as we'll see when Jeremy becomes unwell, reactive. Crucially, it's not an end in itself.

As a starting point of a systematic framework, assessment gives us a baseline from which to plan, implement and evaluate support. Within this process we can consider the best way to offer help. For example, are there any new ideas, services or – ideally – an evidence base for interventions to meet a particular need? Assessment is also part of a dynamic cycle, where reassessment can check progress, identify changes or emergent need.

A variety of assessments, with different emphases, conducted within and between a range of professions, agencies and individuals is illustrated in this chapter using Jeremy's story. They may be holistic or specific, broad or targeted. Some require special training or preparation, others rely on good communication, observation and the ability to interpret information. Figure 10.1 explores this further and highlights some words commonly used in relation to assessment. We recognise the importance of sharing content on a 'need to know' basis with consent to avoid repeated 'story telling' which may increasingly be achieved by use of electronic systems, for example, SystmOne (TPP,

---

The assessment process can be understood in several ways including ...

- Characteristics of the assessor: for example: **self-assessment, non-specialist assessment**.
- Availability of the assessment: for example, *Community Care Assessment (CCA)* should be available to all who may be in need of community care services (**universal**). Such a broad initial assessment may also be referred to as **holistic**, identifying areas where more focused attention is needed.
- Focus of the assessment: for example, **assessment** for employability and independent travel undertaken by field **specialists**, or undertaken by **non-specialists with appropriate training** (see below for use of DisDAT in Accident and Emergency).
- Ability to measure or quantify: for example: use of *Bristol Stool Form Scale*.[1] Standardised tools can produce more **objective** or **quantitative information** (**data**).
- Ability to collect impressions or opinions: for example: while assessment of mood might be considered **subjective**, such **qualitative** data can help us understand people's experiences through use of tools including the *Beck Depression Inventory ®-II*[2] could raise objectivity. This can be self-administered or verbally by a trained administrator.

Figure 10.1 The Assessment Process

Notes: 1 Heaton (1997).
2 Beck, Steer and Brown (1996).

2012). Assessment of risk is also integral. Our key message is that assessment has little worth unless it is used as the basis for intervention.

Self-assessment

Just because Jeremy's assessment of his circumstances has not been formally conducted using a reliable tool or printed tick box format, it should not be dismissed. However, there is evidence that self-reporting of health-related behaviours (for example, smoking in pregnancy, see Shipton *et al.*, 2009) may be inaccurate and that some people with – and without – learning disabilities may tend to try to please others (Banks, 2003), leading in some circumstances to a need for further information. You may experience such issues yourself by undertaking Reader activity 10.1.

Reader activity 10.1 Potential issues with self-reporting

Complete the NHS Choices (2010) 'Healthy eating self-assessment' tool available at: www.nhs.uk/Tools/Pages/HealthyEating.aspx.

If you don't have internet access you could complete any magazine or newspaper quiz that requires you to report on your behaviour.

Then, ask yourself . .

- Was I entirely honest in my answers?
- Would someone observing me answer differently?

- Suppose I was completing this in the presence of a prospective friend or partner, could this further influence my responses?
- In what way?

In his story above, Jeremy recognises he has successfully negotiated the transition between adolescence and adulthood. With his own home and paid employment it is little wonder he wishes to set aside his childhood name. How many of us have chosen to reinvent ourselves as we have moved on from areas, jobs or relationships? Unlike more than half of adults with learning disabilities, he is no longer living in the family home (Emerson and Hatton, 2008). Additionally, Improving Health and Lives (IHAL): Learning Disability Observatory (2007–2012) identifies his tenancy as stable accommodation. Jeremy is also among the 7 per cent of adults with learning disabilities in paid work (Emerson *et al.*, 2012). Above the strapline *changing lives*, the Foundation for People with Learning Disabilities (FPLD) points out this is despite 65 per cent of people with learning disabilities wanting a job.

Case study 10.2   Independent living

Jeremy is able to compare his home with that of his sister Jo; she's in her first year at university and moved into a house with people she didn't even know in an area their mum thinks is even worse than his! Despite what people say about men's and women's approaches to housekeeping, Jeremy maintains his flat is both cleaner and tidier. On the other hand, his cousin lives with his partner and children in a large house outside the city; perhaps something Jeremy would like in the future. An important consideration for him right now is that since successfully completing independent travel training, he can either walk to work – when the mood takes him, he has time or the weather is good – or just to the bus that stops outside the supermarket.

The next logical step from forming a view is to express it - or share it with someone who can speak on your behalf – the basis of self-advocacy and citizen advocacy respectively. By adopting elements such as those in Practice alert 10.1 we can help Jeremy to realise his hopes and dreams.

Practice alert 10.1

In supporting Jeremy we must:

- Use the name he prefers (Jeremy rather than Jem).
- Respect his right to make his own assessment of his circumstances.
- Take care not to expect higher standards, for example, of household cleanliness, from him than would be accepted of others without a learning disability.

Case study 10.3   Non-specialist assessment

Jeremy's move within the supermarket from collecting trolleys to stock control was based on his supervisor's observations of his skills, rather than on a structured assessment administered by a supported employment specialist. That it has been successful is due in part to the skills of the supervisor *in his field*. There are times when people with learning disabilities may benefit from specialist intervention but in this context Jeremy is first and foremost an employee. In common with his co-workers, he is protected by UK legislation including the Health and Safety at Work Act 1974 and the Equality Act 2010. The first applies to all while the second is aimed at those with protected characteristics including disability.

We do not know what led Chris to believe Jeremy might be constipated. The crucial opening is that he listened, having shown himself to be someone with whom Jeremy felt comfortable. According to NHS Choices (2012a), stomach ache and cramps are indeed symptoms of constipation. Perhaps Chris' suggestion was based on a conversation with Jeremy about a change in his bowel habit as constipation can be when passing stools becomes more difficult than it used to be *for the individual* in terms of frequency or efficiency (Hicks, 2008). However, Jeremy may have omitted features such as rectal bleeding due to embarrassment. The Department of Health's *Be Clear on Cancer* campaign (2011) to promote earlier diagnosis of bowel cancer recognises embarrassment as a factor preventing individuals seeking timely advice from their General Practitioner (GP). Jeremy may not differentiate between bleeding from straining to pass a motion and blood *in* the stools as experienced by his granddad prior to the diagnosis of bowel cancer from which he later died. Feeling stressed or being anxious or depressed can contribute to, or exacerbate, constipation. Other relevant areas that may not have been discussed include Jeremy's level of activity, for example, has the move at work from collecting trolleys to the warehouse resulted in less physical exercise? Is the environment busier or the toilet less accessible so he ignores the urge to pass stools or is there less privacy?

A lack of improvement – or even a worsening of symptoms despite taking what would be considered healthy lay dietary advice (for example, Bupa, 2010) – may go undisclosed by Jeremy, particularly once Anne returns and Chris moves on. By Chris observing Jeremy's right to privacy, Anne may be unaware of any difficulties. There may not be a useful system of record keeping or liaison between support workers, even if Jeremy were happy for such information to be shared. While the menu planning remit for his two hours support twice a week might allow for recording the increase in fruit, vegetables and fluids suggested by Chris, without a rationale (*why* have they been increased?) or baseline (how much fruit, vegetables and fluid was Jeremy taking *before* the increase?), this may have limited impact. Additional wholegrain and wholemeal fibre are also indicated in treatment of constipation while more drinks containing caffeine or alcohol could worsen the problem. Jeremy's income and level of skill may also influence his ability to access a healthy diet (World Health Organisation, 2012). To summarise, there are several reasons why if constipation is suspected, more thorough or specialist assessment may be helpful and useful tools are suggested and described in Practice alert 10.2.

Practice alert 10.2

The following are elements used in the constipation toolbox:

- *Assessment of mood.* Self-reported or observed, tailored to individual need, for example, use colour charts or faces to represent agreed moods.
- *Bristol Stool Form Scale.* A well-known chart designed to classify the various forms of human stools into seven categories, available for download as a mobile application (App).
- *Bowel diary.* For example, amounts and times, possibly places. Using the App as above would mean date and time of entry were automatically recorded.
- *Environmental assessment.* Could be undertaken by an Occupational Therapist (OT) or less formally by the individual or supporter. Where is the toilet, is it easily accessible and suitably private? Is it an appropriate height for access and optimum positioning (feet touching floor)?
- *Exercise diary.* Kept by the individual or supporters, greater detail increases usefulness. For example, 'went swimming' could mean 20 lengths of a 25m pool or 20 minutes in the jacuzzi! Jeremy could wear a pedometer on the journey to, or at, work.
- *Food and fluid diary.* Including amounts and types will be most useful. For example, 'meat pie and veg' could be a plate-size pie and a single spoon of peas, or an individual (or slice of) pie with the recommended '5 a day' vegetables (or anything in between). Digital photography enables images of food to be taken. Volume of a favourite mug could be measured.

Community Care Assessment (CCA)

A number of assessments may have been conducted as a prequel to Jeremy's story at the beginning of this chapter. Without them, and the support provided in respect of their findings, the route from living at home without meaningful employment to his current situation may have proved more difficult. The starting point for this process was a Community Care Assessment (CCA) requested by Jeremy while he shared his mother's home. In England and Wales, the NHS and Community Care Act 1990 aims to help people live safely in their local communities by providing the support they need. It obliges the Local Authority Social Services Department to conduct such an assessment when it becomes aware that someone may be in need of community care services, including aids and adaptations in the home, support workers or residential care. Similar arrangements exist in Scotland (Care Information Scotland 2012) and Northern Ireland (nidirect 2010a). Legislation also exists (for example, Carers and Disabled Children Act 2000, Community Care and Health (Scotland) Act 2002) to allow anyone who provides – or intends to provide – a substantial amount of care on a regular basis to have a Carer's Assessment (though Jeremy might dispute his mother's entitlement to this).

The circumstances surrounding the request for assessment included increased tension between Jeremy and his mother relating to his desire for more independence. This was potentially affecting their mutual mental health to the extent that his continued residence in the family home was threatened. Without planned intervention there was a risk the situation would break down irretrievably, necessitating an emergency response and untold emotional cost. However, at the time of referral

Jeremy had a roof over his head and a family member concerned for his welfare; that his mother was stressed was not an unusual occurrence (Carers Trust, 2012). Under *Fair Access to Care Services (FACS)* (DH, 2003), unless Jeremy's needs were identified as critical or substantial, he might not have been eligible for intervention. However, following the findings of *Cutting the Cake Fairly* (CSCI, 2008) there emerged guidance (DH, 2010a) enabling targeted intervention to support those at increased risk, in this case of family breakdown, homelessness and poor health. In addition, according to NHS Choices (2011), assessments for people with learning disabilities should abide by principles set out in *Valuing People* (DH, 2001a), taking an individualised, person-centred approach supporting Jeremy's right to exercise choice and control over his life.

It was within this context that Jeremy's desire for a more independent life was realised. The CCA identified competent personal care and social skills with some domestic housekeeping knowledge, a desire to work and have a place to live. At this time no health concerns were raised, for those with complex health needs, a Continuing Health Care Assessment may be triggered (Age UK, 2012). The resultant Care Plan, arrived at with the support of a Person Centred Facilitator using PATH (Lay and Kirk, 2011), contained the ultimate goals of having a paid job and living alone. In order to achieve these, focused assessment of skills including employability and independent travel was indicated. In Jeremy's case, these were both available from a specialist Local Authority resource which went on to provide the training identified. Other sources of employment support include MENCAP's *Employ Me* programme. The ability to travel freely and easily enhances social inclusion and concessions may be available for individuals, such as Northern Ireland's SmartPass (nidirect 2010b), and companions should they be required. While these may facilitate independent travel training, there are a number of issues that could be identified and managed to minimise risk. Potential dangers to the individual or others are often cited as grounds for not going ahead with skills training but it would also be unwise to proceed without any such consideration. It is important to remember that many people (with and without learning disabilities) are confident in their routine journeys but less so for those that are new or venture further afield, or where mode of transit changes. For example, making the same journey on foot might be an entirely different experience to taking the bus. Reader activity 10.2 is designed to help you consider some of these issues.

Reader activity 10.2   Travel risks

Can you identify any potential risks to Jeremy in learning to travel independently between home and work? You may have identified issues including:

- getting lost;
- becoming flustered;
- mislaying his travel pass and/or money;
- unwanted attention from fellow travellers or members of the public;
- road safety;
- recognising and/or understanding numbers, timetables.

Having identified potential risks, each could be rated in relation to how likely it might be and how serious the consequences, should it occur, using your knowledge of the individual. This information could then be used to form a risk management plan.

What strategies could Jeremy be equipped with to minimise each potential risk?

London Transport provides great tips for supporters online at: http://www.tfl.gov.uk/gettingaround/transportaccessibility/1201.aspx, where you will also find a Guide that can be personalised, and an audio version, including sound effects.

A referral was made to the Local Authority Housing Department for suitable accommodation. This may also have been available via Housing Associations or private landlords. Although Jeremy didn't need ground floor accommodation, the property he was offered wouldn't have been suitable for adaptation for someone with physical disabilities due to limited space. The National Development Team for inclusion (NDTi, 2010, p. 21) confirms:

> Most people understand the basics of a tenancy agreement which come down to having to pay money and look after your home in return for being able to live there in peace and enjoyment. There is no need to have an in depth understanding of tenancy law to have a tenancy as indeed is the case for most of the population.

This Discussion Paper recognises the Mental Capacity Act 2005 (see Figure 10.2 on p. 183) as providing a helpful framework within which to address issues surrounding individuals who may be judged to lack capacity entering into a tenancy arrangement. It would appear that the Adults with Incapacity (Scotland) Act 2000 could also be used in this respect. With so many changes occurring in a short time span, Jeremy chose to accept the sessional support in relation to budgeting and menu planning offered by the Local Authority rather than the alternative of receiving a Direct Payment to arrange the service himself. It just seemed easier and he could always think again later. In any case, he still needed a means-tested financial assessment to assess whether he had to contribute anything towards the cost of services. Citizen's Advice Bureau (2012) explain that in England, Wales and Northern Ireland, an entitlement to community care services leads to the option of receiving Direct Payments – known in Scotland as Self Directed Support – to arrange a service from a voluntary organisation or care agency, or by employing Personal Assistants (PAs), or a combination of both.

Primary care assessment

When moving to a new area, many of us need to acquaint ourselves with local facilities and familiarise ourselves with how we access them. Perhaps Anne, Jeremy's support worker, will have pointed out where he can buy bread and the local shop to buy fruit and vegetables but may have overlooked the need to point out the local pharmacy and explain the services available.

As part of the government's long-term vision for the future of public health in England, it published the White Paper, *Healthy Lives, Healthy People: Our Strategy for Public Health in England* (DH, 2010b). The government's view is that everyone has a responsibility for public health and protecting the nation's health and well-being. This document highlights that community pharmacies are a valuable resource and can help manage minor ailments and common conditions by the provision of advice and, where appropriate, the sale of medicines. Jeremy could have visited his local pharmacy and asked to speak to the pharmacist, who would have then been able to advise on lifestyle changes and, if appropriate, recommend medication. The pharmacist could also have reviewed any other regular medication Jeremy may take (such as painkillers) that may have side effects such as constipation. Additionally the pharmacist may have asked Jeremy more probing questions relating to his bowel habits, for example, if constipation is associated with severe abdominal pain, vomiting or passing blood or mucus in the motions. If appropriate, the pharmacist can keep records of this consultation and recommend that, if his symptoms persist, where Jeremy can seek medical advice if these measures don't help.

Some knowledge of Down's Syndrome within primary care services, for example, the tendency to hypotonia or hypothyroidism, may have been helpful in making tentative connections with Jeremy's concerns, allowing for consideration of whether his symptoms were directly related to his Down's Syndrome. Most infants born with Down's Syndrome have low muscle tone (hypotonia). This means that their muscles are weak and appear 'floppy'. Although hypotonia cannot be cured, muscle tone usually improves with physiotherapy (Fergus, 2009) but may persist into adulthood. Additionally, people with Down's Syndrome have an increased incidence of hypothyroidism (Prasher and Gomez, 2007). Hypothyroidism means that the thyroid gland, located in the neck, is underactive and does not produce enough thyroid hormones. Symptoms include increase in weight, dry skin, constipation, and lethargy. There is a danger that healthcare professionals may make an assumption that these presenting symptoms are associated with Down's Syndrome rather than considering these symptoms independently as a new condition. This is described as diagnostic overshadowing and if these health problems remain unrecognised and therefore untreated, there may be serious consequences for the individual (Sowney and Brown, 2007). To guarantee the best possible long-term outcome for people with learning disabilities, health practitioners should offer routine examinations while simultaneously remaining attentive and suspicious of comorbid conditions more common (in this instance) with Down's Syndrome.

Annual health assessment

If the pharmacist felt that Jeremy's symptoms were more complex, then he might suggest that he makes an appointment to see his GP for an Annual Health Check. Annual Health Checks for adults (over 18 years old) with learning disabilities were introduced in 2008 as a Direct Enhanced Service (DES). As part of contract negotiations the General Practitioners Committee of the British Medical Association agreed five new clinical groups, one of which was people with a learning disability. DESs focus on health and service priorities of the Department of Health that will benefit patients. They are considered to be a 'reasonable adjustment' to address known health inequalities faced by people with a learning disability as highlighted in a number of reports (Disability Rights Commission, 2006; Mencap, 2007; Michael, 2008). The DESs are special services or activities provided by GP practices which in return receive a financial payment for providing additional services to specific groups of people. It is anticipated that Annual Health Checks will begin to address the health inequalities experienced by people with a learning disability (Cumella and Martin, 2000). The Down's Syndrome Association (DSA) recommends that Annual Health Checks should also monitor activity levels as a decrease in activity is often one of the first indicators to a decline in health (DSA, 2012). If Jeremy had received an Annual Health Check and discussed that he was experiencing abdominal pain and nausea, then further investigations might have been recommended and a situation avoided whereby a support worker with limited medical knowledge may have given inappropriate (though well-meant) advice.

Even if Jeremy had an Annual Health Check, his GP might not have been skilled in communicating with him and he may have benefitted from the assistance of Anne or Chris, his support workers, who could have helped prepare him for his appointment and discussed with him health issues he would like to raise with his doctor. In 2011, the DSA conducted a survey. This study investigated the experience of people with Down's Syndrome across the United Kingdom. Previous studies have highlighted that people with Down's Syndrome have poorer health and a higher prevalence of unmet needs than the general population and would therefore benefit from an Annual Health Check. The study revealed that from the sample studied, 48 per cent of adults with Down's Syndrome had not seen a doctor in the last year and 33per cent had not had a medical assessment in the previous three years (Henderson *et al.*, 2007). Additionally, GPs have been advised to use the *Cardiff Health Check* but the study revealed that health checks were not performed with this protocol, and basic checks vital for the health of people with Down's Syndrome were being neglected. The Cardiff Health Check is a comprehensive assessment which includes the physical, behavioural and communication needs of an individual (Kerr, 2001). An updated version, the Cardiff Health Check 2 became available in 2012.

For all adults with learning disabilities who present with complex health needs, it is imperative that a full medical history is undertaken, including a family history. This information will then be included in the individual's Health Action Plan (DH, 2007a). This is a personal individualised plan which lists what needs to happen to keep a person healthy and the support the individual will require.

Some organisations in the UK have employed specialist nurses to work with primary care practitioners whose role is to identify, facilitate reasonable adjustments, and prepare and support adults with learning disabilities through the process of their Annual Health Check. This may include supporting people with communication difficulties, desensitising people to specific health tests or by providing health information in an accessible format.

Case study 10.4   Urgent health assessment

Even with an Annual Health Check, as with Jeremy, people can experience an acute episode of ill health that warrants access to an acute hospital for further investigation and treatment. As Jeremy has arranged his own transport to hospital, on arrival he would be assessed by a triage nurse whose role is to establish the severity of a patient's condition and to decide how quickly they need treatment. It would be hoped that at this stage it is recognised that Jeremy has a learning disability and may need additional support. Although everyone is an individual, with a unique appearance, personality and set of abilities, people with Down's Syndrome do have some common facial features and a degree of learning disability (Scottish Down's Syndrome Association, 2001). Health care professionals working in this environment are expected to respond professionally to everyone who may access the service but they may not all have received appropriate education in the health needs of people with learning disabilities and may be inexperienced in assessing their needs. In research undertaken by Houghton (2001), it was found that a comprehensive assessment of an individual with learning disabilities can take up to four times longer than an average assessment. As Jeremy's additional needs were recognised immediately by the triage nurse, Kate, a staff nurse on duty, was alerted as the Learning Disability Champion for the Accident and Emergency department. In response to a number of reports (for example, Mencap, 2007), some Trusts have facilitated the development of Learning Disability Champions. These are hospital staff with additional training who promote best practice in the care and treatment of people with learning disabilities during their time within a particular department. Kate introduced herself to Jeremy and explained in clear and straightforward language that he would need to be seen by a consultant who specialised in gastroenterology. In the meantime, Kate explained the routine tests that were needed and asked him to clarify his understanding. From her conversation with him, Kate assessed that Jeremy had capacity. This refers to the legal competence of adults to make their own decisions in England and Wales. It is a legal requirement to assume that all people have capacity and only where there is any doubt should a capacity assessment be undertaken in relation to proposed courses of action (Mental Capacity Act 2005). The principles of the Act are shown in Figure 10.2.

While waiting with Jeremy to see the consultant, Kate observes he is profusely sweating, constantly rubbing his stomach and is reluctant to move. She therefore decides to undertake an assessment using the *Disability Distress Assessment Tool (DisDAT)*. This validated tool was designed to help identify indicators of distress in people with severely limited communication due to cognitive impairment or physical illness (Regnard *et al.*, 2007). Although this is not a specific pain assessment tool, it has been found to be very useful when someone is new to a service as it documents current signs and behaviour and therefore acts as a baseline to monitor change. During the assessment Jeremy became very tearful and tells Kate that he doesn't want to die. As Kate has additional training in communication with people with learning disabilities, she gently explores with Jeremy why he thinks he might die and when the consultant arrives, she is able to explain that his granddad died from bowel cancer and Jeremy fears that he might have the same condition.

Mr Roberts, the consultant, sits beside Jeremy's bed and asks if he can touch his stomach so that he can find out a bit more why he is in so much pain. Jeremy consents by lifting up his shirt, implying that he gives his consent (General Medical Council, 2012). As Jeremy's abdomen is extremely tender, Mr Roberts decides to request a blood test and a computerised tomography (CT) scan to see if an infection is present and suggests that in the meantime, Jeremy may be more comfortable on the Acute Assessment Unit. When Mr Roberts leaves, Jeremy again becomes very tearful and Kate asks if he would like her to contact someone, informing him she will not share any information without him knowing.

The following principles apply for the purposes of this Act:

- A person must be assumed to have capacity unless it is established that he lacks capacity.
- A person is not to be treated as unable to make a decision unless all practicable steps to help him to do so have been taken without success.
- A person is not to be treated as unable to make a decision merely because he makes an unwise decision.
- An act done, or decision made, under this Act for or on behalf of a person who lacks capacity must be done, or made, in his best interests.
- Before the act is done, or the decision is made, regard must be had to whether the purpose for which it is needed can be as effectively achieved in a way that is less restrictive of the person's rights and freedom of action.

Figure 10.2 Principles of the Mental Capacity Act 2005

(Chapter 23 also contains a detailed discussion of these principles)

(continued)

(continued)

By the time his mum arrives, Jeremy has already had a blood test and is just about to go for his scan but tells Kate that he's happy for his mum to know what has happened. Kate has already explained that during the scan he will not feel anything and just needs to lie still. He has had some medicine to alleviate his discomfort and would prefer to go for his scan alone rather than have to hear his mum fussing.

Kate has been very clear with Jeremy throughout his admission, informing him what is happening and has always ensured that he has given his consent. People with learning disabilities have the right to complete confidentiality, except if there is a concern about abuse or risk of abuse. They have the right to have their confidentiality recognised and valued. In addition they also have the right to know if any of their information will be shared and with whom and the right to decide whether the information should be shared at all (DH, 2001b). Kate therefore explained to Jeremy that she cannot stay with him on the ward but with his permission will telephone the Acute Liaison Nurse, Jonathan, to inform him that Jeremy may need additional support. The Acute Liaison Nurse supports a person with a learning disability when they are accessing acute physical care either as an inpatient or an outpatient and also offers advice and support to acute services staff. It has been found that this role reduces the impact of health inequalities on people with learning disabilities (Emerson *et al.*, 2012). The role also encompasses training of staff in how to improve the patient journey for people with learning disabilities in the acute sector. Many Acute Liaison Nurses are members of the Access to Acute (A2A) group. This network has become a national forum for people interested in improving access to acute hospital care for people with learning disabilities.

Case study 10.5 Surgery and after

Jeremy's test reveals he has acute diverticulitis. This is a disease which affects the large intestine (colon). Diverticulitis describes infection that arises when a bacterium becomes trapped and small bulges develop on the lining of the intestine that become inflamed or infected. Diverticulitis can lead to complications such as an abscess inside the intestine. In Jeremy's case this is so severe that it necessitates surgery to perform a colectomy. This is where a stoma is made in the lower abdomen and a section of the large intestine is removed and connected to a stoma (NHS Choices, 2012c). This will require Jeremy to wear a pouch to collect waste material following the operation (a colostomy). On the day of his operation, Mr Roberts' Registrar comes to see him and asks his mum to sign a form. However, when Jonathan, the Acute Liaison Nurse explains that Jeremy is able to consent to his operation, the Registrar reluctantly takes him through what will happen in theatre and informs him that without the operation he may develop peritonitis. Fortunately Jonathan is able to explain what this means. The Mental Capacity Act (2005) clearly states that a person must be assumed to have capacity unless it is established that he lacks capacity. Additionally, it is vital that information that informs decision-making must be in an accessible format. The Department of Health (2001b) has published guidance on good practice in this area and acknowledges that all health professionals need to be familiar with consent and capacity guidelines.

Following surgery, Jeremy is transferred to a High Dependency Unit (HDU) for specialised monitoring. Throughout his stay in hospital Jeremy could experience a range of assessments from a number of health professionals working collaboratively within a multi-disciplinary and multi-agency team. How his daily care is compromised may be assessed by a nurse using an assessment model, for example, Roper, Logan and Tierney (2000). Following surgery, a physiotherapist may assess Jeremy's risk of developing pressure ulcers using the *Waterlow* (2005) *Pressure Ulcer Risk Assessment Tool.* He may also have been seen by a dietician to assess dietary needs and advise on a diet to prevent his condition reoccurring. Throughout this process the Acute Liaison Nurse should ensure that Jeremy understands the information made available to him and also support the health care team in providing information in an accessible format.

Discharge assessment

The National Institute for Health and Clinical Evidence (2009) recommends that, when a patient is well enough to be discharged from hospital, they should have a functional assessment to ascertain any physical, sensory or communication problems, emotional or psychological problems, and any social care or equipment needs they may have. The discharge team should judge how the results of the assessment could affect a person's daily life and organise any referrals for further care before the patient leaves the hospital. This networked approach recognises that no one profession has the knowledge, skills and resources necessary to meet the complex and varied needs of individuals (Barrett *et al.*, 2005). As it is good practice to ensure Jeremy is also involved in the process and his views are represented, Jonathan meets with Jeremy and his mum to discuss what may happen once he is discharged from the hospital. At this meeting Jeremy is adamant he wishes to return to his flat, despite his mum's opposition. He argues that he lives in a ground floor flat and has easy access to the toilet whereas at his mum's house the only toilet is upstairs. Jeremy also takes the opportunity to discuss with Jonathan something he has been thinking about for some time. When he initially moved into independent living, he agreed that the Local Authority could organise his support worker. Jeremy now feels it might be better if he could choose who offered him support as he would prefer a male of a similar age. Jonathan agrees to ask the Local Authority to reassess his needs. People are eligible to apply for a personal budget if they receive help from Social Services. This then lets individuals choose and buy the services they need themselves, giving greater choice and control. This process of personalisation is outlined in the government document, *Our Health, Our Care, Our Say* (DH, 2006).

Jeremy is pleased to be home, his mum visits most days and busies herself with washing and cleaning despite Jeremy protesting he can do this for himself. He also receives visits from his colleagues at work who keep him up to date with what's happening in the warehouse. He hopes to go back to work in a few weeks when his GP assesses he is fit. In the meantime he receives regular home visits from the stoma nurse who ensures that he is able to change his colostomy bag correctly and checks that the area around his stoma is not infected. Also, Jonathan has arranged for Rachael, a Community Nurse from the local Community Team Learning Disability (CTLD) to visit. Rachael works with him on healthy eating. She has also suggested he visits the optician after she observed that he was having difficulty finding the handle on his cup and he admitted he'd put salt in the sugar bowl as he couldn't quite read the label on the packet. Both the stoma nurse and Rachael have explained to Jeremy that he will need to return to hospital for a further operation in about six months to reverse his colostomy.

Throughout Jeremy's journey as a patient through services, he feels that he has learnt a lot. During his stay, most health care professionals treated him with respect. However, there were some people who were very busy and forgot to ask if he wanted his bloods taking or assumed that he didn't understand. Rachael has asked if he would like to share his experiences and has offered her support to enable Jeremy to become involved in the Expert Patient Programme. This is designed to assist individuals to develop a better understanding of their health condition and improve confidence in managing long-term health issues (DH, 2007b). Rachael has also suggested that she helps Jeremy put together a Patient Passport (Kent, 2008) for when he is next admitted to hospital. This patient-held document records pertinent personal information relating to an individual's health and includes preferred methods of communication. This passport is endorsed by Mencap (2012) which has promoted use within hospitals and primary care trusts to improve access to services.

In the meantime, Jeremy is looking forward to next week when he will be holding interviews for his new support worker, he hopes he can find a young man who he can talk to and who won't fuss around him.

Conclusion

This chapter has considered a range of assessments that a young man with Down's Syndrome may be exposed to in adulthood. The number of assessments Jeremy is subjected to in order to live an independent life and when his health becomes impaired are both numerous and varied. This chapter has sought to focus on the positive outcomes that can be achieved if people who support individuals with learning disabilities are willing to work in collaboration. Some assessments have been very broad while others have needed to be very individual. What they all have in common is the need to respect Jeremy's wishes and take into consideration the culture, relationships and experiences which are all part of his life. This person–centred approach has become a central value in supporting individuals with learning disabilities. The need to consider potential risk in all assessments has been considered but the need to balance what can go wrong against positive risk taking is a fundamental part of everyday life. Working alongside Jeremy enables him to develop the skills and knowledge to continue to develop a healthy and independent life.

Acknowledgements

With thanks to our colleagues Susan Hannigan (University of Hull), Karen Helbrow (East Riding of Yorkshire Council) and Michaela Marr (Humber NHS Foundation Trust) for their help.

Points to remember

- Assessment is the key in finding a baseline for future intervention.
- Accurate, in–depth assessments help to gather the most useful information.
- Service users and carers should be involved in the assessment process as far as possible.

Resources

Department of Health (2009) *Valuing People Now: A New Three Year Strategy for People with Learning Disabilities* London: Department of Health.
Although it's now more than five years since this was published, the four guiding principles of Rights; Independent living; Control; and Inclusion remain relevant.

Higgins, B. (2009) *Good Practice in Supporting Adults with Autism: Guidance for Commissioners and Statutory Services*. London: National Autistic Society.
While it is important to remember that many adults with autistic spectrum conditions do not have a learning disability, this guide gives examples of local initiatives to overcome some of the challenges experienced when trying to develop support services to meet needs. In particular, it includes sections on employment; supported living options; personalisation and self-directed support.

Housing options: A housing advisory site with General Information, Easy Read and Members areas. The Easy Read area also includes information and resources on money and support options. It has a 'listen' option with video and real-life stories. Photo options show a range of housing options and what to think about when making housing choices.
http://www.housingoptions.org.uk/

Mansell, J. (2009) *Raising Our Sights: Services for Adults with Profound Intellectual and Multiple Disabilities*. London: HM Government.
Some people experience greater disability than Jeremy in this chapter. If this is the case for someone you're supporting, you may find this report by the late Jim Mansell useful. It identifies good services as those that are individualised and person-centred, that treat the family as expert and that focus on the quality of staff relationships with the disabled person.

Website: Understanding Intellectual Disability and Health
Edited by Professor Sheila Hollins, this website is jointly managed by the Down's Syndrome Association and St. George's, University of London. It features contributions on a range of topics by a variety of people, including adults with learning disabilities. Despite the description 'Ideal learning resource for medical, nursing and other health care students', anyone supporting people with learning disabilities can find valuable information on this site.
www.intellectualdisability.info/.

References

Access to Acute (A2A) Access to Acute Hospitals Network. Available at: http://a2anetwork.co.uk/.
Age UK (2012) *NHS Continuing Healthcare and NHS-Funded Nursing*. Available at: www.ageuk.org.uk/health-wellbeing/doctors-hospitals/nhs-continuing-healthcare-and-nhs-funded-nursing-care/ (accessed Oct. 2012).
Banks, R. (2003) Psychological treatments for people with learning disabilities, *Psychiatry*, 2(9): 62–65.
Barrett, G., Sellman, D. and Thomas, J. (2005) *Interprofessional Working in Health and Social Care*. Basingstoke: Palgrave Macmillan.

Beck, A., Steer, R. and Brown, G. (1996) *Beck Depression Inventory®-II*. Available at: www.pearson-assessments.com/HAIWEB/Cultures/en-us/Productdetail.htm?Pid=015-8018-370 (accessed Oct. 2012).

Bupa (2010) *Healthy Eating*. Available at: www.bupa.co.uk/individuals/health-information/directory/h/healthy-eating (accessed Oct. 2012).

Care Information Scotland (2012) *Assessment of Your Care Needs*. Available at: www.careinfoscotland.co.uk/how-do-i-get-care/assessment-of-your-care-needs.aspx (accessed Oct. 2012).

Carers Trust (2012) *Managing Stress*. Available at: www.carers.org/help-directory/managing-stress (accessed Oct. 2012).

Citizen's Advice Bureau (2012) *Community Care*. Available at: www.adviceguide.org.uk/england/relationships_e/relationships_looking_after_people_e/community_care.htm (accessed Oct. 2012).

Commission for Social Care Inspection (CSCI) (2008) *Cutting the Cake Fairly*. London: CSCI.

Cumella, S. and Martin, C. (2000) *Secondary Health Care for People with Learning Disabilities: A Report Completed for the Department of Health*. Kidderminster: British Institute of Learning Disabilities.

DH (Department of Health) (2001a) *Valuing People: A New Strategy for Learning Disability for the 21st Century*. London: The Stationery Office.

DH (Department of Health) (2001b) *Seeking Consent: Working with People with Learning Disabilities*. London: HMSO.

DH (Department of Health) (2003) *Fair Access to Care Services: Guidance on Eligibility Criteria for Adult Social Care*. London: DH.

DH (Department of Health) (2006) *Our Health, Our Care, Our Say*. London: HMSO.

DH (Department of Health) (2007a) *Health Action Planning and Health Facilitation for People with Learning Disabilities: Good Practice Guide*. London: HMSO.

DH (Department of Health) (2007b) *The Expert Patient Programme*. London: HMSO.

DH (Department of Health) (2010a) *Prioritising Need in the Context of Putting People First: A Whole System Approach to Eligibility for Social Care. Guidance on Eligibility Criteria for Adult Social Care*. London: DH.

DH (Department of Health) (2010b) *Healthy Lives, Healthy People: Our Strategy for Public Health in England*. London: HMSO.

DH (Department of Health) (2011) *Be Clear on Cancer. National Campaign to Promote Earlier Diagnosis of Bowel Cancer*. Available at: www.dh.gov.uk/health/2011/11/bowel-cancer-letter/ (accessed Oct. 2012).

Disability Rights Commission (DRC) (2006) *Equal Treatment: Closing the Gap*. London: DRC.

Down's Syndrome Association (DSA) (2011) *Annual Health Checks for Adults with Down's Syndrome*. Teddington: DSA.

Down's Syndrome Association (DSA) (2012) *Adult Annual Health Checks*. Available at: www.downs-syndrome.org.uk/campaigns/annual-health-checks.html (accessed Oct. 2012).

Emerson, E. and Hatton, C. (2008) *People with Learning Disabilities in England*. Lancaster: Centre for Disability Research (CeDR).

Emerson, E., Hatton, C., Robertson, J., Roberts, H., Baines, S., Evison, F., and Glover, G. (2012) *People with Learning Disabilities in England 2011*. Lancaster: Improving Health and Lives (IHAL), Learning Disabilities Observatory.

Fergus, K. (2009) *Medical Problems that Occur More Frequently in People with Down Syndrome*. Available at: http://downsyndrome.about.com/od/featuresofdownsyndrome/a/featurelong_ro_2.htm (accessed Oct. 2012).

Foundation for People with Learning Disabilities (FPLD) Available at: http://www.learningdisabilities.org.uk/ (accessed Oct. 2012).

General Medical Council (2012) *Consent Guidance: Expressions of Consent*. Available at: www.gmc-uk.org/guidance/ethical_guidance/consent_guidance_expressions_of_consent.asp (accessed Oct. 2012).

Heaton, K. (1997) *Bristol Stool Form Scale*. Available for download as a mobile application (App) at: www.bristol-stool-scale.com/.

Henderson, A., Lynch, S., Wilkinson, S. and Hunter, M. (2007) Adults with Down's syndrome: the prevalence of complications and health care in the community, *British Journal of Medical Practice*, 57(534): 50–55.

Hicks, R. (2008) *Constipation*. Available at: www.bbc.co.uk/health/physical_health/conditions/constipation1.shtml (accessed Oct. 2012).

Houghton, B.M. (2001) Caring for people with Down syndrome in Accident and Emergency, *Nurse*, 9(2): 24–27.

Improving Health and Lives (IHAL), Learning Disabilities Observatory (2007–2012) *Categories of Accommodation for National Indicator 146*. Available at: www.improvinghealthandlives.org.uk/numbers/stableaccommodation/categories/ (accessed Oct. 2012).

Kent, A. (2008) *Improving Acute Care of People with Learning Disabilities*. Available at: www.nursingtimes.net/nursing-practice/clinical-zones/learning-disability/improving-acute-care-of-people-with-learning-disabilities/583223.article (accessed Oct. 2012).

Kerr, M. (2001) *Cardiff Health Check*. Cardiff: Welsh Centre for Learning Disabilities.

Lay, J. and Kirk, L. (2011) Person-centred strategies for planning, in H. Atherton and D. Crickmore (eds) *Learning Disabilities: Toward Inclusion*, 6th edn. Edinburgh: Churchill Livingstone.

Mencap (2007) *Death by Indifference*. London: Mencap.

Mencap (2012) Mencap report finds NHS still unsafe for people with a learning disability. Available at: www.mencap.org.uk/news/article/mencap-report-finds-nhs-still-unsafe-people-learning-disability-0 (accessed Oct. 2012).

Michael, J. (2008) *Healthcare for All: The Findings of the Independent Inquiry into the Health Inequalities of People with Learning Disabilities*. London: Department of Health.

National Development Team for Inclusion (NDTi) (2010) *The Real Tenancy Test*. Bath: NDTi.

National Institute for Health and Clinical Excellence (2009) *Rehabilitation After Critical Care*. Available at: www.nice.org.uk/nicemedia/live/12137/43527/43527.pdf (accessed 23 Oct. 2012).

NHS Choices (2011) *Community Care Assessments*. Available at: www.nhs.uk/CarersDirect/guide/assessments/Pages/Communitycareassessments.aspx (accessed Oct. 2012).

NHS Choices (2012a) *Constipation: Symptoms*. Available at: www.nhs.uk/Conditions/Constipation/Pages/Symptoms.aspx (accessed Oct. 2012).

NHS Choices (2012b) *Thyroid – Underactive*. Available at: www.nhs.uk/conditions/Thyroid-under-active/Pages/Introduction.aspx (accessed Oct. 2012).

NHS Choices (2012c) *Treating Diverticular Disease and Diverticulitis*. Available at: www.nhs.uk/Conditions/Diverticular-disease-and-diverticulitis/Pages/Treatment.aspx (accessed Oct. 2012).

nidirect (2010a) *Health and Social Care Assessments*. Available at: www.nidirect.gov.uk/health-and-social-care-assessments (accessed Oct. 2012).

nidirect (2010b) *Free Bus Travel and Concessions*. Available at: www.nidirect.gov.uk/free-bus-travel-and-concessions (accessed Oct. 2012).

Pharmaceutical Services Negotiating Committee (2011) *Changes to the Pharmacy Contract*. Available at: www.psnc.org.uk/pages/changes_to_the_pharmacy_contract_201112.html (accessed Oct. 2012).

Prasher, V. and Gomez, G. (2007) Natural history of thyroid function in adults with Down syndrome: 10 year follow up study, *Journal of Intellectual Disability Research*, 51: 312–317.

Regnard, C., Reynolds, J., Watson, B., Matthews, D., Gibson, L. and Clarke, C. (2007) Understanding distress in people with severe communication difficulties: developing and assessing the Disability Distress Assessment Tool (DisDAT), *Journal of Intellectual Disability Research*, 51(4): 277–292.

Roper, N., Logan, W.W. and Tierney, A.J. (2000) *The Roper-Logan-Tierney Model for Nursing: Based on the Activities of Living*. Edinburgh: Churchill Livingstone.

Scottish Down's Syndrome Association (2001) *What Is Down's Syndrome?* Edinburgh: Down's Syndrome Association.

Shipton, D., Tappin, D., Vadiveloo, T., Crossley, J., Aitken, D. and Chalmers, J. (2009) Reliability of self reported smoking status by pregnant women for estimating smoking prevalence: a retrospective, cross sectional study, *British Medical Journal*. Available at: www.bmj.com/content/339/bmj.b4347 (accessed Oct. 2012).

Sowney, M. and Brown, M. (2007) People with learning disabilities: issues for accident and emergency practitioners, in B. Dolan and L. Holt (eds) *Accident and Emergency: Theory into Practice*. London: Baillière Tindall.

TPP (2012) SystmOne. Available at: http://www.tpp-uk.com/ (accessed Oct. 2012).

Waterlow, J. (2005) *Pressure Ulcer Prevention Manual*. Available at: www.judy_waterlow.co.uk (accessed 23 Oct. 2012).

World Health Organisation (2012) *The Determinants of Health*. Available at: http://www.who.int/hia/evidence/doh/en/ (accessed Oct. 2012).

11 Defining old age in the learning disabled population

Jo Lay

Learning outcomes

After reading this chapter you will be able to:

- define the concept of 'old age' for someone with a learning disability
- consider the range of assessments that can be used to promote independence, and well-being for the older population with a learning disability.

Introduction

> Attitudes can fail "to recognise the humanity and individuality of people concerned and respond to them with sensitivity, compassion and professionalism."
>
> Parliamentary and Health Service Ombudsman (2011 p. 7).

This chapter will consider Jeremy's situation following the Care Programme Approach (CPA) decisions. It will explore the impact that early dementia diagnosis has had on his life and the assessment tools that were involved in this. At the age of 46, Jeremy's needs are similar to those of older adults within the wider population. This has implications for the care Jeremy receives and the services that are available to him. The chapter will identify key areas of assessment that are integral to the health and social care of older adults.

The CPA is the NHS framework which was developed to coordinate effective mental health services through inter-professional working. CPA support is available to individuals who have a severe mental disorder; have a learning disability; are at risk of serious self-harm or suicide; have a history of violence; have a history of substance misuse; or are neglecting themselves or refusing care or treatment. A CPA care coordinator will be appointed. This can be any of the key professionals involved in the individuals care and support. In Jeremy's case it was his Care Manager. This person has responsibility for ensuring all professional assessments are completed and that they contribute to understanding the focus person's situation.

Case study 11.1   The Care Programme Approach

Jeremy is now 46 years old. Five years ago he had significant problems with his mental health. Jeremy's mum contacted his Care Manager because he was refusing to see her and neighbours had expressed concern. He had become increasingly isolated following his refusal to use his contact hours for day support. The Care Manager had been planning to arrange a Community Care Needs Assessment for Jeremy but after hearing concerns felt it more appropriate to instigate the Care Programme Approach. Jeremy refused to participate in this process and was identified as seriously neglecting himself. He became verbally abusive and at times physically aggressive to those around him. Following a number of functional assessments and behavioural checklists undertaken in an NHS specialist residential assessment centre, Jeremy was diagnosed as being in the early stages of dementia. Jeremy never returned to his flat but moved instead to a residential home for older adults. Most of the other residents are in their eighties.

Jeremy seemed very confused when he first moved into the home. He cried a lot and wanted to know when he could go home. Although he talked about home, Jeremy showed little interest or acknowledgement of friends or family when they visited, including his mum, JoJo and JoJo's family. His mum was very distressed at times but continued twice a week visits. Jeremy was underweight when he was admitted but over a 6-month period started to gain weight and at times was more like his old self. He started to show an interest in his new home and developed relationships and friendships with other residents and staff.

Initially Jeremy's mum had concerns about his admittance to the residential service as most of the other residents were older than her! She was very vocal and demanding in making her son's needs clear. Gradually she too started to build relationships and has been happy with the standard of care provided to Jeremy. She introduced the concept of person-centred planning to the service and now staff and residents have a greater awareness of tools such as PATH (Planning Alternative Tomorrows with Hope) and Essential Lifestyles Planning.

Jeremy's emotional and physical health status has gradually decreased but 6 weeks ago he had a fall walking to the bathroom at night. This has shaken Jeremy's confidence and he has become very withdrawn, refusing to walk even with a frame. A physiotherapist has visited on a number of occasions but Jeremy will not speak to her or attempt to walk for her. On the last occasion he lashed out at her, cutting her cheek.

The Home Manager has advised Jeremy's mum that they may soon need to look at nursing home provision to meet Jeremy's needs. His mum is upset by this. She believes that the best place for Jeremy is in his current home where people and his environment are familiar and supportive.

Fast facts 11.1   Assessment of needs

Anyone experiencing mental health problems is entitled to an assessment of their needs with a mental healthcare professional, and to have a care plan that is regularly reviewed by that professional (NHS Choices, 2012).

Life expectancy in the UK has risen significantly in the past 50 years due to increased medical interventions and knowledge. Life expectancy has also increased for people with a learning disability and more specifically people with Down's Syndrome. The Down's Syndrome Association (DSA) (n.d.) identify three possible reasons for this:

1. Better nutrition and living standards (as for the general population).
2. Effective prevention and/or treatment of infectious illness and other serious diseases, such as pneumonia, measles, etc.
3. Improved surgical and medical treatment of congenital heart disease and its consequences.

We need to consider why the life expectancy of people with Down's Syndrome is still less than the wider population. It would appear that there are two main reasons. First, that people with Down's Syndrome age prematurely, and, second, that they are more prone to illnesses and disease that shorten their life expectancy. The most common causes of death through illness in the older population are heart disease, vascular disease and cancers. There is mixed evidence to support the idea that people with Down's Syndrome are predisposed to these. Congenital heart problems are a characteristic that some associate with Down's Syndrome. As we have seen in other chapters, a range of holistic health factors can impact on susceptibility to disease. Some people with learning disabilities reduce their risk of illness and disease due to reduced likelihood of smoking or lower alcohol intake. However, a large number of people are obese due to poor dietary support and lack of leisure and recreation opportunities. The link between Down's Syndrome and dementia is perhaps the most significant disease which can shorten life expectancy. The DSA strongly state that not all people with a learning disability will develop dementia.

Jeremy's placement in an older adult residential home was not ideal because of the large age gap between him and other residents. However, the nature of his dementia meant that many of his care needs were similar to that of older people in the population without a learning disability. This does highlight a lack of suitable services for the increasing population of older adults with learning disabilities. Jeremy's Care Manager identified his residential home as the best available option for Jeremy, based upon current care needs in relation to his dementia diagnosis.

Reader activity 11.1   Dementia assessment

- From your knowledge of the nature of a learning disability, what do you consider may be the barriers to accurate assessment of dementia?
- What do you think the key features of an assessment should be?

Dementia and learning disability

Compared to the general population, Jeremy has been diagnosed with dementia at a young age. However, for an adult with Down's Syndrome, this has become increasingly common. Signs and symptoms in Jeremy's case were withdrawal, behaviour changes and difficulties in communication. Jeremy lived alone and had high levels of independence. Although he was a sociable man, it may have been some time before friends and family recognised these signs. Signs and symptoms may include:

- Loss of memory, the inability to concentrate and a poor sense of time and space, e.g. difficulties with completing simple tasks, solving minor problems or forgetting routines that have been done time and time before.
- Abstract thought becomes difficult, e.g. struggling to find the right words to express themselves or misunderstanding others.
- Appearing self-centred and uninhibited. People can find it difficult to vary responses, seeing only one way of doing things. Their understanding of the actions and feelings of others can decline. For some, there may be a noticeable reduction in moral standards.
- Some people develop the inability to show tenderness to a partner when they are with them and are unconcerned about them in their absence. As part of their memory loss they may lose all recognition of loved ones.
- Depression and mood changes.

A diagnosis of dementia can be particularly problematic for people who have a severe learning disability. Many symptoms may already exist as part of an intellectual impairment. The use of memory tests may have limited value for an individual who already has difficulties expressing themselves. The process of diagnosis should include:

- a detailed personal history;
- a full health assessment;
- psychological and mental state assessment;
- any other special investigations that symptoms suggest are required.

Aylward *et al.* (1997) agree the main impediment to progression in understanding dementia in people with an intellectual disability is the 'lack of standardised criteria and diagnostic procedures'. They identify three key features to look for in assessment:

1. Is there a change in the baseline functioning of the individual? Are there assessment records that current functioning can be compared to?
2. A decline in everyday functioning should be reflected in a decline in cognitive tests.
3. Changes in functioning and behaviour should be greater than those generally associated with 'ageing' in people who have an intellectual disability.

Changes in behaviour are an important consideration. With the onset of dementia, behaviours may increase in aggression or negative old behaviours return. These behaviours will need to be managed in the context of dementia care, not necessarily the same way as previous approaches. For people who have more moderate learning disabilities, symptoms may include apathy, withdrawal, daytime sleepiness and loss of self-help skills.

For many people with Down's Syndrome the neuropathology of Alzheimer's disease is evident by the time they are 50 years old, though not all will show the signs and symptoms already identified (Devenny *et al.*, 2002). There are a number of different diseases that give rise to dementia (see Figure 11.1) but there is now a well-researched link between Down's Syndrome and Alzheimer's disease.

> - Alzheimer's disease
> - Multi-infarct dementia
> - Creutzfeldt Jakob Disease (CJD)
> - Alcoholism
> - Parkinson's disease
> - Picks disease
> - Huntingdon's disease (Huntingdon's Chorea)

Figure 11.1 Dementias

It must be noted that early signs of dementia can easily be confused with Acute Confusional State (ACS) usually brought on by acute infection. It is important that healthcare professionals rule out ACS as part of their initial assessment and diagnosis. Table 11.1 highlights the similarities and differences between these conditions.

Recognising the signs and symptoms of dementia illnesses is clearly an essential part of early assessment, as is the ruling out of other causes for these symptoms. Dementia will be diagnosed by a doctor and should include the input of the inter-professional team. The doctor may be a GP or a specialist, i.e. a psychiatrist, neurologist or gerontologist. Holistic assessment is essential to review a person's strengths as well as needs. This enables care plans to be written which promote skill maintenance (Bush and Holmes, 2001). There are a number of tests that can be carried out to aid diagnosis that are based on memory and ability to manage functions of daily living. Two tests that can be used are the AAMD Adaptive Behaviour Scale (part 1) (Nihra *et al.*, 1974) and the (MMSE) Mini Mental State Examination (Cockrell and Folstein, 1988, cited in Smith, 2001). Examples of questions that may be included in the Mini Mental State Examination are:

1. What day of the week is it?
2. The questioner identifies three objects and asks the person to name them.
3. Start at number 25 and count backwards in 5s.
4. Spell the word 'prime' backwards.
5. What were the three objects in question 2?

The Growing Older with Learning Disabilities (GOLD) programme (Thompson, 2001) identifies some of the significant links between Down's Syndrome and dementia that impact on service provision.

- At least 36 per cent of people with Down's Syndrome aged 50–59 years and 54.5 per cent aged 60–69 are affected by dementia (compared to 5 per cent of the general population aged over 65 years). The prevalence increases significantly with age.
- The life expectancy of people with Down's Syndrome continues to increase.
- Between 15–20 per cent of the learning disabilities population have Down's Syndrome.
- The majority of people with Down's Syndrome have Trisomy 21 (they have three chromosomes 21 rather than the usual two). Research into Alzheimer's disease has shown that three of the genes implicated in its development are found on chromosome 21.
- There is a current lack of appropriate residential and day services for people with Down's Syndrome and dementia.

Table 11.1 Characteristics of dementia and ACS

Characteristic	Dementia	ACS
Physical illness	Rarely present	Usually present
Awareness of surroundings	Usually impaired	Usually impaired
Onset	Progressive	Sudden
Development over time	Progressive	Fluctuating, can be worse at night
Understanding	Impaired	Disordered
Speech	Difficulty in finding words	Usually extremes, i.e. slow or rapid
Involuntary movement	Usually absent	Tremors are common
Hallucinations	Rarely apparent	Can be visual and auditory

Fast facts 11.2   Down's Syndrome trends

- People with learning disabilities have a higher risk of developing dementia compared to the general population, with a significantly increased risk for people with Down's Syndrome and at a much earlier age.
- Life expectancy of people with Down's Syndrome has increased significantly.
- The incidence and prevalence of Down's Syndrome are not decreasing.

(The British Psychological Society and
the Royal College of Psychiatrists, 2009, p. 11)

It is important to consider a differential diagnosis which acknowledges all the potential causes of decline in functional skills and behaviours/emotional distress. This is more likely to occur in the wider population for older adults, particularly in in-patient placements for this age group. As life expectancy grows, it is not untypical to find older adult services limiting their service to those over the age of 80 years. If we accept that people with Down's Syndrome age prematurely, then services must assess the causes of decline. These may include physical problems (including epilepsy, nutritional decline, etc.), sensory impairment, impact of high dose or long-term anti-psychotic or anti-convulsant medication, life events such as loss and bereavement, poor environment, and dementia. This is not an exhaustive list and these conditions can coexist, i.e. one individual may be experiencing a number of them simultaneously and in addition to dementia. Figure 11.2 identifies the wide range of different assessment tools which can be used to support a dementia diagnosis. Many more profession-specific tools will be available to members of the inter-professional team. They will be able to advise on and discuss assessment strategies.

Reader activity 11.2   Assessment tools

Identify one of the assessment tools in Figure 11.2. Using an internet search and/or other search opportunities at your disposal e.g. NHS libraries, find out what you can about its purpose, structure and practical application.

Neuropsychological Assessment

- Neuropsychological Assessment of Dementia in Adults with Intellectual Disabilities (NAID). (Crayton *et al.*, 1998)
- Severe Impairment Battery (SIB) (Saxton *et al.*, 1993)
- Test for Severe Impairment (Albert and Cohen, 1992)
- Dalton Brief Praxis Test (Sano *et al.*, 2005)

Depression Assessment

- Glasgow Depression Scale (GDS-LD) (Cuthill *et al.*, 2003)

General Dementia Screening Tools

- Dementia Questionnaire for People with Learning Disabilities (DLD formerly known as DMRR) (Evenhuis *et al.*, 2007)
- The Dementia Scale for Down's Syndrome (DSDS) (Gedye, 1995)
- Dementia Screening Questionnaire for Individuals with Intellectual Disabilities (DSQIID) (Deb *et al.*, 2007)
- Adaptive Behaviour Dementia Questionnaire (ABDQ) (Prasher *et al.*, 2004)

Assessment of Daily Living

- AAMD Adapted Behaviour Scales (ABS), 1974 revision (Nihira *et al.*, 1974)
- Hampshire Social Services – Staff Support Levels Assessment (Hampshire Social Services, 1987)
- Vineland Adaptive Behaviour Scales: Second Edition (Sparrow *et al.*, 2007)
- Adaptive Behaviour Assessment System-II (ABAS-II) (Harrison & Oakland, 2003)

The British Psychological Society (2009)

Figure 11.2 Diagnostic assessment tools

Quality of life

The prevalence of dementia in the Down's Syndrome population is difficult to estimate but services need to consider screening in order to provide the services required to meet their needs. Health Needs Assessment (HNA) provides one way of measuring this. HNA was introduced to UK health policy at the beginning of the twenty-first century as part of a wider strategy in reducing health inequality. It involves a five-step process (Cavanagh and Chadwick, 2005):

1. Identifying the population of interest.
2. Identifying health priorities.
3. Identifying a health priority for action.
4. Planning for change.
5. Moving on/Review.

Practice alert 11.1

Health Needs Assessment provides a systematic framework for improving the efficiency and effectiveness of health services. It uses epidemiological, qualitative, and comparative methods to identify particular populations; consider inequalities in health experienced by this group and prioritise the services needed.

The British Psychological Society and the Royal College of Psychiatrists (2009) advocate a three-stage screening process which starts with a baseline assessment of every adult with Down's Syndrome while they are in good health. This should be followed by reactive screening, i.e. assessments which pick up on any of the triggers that may lead to future health difficulties, as opposed to waiting for a problem to occur. Because we know of the increased risk of dementia in the Down's Syndrome population, this should then be followed by appropriate dementia assessment at regular intervals to be pro-active in identifying health needs. Sims (2002) explores debate on the criticisms of undertaking baseline assessments which Jervis and Prinsloo (2007) summarise as:

- Does seeking consent for the assessment cause undue stress to the person with learning disabilities and their carers?
- What is the real value of screening for early diagnosis of dementia?
- Is there a balance between the information gathered from screening with the distress of the individual, i.e. does one outweigh the other?
- Are assessments contrary to the philosophy of normalisation and inclusion?
- Is the high opportunity cost of evaluations unacceptable?

Sims (2002) concludes that the positive outcomes of screening and assessment outweigh the negative ones, however, it is useful to consider these arguments in determining best care practice for the individual and wider service provision.

Reader activity 11.3 Normalisation

Consider the question above: 'Are assessments contrary to the philosophy or normalisation and inclusion'? Wolfensberger (1972) developed the ideology of 'normalisation' which sought to consider how the learning disabled could adapt to meet the norms of society. He developed this in contrast to the theory of 'social role valorisation' in 1983. This change recognised that it was difficult to determine what is a 'norm' and the important part of being respected within a society is having a valued social role. Current philosophy focuses on the principles of person centredness which advocate inclusion and celebrate difference. While evidence of these principles can be found within specialist learning disability services, the training and support that varied healthcare professionals have in understanding and interpreting these principles are unclear.

How might early screening for dementia in adults with Down's Syndrome be contrary to the policy and philosophy of inclusion?

There is a tension between generic and specialist services when vulnerable groups have specific needs. People who have Down's Syndrome and dementia are one of these groups. As carers we must consider our values and expectations for this group of people in line with quality indicators and service outcomes.

In 2009, the Department of Health (DH) published a dementia strategy which made 17 recommendations to improve services. These were based on three broad aims:

- to raise public and professional understanding and awareness of dementia;
- to implement early diagnosis and support in managing the disease;
- to support the well-being of people with a dementia diagnosis. This recognises the importance of quality of life in care management plans.

Jeremy's mother is concerned about future residential/nursing placements for him. One of the dementia strategies' recommendations is that services will work to ensure:

- better care for people with dementia in care homes;
- clear responsibility for dementia in care homes;
- a clear description of how people will be cared for;
- visits from specialist mental health teams;
- better checking of care homes.

The Dementia Strategy was updated in 2010 with additional emphasis on reducing anti-psychotic medication as a management strategy. This questions the therapeutic value applied to some medication and challenges service to find more therapeutic supporting strategies.

Inclusion is a priority in current health policy. Inclusion is also the key to person centred philosophies and the current trend is for organisations to be explicit in how they are involving service users in planning and service delivery. This is true with the needs assessment process. This is a key feature of the NHS Quality Assurance programme also known as Clinical Governance. The NHS Centre for Public Involvement was established in 2008 in response to a parliamentary assessment that suggested a model of user involvement which bridged all public services (NHS Centre for Public Involvement, 2008). Prior to the community care initiatives in the 1980s, people with a learning disability had little opportunity to make decisions or have any control over decisions in their lives, let alone a voice within the services they used. Quality assurance formed a key component of community care and organisations were encouraged to consider the level of choice and involvement that service users had. Emerson and Ramcharan have written extensively on the tensions between community care, cost and quality, and suggest that there remains 'a marked gap between what is being delivered and the aspirations of social inclusion and empowerment that underlie current policy' (2010, p. 65). There is still little research that addresses the views and opinions of people with a learning disability and their families (Gale *et al.*, 2008). One such study conducted by Emerson *et al.* in 2005 highlighted the importance of involving people with a learning disability in research about them. As respondents they had very different views of their health status and definitions of health compared to the professionals and organisations that provided the health service to them. In the main, respondents viewed health as something that allowed them to live the life they chose, e.g. going out independently, having friends, etc. Fender *et al.* (2005) promote this point of view. They undertook research to assess the understanding of the concept of 'health' of a group of older adults who had Down's Syndrome. They particularly looked at what role the participants believed should be played by a doctor. The participants were able to identify their thoughts with the support of small group work. They described what health meant to them (see Figure 11.3) and recognised signs and symptoms of illness such as vomiting and having limited movement.

While a move away from the medical model of health has led to more holistic definitions of health that recognise the bio-psycho-social impact on well-being, the professionals involved have not always recognised health in respect of these quality of life indicators.

```
Diet
  • Eating fruit and vegetables
  • Not having sugar
  • Not eating chocolate
Activity
  • Ironing
  • Hoovering
  • Keeping busy
  • Shopping
Body
  • Look after yourself
  • Brushing teeth
  • Keeping fit
  • Keeping clean
  • Not smoking
```

Figure 11.3 What does health mean?

Reader activity 11.4   Quality indicators

Imagine that you are using a health service for the first time. As part of local user involvement initiatives, you are invited to join other patients within the service to identify quality indicators for the service. These are the criteria that patients think the service should be measured on. Think about what your expectations of a service might be.

The rights and expectations of people with learning disabilities are likely to be the same as anyone else but previous experience of inequality may make them more focused on particular issues such as long enough appointments, accessible information, etc. Figure 11.4 summarises the barriers to health experienced by the learning disabled and therefore the issues that should be considered in the assessment process.

In 2013, the National Institute for Health and Care Excellence (NICE) published a new quality standard for supporting people to live well with dementia (QS30). Quality standards are statements of intent that all health services are expected to adhere to. They work in tandem with other strategies and frameworks such as the Adult Social Care Outcomes Framework. NICE (2013) provide the following summary of the new standard:

1. People worried about possible dementia in themselves or someone they know can discuss their concerns, and what having dementia confirmed might mean, with someone with knowledge and expertise.
2. People with dementia are involved in making choices and decisions about their care and support.
3. People with dementia take part in a review of their needs and preferences when their circumstances change.
4. People with dementia can choose to take part in leisure activities, during their day, which match their interests.

- Not enough people to support with health
- Sometimes it is difficult to understand what has been told by doctors/nurses
- People are not getting the health treatment they need
- Lots of people said their GP did not talk to them
- Appointments are too short – there is not enough time to explain things
- Some people want a carer or a family member to stay with them in hospital
- We (people with learning disabilities) have more health problems
- Not treated fairly
- Lots of people are unhealthy and overweight
- There is not enough information about staying healthy
- Carers need to be listened to by health workers
- Lack of easy-to-read information
- Lack of knowledge among hospital staff about learning disabled patients
- Jargon

Figure 11.4 Barriers to effective health care

5. People with dementia can continue to meet their friends and family and can make new relationships.
6. People with dementia can have routine check-ups of their physical and mental health and can see healthcare professionals when they have concerns.
7. People with dementia live in housing that is adapted to help them maintain their independence.
8. People with dementia are given the opportunity to be involved in and influence the design, planning, evaluation and delivery of services.
9. People with dementia can have help from independent advocacy services to present their views.
10. People with dementia can continue to be involved in and contribute to their community.

These standards are applicable to all people diagnosed with dementia or other cognitive decline with similar symptoms.

Age appropriateness

Age-appropriate care has been a long-term concern for many in learning disability services. This has, in part, been connected with diagnostic criteria that measure Intelligent Quotient (IQ) in order to classify learning disability. The lower a person's IQ is, the more severe their learning disability. Many people have experienced being treated like a child because they have been identified as having the 'mental age' of a young person. Others have been prevented having things that they want, e.g. a toy or a comic book, because it is deemed to be too childish for an adult and against the principles of normalisation. Inclusion asks us to accept difference and diversity but the realistic experience of many societies and cultures is that often we want others to 'fit in' and conform. Considering quality of life indicators, the focus for care-givers is to meet the needs of the patient. Research suggests that some skills-based children's games such as threading beads or jigsaw puzzles can be therapeutic activities for a dementia patient. However, these need to be based on individual need and preferences and supported by a carer who recognises the therapeutic nature of the activity.

We have identified that people with Down's Syndrome and dementia are usually younger than others with dementia. This does not mean that other younger adults do not suffer from this condition.

Fast facts 11.3 Age and dementia

The Alzheimer's Society (2012) estimates that there are 17,000 people in the UK diagnosed with dementia, under the age of 65 years.

The Alzheimer's Society believes their dementia prevalence in younger people figure is a low estimate as the numbers are taken from referrals to GPs. Many people live with the condition or are misdiagnosed before health services are sought. Symptoms of dementia are the same as in older people but generally there are different environment and socio-economic concerns. People may be carers themselves; have jobs, mortgages and other commitments. If someone has a learning disability, we cannot make the assumption that this is not true for them too.

Functional decline

As all adults age, they experience varying degrees of functional decline in all aspects of holistic health-care. Generic older adult services identify mobility and pressure area care; nutrition and assessment of falls and accidents as particular areas of concern. Difficulties in these areas can impact on independence and confidence and the person can take a long time to recover from these. It is therefore essential that carers of older adults have some knowledge and skill in recognising concerns and highlighting these to relevant health and social care professionals. Research suggests that people with learning disabilities have, on average, more physical and mental health needs than the wider population, however, they use GPs and preventative health services less frequently. This poses a significant challenge for future services, particularly in the area of public health. Higgins and Mansell (2009, p. 208) state that:

> The current cohort of older people with intellectual disabilities is the first sizeable group to have survived into later life and have lived through a period during which policies have shifted from institutional to community care, presenting service providers and policy makers with significant challenges.

Malnutrition refers to any deviation from a healthy, balanced diet. It could mean that a person is not having enough to eat or too much of the wrong things. Factors that impact on nutritional status in older adults can be hospital stays; decrease in physical skills and/or physical strength, e.g. ability to open jars or use other kitchen equipment; poverty; and decrease in appetite. This is not an exhaustive list. There are many nutritional assessment tools available including the Malnutrition Universal Screening Tool (MUST). Assessment tools should all include the following comprehensive criteria:

* A measurement of physical characteristics such as weight and height. This provides a baseline for comparison.
* Likes and dislikes. These are an important motivating factor.

- Any allergies or medical conditions.
- Cultural/ethnic/religious needs and requirements.
- Any physical difficulties, including assistance required.

It is important that the outcomes of this assessment are detailed in a care plan that carers can access. This applies to all assessments undertaken in functional decline. As older people develop a more sedentary lifestyle, their risk of pressure area problems increases. This is of particular concern for wheelchair users or people experiencing long hospital stays. Pressure areas risk assessments, including the Norton scale and Waterlow assessment, provide a screening tool for an individual susceptibility to pressure ulcers.

Fast facts 11.4 Pressure ulcers

- Screening of people who are at risk of developing pressure ulcers is the first key to prevention.
- Risks are most often assessed using tools specifically for this. Information on these will be available from GPs, district nurses or local health centres.
- Tools must be used alongside clinical judgement, skin assessment and consideration of support surfaces.
- Any skin damage should trigger a re-evaluation of preventive strategies.
- Nurses, patients and relatives need to accept that some pressure ulcers are unavoidable (Guy, 2012).

Difficulties with mobility can have the biggest impact on confidence and independence in older adults. Accidents can be caused by obstacles; being in a hurry; problems with medication; infection that leads to dizziness or imbalance; tiredness; poor eyesight; poor lighting, etc. The following tips are extremely useful in the risk assessment of falls in older adult services and can be built into handovers or shift checks:

- Look around for anything that may cause an accident, obstacles or uneven floors.
- Decide who is most at risk and then take preventative measures.
- Keep a record of what you have changed and why. Build this into a risk assessment and care plan for those most at risk.
- Continually check the living space – keep a note of all potential hazards.

Practice alert 11.2

'Physical exercise should be facilitated and encouraged where possible, with assessment and advice from a physiotherapist when needed. Exercise is thought to help improve continence, slow loss of mobility and improve strength, balance and endurance. It is also used in falls prevention' (Taylor et al., 2009).

Conclusion

For Jeremy and other people in his situation, it is essential that there is good care management to coordinate the input of the inter-professional team, family members, friends and other informal carers. The care manager should ensure that:

- assessments are accurate and up to date so that plans are current and relevant;
- the importance of person-centred risk assessment and its place within mental capacity legislation is understood;
- there is effective communication and liaison between all members of the inter-professional team;
- financial plans take into account actual need.

Commissioners of services need to continue to weigh the balance between use of generic services and specialist resources for individuals with dementia and learning disability. In relation to Jeremy's situation, Thompson (2001) commented: 'Often the only alternative is placement within generic older people's services, where staff may have no experience of caring for people with learning disabilities. At a time when they most need an established routine, people's lives are being destabilised.' It is worrying to note that a recent paper from the Parliamentary and Health Service Ombudsman (2011, p. 7), investigating NHS care provided to 10 older adults, identified that their findings were difficult and distressing to read, stating:

> They illuminate the gulf between the principles and values of the NHS constitution and the felt reality of being an older person in the care of the NHS in England. The investigations reveal an attitude – both personal and institutional – which fails to recognise the humanity and individuality of the people concerned and to respond to them with sensitivity, compassion and professionalism.

This report was not specific to people with a learning disability but identified poor care practice in all of the 10 cases identified. A study into the needs of older adults with intellectual disabilities in Eire (Doody *et al.*, 2011) identified that although Registered Nurses in Intellectual Disability (RNID) were the one health professional group specifically trained in assessing and meeting the health needs of the intellectually (learning) disabled, most of these nurses were employed in residential settings as opposed to nursing homes. Similar concerns have been noted in the UK. While many nurses play an important role in residential settings, the variety of employers across the public, private and voluntary sectors do not always employ the individual as a nurse, limiting their scope of practice. This also can result in the individual with learning disabilities having to move on once their needs become classified as 'nursing'. To conclude, Higgins and Mansell's (2009) research found that:

- People who lived in homes specifically for those with an intellectual disability undertook more activities in the home compared with people living in older people's homes.
- People who lived in homes specifically for those with an intellectual disability went out more compared with people living in older people's homes.
- Where people live as they get older makes a big difference to their lives.

Points to remember

- Dementia becomes prevalent in many cases in adults with Down's syndrome from as early as 40 years old.
- Skilled assessment will enable a correct diagnosis to be made.
- Steps should be taken to breakdown barriers that exist so enabling people with learning disabilities to have their health needs met.
- Individualised, person centred care is essential.

References

Albert, M. and Cohen, C. (1992) The Test for Severe Impairment: An instrument for the assessment of people with severe cognitive dysfunction, *Journal of the American Geriatric Society*, 40: 449–453.

Alzheimer's Society (2012) Young people and dementia. Available at: http://www.alzheimers.org.uk/site/scripts/documents_info.php?documentID=164 (accessed 29 April 2013).

Aylward, E.H., Burt, D.B., Thorpe, L.U., Lai, F. and Dalton, A. (1997) Diagnosis of dementia in individuals with intellectual disability, *Journal of Intellectual and Disability Research*, 41(2):152–164.

British Psychological Society and the Royal College of Psychiatrists (2009) *Dementia and People with Learning Disabilities*. Leicester: The British Psychological Society.

Bush, T. and Holmes, J. (2001) Slowing the progression? *Nursing Times*. Available at: www.nursingtimes.net.

Cavanagh, S. and Chadwick, K. (2005) *Health Needs Assessment: A Practical Guide*. Available at: www.nice.org.uk/media/150/35/Health_Needs_Assessment_A_Practical_Guide.pdf (accessed 10 Feb. 2013).

Crayton, L., Oliver, O., Holland, A., Bradbury, J. and Hall, S. (1998) The neuropsychological assessment of age-related cognitive deficits in adults with Down's syndrome, *Journal of Applied Research in Intellectual Disabilities*, 11: 255–272.

Cuthill, F.M., Espie, C.A. and Cooper, S.A. (2003) Development and psychometric properties of the Glasgow Depression Scale for people with a learning disability, *British Journal of Psychiatry*, 182: 347–353.

Deb, S., Hare, M., Prior, L. and Bhaumik, S. (2007). The dementia screening questionnaire for individuals with intellectual disabilities, *The British Journal of Psychiatry*, 190: 440–444.

DH (Department of Health) (2009) *Living Well with Dementia: A National Dementia Strategy*. London: The Stationery Office.

Devenny, D. A., Krinsky-McHale, S. J. and Silverman, W. P. (2002) Changes in explicit memory associated with early dementia in adults with Down's Syndrome, *Journal of Intellectual Disability Research*, 46(3): 198–208.

Doody, C., Markey, K. and O Doody, K. (2011) Future need of ageing people with an intellectual disability in the Republic of Ireland: lessons learned from the literature, *British Journal of Learning Disabilities*, 134: 1–9.

Down's Syndrome Association (n.d.) *Down's Syndrome and Alzheimer's Disease: A Guide for Parents and Carers*. Middlesex: DSA.

Emerson, E., Malam, S., Davies, I. and Spencer, K. (2005) *Adults with Learning Difficulties in England 2003/4*. London: HMSO.

Emerson, E. and Ramcharan, P. (2010) Models of service delivery, in G. Grant, P. Ramcharan, M. Flynn and M. Richardson (eds) *Learning Disability: A Life Cycle Approach*, 2nd edn. Maidenhead: Open University Press.

Evenhuis, H.M., Kengen, M.M.F., and Eurlings, H.A.L. (2007) *Dementia Questionnaire for People with Learning Disabilities (DLD): UK Adaptation*. San Antonio, TX: Harcourt Assessment.

Fender, A., Marsden, L. and Starr, J. (2005) What do older adults with Down's Syndrome want from their doctor? A preliminary report, *British Journal of Learning Disabilities*, 35: 19–22.

Gale, L., Lesley, R. and Habib, N. (2008) *The Health of People with Learning Difficulties in Bristol. A Survey of More than 1000 Patients from 28 Primary Care Practices within Bristol PCT*. Bristol: Bristol Public Health Department.

Gedye, A. (1995) *Dementia Scale for Down's Syndrome: Manual*. Vancouver: Gedye Research and Consulting.

Guy, H. (2012) Pressure ulcer risk assessment, *Nursing Times*, 108(4): 16–20.

Hampshire Social Services (1987) *Hampshire Social Services: Staff Support Levels Assessment*. Winchester: Hampshire Social Services.

Harrison, P.L. and Oakland, T. (2003) *Adaptive Behaviour Assessment System (ABAS-II)*, 2nd edn. New York: The Psychological Corporation.

Higgins, L. and Mansell, J. (2009) Quality of life in group homes and older person homes, *British Journal of Learning Disabilities*, 37: 207–212.

Jervis, N. and Prinsloo, L. (2007) How we developed a multi disciplinary screening project for people with Down's Syndrome given the increased prevalence of early onset dementia, *British Journal of Learning Disabilities*, 36: 13–21.

NHS Centre for Public Involvement (2008) *Public Administration Select Committee Press Notice*. Available at: www.nhscentreforinvolvement.nhs.uk/index.cfm?action=PREandPressID=96 (accessed 20 July 2010).

NHS Choices (2012) Care Programme Approach. Available at: www.nhs.uk/CarersDirect/guide/mental-health/Pages/care-programme-approach.aspx (accessed 18 April 2013).

NICE (2013) *NICE Quality Standard for Supporting People to Live Well with Dementia: Information for the Public*. Manchester: NICE.

Nihra, K., Foster, R., Shellhaas, M. and Leyland, H. (1974) *AAMD Adaptive Behaviour Scale 1974 Revision*. Austin, TX: American Association on Mental Deficiency

Parliamentary and Health Service Ombudsman (2011) *Care and Compassion? Report of the Health Service Ombudsman on Ten Investigations into NHS Care of Older People*. London: The Stationery Office.

Prasher, V.P., Holder, R. and Asim, F. (2004) The Adaptive Behaviour Dementia Questionnaire (ABDQ): screening questionnaire for dementia in Alzheimer's disease in adults with Down's syndrome, *Research in Developmental Disabilities*, 25: 385–397.

Sano, M.C., Aisen, P.S., Dalton, A.J., Andrews, H.F., Tsai, W., and the International Down's Syndrome and Alzheimer's Disease Consortium (2005) Assessment of ageing individuals with Down's syndrome in clinical trials: results of baseline measures, *Journal of Policy and Practice in Intellectual Disabilities*, 2: 126–138.

Saxton, J., McGonigle, K.L., Swihart, A.A. and Boller, F. (1993) *The Severe Impairment Battery*. Harlow: Pearson.

Sims, J. (2002) The ethics of prospective assessment for dementia in people with Down's Syndrome, *Clinical Psychology*, 13: 30–33.

Smith, P. (2001) Let's stand up for people with dementia, *Nursing Times*. Available at: www.nursingtimes.net.

Sparrow, S.S., Cicchetti, D.V. and Balla, D.A. (2007) *Vineland-II: Vineland Adaptive Behavior Scales*, 2nd edn. Harlow: Pearson.

Taylor, C., Harrison, K., Dening, H., Duncan, A. and Kendall, T. (2009) Therapeutic interventions in dementia 1: cognitive symptoms and function, *Nursing Times*, 105(1): 16–17.

Thompson, D. (2001) *New Guidelines on an Overlooked Need: Services for Down's Syndrome and Dementia. GOLD Programme*. London: Mental Health Foundation.

Wolfensberger, W. (1972) *The Principle of Normalisation in Human Services*. Toronto: National Institute on Mental Retardation.

12 Assessment at the end of life

Isabel Quinn

Learning outcomes

After reading this chapter you will be able to:

- explore the changing care needs of an individual with deteriorating health
- identify the principles of holistic assessment in end-of-life care and support
- review a range of assessment tools which assist staff in assessing needs of people with intellectual disabilities and/or dementia
- discuss the impact of end-of-life care on the family and carers
- recognise the importance of person-centred values in end-of-life care.

Introduction

> You matter because you are you. You matter to the last moment of your life, and we will do all we can not only to help you die peacefully but to live until you die.
>
> Dame Cicely Saunders, founder of the modern hospice movement)

This chapter continues Jeremy's story with a focus on assessment in his end-of-life care. The associated discussion will cover a range of issues around holistic assessment which will incorporate physical, psychological, social and spiritual aspects. There will also be discussion about the values and limitations of assessment tools to assist staff in assessing needs of people with intellectual disabilities who also have developed dementia. This will raise discussions about developing person-centred management plans and multidisciplinary assessment and discussion. Other issues will include equality and access to services.

This chapter will also consider assessing and supporting Jeremy's family and the care staff who look after him at this difficult time.

Case study 12.1 Jeremy's deterioration

Over recent months, the care staff who support Jeremy have noticed that there has been a deterioration in his functional and cognitive abilities, resulting in him now requiring more verbal and physical prompts for all tasks of daily living.

Jeremy does not now finish meals that he previously enjoyed and he is obviously losing weight as his clothes appear looser. He is often noticeably withdrawn and does not interact with other residents.

On a routine GP visit, the staff expressed their concern and the GP initially suggested trying some softer diet and increased assistance at meal times. On a follow-up consultation there was no improvement and it was suggested by the GP that at this stage 'it would be too distressing for him to have further assessments or investigations'. Staff remain concerned that he is continuing to lose weight and often appears distressed at mealtimes.

Jeremy tends not to engage with staff and when his mother and sister visit he does not speak to them. He previously used to enjoy the company of others and was always smiling and chatty. Jeremy no longer communicates using full sentences. Instead he only uses some occasional words and gestures such as turning his head away when people speak to him. Lately he has become agitated and distressed when strangers and new staff have been introduced to him.

Over the next few months, Jeremy's mobility continued to decline to the extent that he required assistance with all transfers and was essentially chair-bound during the day. He also needed full assistance with personal care and has become doubly incontinent. His family were upset when he had 'an accident' which is causing some issues with staff–family relationships.

As his condition continued to deteriorate, he had episodes where he has choked on food and fluids and has had recurrent chest infections, forcing him to spend longer episodes in bed. His chest sounded very moist and the GP suggested that Jeremy had probably developed pneumonia.

The staff were anxious that Jeremy is now approaching the end of his life and expressed concern that they would not be able to do the best for Jeremy and are frightened of what might happen. The Home Manager has asked for help from the district nurses but is unsure who else to contact for advice and support.

Jeremy's Care Manager suggested that Jeremy may need to be moved into another care setting as his current home may be unable to continue to meet his needs but his family and the care staff strongly feel that this is Jeremy's home and moving him would cause great distress for everyone.

Reader activity 12.1   Key issues

- What are the key issues identified from the case study above?
- Make a list of the issues you think will require further assessment and suggest who needs to be involved in this.

Holistic assessment

Holistic assessment is at the core of good palliative and end-of-life care and this should acknowledge that the physical, psychological, social and spiritual dimensions of the person and their family are intertwined (Read and Thompson-Hill, 2008).

It is recommended that when someone is acknowledged to be approaching the end of their life, structured holistic assessments will be undertaken at each of the following *key points* in the individual's care pathway (National End of Life Care Programme, 2010):

- identification of the end-of-life phase;
- the point at which dying is diagnosed;
- at any other time that the individual may request;
- at any other time that a professional carer may judge necessary.

Practice alert 12.1

1. Holistic assessment is about the physical, social, psychological and spiritual needs of a person at the end of their life.
2. Holistic assessment can result in a plan which records the wishes and decisions of a person at the end of life. This may be useful for family and everyone involved in their care.
3. Holistic assessment is an *ongoing* process which can be updated and changed as the person's choices and preferences change.
4. The process of making a holistic assessment may increase the confidence and trust of a person at the end of life.

When is the end of life?

As someone approaches the end of life, there is usually a decline in their physical health. This can be quite apparent in people with a cancer diagnosis where there is a marked reduction in function in a relatively short period of time. In frailty and dementia cases, individuals can have a prolonged period where there is a gradual decline in function with intermittent episodes of acute illness and this presents a challenge to identifying when we should start to consider end-of-life care. Using guidance from the End of Life Care Strategy (DH, 2008), this period usually refers to the last 6–12 months of someone's life. When end of life is less clear, the End of Life Care Strategy advocates that the 'surprise question' should be used as part of the assessment process.

The surprise question asks:

Would you be surprised if this person died in the next 6–12 months?

If the answer is no, then it should be considered that the individual could be approaching the end of their life. However, the determination of someone's life expectancy is variable and unpredictable and doctors often look for other signs or factors to inform a timescale or prognosis. Healthcare practitioners are often asked to predict how progressive a condition is and whether someone is approaching the end of life. The process of anticipating how long someone is expected to live, or whether they are expected to respond to a treatment or intervention, is often referred to as prognostication.

Fast facts 12.1   Prognostication

In less than a year. This is often accompanied by the person not communicating or retaining only a few words. There is also an increasing likelihood of people being unable to carry out their own care needs. Many people are often doubly incontinent at this stage.

Instead of the use of the surprise question, where many professionals are unsure about committing themselves to a specific prognosis, it is often very useful to use a variation of the original question and ask health professionals to consider

Would you be surprised if this person *DID NOT* die in the next 6–12 months?

This might lead to professionals preparing families and carers that the future is uncertain and unpredictable, and hopefully to begin to prepare themselves that the person may be approaching the last months of their life. This still allows the healthcare staff to identify that everyone is different and that it is difficult sometimes to predict how long this process will take. This is also a useful time to initiate discussions about any future care preferences. If the person who is approaching the end of their life is unable to communicate their wishes and preferences, and there is no appointed lasting power of attorney for healthcare decisions, then the views of family members should still be taken into account.

Recognition of advanced illness

Care staff may need further training about the needs of people with intellectual disability who develop complex health needs. This is supported by Wilkinson *et al.* (2005) who identify that staff in care home settings need additional support to effectively care for people with intellectual disabilities who develop dementia.

A recognised tool such as FAST (the Functional Assessment Staging Tool) (Reisberd, 1988) (Figure 12.1) may be useful in improving recognition of advanced disease when someone has a dementia illness. This allows proactive approaches to care to be initiated, following discussion with family members and care staff. At each stage there are specific indicators which may identify the extent of the dementia; these include when someone becomes less mobile and when they no longer smile or interact. It is apparent that Jeremy has a severe dementia, given that he was no longer mobile or able to communicate or interact. This indicates that it is often difficult to predict the end of life in people with advanced dementia and there is a reluctance to recognise that dementia is a terminal condition which requires a palliative approach to care (Mitchell *et al.*, 2009; Sachs *et al.*, 2004).

End stage dementia is frequently characterised by recurring infections, including urinary tract infections (UTIs) and chest infections, which may lead to the development of pneumonia, and

The FAST scale has seven stages:

1. Normal adult
2. Normal older adult
3. Early dementia
4. Mild dementia
5. Moderate dementia
6. Moderately severe dementia
7. Severe dementia

Figure 12.1 Functional Assessment Staging Tool (FAST scale)

Source: Reisberg (1988).

reduction in oral intake (Lamberg *et al.*, 2005). In the case study at the beginning of this chapter, Jeremy had frequent chest infections in the last months of his life and ultimately he developed a pneumonia. At this point the care staff were able to see the rapid deterioration. Jeremy was unable to take antibiotics which highlighted the severity of the situation. In fact, care staff are often well placed to recognise many of the changes that occur in advanced disease and they often are the ones who notify the doctor of their concerns.

Unfortunately a reluctance to recognise the terminal stages of dementia often results in people being treated as acutely ill when they are in the final weeks of life. This means that many individuals will not receive the appropriate assessment of their palliative and end-of-life care needs.

In addition to the surprise question, the Gold Standards Framework (2005) has also identified some specific prognostic indicators for people with dementia that indicate that someone may be approaching the end of life. These are equally applicable when someone with a learning disability has developed dementia. These are presented in Figure 12.2.

Assessment of common symptoms as end of life approaches

A range of other assessment tools have been devised for use in palliative care to assess a range of symptoms. Most of these involve asking questions about the symptoms, and asking the patient to rate the severity or impact of the symptom on their quality of life. The problem with using many of these tools is that they are reliant upon the individual being able to convey accurate verbal information regarding their symptoms.

When working with people with intellectual disabilities, it must be acknowledged that some of these assessment tools may only be suitable if the person can understand what is being asked and if they have sufficient communication and language to respond. However, on many occasions, such as with Jeremy, some of the language and terminology found in assessment tools may not be appropriate to use.

There are some limited modified versions of symptom assessment tools available that may include pictures and images and the use of these should be considered when caring for people with learning disabilities however, even these may be unsuitable for some individuals.

Elderly/Frailty

Multiple co-morbidities with signs of impairments in day-to-day functioning:

- Deteriorating Karnofsky score
- Combination of at least three symptoms of: weakness, slow walking speed, low physical activity, weight loss, self-reported exhaustion

Specific to dementia

- Unable to walk without assistance
- Urinary and faecal incontinence
- No consistently meaningful verbal communication
- Unable to dress without assistance
- Barthel score < 3
- Reduced ability to perform activities of daily living

Plus any one of the following:

- 10% weight loss in previous six months without other causes
- Pyelonephritis (kidney infection) or urinary tract Infection
- Serum albumin 25 g/l – a protein found in blood plasma.
- Severe pressure scores e.g. stage III/IV
- Recurrent fevers
- Reduced oral intake/weight loss
- Aspiration pneumonia

Figure 12.2 Gold Standards Framework 2005 Prognostic Indicator Guidance

Source: GSF (2005).

It is important to have a mechanism to assess the impact of any intervention and treatment. This is particularly useful for people whose communication is so compromised that carers feel that this is difficult to assess. In these situations it is essential to explore every possible method available which will help to facilitate and maximise assessment of symptoms. In these circumstance multidisciplinary/ collaborative working should be encouraged. It is also good practice to share with others involved in the person's care which assessment tool has been used in order to ensure consistency of care and approach.

It is important to ensure that assessment at the end of life, regardless of the person's diagnosis, should ensure that the needs of the individual and their families are at the centre of all interventions.

As Jeremy's condition deteriorates, reaching the end phase of his illness, his care and support must focus on the continuity of symptom control, psychological, emotional and spiritual support.

Reader activity 12.2   Tools in holistic assessment

What assessment tools can you find that may be useful in the holistic assessment of individuals with intellectual disabilities or dementia?

You may have identified some tools from reading Chapter 11 but it also useful to consider what resources you can access to improve holistic assessment. When assessing Jeremy's needs, we should consider the following areas.

Physical assessment

Assessment of physical aspects of end-of-life care is an ongoing process. The case study highlights that as an individual's illness progresses, their functional status declines, resulting in a significant change in care needs. Staff require education, training and support to enable them to continue to assess need and deliver care that is appropriate and responds to changes in condition.

The routine care delivery can continue to be provided by care staff. However they may need some specialist advice and support on assessing and managing symptoms and problems that may arise. Research indicates that staff who work with people with intellectual disabilities often feel inadequately trained to assess and deliver end-of-life care (Bekkema *et al.*, 2014). In some care homes, there may be input from district nurses and palliative care teams who can advise staff. However, in many areas there is a lack of collaborative working and there is a need to establish links with palliative care services (Todd, 2004).

Eating and drinking

Significant weight loss is not uncommon in people with dementia, particularly during the stage where they walk around a lot and lose focus on tasks such as eating or drinking. However, Jeremy is now past this stage of his illness. He is having difficulties with the basic mechanics of getting food and drink into his mouth without external support; he has lost his 'sequencing skills'. He has also possibly lost his ability to 'feel hungry' or is unable to recognise if he is full or thirsty. He may now require his diet to be modified to make eating and drinking easier and safer.

In the early stages of eating difficulties, there are some things that may help. These include:

- the use of specialised/adapted cutlery or plate guards;
- ensuring that noise and distraction are minimised;
- providing appropriate seating which may require additional external support;
- allowing more time for meals;
- changing the timing of mealtimes;
- increased assistance/support, including verbal and physical prompts;
- frequent snacks and desserts throughout the day are sometimes better tolerated than large meals;
- finger foods and convenient snack bars may be appropriate for the person who will not sit at a table or use cutlery. It is still possible to introduce a variety of food groups such as fruit and vegetables in this way.

It is necessary to maintain an adequate fluid intake as dehydration can cause people to become very unwell. Some of the problems associated with dehydration are:

- lethargy and confusion;
- dry mouth/mouth problems;

- increases the risk of infection, i.e. urinary tract infection;
- affected skin integrity which increases the risk of pressure problems.

There may be a need to assess for any reversible causes which may affect Jeremy's eating or contribute to his weight loss. These may include medication changes, metabolic disorders or changes in mood. Anxiety, depression and low mood are often present in people with dementia and can affect interactions with others and also may affect appetite. Staff can observe and report any identified problems to the doctor or other health professionals to assist with the overall assessment of eating problems.

There needs to be recognition that swallowing difficulty (dysphagia) should not be ignored. The National Patient Safety Agency (2007) identifies that this is a 'serious problem' for many adults with learning disabilities. It is important to raise awareness that this can lead to serious problems and even death in some circumstances.

While the advice given by the GP to Jeremy's carers may be appropriate in some cases, the ongoing persistence of the care staff in raising their concerns should result in Jeremy receiving the appropriate assessments he requires. Table 12.1 shows the people and features of an eating and drinking assessment.

As discussed in Chapter 6 the Mencap report *Death by Indifference* (Mencap, 2007) highlights five people with a learning disability who died as a consequence of inadequate healthcare, including delays in assessing and treating severe swallowing problems. Despite Mencap's report, Duffin (2010) identifies that there are still issues with providing appropriate interventions to manage swallowing difficulties.

Mobility issues

As people get older, their ability to move around changes, they can get slower, be less flexible and can fall for no apparent cause. This is usually the case for people reaching the later stages of their life

Table 12.1 Eating and drinking assessment

Assessments required	People who can help
- Mouth care:- Observation of oral status e.g. thrush, infections - Check for dental problems or loose-fitting dentures - Food diary. Record specific foods that cause most difficulty - Record and monitor amount of food/drinks offered and taken/refused - Monitor any presence of distress associated with eating - Coughing chart. Monitor if when Jeremy coughs at mealtimes in the context of what he is eating - Check for the presence and frequency of vomiting, choking or regurgitation	- The care team who look after Jeremy - District Nurse - Dentist - Speech and language therapist for swallowing problems - Dietician - Physiotherapist for posture - Occupational therapist for equipment, e.g. cutlery

but can be especially a problem for people with dementia due to the physical problems associated with this disease (Oddy, 2011). As the brain becomes more damaged by the dementing process, this affects the way the messages are conveyed to the joints and muscles, resulting in an altered gait pattern and compromised balance reactions for the person (Waite *et al.*, 2000). In the early stage of dementia there may be an increase in walking around, unable to settle which is sometimes described as wandering. There may be episodes of bumping into things, 'falling over their own feet' or generally becoming disorientated. At this stage, though mobility is slightly affected, it is not usually an issue. In the mid-stage of dementia, mobility is a major concern resulting in an increase in falls and loss of gross motor skills such as standing up from a chair, climbing stairs, negotiating kerbs, inclines and rough ground. What also compounds mobility problems at this stage is a loss of spatial awareness, that is, where our body is in space, for example, 'am I sitting straight on this chair?' as well as perception problems such as 'how deep is that step?'.

The environment can have a significant impact upon mobility but problems due to this can usually be overcome. Increased noise levels and sudden sounds can startle individuals causing them to 'jump' and subsequently increase the risk of falls. There may be obstacles that can become trip hazards along frequently used pathways such as to the dining room. Chairs may not be at the best height for the person at the table or it may be the table that is too high. Lack of appropriate lighting and signage can affect orientation and mobility. The case study indicates Jeremy was now in the end stage of his illness and as he is no longer able to walk independently around the home and is reliant upon a wheelchair for his mobility, his falls will have decreased but other issues emerge. For people with end stage dementia, there will be little active functional movement and in the very end stage of their illness, they may need full assistance for every movement, even turning in bed or holding their head up.

Jeremy will need to have a moving and handling assessment to determine the best slings/hoist to cater for his deteriorating skills. This will inform a moving and handling care plan which should be reviewed regularly. At the point when Jeremy still had some sitting balance, he was able to sit in his wheelchair armchair, however, because of his lack of movement, other problems need to be assessed for and monitored, such as skin integrity/postural management. Inability to change position when sitting can lead to stiffness and discomfort, but if this is a permanent situation, such as in Jeremy's case, and not addressed, it can lead to other physical problems. One of the main issues that result from loss of mobility and which requires careful assessment is skin integrity/pressure problems. When sitting, our weight is distributed through the points that are supported by the chair surface such as bottom, hips or elbows. We are able to shift our weight, therefore altering the places that weight is distributed through. We know Jeremy is unable to do this, so if he is in the same position in his chair for a long period of time, he will be susceptible to pressure problems. This is even more important if people are unable to maintain a symmetrical posture which we know Jeremy cannot, so the chances of him having weight going through one side more than the other is high, thus increasing the risk of skin damage. For skin integrity to be maintained, there needs to be regular assessment using pressure risk assessment tools, such as the Waterlow pressure ulcer risk assessment, with protocols in place to act upon if the assessment identifies an issue or deterioration. District nurses can help with the provision of pressure relief equipment in some cases and give advice on pressure area care and wound care.

Practice alert 12.2

Risk of pressure sores can be influenced by the following intrinsic factors:

- reduced mobility/immobility
- sensory impairment
- acute illness
- level of consciousness
- age
- vascular disease
- previous history of pressure damage
- malnutrition and dehydration.

More information on the Waterlow assessment tools can be found at www.judy-waterlow. co.uk/waterlow_score.htm.

Another complication of deteriorating gross motor skills such as sitting balance is the increasing need for specialist equipment so Jeremy's posture can be maintained. For example he may need a specialist wheelchair or armchair that has side supports; head supports or Tilt in Space facilities to help keep him in an upright position. He may also need special mattresses with pressure-relieving properties and perhaps a profiling bed. The need for equipment requires regular monitoring in conjunction with postural assessments. In accordance with other aspects of care for posture and mobility, Jeremy will require on-going assessments from a range of people, including external professionals. Table 12.2 shows probable issues with mobility at each stage of the dementia journey

As Jeremy's illness progresses, and he continues to lose his skills and abilities, he will become more dependent on the staff team who will then have to adapt to his deteriorating needs. There are a range of assessment tools which can be used to identify what help is required with Jeremy's personal care and this information can be used to develop a person-centred care plan for staff.

Within a nursing context the best-known assessment is Activities of Daily Living which incorporates a range of personal care tasks. This allows staff to record what assistance is required for each activity and provides a useful ongoing assessment mechanism.

There is a range of other functional assessment tools available. Consideration must be given as to whether these are appropriate to use in an End of Life Care context and/or with people with learning disabilities. For example, are they accessible? Are they relevant to the environment? Does it focus on present needs or futures planning?

Dignity should be at the centre of care delivery and this will focus on ensuring privacy and dignity for Jeremy during all care procedures. At all times staff should aim to ensure that Jeremy is cared for in response to his assessed needs rather than suiting the needs of the staff routine. There are many recent adverse reports about poor quality care of individuals in hospitals and in care homes. There will be many recommendations to follow, but there is also some very useful information about dignity found in the End of Life Care guide produced by Mencap (2008).

The Commission of Dignity in Care for Older People (2012) identified that 'care homes must help older people to understand their health and care needs, work with them and their families to

Table 12.2 Probable issues with mobility at each stage of the dementia journey

Mobility – First stage of dementia	Mobility – Mid stage dementia	Mobility – End stage dementia

• Loss of self help skills
• Confusion
• 'Start wandering'
	• 'Wandering' – can be big issue
	• Problems with sequencing – cannot remember the pattern of walking
	• Altered gait pattern
	• Compromised balance
	• Decreased gross motor skills
	• Increased falls
	• Problems with 'initiation' – cannot start the action – suddenly stops still
	• Problems with spatial awareness – 'slips off chairs'/'bumps into door frames'
	• Problems with perception – 'stops at thresh holds'/'walks around patterns in carpets'/'stairs'
	• Wheelchair considered
	• Hoisting can start
		Now requires full hoisting
		• No functional active movement
		• Sitting balance deteriorates, eventually resulting in unable to maintain sitting
		• Full assistance required for all actions including:
		  • All transfers – bed to chair, etc.
		  • Moving within the bed
		  • Maintaining upright posture in chairs

help them manage these needs, and support them physically and emotionally to live as well as possible if they cannot get better', see http://www.nhsconfed.org/Publications/Documents/Delivering_Dignity_final_report150612.pdf. If this approach is adopted by the care team it will help to alleviate any concerns that Jeremy's family may have.

Practice alert 12.3

Ensuring dignity is of paramount importance during all aspects of care delivery. Further information about dignity in care can be accessed on the National Dignity Council website, www.dignityincare.org.uk/.

Communication

Communication difficulties are frequently identified as a 'major obstacle in supporting people with learning difficulties at the End of Life Care' (Tuffrey-Wijne and McEnhill, 2008). Issues with communication can be found in many situations. For example, we can all have problems communicating with our peers, colleagues and friends, where our formal speech is a highly developed skill but by using the wrong words or a different tone of voice, our intentions can be misinterpreted. In other cases there can be misunderstanding and poor communication between professionals and families where barriers are formed by using jargon or platitudes, or just by not communicating. Then there are the problems experienced by people like Jeremy who have lost their ability to communicate with others and are often deemed incapable of communicating at all.

Communication difficulties can occur in a wide range of conditions and people, including those with a learning disability and people with dementia, and this is often the descriptive term used when someone is unable to use formal speech. Compared to any formal spoken language, the vocabulary used by people with cognitive problems, like Jeremy, is smaller and some may not participate in a formal language system at all, resulting in difficulty recognising what their actions, signs and expressions mean.

Meaningful communication in these circumstances is often referred to as alternative or augmentative communication. This is dependent on the ability of the people close to them, including the carers, to recognise and translate the many different cues available and not just those verbally expressed. Jeremy's family have described how he no longer engages with them. However, in his way he is still demonstrating how he is communicating with them as he accepts their presence and is comfortable to be close with them.

> ### Reader activity 12.3   Communication problem
>
> Who should we involve when assessing the needs of individuals who may no longer use speech to communicate their needs?

Assessing distress

In common with other progressive life-threatening conditions, the principles of palliative and supportive care should apply to people with intellectual disabilities throughout the course of the disease, including the need to treat pain and distress. Research also suggests (Morse *et al.*, 1994) that comfort remains central to effective care and is achieved by easing and relieving distress.

However, when an individual with communication difficulties is agitated and distressed (as Jeremy was in the case study), it is important not to single out the symptom of pain (physical distress) from other forms of distress such as emotional, psychological and spiritual ones. The relationship between pain and distress is complex and there is no published evidence to support assumptions that signs or behaviour caused by a physical cause such as pain are different to the signs or behaviour caused by psychological distress such as anxiety. Many people with dementia have painful conditions, which in people with impaired language and abstract thinking may manifest as agitation (Husebo *et al.*, 2011).

Jeremy cannot communicate his distress and/or discomfort effectively, therefore recognition of this problem can be difficult and is reliant upon the ability of his carers to recognise and translate his different verbal and non-verbal cues, such as expression and gesture. His carers can be intuitively skilled at picking up the distress cues but sometimes have little confidence in interpreting them.

It has already been stated that Jeremy can show distress when meeting strangers, therefore by recognising the 'language' he uses in those situations carers can transfer that knowledge into different situations. Once distress has been identified, it needs to be put in context and then clinical decisions will have to be made by the team caring for Jeremy to decide the most appropriate intervention to proceed with. Therefore, to achieve effective dementia care, there needs to be careful assessment and documentation of the signs and behaviours of distress, which is only the start when identifying the cause. For example, if Jeremy is emotionally upset because his family have just left, it would be wrong to give him a painkiller.

There are a range of tools that have been developed to assess pain and/or distress in people with intellectual disabilities, such as Disability Distress Assessment Tool (Dis DAT) and staff who work in care settings should be familiar with them and confident in using them (Regnard *et al.*, 2006). Jeremy will need on-going assessments of his distress throughout the end stage of his disease which will inform his symptom management and other aspects of his holistic care.

Reader activity 12.4   Pain assessment tools

Undertake an internet search to find different pain assessment tools/scales. Evaluate how effective you feel these scales would be for someone with impaired communication. Are there strategies you can use to overcome these difficulties?

Partnership working between professionals, families and carers is essential to ensure a full assessment of need for Jeremy and others in his situation. It is vital that professionals recogise any impact that his learning disability has on his ability to communicate and be involved in planning his care. The on-going support and comfort from family members and friends of people with intellectual disabilities have been the focus of many studies which demonstrate that even when individuals suffer progressive decline in their physical and mental status, the presence of family members has been shown to be beneficial in reducing distress and anxiety. We also need to acknowledge the contribution of staff working to address factors which may contribute to physical and psychological distress. There is also a need to value the contribution of family carers and reinforce the positive impact they make.

Managing recurring infections

There should be joint working between professionals to make a treatment plan for the prompt management of infections. Simple care measures to promote comfort are also important. Care staff can monitor Jeremy's temperature and use of a fan may help manage a fever. Gentle bathing with room temperature cloths can also help with temperature control and comfort if Jeremy's skin is clammy or sweating. Maintaining a semi-upright position can help breathing and reduce the effect of troublesome secretions. Having antibiotics available to commence as soon as the infection starts is helpful to avoid delays but only if Jeremy is able to swallow the medication. The use of paracetamol and ibuprofen may also help with managing a raised temperature. There needs to be support and advice from district nurses, GP and local pharmacy staff to make sure the medication is prescribed and dispensed in the most suitable form, e.g. solutions or syrup form, as this may be easier to take than large tablets.

Practice alert 12.4

We should encourage carers to participate in any aspect of care delivery that they want to be involved in. Staff should provide positive support and feedback.

Place of care and advance care planning

Preferred Priorities for Care (PPC) is a a document where people can identify choices about their future care, including saying where they would like to be cared for at the end of their life. This can be found at www.cancerlancashire.org.uk. There are many adaptations of this document available to allow it to be used with people with learning disability and some positive case studies which highlight the benefits to individuals in enabling them to be cared for in their place of choice. Gaining an under-standing of the person's wishes and needs requires careful listening, plus consideration of the realistic options, with constant adjustments to a changing situation. This is particularly challenging when the care needs cannot be met in the person's own home. Features of a good place of care included being in safe surroundings with familiar people, being free from pain and anxiety, and having family carers who are well supported (Tuffrey-Wijne, 2009).

The process of helping people with learning difficulties and/or dementia identify their wishes and preferences about care should ideally be undertaken while the person still has capacity to make such a decision and the necessary language to communicate their decision. We know Jeremy has Down's Syndrome and a learning difficulty, therefore may never have had capacity to identify his wishes and preferences using the legal framework. However, even people without capacity can still express their preferences using a variety of approaches. Many people with a learning disability have been involved in developing their own person-centred plan which documents what they would like to happen at certain times in their lives and who they would like to help them achieve this. This may include where they would like to be cared for at the end of their life as well as practical aspects such as funeral arrangements.

Fast facts 12.2   The Mental Capacity Act

The Mental Capacity Act provides guidance for all health and social care staff to ensure that all care delivered is in the best interest of the individual, if the person is unable to give consent (Department of Constitutional Affairs, 2005).

Where do people die?

In the UK, around 20 per cent of people will die in nursing and care home settings. The majority of people will die in hospital. When people with learning difficulties are admitted to general hospital wards, this can increase their distress as they are not in familiar surroundings. Unfortunately people still have some negative perceptions regarding care homes where these are not always considered in the same way as the individual's own home, even if the person has lived there for a long time. In Case study 12.1, there was some discussion about whether Jeremy's care needs could still be met in the care home. If he was admitted to hospital, he might be placed on a busy ward where staff do not know him and he does not know the staff caring for him. There remains a lack of recognition that care homes can be an end-of-life care environment.

The End of Life Care Strategy (DH, 2008) specifically identified the need for education and training of all health and social care staff and acknowledges that many care home staff often are not given access to end-of-life care education despite the fact that they frequently deal with people who are at the end of their life. To address these situations there is a range of resources such as those developed by the National End of Life Care Programme working in collaboration with others, e.g. Skills for health/ Skills for care. Common core principles and competences to support the end-of-life care workforce are a good example of the type of resources available (National End of Life Care Programme, 2009).

A range of learning materials can be obtained from the Social Care Institute for Excellence (SCIE), available at: http://www.scie.org.uk/.

Care in the dying phase

A point comes when an individual enters the dying phase. For some, this may appear to happen suddenly and without warning but for many others it can be a gradual process. There is often reluctance to make a diagnosis of dying when someone has dementia because of the uncertainty, and sometimes people do get better. It is always good practice to identify to relatives and staff that there is often uncertainty. If an individual is considered to be approaching the end of their life, they may be included in a local palliative or end-of-life care register. The decision to do this would be made by medical staff following discussion with those involved in the individual's care. This would also be accompanied by regular discussions of the individuals who are on the register to identify and manage any problems.

Froggatt (2001) highlighted the importance of care staff relationships in providing care at the end of life. If staff have been closely involved with an individual, this should enable them to perceive the person's needs even when the latter is unable to communicate and respond to them. Care staff, who have developed good relationships with the person, are able to perform the caring tasks smoothly at the end of life.

Hanson et al. (2002) identified that death in a residential home may often be characterised by psychological suffering. It is suggested that this may be alleviated by the provision of 'individualised' care to compensate for social isolation and other factors which may contribute to psychological distress. Katz (2003) has listed three inter-related principles for good end-of-life care. The first is to enable the dying person to die with dignity. The second is to retain the dying person in his/her familiar surroundings till death, if at all possible, and the third is that the dying person is entitled to good pain control and nursing care. It has never been an easy task to adopt the first principle since physical deterioration and decline, such as immobility and incontinence, may create a loss of dignity for dying people. So we tend to define dying with dignity more in terms of being treated well and respected as a person.

Practice alert 12.5

The nature of the uncertainty and difficulty in predicting when death may be imminent should be conveyed to relatives and carers. The important thing is to ensure there is ongoing communication and clear explanations about any changes which may occur.

When the possibility of a person's death is acknowledged by the care team to be imminent (by this, we mean hours or days), a senior staff member should discuss this with the family. Staff should be prepared that conversations at the end of life can be very emotional and relatives and carers should be given time and space to express their concerns and emotions. If possible, this conversation should be in a private space away from the bedside. The family should be informed about the changes that may occur when someone is dying, such as irregular breathing and changes in circulation. Relatives should be offered an opportunity to stay with the person or identify how they wish to be contacted if there is any change in conditions.

When someone becomes semi-conscious, they are often unable to swallow fluids, so issues such as this must be explained to relatives so that they can understand why staff are no longer giving oral diet and fluids. Sensitive discussions are needed to highlight that this may be an indication that the person may be approaching death. Relatives can still be involved in providing comfort care and mouth care of the person if they wish. Relatives will be reassured that the person will continue to be assessed regularly and that if there is any improvement noted or swallowing improves, or the person becomes more alert, then eating and drinking may be resumed.

The focus is on providing optimum comfort at this time, therefore regular assessment is required to ensure there are no distressing symptoms present. The ability to assess and manage the physical symptoms can only be achieved by good collaborative working involving those who know the person well (Regnard et al., 2006).

The most common symptoms at the end of life are pain, breathlessness, agitation, respiratory secretions and nausea and vomiting. Medication is often given using a syringe driver (small pump) with a needle placed under the skin. If symptoms do not settle, then advice should be sought from palliative care professionals. Carers and families should be informed about the side effects of any medications used to alleviate these symptoms, such as increased sedation. All discussions including discussions about resuscitation should be recorded in care plans.

Spiritual assessment

This is a topic which is very difficult to define as it is not tangible and therefore very difficult to assess. In reality, spirituality and religion are often mixed up. Spirituality has to do with the search for a meaning and purpose in life whereas religion is any specific system of belief worship and conduct. Although in the current climate there is increased focus on managing healthcare as a business, within limited resources, staff have a responsibility to address the spiritual needs of the people they care for. This must include people with a learning disability, whose spiritual needs may go unrecognised as they are not able to express them. As Jeremy is unable to tell people what is important to him, staff must strive to maintain previous contacts in his life. As well as the family, this may include pertinent people in his life, such as people from various groups Jeremy has attended in the past, and any friends/mentors.

Good spiritual care is associated with health and well-being, and it is important therefore to try and ensure an individual's spiritual needs are addressed, however difficult this may be (Figure 12.3). A study by Hatton et al. (2004) found that spiritual care needs were given a low priority by many services and many staff did not consider that meeting religious and spiritual needs was within their remit.

Care after death

Every organisation should have guidance on what to do when someone has died. There is also useful practical guidance for families produced by the Department of Work and Pensions. This is a very

The National End of Life Care programme (2010) suggests that assessment should consider the following. However, these may be difficult to ascertain in someone with dementia:

Identify practical support or other needs related to religion or spiritual matters

- Religious items (e.g. religious texts or books, prayer mat, religious objects, holy water).
- Someone to speak to: faith leader or minister (e.g. minister, chaplain, vicar, priest, imam, rabbi, spiritual leader, church leader), or other person.
- Help. Things to help you practise your faith e.g. space to pray, quiet environment, privacy.

Practical support or other restrictions related to person's cultural or ethnic background, or belief system.

- Requirements
- Restrictions
- Diet
- Medicines

Person's concerns or desires regarding a 'goal' they want to achieve in their life.

- Important occasions
- Family gatherings
- Holidays
- Big events

Figure 12.3 Spirituality

difficult time and staff have to ensure that they continue to offer time and space for relatives and provide support. Belongings and possessions should be treated with respect.

Staff should also be aware of their own feelings following the death of an individual:

1. When a resident in a care homes dies, care staff are very likely to feel affected and bereaved.
2. Good practice lies in acknowledging staff may be affected by a death and need time to reflect on and deal with feelings of bereavement.
3. Staff need to be able to talk openly about their feelings and emotions. Managers can support staff to do this in one-to-one meetings as well as group settings.
4. This acknowledges the importance of staff to the care and confirms how important and valuable their contribution to good care is.
5. It is important to recognise that grief may take some time to surface in staff following a death.

Practice alert 12.6

Staff should support each other and other residents and recognise signs of distress as early as possible.

Ongoing care and support for relatives may be difficult after someone has died in a care home, However, some simple things like sending condolence cards and allowing staff and residents to attend the funeral service are very important to family members. Some care homes have an annual memorial service where families and friends can come and meet staff and residents. These events are often valued by families and carers especially if they have previously spent a lot of time at the care home. Many family members may be socially isolated following the death of a loved one. Meeting other people in the same situation is sometimes a helpful way for families to support each other. Some family members also like to take up volunteer roles in the care home where this is appropriate.

Carrying out end-of-life care for someone with intellectual disability and dementia can be a difficult experience. However, by working together with other colleagues, and using their knowledge and expertise, it is possible to achieve good quality end-of-life care in most care settings (Read, 2005).

Points to remember

- The 'end-of-life' stage is acknowledged by a multidisciplinary team.
- Skill is needed to pick up on any non-verbal indications of pain, distress, discomfort and anxiety.
- Care should be person centred.
- Specific assessment tools are useful in helping to understand a person's changing needs.
- Everyone has a role in end-of-life care. If any staff need support or guidance it is available.
- Dignity is the good treatment of someone at the end of their life.

Acknowledgements

Thank you to contributors Lynn Gibson and Dorothy Matthews.

Resources

Disability Distress Assessment Tool (Dis DAT). Available at:
www.DisDAT.co.uk.

Mencap (2008) *Living and Dying with Dignity*. Available at:
www.mencap.org.uk/sites/default/files/documents/2009-04/best_practice_guide.pdf.

NHS North East End of Life Care Resource Guide. Available at:
http://a2anetwork.co.uk/wp-content/uploads/2010/01/EoL-resource-pack-N.-East.pdf.

References

Bekkema, N., de Veer, A.J.E., Albers, G., Hertogh, C.M.P.M., Onwuteaka-Philipsen, B.D. and Francke, A.L. (2014) Training needs of nurses and social workers in the end-of-life care for people with intellectual disabilities: a national survey, *Nurse Education Today*, 34: 494–500.

Commission on Dignity in Care for Older People (2012) *Delivering Dignity: Securing Dignity in Care for Older People in Hospitals and Care Homes*. London: NHS Confederation. Available at: www.nhsconfed. org/Publications/Documents/Delivering_Dignity_final_report150612.pdf.

Department of Constitutional Affairs (2005) *Mental Capacity Act*. London: HMSO.

DH (Department of Health) (2008) *End of Life Care Strategy: Promoting High Quality Care for All Adults at the End of Life*. London: Department of Health.

DH (Department of Health) (2009) *Living Well with Dementia: A National Dementia Strategy*. London: Department of Health.

Duffin, C. (2010) Raising awareness of dysphagia among health care professionals, *Learning Disability Practice*, 13(4): 21–24.

Froggatt, K.A. (2001) Palliative care in nursing homes: where next? *Palliative Medicine*, 15: 42–48.

Gold Standards Framework (2005) Prognostic Indicator Guidance. Available at: http://www.goldstandards framework.org.uk/.

Hanson, L.C., Henderson, M. and Menon, M. (2002) As individual as death itself: a focus group study of terminal care in nursing homes, *Journal of Palliative Medicine*, 5: 117–125.

Hatton, C., Turner, S., Shah, R., Rahim, N. and Stansfield, J. (2004) *What About Faith? A Good Practice Guide to Meeting the Religious Needs of People with Learning Disabilities*. London: Foundation for People with Learning Disabilities.

Husebo, B., Ballard, C., Sandvic, R., Nilsen, O.B. and Aarsland, D. (2011) Efficacy of treating pain to reduce behavioural disturbances in residents of nursing homes with dementia: cluster randomised clinical trial, *British Medical Journal*, 43: 1–10.

Katz, J. S. (2003) Managing dying residents, in J.S. Katz and S. Peace (eds) *End of Life in Care Homes: A Palliative Care Approach*. Oxford: Oxford University Press.

Lamberg, J., Person, C., Kiely, D. and Mitchell, S. (2005) Decisions to hospitalize nursing home residents dying with advanced dementia, *Journal of American Geriatrics Society*, 53: 1396–1401.

Mencap (2007) *Death by Indifference*. London: Mencap.

Mencap (2008) *Living and Dying with Dignity: Best Practice Guide to End of Life Care for People with a Learning Disability*. Available at: www.mencap.org.uk.

Mitchell, S., Teno, J., Kiely, D., Shaffer, M., Jones, R., Prigerson, H., Volicer, L., Givens, J. and Hamel, M. (2009) The clinical course of advanced dementia, *New England Journal of Medicine*, 361: 1529–1538.

Morse, J.M., Bottorf, J.L. and Hutchinson, S. (1994) The phenomenology of comfort, *Journal of Advanced Nursing*, 20: 189–195.

National End of Life Care Programme, Skills for Health, Skills for Care (2009) *Common Core Competences and Principles for Health and Social Care Workers Working with Adults at the End of Life*. London: DH.

National End of Life Care Programme (2010) *Holistic Common Assessment of Supportive and Palliative Care Needs for Adults Requiring End of Life Care*. Available at: http://www.nhsiq.nhs.uk/resource-search/publications/eolc-hca-guide.aspx.

National Patient Safety Agency (2007) *Ensuring Safer Practice for Adults with Learning Disabilities Who Have Dysphagia*. Available at: http://www.nrls.npsa.nhs.uk/resources/?entryid45=59823.

Oddy, R. (2011) *Promoting Mobility for People with Dementia: A Problem-Solving Approach*. London: Alzheimer's Society.

Read, S. (2005) Learning disabilities and palliative care: recognising pitfalls and exploring potential, *International Journal of Palliative Nursing*, 11(1): 15–20.

Read, S. and Thompson-Hill, J. (2008) Palliative care nursing in relation to people with intellectual disabilities, *British Journal of Nursing*, 17(8): 506–510.

Regnard, C., Clarke, C.L., Gibson, L. and Matthews, D. (2006) Pain and symptom management, in S. Read (ed.) *Palliative Care for People with Learning Disabilities*, London: Quay Books, pp. 39–57.

Regnard, C., Reynolds, J., Watson, B., Matthews, D., Gibson, L. and Clarke, C. (2007) Understanding distress in people with severe communication difficulties: developing and assessing the Disability Distress Assessment Tool (DisDAT), *Journal of Intellectual Disabilities Research*, 51(4): 277–292.

Reisberg, B. (1988) Functional Assessment Staging (FAST), *Psychopharmacology Bulletin*. 24: 653–659. Available at: http://geriatrics.uthscsa.edu/tools/FAST.pdf.

Sachs, G., Shega, J. and Cox-Hayley, D. (2004) Barriers to excellent end-of-life care for patients with dementia, *Journal General Internal Medicine*, 19: 1057–1063.

Todd, S. (2004). Death counts: the challenge of death and dying in learning disability services, *Learning Disability Practice*, 7(10): 12–15.

Tuffrey-Wijne, I. (2009) The preferred place of care for people who are dying, *Learning Disability Practice*, 12(6): 16–21.

Tuffrey-Wijne, I. and McEnhill, L. (2008) Communication difficulties and intellectual disability in end-of-life care, *International Journal of Palliative Nursing*, 14(4): 189–194.

Waite, L., Broe, A., Grayson, D.A. and Creasy, H. (2000) Motor function and disability in the dementias, *International Journal of Geriatric Psychiatry*, 15: 897–930.

Wilkinson, H., Kerr, D. and Cunningham, C. (2005) Equipping staff to support people with intellectual disability and dementia in care home settings, *Dementia*, 4(3): 387–400.

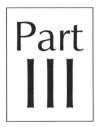

Part III

Health throughout life

Statistically, a person with a learning disability:

- is four times more likely to die of preventable causes;
- is 58 times more likely to die before 50;
- does not have the same access to health support;
- has higher levels of unmet need;
- will be discriminated against.

(Michael, 2008)

In order to promote the reader's aim to support people with learning disabilities, Part III addresses lifelong health needs in relation to people with learning disabilities. It begins by introducing some key factual information and statistics about the health of people with learning disabilities (Tables III.1 and III.2).

Each chapter in this part presents case studies that shed light on some of the health support that people with learning disabilities need at varying life stages. These case studies support best practice by addressing a range of the barriers that may be encountered and strategies that aim to support people to overcome those barriers. All of the case studies are based upon the real lives and experiences of people with learning disabilities, some of whom express their views directly in these stories. The case studies are supplemented by health-related tables, fast facts and activities to support the reader's personal reflection and learning.

The chapters that make up Part III are:

Chapter 13 Supporting people with severe epilepsy: a case study in diagnostic over-shadowing
Chapter 14 A life with cerebral palsy: Neil's story and Jose's case examples
Chapter 15 Supporting people with an autistic spectrum disorder
Chapter 16 Specific health needs and conditions
Chapter 17 Emotional difficulties

Table III.1 General health status of people with learning disabilities in relation to the non-disabled population

Mortality of people with learning disabilities	Shorter life expectancy; increased risk of early death	Life expectancy increasing, especially people with Down's Syndrome and people with milder learning disabilities	Three times higher for people with moderate to severe learning disabilities, especially young adults, women and people with Down's Syndrome	People with moderate to profound learning disabilities are more likely to die from congenital abnormalities
General health of people with learning disabilities	Fair to poor 2.5–4.5 times greater for children	1 in 7 adults with learning disabilities rate their general health as not good	Tendency for carers to underestimate poorer health than suggested by medical examination	Health screening via General Practitioners reveals high levels of unmet physical and mental health needs
Cancer	Overall lower incidence than in general population 12%–18% vs 26%	Higher rates of gastrointestinal cancer than general population 48%–59% vs 25% partly associated with higher incidence of helicobacter pylori, a class 1 carcinogen	Cancer rate increasing as life expectancy increases;	Children with Down's Syndrome at higher risk of leukaemia
Coronary heart disease	A major cause of death 14%–20% among people with learning disabilities	Rate expected to rise as a consequence of community lifestyle changes and increasing life expectancy	Approximately 50% of people with Down's Syndrome have congenital heart abnormalities	
Respiratory disease	A major cause of death 46%–52% among people with learning disabilities vs 15%–17% in general population	People with asthma and learning disabilities twice more likely to be smokers than non-asthmatics with learning disabilities	More than 50% of women with asthma and learning disabilities are also obese	

Mental health	Higher incidence of childhood psychiatric disorders 36% vs 8% in children without a learning disability	Children with learning disability represent 14% of all children with a diagnosable psychiatric disorder	Psychiatric disorder raised among people with autistic spectrum disorder, ADHD/ hyperkinesis and conduct disorders	Psychotic illness three times higher in adults especially among South Asian population. Also higher incidences of psychiatric disorder in adults
Challenging behaviour	Aggression, destruction, self-injury and others occurs in 10%–15%	Some challenging behaviours are the result of untreated/undiagnosed pain		
Dementia	Higher incidence in older adults with learning disabilities 22% vs. 6% aged 65+	Associated with a range of challenging behaviours and health problems	Onset in people with Down's Syndrome occurring 30–40 years sooner than in the general population	Related deaths are more common among men with moderate to profound learning disabilities than women
Epilepsy	Prevalence conservatively estimated at 20 times higher than for the general population	Tonic–clonic and absence types of seizures, often multiple and resistant to medical treatment for many of those affected	Lack of control of epilepsy can seriously reduce an individual's quality of life and mortality.	
Sensory impairments	8–200 times more likely to have a visual impairment	Approximately 40% have a hearing impairment	People with Down's Syndrome more likely to develop vision and hearing loss	Eye testing less prevalent if living with family or independently; carers often failing to indentify significant sensory impairments

(continued)

Table III.1 *(Continued)*

Physical impairments	Adults with learning disabilities who are non–mobile at seven times greater risk of death than those who are fully mobile	Adults with learning disabilities who are partially mobile at two times greater risk of death than those who are fully mobile	One study (cited by Emerson and Baines, 2010) reported that people with learning disabilities are 14 times more likely to have musculo–skeletal impairments	
Oral health	1 in 3 adults with learning disabilities have unhealthy teeth and gums	4 out of 5 adults with Down's Syndrome have unhealthy teeth and gums	Adults living with families have more untreated decay/poorer oral hygiene	Adults living in residential services had more missing teeth
Dysphagia (difficulties eating, drinking and swallowing)	Significant implications for health and well–being	40% of people with dysphasia suffer frequent respiratory tract infections	Danger of asphyxia, difficulty maintaining a balanced diet and nutrition which effects physical wellbeing, weight maintenance, health, energy levels, hydration and constipation	
Diabetes	There is very little published information on rates of diabetes among people with learning disabilities	One study in the Netherlands indicated an increased rate of diabetes in people with learning disabilities		
Gastro-oesophageal reflux disease (GORD)	More common in children and adults with cerebral palsy (Bower, 2009)	Almost half of a sample of people institutionalised in the Netherlands were reported to have GORD	Causes irritation and pain in the digestive tract, leading to sleep disturbance, potential problem behaviour, anaemia and risk of oesophageal cancer. Anecdotal evidence from experienced carers, dieticians, nurses and physiotherapists who regularly work with people who have complex physical and sensory impairments report that reflux problems are not uncommon due to muscle contractions which can result in postural changes compressing stomach and its contents.	
Constipation	Constipation is a common problem among people with complex physical impairments such as cerebral palsy which is often combined with sensory impairments and affects a large proportion of people with learning disabilities, including individuals with severe to profound learning disabilities (Bower, 2009).			

Some individuals are especially prone to severe constipation which is highly painful and distressing as well as potentially life-threatening. Constipation is exacerbated by poor or inappropriate nutrition, dehydration and lack of mobility. It requires careful management of fluid intake, diet, soluble roughage, exercise and movement and may require manual and medical intervention to manage individuals who are most affected to enable regular evacuation of bowel contents. Where epilepsy is also a factor, constipation is associated with an increased incidence of epilepsy. Similarly the discomfort caused by constipation may be expressed in challenging behaviour.

Osteoporosis	Emerson and Baines (2010) point to Australian and US studies that indicate increased prevalence and a lower bone density than the general population	Contributory factors: lack of weight-bearing exercise, delayed puberty, earlier menopause, poor nutrition, being underweight
Endocrine disorders	9–19% of children with Down's Syndrome have hypothyroidism with a further increase in prevalence associated with ageing	
Injuries, accidents and falls	Higher rates for all of these (some leading to death) are reported among people with learning disabilities	
Socio-economic factors	A person with a learning disability is more likely to experience poverty, poor housing, unemployment, social isolation and overt discrimination	
Communication difficulties	Increased incidences of impaired communication, reading and language difficulties which reduce the individual's health 'literacy'. For example, reducing the ability of people with learning disabilities to convey health needs to people who could support their health needs such as relatives, friends or paid support workers. As a result, carers are important in identifying health needs for many people with more severe learning disabilities but may also have difficulty recognising expressions of need. People with learning disabilities may be less likely to obtain and act upon health promotion information.	
Access to health services	Impeded access to health support due to disabling barriers in the physical layout or location of services, informational barriers, services failing to make 'reasonable adjustments' to compensate for disabilities, attribution of the symptoms of physical ill health to being integral to the learning disability or to mental health or behavioural problems (diagnostic over-shadowing); disablist attitudes within health service staff.	

Sources: Emerson and Hatton (2007); Beresford and Rhodes (2008); Robertson *et al.* (2010); Emerson and Baines (2010).

Table III.2 Some syndromes associated with learning disabilities pose specific health risks

Health risk	Syndrome
Obesity	Prader–Willi syndrome; Cohen syndrome; Bardet–Bedle syndrome
Heart problems	Down's syndrome; William's syndrome
Early onset dementia	Down's syndrome; severe epilepsy, e.g. Tuberous Sclerosis (Epiloia)
Hypothalamic disorder	Prader–Willi Syndrome
Mental health problems and challenging behaviours	Autistic spectrum disorders; Rett syndrome; De Lange syndrome; Riley–Day syndrome; Fragile X syndrome; Prader–Willi syndrome; Velocardiofacial syndrome; Williams syndrome; Lech–Nyhan syndrome.

Sources: Emerson and Hatton (2007); Beresford and Rhodes (2008); Robertson *et al.* (2010); Emerson and Baines (2010).

References

Beresford, B. and Rhodes, D. (2008) *Housing and Disabled Children*. York: Joseph Rowntree Foundation.

Emerson, E. and Baines, S. (2010) *Health Inequalities and People with Learning Disabilities in the UK: 2010, Improving Health and Lives*, Durham: Learning Disabilities Observatory, University of Durham.

Emerson, E. and Hatton, C. (2007). The mental health of children and adolescents with intellectual disabilities in Britain, *British Journal of Psychiatry*, 191: 493–499.

Michael, J. (2008) *Healthcare for All: Report of the Independent Inquiry into Access to Healthcare for People with Learning Disabilities*. London: Department of Health.

Robertson, J., Roberts, H. and Emerson, E. (2010) *Health Checks for People with Learning disabilities: A Systematic Review*. Durham: Improving Health and Lives, Learning Disability Observatory. Available at: www.improvinghealthandlives.org.uk/uploads/doc/vid_7646_IHAL2010-04HealthChecksSystemtic Review.pdf.

13 Supporting people with severe epilepsy: A case study in diagnostic over-shadowing

Malcolm Richardson

Learning outcomes

After reading this chapter you will be able to:

- understand how epilepsy affects people
- know how to support people who have epilepsy
- realise the importance of correct health support when required
- spot the dangers from diagnostic over-shadowing
- understand how some conditions associated with learning disabilities may be life-threatening but can be successfully managed within a rich and diverse lifestyle
- recognise that some conditions associated with learning can lead to premature death
- identify the importance of making reasonable adjustments.

Introduction

About a third of all people with learning disabilities will have epilepsy.

(Michael, 2008)

This chapter begins by considering the nature of epilepsy, how it affects people and how to give appropriate support to people who have epilepsy. The reader will then be introduced to Roger, who had a severe form of epilepsy. Some aspects from Roger's life are considered in order to demonstrate not only the importance of correct health support for people who have learning disabilities and epilepsy, but also some harmful effects that stem from diagnostic over-shadowing. Roger's case study is also employed to assist the readers to think about their own work or practice context and how they may support people who have epilepsy. It also demonstrates that some causes of learning disability can be life-threatening, require skilled support and may yet cause death. Roger's story also reflects some of the celebratory aspects from his life, including that a person with a learning disability has a life and personality that is just as complex, idiosyncratic, humorous, serious and ultimately as fragile as anyone else's, and whose death is mourned just as much by those closest to him, as would befit any human being.

> ## Reader activity 13.1   Many famous and highly successful people have epilepsy
>
> The website below presents a list containing hundreds (and that's only a tiny fraction) of highly successful people throughout all walks of life and throughout history, as well as right now, who have something in common – all of them have epilepsy. http://en.wikipedia.org/wiki/List_of_people_with_epilepsy.

Fast facts 13.1   Epilepsy: general information

- Epilepsy is typically due to abnormal disturbances in the brain as result of lesions causing abnormal neurological disturbances which result in seizures or convulsions (jerking movements).
- Epilepsy is typically described in either of two ways: first, by the type of epilepsy, and, second, by the type of seizure.
- Anyone can have a seizure/convulsion at some point in life.
- Not all seizures are due to epilepsy, some may be due to a temporary cause, such as: high fever; the effects of a drug, abnormal levels of glucose, electrolyte imbalances, alcohol poisoning and other physiological disturbances that can precipitate a convulsion or seizure. Convulsions due to these causes will not repeat once the underlying cause is corrected and therefore these types of convulsions are not epilepsy.
- Similarly, febrile convulsions which arise from a high temperature in a young child are not epilepsy (Epilepsy Society, 2012a, 2012c; Medline Plus, 2012).

How seizures affect a person varies widely between people and knowing the type of epilepsy someone has will not, of itself, tell you much about how that person's epilepsy presents. Some people have more than one type of epilepsy, so even knowing that a person has both major and minor seizures does not tell you what happens to that person during either of these types of seizure. How long a seizure lasts and how frequently they occur tend to be constant for an individual, but can change over time. Not all seizures involve convulsive jerking (sometimes called tonic–clonic convulsions). Some people's seizures occur during the day or can happen at night, some only at night (Epilepsy Society, 2012a, 2012c; Medline Plus, 2012).

Fast facts 13.2   Types of epilepsy

- *Idiopathic epilepsy* – This refers to an obscure or unknown cause which results in chronic seizures usually commencing between ages of 5 and 20 . Sometimes there may be a family history of epilepsy (Epilepsy Society, 2012 a, 2012c; Medline Plus, 2012)
- *Triggers* – Some people's epilepsy can be triggered by specific situations, for example flashing or strobe lighting or lack of sleep, so knowing a person's triggers can help them avoid those situations.
- *Symptomatic epilepsy* – Symptomatic epilepsy arises from a known cause such as:

  - brain tumour or other brain lesions (such as bleeding in the brain);
  - brain injury, damage or defect at any time after conception, during labour, at birth or in later life;
  - stroke, lack of oxygen, transient ischemic attack, Alzheimer's disease;
  - sudden withdrawal from a long period of heavy alcohol consumption;
  - infections that reach the brain, e.g. encephalitis, meningitis, brain abscess, neuro-syphilis and due to auto-immune deficiencies;
  - metabolic disorders such as low blood sugar or an electrolyte imbalance;
  - kidney or liver failure;
  - drug misuse, e.g. cocaine, amphetamines and some other recreational drugs;
  - sudden stoppage of some drugs, such as barbiturates, morphine, sleeping pills, after taking them for a period of time;
  - phenylketonuria (a genetically inherited condition) sometimes causes seizures in infants.

  (Epilepsy Society, 2012a, 2012c; Medline Plus, 2012)

Absence seizures

Absence seizures (sometimes called petit mal) present as a momentary disturbance of brain function due to abnormal electrical activity in the brain, usually of less than 15 seconds. Typically characterised by a vacant staring, it can be so brief as to be almost imperceptible to an onlooker. Absence seizures are commonest in children aged 6–12, usually becoming less common beyond age of 20. An affected individual may have only absence seizures, or can have other types of epilepsy as well, such as generalized tonic-clonic seizures (also termed grand mal seizures), myoclonic seizures where the limbs twitch or jerk, or sudden loss of muscle strength (atonic seizures) (Epilepsy Society, 2012a, 2012c; Medline Plus, 2012). Symptoms of absence seizures may include:

- alterations in consciousness, may be either sudden or gradual, lasting a few seconds to minutes;
- unintentional staring absences;
- sudden cessation of conscious activities such as movement and talking;
- lack of awareness of surroundings;
- may be provoked by stimuli specific to the individual such as flickering images;
- each seizure lasts no more than a few seconds;

- can be full recovery of consciousness with no residual confusion or sometimes recovery may be slower e.g. a short period of confusion or bizarre behaviour;
- no memory of seizure;
- may progress into a different form of seizure (e.g. as a tonic-clonic or atonic);
- muscle activity changes;
- cessation of movement;
- fumbling (commoner with longer absences);
- lip smacking or chewing (especially with longer absences);
- fluttering eyelids.

Tonic-clonic seizures

Tonic-clonic usually arrive suddenly, they last from seconds to a few minutes, they may include an aura (a sensation of some kind that sometimes acts as a warning of an imminent seizure) or there may be a simple partial seizure during which the person has some conscious awareness but which may also include one or more of the following examples (Epilepsy Society, 2012a, 2012c; Medline Plus, 2012):

- change in consciousness, so that the individual is confused or cannot recall a particular period of time;
- emotional states such as fear, panic, joy, or laughter with no external causation;
- sensory hallucinations such as tingling or numbness of the skin, sounds, smells, bright flashes in the eye, tasting a bitter or metallic flavour;
- picking up objects, fiddling with an item for no reason, mumbling;
- wandering around in a confused way, possibly unaware and unable to respond normally to you if you speak to them, if you speak loudly to them they may misinterpret that as aggression and respond aggressively;
- making a loud vocal sound;
- making repetitive movements of face, or limbs.

For some individuals one or more of these kinds of symptoms, such as in the examples above, can be experienced consciously and may act as a warning or aura which indicates that a tonic-clonic seizure is shortly to occur and the person may prepare, by, for example lying down. This may be followed soon by:

- *Tonic seizure* – sudden stiffening and rigidity of muscles, a standing person usually falls backwards and may injure themselves. This often occurs without a warning or aura, is usually brief and the person recovers quickly;
- *Atonic seizure* – A sudden loss of consciousness with accompanying loss of muscle tone which causes the person to fall suddenly, by which the person may be seriously injured;
- *Myoclonic seizure (muscle jerk seizure)* – The person does not usually lose consciousness but jerking movements affect one or more limbs and may spread to other limbs. It can progress into clonic seizures;

- *Clonic seizure – can include the following:*
  - loss of consciousness and a fall accompanied by sudden muscle tension which results in a sudden cry or the person may bite their tongue;
  - rapid alternating rhythmic relaxation and contractions of muscles causing shaking;
  - breathing might be difficult and noisy;
  - skin may change and go pale, then bluish as breathing is impaired;
  - they may wet themselves or involuntarily urinate;
  - the seizure should last only few minutes and stop within 5 minutes. After the seizure the person may feel tired, confused, have a headache, want to rest or sleep.

- *Status epilepticus* – a medical emergency–- any type of seizure normally stops after a few minutes at most. Any type of seizure may also progress into status epilepticus where the seizure continues indefinitely or one seizure is quickly followed by another soon after. If a tonic–clonic seizure continues up to 5 minutes, it should be treated as status epilepticus, which is life-threatening and constitutes a medical emergency. Similarly, if there are repeated seizures one after another, this also constitutes status epilepticus and must be treated as a life-threatening medical emergency.

How you may support an adult who has epilepsy

- *Absence seizure* – though the absence may not always be noticeable, once the absence has ended, you may explain to the person what you noticed, and how long it lasted. If you are a nurse or other person supporting a person with a learning disability, you will also need to record when the absence occurred, how the absence affected the person, how long it lasted, any triggers that may have induced the seizure, and what steps you are taking to support and monitor the person's recovery following the absence seizure.
- *Focal and generalized seizures* – sometimes the individual will have a warning sign that they are about to have a seizure and they may wish to lie down, so far as possible assist/allow them to follow their preferred procedure.

Before and during the seizure, try to ensure the area surrounding the person having a seizure is safe and clear of objects that they might knock themselves against. Note how long the seizure lasts and if it has not ended after 3 minutes, call for medical assistance as this may be status epilepticus. If the seizure lasts as long as 5 minutes, it has become a medical emergency. If you are the person's support carer with access to the individual's anti-convulsant medication for status epilepticus, then administer prescribed medication as required. If, however, the person's seizure ends after a shorter time, ask them if they would like your assistance. Many people with epilepsy will not appreciate you sending for an ambulance or medical help if their seizure has ended without undue harm. They will usually know what to do for their own recovery and have a strategy that they use, so follow their lead whenever possible. If the person has a learning disability, they may need additional support to assist them to recover, for example, they may feel unwell, disorientated, tired and confused. If you are a nurse or other person supporting a person with a learning disability, you will also need to record when and how the seizure began (including if there was any kind of warning sign), how long it lasted and what form it took. Note also any triggers that may have induced the seizure and what steps you are taking to support and monitor the person's recovery following the seizure, including how well and how quickly the recovery progresses.

You can find further general information at Epilepsy Action (2012); Epilepsy Society (2012a, 2012b, 2012c) and Medline Plus (2012).

Case study 13.1   A life with a severe form of epilepsy: Roger's story

Roger was born with a rare genetic condition called Epiloia or Tuberous Sclerosis. This condition is caused by an autosomal dominant gene of poor penetrance, i.e. it can take a few or many years before it becomes apparent and the severity can vary from being imperceptible to causing learning disability with severe epilepsy. About 50 per cent of people with this condition present with a learning disability (Fryer, 1991; Webb *et al.*, 1991; Patient.co.uk 2012). The tuberous growths (harmatomas) that this condition induces within internal organs and the central nervous system can sometimes result in significant health issues.

Roger experienced a normal childhood until the age of 3 when he started to have frequent tonic-clonic seizures. Numerous medical and neurological tests and scans were undertaken to determine the underlying cause of his epilepsy and eventually he was diagnosed with Epiloia.

For the remainder of Roger's childhood his epilepsy was expertly managed by his parents with additional careful monitoring of his condition and anti-convulsant therapy by Roger's consultant physician. Thus his seizures were kept as infrequent as possible. Nevertheless, when they did occur, they were often very severe and sometimes took the form of status epilepticus, which is a life-threatening form of seizure, requiring medical intervention to halt the seizure and thereby prevent death from cardio-respiratory arrest. Roger was also found to have moderate learning disabilities and he attended a special school from ages 4–19.

By his mid-twenties Roger's epilepsy was becoming more frequent and more severe and he left his parents' home to live in a group home where his epilepsy could be carefully monitored and managed by a learning disability nurse who understood his health and social needs. His consultant physician continued to monitor Roger's medical needs arising from epiloia. These arrangements continued for many years.

Reader activity 13.1   Advice and support for epilepsy

Using the information about epilepsy that you have read earlier in this chapter, imagine that you witness a young woman using the services where you work having a tonic-clonic seizure. During the seizure you can assist her by removing any hard or sharp objects close by that she might knock against during the seizure.

- What advice should you give to other people who are not sure what to do?
- What support might the young woman need immediately following the seizure?

Case study 13.2   Roger's active life

At the group home Roger lived with three other people who had learning disabilities. He attended a day centre five days per week where he enjoyed many of the activities and the company of the other people at the centre. He enjoyed living at the group home where he was supported to keep in touch and see his friends and relatives and he quickly formed new friendships with other residents, enjoying the busy social life, as well as his hobbies which included singing and music. In fact, Roger had a fantastic musical memory and despite his learning disability, he could sing the words to almost any pop song from the 1980s, his favourite music era.

Throughout his twenties and thirties and early forties, Roger's anti-convulsant medication was adjusted to compensate for his seizures which became more severe and more frequent. Overall it proved possible to limit his tonic-clonic seizures to about two to three grand mal seizures per month. However, during his twenties, Roger became increasingly susceptible to a form of life-threatening epilepsy called status epilepticus (see above) in which Roger would repeatedly have several tonic-clonic seizures, one immediately after the other, or have seizures lasting more than 3 minutes. Some of these status epilepticus episodes occurred in the middle of the night and as often as five or six times in a year. The staff at the home knew exactly how to monitor and manage status epilepticus attacks both day and night, including access to his medication that normally ends an episode of status epilepticus. Consequently Roger spent about 20 happy years living at the home.

Reader activity 13.2   Support team

People with learning disabilities who have epilepsy and require anti-convulsant medication need support to minimize and manage the frequency, type and severity of their epilepsy.

- If you support a person who has a learning disability and epilepsy where can you find out about their anti-convulsant medication?
- Who in the support team is responsible for administering anticonvulsant medication?
- Do you know how to contact that person in an emergency?
- If you support someone who has severe epilepsy, is that person's anti-convulsant medication accessible at any time of the day/night if needed?
- Who in the support team is responsible for arranging medical reviews to ensure that the epilepsy support to the person with a learning disability remains effective and is reviewed at least annually and whenever there is an adverse change in the person's pattern of epilepsy?
- What examples of changes in a person's epilepsy would lead you to seek a specialist review of their epilepsy or report your observations to someone who can arrange that review?

Case study 13.3 Roger's 45th birthday party

Roger decided that for his 45th birthday he wanted to celebrate by inviting all his family and friends to the local pub for a meal, lots of music, dancing and karaoke. Roger's party was a great success, he and his friends had a great time and Roger was in top form singing his favourite songs from the 1980s on the karaoke. His personal worker videoed much of the party and during the following weeks Roger and his friends enjoyed looking at these video recordings.

Sadly about six weeks after Roger's birthday party, he became very unwell. Initially he suffered several events of daytime and nocturnal status epilepticus within a single week. His learning disability nurse administered Roger's supplementary medication in the usual way, bringing each individual bout of status epilepticus to an end. Nevertheless, by the end of that period, Roger was unable to stand and walk without assistance. Roger's coordination had become noticeably impaired and his speech had become slurred. His learning disability nurse arranged for Roger's doctor to see him. Subsequently the doctor arranged for Roger to be admitted to the local hospital for further medical investigations.

Case study 13.4 Diagnostic over-shadowing of Roger's medical condition

Hospital day 1: Roger was admitted at 10.00 a.m. and given a room to himself. Throughout the day he was very drowsy. The support worker from Roger's home stayed with him until 5 p.m. At various points during that day Roger was visited by different hospital personnel such as doctors and nurses who took the history of Roger's recent illness from his support worker and did tests such as urinalysis, full blood count, blood pressure, temperature, pulse and respiration. Roger was assisted to eat his lunch by his home support worker, but Roger had very little appetite and only ate about half of the food. Roger's home support worker left at 5 p.m.

Hospital day 2: morning: Roger's support worker from his home arrived at 9.00 a.m. to find that Roger's condition had deteriorated. Roger was awake but only able to speak weakly. He asked for a drink and said that he had a bad headache and that he had not had a drink since the previous afternoon. The support worker assisted Roger to take a drink before seeking the nursing staff to find out why Roger had not been assisted with his breakfast and to ask for something for the headache.

The nurse explained to Roger's support worker that Roger had not been cooperative, for example, he would not sit up to take his meal or drink, nor get out of bed to walk to the toilet, so they had 'padded him up' during the night.

Reader activity 13.3 Reasons for dehydration

List some possible reasons why Roger had been left to become dehydrated after his support worker left him on day one through to the following morning.

Fast facts 13.3 Diagnostic over-shadowing

Diagnostic over-shadowing occurs when a real medical condition is misunderstood and ascribed to something different. For example, if a person with a learning disability became ill and that illness produced symptoms of lethargy and apathy, a health worker might assume that these are just aspects of the person's learning disability and fail to recognise these as symptoms of an illness. Or the health worker may assume that the life of a disabled person is not worth living and therefore chooses not to intervene but rather to allow an illness to take its course (Davies, 1987; Mencap, 2007, 2012). See Chapter 21 for more on over-shadowing.

Reader activity 13.4 Explanations

- Can you identify some of the reasons why some aspects of our society lead some people to believe that the lives of disabled are less worthwhile?
- It is becoming more common for disabled people to be depicted positively in the media, can you identify any positive ways that you have seen disabled people in the media? Can you also identify any negative depictions?
- In relation to Roger's hospitalisation, though you may not be a health worker, do you think that all of his medical needs were correctly determined and met when he was admitted and in the hours that followed? What was overlooked?
- Why might it have appeared to the nurses that Roger was not cooperating?
- Could there be other explanations for Roger's apparent lack of cooperation?
- What do you think could have been done differently to ensure that Roger took some food and drink and did not become dehydrated and weak from lack of food?

Case study 13.5 Deterioration

Hospital day 3, afternoon: Roger has taken some food and drinks at regular intervals over the past 24 hours, assisted by his support worker from home during the day and by hospital staff in

(continued)

(continued)

the evenings and early morning. Roger is feeling less drowsy, his headache has cleared but he remains unsteady on his feet and his speech remains slurred. The medical investigations and laboratory reports on Roger's blood and urine have not reported any abnormalities.

At 2 p.m. the physiotherapist calls in to begin assessing Roger's physiotherapy needs with a view to helping Roger regain his mobility. The physiotherapist calls on Roger each day for the next two days.

Hospital day 6, afternoon: Roger's home support worker has returned after taking his two days off during which he left Roger in the capable hands of the hospital staff. Roger appears to be no better, but no worse either. His physiotherapist arrives in the afternoon and tries to coax Roger into some exercises. Roger shows no interest, neither does he show any interest in getting out of bed. He attempts half-heartedly to stand but resists any attempt to make him walk. The physiotherapist tells Roger and his support worker that she can do nothing while Roger refuses to cooperate and try the exercises. The physiotherapist says to the support worker that she thinks Roger is lazy, difficult and uncooperative and that this view is supported by the nursing and medical staff too.

Reader activity 13.5   Views of Roger

Why do you think the physiotherapist or any other staff may hold such views about Roger, might they be accurate, if, so why, if not why not?

Case study 13.6   The real Roger

The physiotherapist was surprised to hear the home support worker assert that Roger's behaviour in hospital is purely due to whatever illness has overcome him recently and that Roger is normally not at all lazy but full of energy and 'the life and soul of the party'. The support worker decides to bring the video of Roger at his last birthday party into the hospital. He hopes it might cheer Roger up a little to see it again and showing it to the hospital staff may convince them of what Roger is like when he is well – and he hopes that maybe then they will appreciate that Roger is actually ill.

Hospital day 7: Roger's home support worker brought the video of Roger's 45th birthday party and some others that he thought Roger might like to see. He also brought some of Roger's favourite music. He played the video to Roger on the TV in his room, Roger smiled a little. Throughout the day the video was replayed to the nurses, doctors and physiotherapist. It was soon apparent to them all that they had no idea that Roger was so different now to how he normally was and that clearly he must be very ill, though as yet they could not be sure of the cause.

Very sadly, Roger did not get well. His rapid health deterioration was found to be entirely due to the tuberous sclerosis with which he had been born and which had entered a terminal phase. Roger returned home to spend the remaining weeks of his life among his friends and with the staff he had known for many years. At home he was visited by other friends and family. Eventually Roger lost consciousness and fell into a coma. He died with family, friends and his support staff with him. His funeral was attended by more than a hundred friends, relatives, neighbours and people who had known and cared for Roger and about him during his life and they watched the video taken at his birthday party with fond memories, some tears and some laughter too, recalling many happy times with Roger.

Reader activity 13.6 Personal record

- Why is it important to help hospital and other staff to know what a person with a learning disability is normally like?
- Have you encountered a personal record held by a person with a learning disability? These records typically inform readers about the person, their likes, dislikes, people who are important and matter to them, some parts of that person's life story, photographs and other things that help people to understand 'who this person is'. If you work to support a person with a learning disability, how can such a record held by the person with learning disabilities be useful?
- How can you help someone create a similar type of record special to that person?
- Do you think most people would understand why people would wish to celebrate the life of a person, like Roger, who has a learning disability? If so why, if not why not?
- Do you think the other residents at Roger's group home should have been allowed to have Roger come home to die where they felt he belonged?
- How should those residents have been consulted about Roger returning home?

Reasonable adjustments

In your work you may come across people who have epilepsy, most people with epilepsy can and do enjoy life doing much the same jobs, roles and activities that they could do without epilepsy and just as successfully. There are somethings that people may not be permitted to do in law if they have epilepsy, for example, driving is prohibited in people with uncontrolled seizures and there are minimum periods of freedom from seizures stipulated before people who have had seizures previously are allowed to drive.

Jobs that involve working at heights or around dangerous machinery or under water may pose real risks to people with epilepsy, but many people with epilepsy do choose to undertake leisure activities that include some of these same risks. People with learning disabilities often wish to engage in the same exciting and risk taking hobbies and activities that many other people choose. Having epilepsy can complicate the choices and opportunities open to them, but with proper risk assessment and support, such choices can often be realised rather than denied.

For example, at the home living level, showering may be thought preferable to taking a bath because of the risk of drowning during a seizure, however, the risk of head injury from falling in the shower may be as great. If the person with a learning disability lacks the capacity to decide this risk for themselves, then someone with capacity has to assist in decisions of this type. That person will often be an individual relative or carer, or in more complex instances a multi-disciplinary team that includes the wishes of the person with the learning disability whenever possible. So someone with a learning disability who has epilepsy will require either a care person to be in the bathroom with them all of the time or just outside a partially open bathroom door that allows the individual privacy but enables constant, watchful help to intervene in the event of a seizure happening in the bath. Even a person who has capacity but whose epilepsy is not currently under full control, may choose to bathe or shower alone or might prefer someone close by to check on them while in the bath to make sure that they have not had a seizure.

Similarly, in the leisure context when swimming, other people (friends, support workers, relatives) should be aware of the person's epilepsy and be attentive while they are in the water. People with epilepsy not only like to enjoy normal, everyday activities, like many other people, some will wish to pursue and enjoy extreme sports or go rock climbing, sailing, cycling and undertake many other so-called 'risky' leisure pursuits. However, if they have a learning disability, they will need additional support to assess the risk to themselves and others and then proper strategies will be arranged and supported that will enable them to undertake their chosen activity in light of the assessed risks.

If your work involves supporting people with learning disabilities to engage in leisure and work opportunities, you should obtain proper training in risk assessment and management so that you can support disabled people to engage in activities that might pose a risk in such a way that the risk is reduced at least to that of a non-disabled person undertaking the same activity. People with learning disabilities may need support to make informed choices about activities and associated risks, even if they have capacity to make the choice.

Mental capacity can be affected by a number of variables, including learning disabilities, so assisting people with learning disabilities to make informed choices about risk requires an understanding of the Mental Capacity Act 2005 (Justice, 2012: legislation.gov.uk).

Essentially, therefore, assessing risk, enabling people to make informed choices and give their consent when they want to choose exciting but risky activities are largely about the people who are supporting those activities making reasonable adjustments. Those reasonable adjustments should ensure that people with physical, neurological, learning or psychological impairments may undertake those activities at no greater risk than anyone else. The right to reasonable adjustments similarly extends into employment and are enshrined in the Equality Act (2010) and in Northern Ireland in the Disability Discrimination Act 1995 (Northern Ireland Direct 2012). You can find out more about reasonable adjustment in Chapter 3.

Reader activity 13.7 Reasonable adjustment

- Make a note of some examples of reasonable adjustment that your workplace has in place already to enable better access and participation by disabled people.
- Are there any additional adjustments that may be necessary to enable people with epilepsy and a learning disability to access and participate effectively in your workplace?

Conclusion

This chapter considered how epilepsy presents in its most common forms and some strategies for supporting people with learning disabilities who have epilepsy. A case study explores diagnostic over-shadowing. Epilepsy may strike any of us at any time, so if it strikes someone with a learning disability, they will need someone to explain all about their particular epilepsy to them, perhaps using easy-to-read information and pictures to enable them to choose the best ways to manage their epilepsy. The Epilepsy Society and a number of other organisations provide information in a format helpful to people with learning disabilities (e.g. Epilepsy Society, 2012b; 2012c).

Points to remember

- Epilepsy affects about one third of all people with learning disabilities.
- People experience different seizures. It is important to know their seizure type and pattern so their needs can be met.
- People's epilepsy can change, so on-going needs should be reassessed
- Risk assessment should enable people to lead active risk-assessed lives.

References

Davies, A. (1987) Women with disabilities: abortion or liberation? *Disability, Handicap and Society*, 2(3): 275–284.

Epilepsy Action (2012) Epilespy Action: advice and information. Available at www.epilepsy.org.uk/info (accessed 18 Oct. 2012).

Epilepsy Society (2012a) Epilepsy Society. About Epilepsy. available at www.epilepsysociety.org.uk/AboutEpilepsy/Whatisepilepsy/Seizures#k (accessed 18 Oct. 212].

Epilepsy Society (2012b) Epilepsy Society. Epilepsy and Learning Disability. Available at http://www.epilepsysociety.org.uk/AboutEpilepsy/Epilepsyandyou/Epilepsyandlearningdisability-1 (accessed 5 Oct. 2012).

Epilepsy Society (2012c) Epilepsy Society. Easy Read Information. Available at http://www.epilepsy-society.org.uk/AboutEpilepsy/Epilepsyandyou/Easyreadinformation (accessed 5 Oct. 2012).

Equality Act (2010) Available at:www.legislation.gov.uk/ukpga/2010/15/section/6 (accessed 18 Oct. 2012).

Fryer, A.E. (1991) Editorial: tuberous sclerosis, *Journal of the Royal Society of Medicine*, 84: 699–701.

Justice (2012) Justice: Protecting the vulnerable. Mental Capacity Act. Available at www.justice.gov.uk/protecting-the-vulnerable/mental-capacity-act (accessed 18 Oct. 2012).

Medline Plus (2012) Epilepsy. Available at: www.nlm.nih.gov/medlineplus/ency/article/000694.htm (accessed 5 Oct. 2012).

Mencap (2007) *Death by Indifference*. Available at www.mencap.org.uk/campaigns/take-action/death-indifference (accessed 18 Oct. 2012).

Mencap (2012) *Death by Indifference: 74 Deaths and Counting*. Available at: www.mencap.org.uk/news/article/74-deaths-and-counting (accessed 18 Oct. 2012).

Mental Capacity Act 2005. Available at:www.legislation.gov.uk/ukpga/2005/9/contents (accessed 26 Oct. 2012).

Michael, J. (2008) *Healthcare for All: Report of the Independent Inquiry into Access to Healthcare for People with Learning Disabilities*. London: Independent Inquiry into Access to Healthcare for People with Learning Disabilities.

Northern Ireland Direct (2012) The Disability Discrimination Act. Available at: www.nidirect.gov.uk/index/information-and-services/people-with-disabilities/rights-and-obligations/disability-rights/the-disability-discrimination-act-dda.htm (accessed 18 Oct. 2012).

Patient.co.uk (2012) Tuberous sclerosis. Available at: http://www.patient.co.uk/doctor/Tuberous-Sclerosis.htm (accessed 4 Oct. 2012).

Webb, D.W., Fryer, A.E. and Osborne, J.P. (1991) On the incidence of fits and mental retardation in tuberous sclerosis, *International Journal of Medical Genetics*, 28: 395–397.

14 A life with cerebral palsy: Neil's story and Jose's case studies

Malcolm Richardson, Bronwyn Roberts and Anne Lyons

Learning outcomes

After reading this chapter you will be able to:

- understand the nature and main features of cerebral palsy and how biological, psychological and social development may be fostered
- appreciate the importance of postural management
- appreciate how adjustments to the environment and strategies of support may promote and facilitate citizenship in relation to people with complex physical and sensory impairment.

Introduction

Seventeen million people are living with cerebral palsy worldwide

(CPA 2013)

This chapter draws on some parts of the life experiences of Neil, who was born with cerebral palsy, and Jose, who has sensory impairments. In so doing, it assists the reader to gain an awareness of the wide range of health and social features surrounding cerebral palsy and sensory impairments, as well as supportive strategies.

Fast facts 14.1   Famous people

- Did you know? There are many people with cerebral palsy and many famous people have cerebral palsy.

- In the London 2012 Paralympics at Greenwich Park, Sophie Christiansen became Britain's first triple gold medalist. Sophie has cerebral palsy (see: http://www.equestrianteamgbr.co.uk/rider.aspx?rider=Sophie-Christiansen).
- Here you can find details of other famous people with cerebral palsy: http://www.disabled-world.com/artman/publish/cp-famous.shtml.
- Also: http://cerebralpalsyworld.com/cp_celebrities.aspx.

Case study 14.1   Neil's story and cerebral palsy

Neil's scenario includes some key health issues at the time of Neil's birth and then supporting Neil through infancy, childhood, adolescence and into adulthood, particularly demonstrating the positive outcomes of having multidisciplinary health support commencing early in life.

Neil is 36 years of age. He works in a garden centre where he tends the greenhouse plants and other horticultural work. Neil was born with cerebral palsy and therefore, at the time of his birth, any notion that Neil might one day find adult employment was far from certain.

His birth was overdue by almost two weeks. At first, it appeared that the delay heralded nothing untoward but then a routine check by the GP indicated the foetus was in distress and subsequently an emergency Caesarean section followed. Immediately after Neil's birth there were serious medical concerns. Although of normal birth weight, Neil was very jaundiced and showing minimal response to stimuli. As the weeks went by it became evident that Neil was floppy, not achieving developmental milestones and was having fits (see Chapter 13).

Cerebral palsy (CP) is the commonest physical impairment in childhood (Scope, 2014). It affects the development of movement and posture and is caused by a non-progressive disturbance in the developing brain, which can result in different forms of cerebral palsy involving one or more limbs and frequently the trunk (Table 14.1). Cerebral palsy is not necessarily associated with having a learning disability, but if other functional areas of the brain are affected, combined physical, sensory and intellectual impairments may result (Scope, 2013a). About a third of people with learning disabilities have a physical disability such as cerebral palsy (Michael, 2008). Different types and combinations of cerebral palsy (Table 14.1) can, to the casual observer, appear the same. The reality, however, is that each individual's cerebral palsy differs in important respects. Therefore, each individual needs a treatment plan tailored to their personal needs. There is no cure for CP and the condition will affect the person throughout their life. Various therapies can and should be used to maximise each person's independence. Current guidelines recommend a network of care team should be evolved around the individual with cerebral palsy, this is defined as 'A multidisciplinary group of healthcare and other professionals working in a network of care to deliver a clinical service' (NICE, 2012, p. 10). Due to the varying levels of severity in cerebral palsy a number of classification systems to promote communication between clinicians are used in practice (Dodd *et al.*, 2010).

A similar group involved with a child might be called the TAC (team around the child) (CWDC, 2009). It is important that these teams work collaboratively, develop effective relationships and implement interventions in partnership with the child, young person or adult, their parents, carers and friends.

Table 14.1 Forms of cerebral palsy

Type of cerebral palsy	Associated characteristics
Dyskinetic (dystonia or choreoathetosis)	Dystonia: involuntary, sustained or intermittent muscle contractions causing twisting or repetitive movements, abnormal postures. Characterised by hyperkinesia (increased activity) and hypertonia (low muscle tone).
Ataxic (rarest from of CP but sometimes appears combined with other forms of CP)	Characterised by an inability to produce smooth coordinated movements in the trunk or limbs, and a lack of balance, for example, when walking, result in an unsteady gait
Spastic bilateral or spastic unilateral cerebral palsy	Spasticity is present in 75–85% of people with cerebral palsy (Krageloh-Mann and Cans, 2009). The limbs of the person resist movement and are stiff. Movements tend to be awkward and difficult to varying degrees depending upon severity. Exaggerated reflexes are present. The spasticity can lead to changes in the soft tissues. Hypotonia or low muscle tone is more common in infants with total body involvement CP; these infants appear very floppy in early life, but this pattern changes and some muscles eventually become overactive, pulling the body into an asymmetrical outline.
Mixed cerebral palsy	Two or more forms of cerebral palsy and may be of varying degrees of severity

Fast facts 14.2   Causes of CP

There may be no obvious explanation for why the person has CP but the main contributory reasons are:

- the mother contracting an infection during pregnancy.
- unusual brain formation of the foetus.
- bleeding in the baby's brain.
- a genetic link which is considered a rarer cause.

There are also some other factors which can contribute to increasing the chances of a person having cerebral palsy:

- premature birth (early birth);
- low birth weight;
- a difficult birth;
- increased numbers of foetuses, i.e. twins and multiple births;
- lack of oxygen during the birth either pre (before birth), peri (during birth) or post (after birth);
- the age of the parents, young or older mums and/or younger fathers.

Cerebral palsy and health

The health issues associated with cerebral palsy are wide-ranging, can differ significantly in their severity between individuals and, like cerebral palsy, require individualised treatment (Bower, 2009; Emerson and Baines, 2010), see Table 14.2.

Impaired muscle control and contractures in hands, limbs and body gradually draw the person's limbs and body outline into tight asymmetrical positions and postures. This may eventually cause pain and compromise internal organs, care, functional mobility and cardio-respiratory function.

Physiotherapists use exercise, and other physical treatments to assist people with cerebral palsy to optimise posture and improve mobility and gross motor skills. They may also recommend mobility devices to aid walking, splints, casts or orthoses (supports for the feet). The physiotherapist monitors the joint range of movement and muscle stiffness, and uses techniques to help prevent secondary impairments associated with contractures or minimise the progression of existing limitations (Dodd et al., 2010).

Occupational therapy supports speech and language acquisition, and plays a key role in the development of fine motor skills such as chewing, swallowing and using a spoon. The techniques employed are determined by the degree of physical and sensory impairments present and what programme of therapy will be advantageous in maintaining and improving the range and extent of gross and fine motor skills and maintenance of body symmetry. Medical treatments with muscle relaxants may also be beneficial (Scope, 2013a, 2013b, 2013c, 2013d), for example, intrathecal baclofen therapy comprises a muscle relaxant used to relieve severe spasms in the limbs, which may interfere with personal care. Similarly, Botulin Toxin A (BTA) has been used to reduce over-activity (spasticity) in

Table 14.2 Health and social issues associated with cerebral palsy

- Motor function skills, such as walking, will be affected.
- Muscle imbalances can lead to hip dislocation and spinal curvature and muscle contractures, resulting in unusual body shapes. These can cause compression of internal organs and exacerbation of conditions such as cardiovascular and respiratory problems.
- Poor cardiovascular circulation.
- Individual eating, chewing and swallowing difficulties require significant assistance with eating and drinking.
- Gastrointestinal problems, such as oesophageal reflux, chronic constipation or even malnutrition weakness in the leg muscles resulting in reduced weight bearing, cause a reduction in bone density with proneness to bone fracture.
- Learning difficulty (although children with cerebral palsy cover the same range of intelligence as other children).
- Epilepsy (up to a third of children with cerebral palsy).
- Hearing impairment (only 8% of children).
- Difficulties with sleeping.
- Communication difficulties require the use of various communication strategies to support verbal or replace verbal communication.
- Needing help with personal care such as going to the toilet.
- Difficulties with spatial awareness and perception.
- Behavioural issues (one in four children with cerebral palsy).
- Pain and discomfort.

selected muscles. Selective dorsal rhizotomy, a neurosurgical procedure, can reduce the effects of spasticity in the lower limbs in people with cerebral palsy.

Thus, physiotherapy and occupational therapy are important to enabling children, young people and adults with cerebral palsy to be more active and better able to participate in play, study, work, recreation, relationships and citizenship (Dodd *et al.*, 2010). Carers can also be trained by these therapists to deliver this type of support on a daily basis.

Complex physical and sensory impairments are sometimes accompanied by profound learning disabilities and epilepsy that is often severe and difficult to control by medication without inducing other problems. As previously mentioned, the presence of any one of these health factors in an individual's life may result in significant health needs.

People with profound learning disabilities and complex physical and sensory impairment therefore represent one of the most vulnerable groups of people whose health and well-being throughout their lifespan will be determined almost entirely by the kind of society in which they live and the people who support their daily living. Therefore, supporting people who have complex physical and sensory impairments demands a wide range of competences in the lifelong management not only of a range of physical and sensory difficulties but of the combined health-related complexities that arise. Let's begin considering how to achieve this support by looking more closely at the health implications arising from Neil's cerebral palsy.

Reacting to a diagnosis

Reader activity 14.1 Immediate questions

- How soon and where (a private office or room, in the corridor, at the bedside, other locations) would be appropriate to giving difficult news such as informing Neil's parents about their newborn baby's health frailties? (Chapters 7 & 8 may help you when considering this point)
- What should Neil's parents be told about Neil? How can this be done in a supportive way?
- Which locations would be less appropriate for talking with parents about potentially serious issues and why?
- Parents on first hearing that their child has cerebral palsy are likely to suffer quite a degree of shock, fear and panic. They will have both emotional and practical needs and may not initially be able to process any information given to them. Also, they will probably seek answers to many questions, for example,

  ○ What is CP?
  ○ 'How can I help my child? I don't know anything about it, what can we expect?' (Bower, 2009).
  ○ Why has this happened to us? What have I/we done wrong?

- If you work in child health, could you answer any of these questions or would you be able to help the parents make contact with someone who can?
- Make a brief network outline of potentially helpful people, sources of help and information about CP that you currently know of. Make a plan to address any gaps in your knowledge.
- Identify a list of positive behaviours you might use with the child.

Parental participation in the care and development of their children is fundamental. In relation to Neil's birth, his parents described how they were informed within half an hour of Neil's birth that Neil might not survive. Neil's parents recall their anxiety surrounding the events leading up to his birth, their worry about his birth being so much overdue and then the difficulties surrounding the birth and for a very long time afterwards. High quality support to parents is crucial to their coping with such questions as those above and the emotional and personal barriers that could otherwise prevent their participation.

In Neil's case, the midwife and doctors involved probably handled the events and breaking the news to Neil's parents as well as possible. Neil's mum describes how the midwife came to her immediately when Neil was delivered to inform her that he was having breathing difficulties which they were dealing with and as soon as possible she could see and hold him. Later Neil's parents did get to hold him briefly and shortly afterwards the consultant came and explained to them that, though Neil was now breathing quite well, he was still very weak indeed and though they would do all they could to help him pull through, it was going to be a close call, especially in the immediate hours and days ahead. Neil's parents say they appreciated the hospital staff's honesty, sympathy and kindness. It helped them to cope with the unthinkable knowledge that their baby might not survive and, much later, that he would have cerebral palsy all of his life.

Reader activity 14.2   Medical sensitivity

If the midwives, doctors and other hospital staff who knew how poorly Neil's condition was, had been evasive, insensitive or dismissive in handling the news to Neil's parents, how might that have affected the parents?

Respiration problems

Respiratory disease is the leading cause of death in people with learning disabilities (Emerson and Baines, 2010; Table 14.2). Where cerebral palsy is a factor, this is partly due to absent or reduced reflexes for coughing and swallowing, a sedentary life and muscle contractures that produce marked changes in body symmetry and can lead to compression of the chest cavity and lungs therein. Health support therefore necessitates, among other things, that carers be proficient in several areas (Bower, 2009), see Table 14.3.

Reader activity 14.3   Breathing exercise

- Restrict your breathing by deliberately taking shallow, less than adequate breaths for one minute (time yourself).
- What did you notice?
- Now try to imagine if your body had cerebral palsy and your respiratory muscles were not strong, if your posture and body symmetry were out of alignment, constricting your lungs and other internal organs. How would this affect your health, your skin, your energy levels, your ability to relax?

On-going health needs

Table 14.3 Health support to people with CP necessitates a wide range of proficiencies

- Supporting breathing
- Airways maintenance
- Daily postural care to support a symmetrical body outline and ease of respiration
- Postural drainage to help maintain clear airways
- Supporting nutrition and hydration
- Supporting general physiotherapy
- Supporting skin care
- Supporting exercise and rest
- Supporting social engagement

Source: Bower (2009).

As you will see later, Neil proved to be quite a resilient fellow. Reader activity 14.4 contains some examples of the things you would need to consider in order to support a person like Neil.

Reader activity 14.4   Supporting people with CP

If you support a person with cerebral palsy, like Neil, you will need to develop, maintain and update your knowledge and skills as that person develops and progresses through childhood, adulthood and into older age.

You would need to consider:

- When was Neil's physiotherapy and occupational therapy last assessed, are both up to date?
- Do I have contact details for physiotherapy and occupational therapy support?
- When is the next review due?
- What daily activities and actions should I and others take to support Neil with regards to the following?
  - posture
  - movement
  - mobility
  - weight bearing
  - breathing
  - mealtimes
  - recreation/leisure/play
  - skin hygiene
  - dental and oral hygiene
  - communication
  - personal choices and autonomy
- What training do I need to help me understand and support Neil with all of the above?
- How will this differ for children/adults and older people?

Neil's cerebral palsy was identified early and his paediatrician ensured that Neil was referred to a physiotherapist who specialised in working with cerebral palsy. Not every town had access to such a specialist but Neil was fortunate in this regard because of where his parents lived. Neil's physiotherapy began in his infancy and was of several types to help promote his development, his posture, breathing, gross motor skills (i.e. the larger muscles such as those in his trunk, arms and legs) and also to help Neil with his fine motor skills. As a consequence, over time Neil's balance and movement improved considerably as did his fine motor skills like using a spoon to eat his meals. To attain and maintain this gradual improvement, his physiotherapist coached Neil and his parents and carers at his schools to undertake his daily physiotherapy. In this way some of Neil's muscles were exercised actively using goal-directed tasks in order to strengthen muscles, and his limbs were passively moved to prevent the muscles tightening up. In infancy Neil was prone to respiratory infections, and daily postural drainage undertaken with Neil lying face down on a foam rubber wedge, helped to drain excess fluids from Neil's chest (Physiotherapy Treatment, 2010 online). Gradually as Neil got older, it was possible to reduce the frequency of these chest clearance techniques.

Daily physiotherapy, throughout Neil's childhood, helped him achieve some important developmental motor milestones. His muscles strengthened and Neil learnt to sit with less and less support so that he progressed from supported sitting, gradually to balancing his body sitting on a floor mat. As his balance and muscle coordination improved, Neil learnt how to roll from sitting, thus building his confidence as he progressed towards learning to crouch and crawl and then to stand with aid and later still to make some walking steps. He also learnt how to sit independently on a stool.

Reader activity 14.5   Daily support

- If you work in an area where you support people with cerebral palsy, are all staff aware of the importance of daily physical support such as Neil was accustomed to and outlined above?
- Is such support, when needed, available and accessible to service users who need it in your area?
- Are any reasonable adjustments to the organisational set-up necessary to enable such supports to be readily accessible when required? If not, how can this be remedied?

Using a wheelchair, other adaptive equipment and other movement and communication skills were all aspects of Neil's therapy and learning. Always it was Neil, together with his carers, who put in the work and made the progress. Much of this was done as part of Neil's structured play and was made into fun activities (see Table 14.4).

Occupational therapy was combined with physiotherapy to aid the development of his fine motor skills and his ability to use both his hands together. The occupational therapist always focused on activities of importance to Neil, for example, as an infant and toddler, they helped Neil's family select suitable toys for play. At school, they focused on his self-care and goal-directed tasks, using tools and technology to advance his learning. Neil's occupational therapist and physiotherapist worked together

Table 14.4 Some examples of play activities that supported Neil's biological, psychological and social development

- Putting Neil onto the floor to let him explore the surroundings at his own pace. If he tended to lie still in one spot, he was helped to change positions often.
- Taking Neil to parks, gardens, zoos, playgrounds, markets and so on, to help with his sensory, motor, social and psychological development.
- Playing games that encourage crawling. Weight-bearing on one hand or both hands and on legs to promote the development of good muscle tone.
- Placing toys that are stimulating in colour, shape, texture and smell, as well as easy to play with, at a distance for Neil to reach out to touch/pick up or crawl towards them.
- Encouraging Neil to put away his toys by himself even if that is slow and time-consuming.
- Encouraging Neil to make friends with other children and ensure so far as possible that he was included in their play. For example, Neil attended an ordinary day nursery from ages 3–5. At age 9, he enrolled in cub scouts, and tried out a few other children's clubs, children's gym classes and other physical exercise programmes that also cater to special needs children. These helped him to meet new friends as well as promote Neil's general physical and social well-being.
- Taking Neil on bicycle rides and, when a bit older and stronger, helping him pedal and then to ride his own tricycle.
- Swimming was especially good for increasing or reducing muscle tone and also helped improve Neil's lung capacity, breathing and cardiovascular strength.
- Playing games with balls to develop good coordination and motor skills.
- Placing a well-anchored, wide, strong plank at a small height from the ground and playing a game of walking from one end to the other without falling off helped improve Neil's balance.
- Neil was encouraged to draw and paint, with his hands and fingers initially and brushes later. This helped instil a feeling of creative achievement as well as the ability to hold objects.
- Neil enjoyed playing with bread dough, plasticine or clay which he could roll and mould and was excellent exercise for his hands.
- Neil liked to look at picture books with his mum and dad and to talk about the pictures and they encouraged Neil to identify the different objects in them.
- Because Neil had speech difficulties, a game was created using signs and picture boards to aid communication. This improved Neil's confidence in communicating his wishes, likes and dislikes so that as his speech developed and his verbal articulation improved, he became less reliant upon signing and other communication aids.
- Neil was afforded many opportunities to have fun, laugh and feel good about himself.

and with Neil and his carers to choose the right type of adaptive equipment that would improve Neil's motor skills. These included wheelchairs, walkers, special eating utensils and other equipment to provide Neil with the freedom to accomplish some tasks on his own, such as holding a spoon, eating, dressing, drawing, and so on.

Speech and language therapy helped Neil to communicate more easily with other people by developing his facial and jaw muscles, improving his speech and sign language, and introducing communication tools such as computers and other visual aids.

- For Neil to attend a pre-school day nursery, what reasonable adjustments do you think would need to be in place to facilitate Neil's daily physiotherapy, postural care, assistance with meals and social engagement?
- Non-disabled children at Neil's day nursery simply accepted a child who used a wheelchair, but as Neil grew older such acceptance was harder to win. How might older school children and adolescents be better informed about CP so that they are more likely to be accepting and inclusive of their peers with physical impairments and/or learning disabilities?
- In your workplace, what is done to foster acceptance and inclusivity of people who are different and in particular people who, like Neil, have physical and sensory impairments and a learning disability?

Neil and epilepsy

During Neil's infancy it became apparent that occasionally Neil would appear to become vacant, and lose both concentration and focus on any activities in which he was engaged. His paediatrician suspected that Neil might be experiencing a form of epilepsy known as absence seizures (see Table 14.5 and Chapter 13 in this volume). Some medical tests were conducted, including an EEG (electroencephalograph) which records electrical rhythms in the brain. These confirmed that Neil was experiencing regular absence seizures lasting up to 0.25 seconds and up to ten times in 24 hours. Each absence meant that for a brief moment of time Neil lost consciousness, not long enough or sufficiently to fall over, but long enough to interrupt his concentration and therefore adversely affect his activities of living.

Anti-convulsant medication especially suited to the treatment of absence was commenced during Neil's infancy and proved effective in eliminating Neil's absence events almost completely. By about the age of 13, Neil became completely free of absence episodes and gradually his medication for this was reduced and eventually ceased. Neil has now been free of absence for more than 20 years. It is not unusual for childhood epilepsy, such as Neil experienced, to disappear eventually. Potentially,

Table 14.5 Absence epilepsy characteristics

Absence seizures or absence epilepsy are terms used to describe a momentary disturbance of brain function due to abnormal electrical activity in the brain, usually of less than 15 seconds. Typically characterised by a vacant staring, it can be so brief as to be almost imperceptible to an onlooker.

Absence epilepsy is commonest in children ages 6–12, usually becoming less common beyond age 20. An affected individual may have only absence epilepsy or can have other types as well, such as generalized tonic-clonic seizures, myoclonic seizures where the limbs twitch or jerk, or sudden loss of muscle strength (atonic seizures).

Symptoms of absence seizures are included in Chapter 13.

Source: Medline Plus (2013).

epilepsy can arise unexpectedly in anyone at any time of life. Sometimes it remains and has to be controlled by medication, and sometimes it disappears of its own accord, never to return. We cannot know for sure that Neil's epilepsy is gone forever, but more than 20 years without is a good sign (Medline Plus, 2012).

Cerebral palsy: incontinence and constipation

Another factor in supporting the health of a person with cerebral palsy is incontinence and constipation. Urinary incontinence arises from palsy in the bladder sphincter muscles or inability to control this sphincter. This can lead to urinary tract infections due to a condition called vesico–ureteral reflux. This can occur when the bladder attempts to empty. Some urine leaves the body via the urethra, as it should, but occasionally some urine is pushed back up the ureters towards the kidneys and can cause kidney damage. The bladder may not empty completely, leaving urine in the body where bacteria can multiply, causing an infection. These problems are most prevalent in individuals for whom their motor neurone damage has led to poor bladder functioning. Similarly, bowel incontinence arises primarily from neuromuscular anomalies in the bowel sphincters and the muscles controlling peristalsis.

Faecal soiling can result when there is a blockage in the bowel, for example, due to faecal impaction (a hard mass of dry stool which is difficult to pass). As a consequence some liquid faeces sometimes escape around the blockage.

Children with CP may be fearful of using the lavatory if they are unsteady in gait or balance. For example, the child may worry about falling into the toilet or falling off it. Although cerebral palsy by itself is not necessarily the cause of incontinence, it was, however, a major contributor to Neil's incontinence.

Both urinary and bowel incontinence require careful, lifelong management not only to promote health, minimise the risk of urinary infections and maintain the health of skin which is coming into frequent contact with the body's astringent waste products, but also to promote the personal dignity of the individual.

Neil's cerebral palsy never stopped him from trying to explore his environment, for example, during his infant years he would shuffle across a room or the ground on his bottom, later he would crawl and roll and later still stand and walk with a walking aid. Neil therefore required a diet similar to that of any active youngster, balanced, nutritious and containing plenty of calories for him to burn up during his activities. However, having CP requires special attention to dietary and nutritional needs (see Table 14.6). For more detailed information on eating with CP, see The Cerebral Palsy Alliance, ParentWise Podcast Series, Making the Most of Your Child's Mealtimes (CPA, 2013).

Neil's facial muscles that controlled his lips, chewing and swallowing were affected by his cerebral palsy. This made chewing hard solid food like a piece of fresh apple impossible, as he would have been unable to chew and swallow it. The consequence of attempting to eat such foods would put Neil's life at risk from choking, so all of Neil's food has to be made soft, as well as appetising and appealing to look at. Additionally, prior to assisting Neil to take his meal, his parents needed to stimulate Neil's lips, cheeks and throat muscles by gently massaging them, which helped Neil to relax and prepare for chewing and swallowing. They placed a small spoonful of food in the centre of Neil's tongue so that he was least likely to push his tongue forward reflexively and thereby push food back out of his mouth.

Table 14.6 Supporting mealtimes with a child who has cerebral palsy

- CP can affect the neuro-muscular functioning, sensation and reflexes in the face, lips and throat that are involved in eating, chewing and swallowing. It is important therefore to ensure that a child's fluid, nutritional and calorie intake is adequate in order to ensure healthy growth, development and fluid intake. Often foods will need to be made soft or semi fluid in order to aid swallowing and thus prevent dehydration, malnutrition, coughing, choking and to promote foodstuffs entering the stomach rather than aspiration into the airways and lungs which can result in potentially fatal choking or lung infection (pneumonia).
- Making mealtimes safe and enjoyable is therefore crucial and should enable the child to anticipate and enjoy mealtime routines, also providing an opportunity for social interaction and for the child to express emotions as well as his food preferences.
- All carers should be trained in how to support mealtimes, including correct posture and positioning of the child, food preparation, the appropriate technique for feeding a meal, the child's preferences and of course making mealtimes an enjoyable social event.
- CP can also create or exacerbate stomach and intestine disorders such as GORD which may adversely affect mealtime enjoyment and comfort after taking food or drink.

Because Neil's intestinal and bowel muscles were affected by cerebral palsy, the peristalsis by which these muscles convey food from his stomach through his digestive passages and out via his bowel was slow and Neil was very prone to constipation. To minimise this, Neil's diet has to contain sufficient fluids, soluble fibre (from fruit and vegetables) and a minimal amount of non-soluble fibre (such as wheat bran) to give some bulk, but not too much to his stools, to help the process of peristalsis. His diet also includes some prescribed supplements to help keep moisture in his stools and avoid constipation. Nevertheless, Neil remains prone to severe and painful constipation which has to be monitored and treated when necessary.

The dietician regularly assessed Neil's diet throughout his childhood. Even so, Neil would sometimes very rapidly develop a severe constipation which became quickly impacted. Laxatives did help prevent constipation, but frequent use eliminates much of their effectiveness. Occasionally manual evacuation aided by an enema was necessary to prevent or alleviate the discomfort of the constipation which would, if untreated, become life-threatening.

Today Neil is able to manage his own diet. He still sees the dietician from time to time to make sure he has the right dietary balance and to minimise constipation. He enjoys food and likes a varied diet, his meals still need to be made soft, for example, by putting them through a blender or by liquidising them.

Reader activity 14.7   Mealtimes

You are helping a person with cerebral palsy to take their meal and you are fully aware that she has some chewing and swallowing difficulties. Today's meal comprises chicken, peas, carrots, cabbage and potato.

- How would you prepare the plate of food so that this girl can experience the different colours, textures and flavours of the different foods on her plate?

- What stimulation of lips, neck, cheek and throat muscles may be required before commencing the meal?
- In this example, choking is a potential hazard so food needs to be liquidised. Even so, the aspiration of food (inhalation into the air passages leading to the lungs) remains a potential hazard. If you assist with meals in this type of context, you must follow the guidance and instructions of a speech and language therapist or occupational therapist who can assess the risk and plan an appropriate mealtime strategy.
- Do you know how to deliver first aid to someone with CP who is choking? If not, find out.

Case study 14.2   Neil's story – in conclusion

Many people with cerebral palsy are able to make similar progress to Neil's. Much depends upon the extent of the cerebral palsy and whether or not there is a severe or profound learning disability and/or additional sensory impairments. People whose impairments turn out to be much more severe than Neil's may not progress to the same extent as was possible for Neil, i.e. all the way from supported sitting to walking, being able to articulate speech and develop fine motor skills.

Today Neil works in a garden centre. He can walk unaided though his gait is affected by the spasticity in his leg muscles, so when necessary he will also use an electric scooter to get about. His speech is a little slow and slightly slurred. He is continuing to make progress in learning to read, swims regularly and hopes to set up home with Jenny, his girlfriend.

It is evident that each individual's cerebral palsy has to be determined and treated according to the individual's differences in the presentation of CP. Although CP alters over time, it is amenable to treatment. Therefore, a person with CP is as unique as anyone else with tremendous capacity for growth and development. A casual encounter or acquaintanceship with a person who has cerebral palsy may give you lots of clues about the person, their personality, likes, dislikes, problems and personal strengths, for example. However, many of these clues can be occluded when an individual is ill or has communication difficulties.

Reader activity 14.8   Learning about CP

- In relation to your area of working, how might you obtain a clearer, more holistic picture of a person with CP whom you do not know well and whose communications you do not understand? Who might know more about the person and can tell you?
- How can you record for future reference and pass on that clearer 'picture', once you have obtained it, to your colleagues so that they will be better informed in their support to this individual?
- What will you need to know about the person with CP?

Some areas of potential interest may include one or more of the following depending upon the circumstances:

- how the individual's day normally starts and their daily routines;
- viewing a video/home movie clip to understand the individual's normal kinds of activities, behaviours and ways of communicating;
- the type of CP, movement disorder and effects on different parts of the body;
- emotional support.

Find out about the person's problems with:

- hearing;
- vision;
- epilepsy;
- speech and language;
- learning disability;
- perception, e.g. judging size and shape of objects.

Find out about their general health including:

- nutritional and dietary needs;
- management of bowel/constipation, incontinence and urinary bladder function;
- weight/obesity;
- dental care;
- osteoporosis, orthopaedic treatment;
- GORD (gastro oesophageal reflux disease);
- respiratory health or lung disease.

Go back to Reader activity 14.3 and add some more points here.

Supporting people with multiple/complex needs using postural management equipment

All people with cerebral palsy have impaired motor function, and some have physical and sensory impairments that restrict movement and posture severely. For example, an individual may have severe physical, learning and communication difficulties and therefore is unable to walk or stand unaided, and is unable to sit in a standard chair without additional postural support. The person may also have difficulties holding the head upright, maintaining their trunk position or controlling their limbs.

Without postural support, people with this level of cerebral palsy cannot maintain a normal body posture, such as keeping the head, neck and trunk in mid-line while seated. Unsupported, their bodies appear to bend and buckle, under their own weight (Pope, 2007). Personal care handling can be difficult for family and other caregivers but, with external body support, safety in sitting becomes possible. A seating intervention is a deliberate physical adjustment of an individual's position to improve his or her seated posture (Costigan and Light, 2011). Maintaining optimal postural positioning is fundamental to promoting health and well-being. See Fast facts 14.3.

Fast facts 14.3 Creating the optimal sitting position

Correct sitting and seating are important for many reasons, such as:

- It provides a platform to enable practical access to transportation.
- It should enhance alertness, task participation (feeding, switch access for a toy or communication device) and performance.
- It allows enhanced opportunity for participation in life situations, access to contemporary educational strategies and social skills training.
- It provides an opportunity for quality one-to-one communicative interactions with a parent, teacher or support worker.
- It supports therapeutic goals as an adjunct to direct treatment interventions.

Unfortunately, people with this severity of physical and sensory impairments are at high risk of secondary health conditions. Their disordered muscle tone and muscle imbalances may lead to soft tissue and body contractures, joint subluxations or dislocation and atypical alignment of the body parts. Sitting postures can deteriorate, significantly affecting thoracic and pelvic structures and the risk of respiratory complications and pressure sores increase. Positioning may become uncomfortable or even painful, making caregiving more difficult.

Therapists, who function within a wide social context but with sound knowledge of these common health issues related to musculoskeletal health conditions, are in a key position to ensure that people with these complex needs receive preventative healthcare. In contributing to an individual's care plan, these professionals seek to achieve the person-centred functional aims described above, while optimising current evidence and positioning principles to prevent deterioration of body shape. The interventional approach is referred to as postural management; in addition to the provision of customised seating (Figure 14.1), other items of positioning equipment, including night-time positioning, as listed in Table 14.7 may also be recommended.

Standing devices may also be useful. The individual is secured in an aligned position, and then the angle of the device is adjusted. This item of equipment allows the individual to perceive and interact with the environment from a more upright position

The individual may be prone, supine or upright. These devices have pelvic, chest, leg/knee and foot positioning support and head support if required. They often have a mobile chassis and an activity tray. Not all individuals are suitable for this type of equipment.

The night-time position is very important in postural management, most of us spend many hours in bed each night (Figure 14.2). Children, for example, spend four times longer in bed than at school (Hill and Goldsmith, 2009). Early provision of a child- and family-centred postural management care

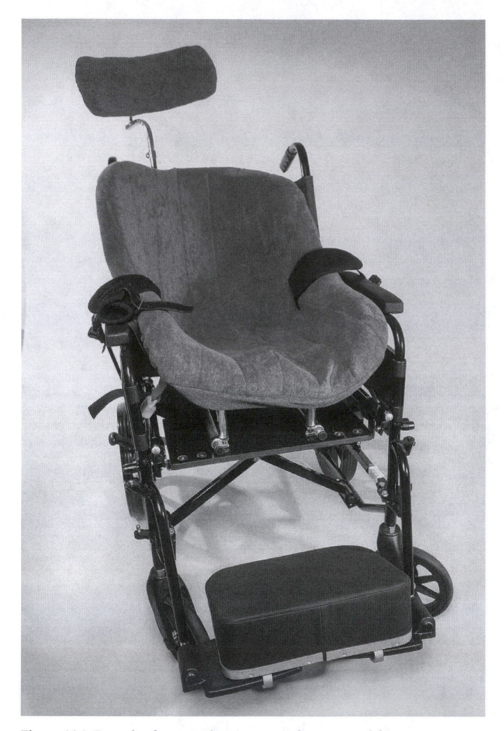

Figure 14.1 Example of contoured seating system for a young adult

Source: Reproduced with permission of Peacocks Posture Care.

Table 14.7 Postural management

Type	Features
Seating systems	Alignment in sitting is considered important for function. Seating systems often have contoured cushioning to support the pelvis
See Figure 14.1	Seating systems may have different seat surface inclinations
	Seating systems have a pelvic positioning harness
	Seating systems often have a contoured back and lateral supports
	Seating systems may have contoured headrests
	Footplates often have sandal straps
	A chest harness may be necessary
	Activity tray
	The seating system may interface with a wheelchair, a pushchair, a stroller, or a Hi Low chassis
	Seating systems may tilt in space and have angled adjustment to allow active and relaxing positions for the user
	Floor sitters allow young children to be involved in floor activities with their peers
Night-time support or sleep systems and side lying devices	These support the individual in an aligned position. Systems can be used for supine, prone or side lying
	Some positioning straps will be necessary

plan is the first step and some infants are less than 6 months old when a postural management programme begins. This should, however, be re-evaluated regularly with the family and across the lifespan.

Postural management is

a planned approach encompassing all activities and interventions which impact on an individual's posture and function. Programmes are tailored specifically for each child and may include special seating, night-time support, standing supports, active exercise, orthotics, surgical interventions, and individual therapy sessions.

(Gerricke, 2006, p. 224)

Over several decades, significant effort has gone into developing multisensory teaching approaches, sensory learning environments, hydrotherapy, physiotherapy, and physical care routines (Aird, 2012). All of these are vitally important to the success of any postural management programme, as they allow the individual to have time out of adaptive equipment such as leg braces and postural supportive wheelchairs. Equipment does, however, remain important as it provides the external postural support to help to maintain body alignment when the individual cannot maintain their own posture through automatic muscle activity. For these individuals, limited positioning options are available, and without the use of adaptive equipment, the unsupported lying position becomes a real and hazardous possibility by increasing the risk of secondary complications due to poor positioning.

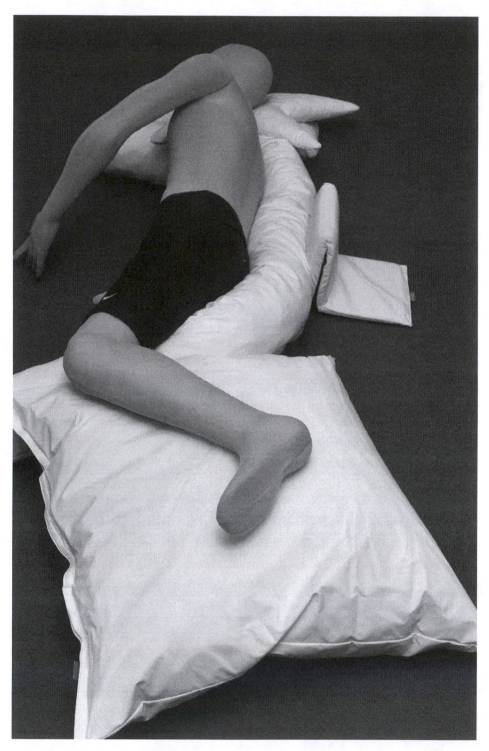

Figure 14.2 The night-time position

Equipment should, however, positively impact on the individual, the family and other caregivers, and it should not be seen as a burdensome barrier to daily routines. Hastiness of care tasks can produce positioning errors. Those responsible for positioning should be mindful of the barriers to successful implementation and accept responsibility for ensuring the individual's optimal level of comfort while using the equipment. Used excessively or inappropriately, well-designed equipment will produce experiences of an adverse physical nature, including discomfort and fatigue. It may also limit any spontaneous movement the individual may possess. Given the social and interactional world in which people with multiple needs live and learn, and the complex nature of their difficulties, successful use requires the combined efforts of parents, teachers, key workers, nurses, therapists and other multi-agency team members to help and support the correct type and use of any equipment, recommended within his or her education, health and care plan effectively (Department of Education, 2012).

This is more likely to occur if:

- the equipment is customised to user requirements;
- the person is positioned without errors;
- an agreed, individual care plan with time restrictions on equipment use is in place and constant, unchanging postural positions are avoided;
- attention is given to the mode of engagement, task or activity being undertaken by the child or young person while using the equipment;
- all caregivers gain an understanding of the issues surrounding postural care;
- communicative partners can affirm the categorical nature of the individual's expressive non-verbal behaviours;
- the professionals with seating/positioning expertise who provide the service communicate effectively and work collaboratively with all those who have positioning/repositioning responsibilities.

Reader activity 14.9   Imagining living with CP

Think about the following experiences:

- Your shoes are placed on the wrong feet and you are compelled to continue with your daily tasks, unable to swap them over.
- On an 8-hour flight, instead of a seatbelt, you have a harness and your feet are strapped to the floor. The flight attendant informs passengers they cannot vacate their seat due to turbulence.

Having thought about the above, you can perhaps better appreciate the importance of people who need it having support to change their posture at regular intervals.

As postural management must be intrinsically combined with attentive care-giving, all staff working with this client group need to gain an understanding of the issues surrounding postural management, and have the confidence to reposition the individual when required.

Guidelines for positioning in this chapter can only be very general as, by definition, the postural programme is individualised, and the process of selection is dependent upon the assessment of a multitude of criteria. Occupational therapists and physiotherapists use the World Health Organisation's International Classification of Functioning, Disability and Health as a framework to assist in the decision-making surrounding equipment provision as this allows appreciation of the complex inter-actions between the person's primary impairments of body function, their environment, the activities they undertake and the life areas in which they participate (McDonald *et al.*, 2004).

With optimum positioning of the pelvis (Table 14.8), consideration can be given to alignment of the trunk, head and neck. Lateral trunk supports are often necessary, and if *in situ* should not be removed. The person should not tilt over the lateral supports, but neither should they be high up in the axilla (armpit). Any front harness should be correctly located to avoid any chance of it slipping up under the chin. If the system has a number of straps, numbering or colour coding may help.

Security comes from the feet on the footrests. The height relationship between the seat and the footrests must be correct. Some individuals may wear splints to help maintain the position of the feet.

It is important to create opportunities for task engagement and participation while the individual uses the equipment in order to make the experience pleasant and engaging, so a range of interesting activities from which to choose are vital. An occupational therapist can help to identify suitable activities.

Table 14.8 Key positioning messages for positioning a person in his/her adaptive seating

- Always gain familiarity with the equipment, inspect the features and accessories
- The individual needs to be positioned correctly on each occasion, with accessories and harnesses secured to achieve the desirable position
- If a hoist is used for the transfer, some repositioning may be necessary
- Pelvic position for sitting: this is most important and an appropriate weight-bearing surface is necessary to adequately position the pelvis for stability
- Focus attention on the seated surface and aim to locate the pelvis and hips square (symmetrical alignment) and at the rear of the seat surface
- NB the pelvis may not always be symmetrical; some individuals cannot sit with their pelvis square, and the pelvis may be rotated and/or tilted. If this is the case, seek guidance from those with experience, aim for the alignment but do not over-stretch the limbs.
- Secure the pelvis with the pelvic positioning belt. It should be secure, not slack or restrictive, and if pelvic guides (supports on either side of the hips) are present, leave *in situ*. Also do not remove the guide at the lower part of the backrest (sacral), if this is present
- If the pelvis is well supported, thigh support from the seat should extend to just behind the knees, but there should be no pressure on the back of the knees.
- With the pelvis square, there should be space between the thighs, and an accessory might be used to maintain this position
- Length of time: how long should be spent in a given position should be clearly indicated in the individual postural care plan, but do look out for warning signs of discomfort or fatigue, and reposition if necessary.

Sensory impairments

If you wear a pair of spectacles with dirty, smudgy, scratched lenses, seeing becomes impaired, light refracts off the dirt and scratches, sometimes making it impossible to see. Something similar happens when driving a car with a dirty windscreen into bright sunshine or oncoming head lights. So even if we do not wear spectacles, many of us do appreciate the importance of having a clean windscreen or clean glasses! People with learning disabilities have a higher level of sensory impairment (Emerson and Hatton, 2007; Beresford and Rhodes, 2008; Robertson *et al.*, 2010; Emerson and Baines, 2010).

Fast facts 14.4   Sensory impairments

- People with sensory impairments are some 8–200 times more likely to have a visual impairment.
- Approximately 40 per cent of them have a hearing impairment.
- People with Down's Syndrome are more likely to develop vision and hearing loss.
- Eye testing is less prevalent if living with family or independently.

Reader activity 14.10   Jose's visual impairment

Jose has a visual impairment and she wears glasses, but her cerebral palsy makes it impossible for her to clean the lenses herself.

- How often should her support worker clean her lenses?
- How often should Jose receive an eye test?
- What reasonable adjustments may be necessary to enable Jose to attend an eye test at the local opticians?

Hopefully Jose's glasses will be cleaned as soon as they become smeared, but will be cleaned at least daily and her eye testing should follow the normal pattern of at least every two years.

Even with the aid of spectacles, Jose needs to have her living environment adjusted so that she may identify the shapes of doorways, stairs and perceive room shapes more clearly. For Jose, this also requires stronger than normal lighting and/or door frames being painted in bright colours that contrast strongly with the colour of the surrounding walls. In this way a person with visual impairment can more readily identify the shape and location of doors or open doorways. Similar colour and lighting schemes can help to contrast walls, stairways, doors, cupboards, drawers, and so on, making these clearer for people with visual impairment.

Unfortunately bright lighting will not suit everyone with a visual impairment. Some people's vision is obliterated by moderately bright lighting, rather like when a bright torch is shone into one's eyes. For people whose vision is impaired in this way, softer, lower levels of lighting are usually more helpful.

Jose has some degree of hearing impairment too, and she wears a hearing aid in each ear. Hearing aids require special batteries that deliver a steady level of power throughout their lifetime. Consequently they go from being effective to completely dead in a very short time. Some batteries last up to 4 days, some last more than 30 days, depending upon variables such as cost and quality. Jose needs assistance to check and replace her hearing aid batteries at regular intervals, in accordance with the manufacturer's guidance on battery life. Similarly her hearing aids need occasional servicing and again this must be in compliance with the manufacturer's recommendations. Hearing aids are sometime purchased under a maintenance contract and Jose requires assistance to comply with that contract.

Reader activity 14.11   Ear plugs

If you have never worn ear plugs, try putting some purpose-made foam rubber ear plugs into each ear. You will probably notice immediately that sounds are deadened significantly. When you speak, you will not 'sense' your own voice in the same way and it becomes difficult to speak in the normal pitch, cadence and tone. The longer you wear the plugs, the more uncomfortable speaking becomes, and removing the plugs gives a sense of relief!

So now you should have some idea of what it feels like to wear a hearing aid with flat batteries!

Because Jose's vision and hearing are both impaired, her home is adapted with a loop to enhance her hearing aid and is well lit with the use of contrasting paints on doorways and stairwells, as outlined above. Additionally Jose's home has some tactile adaptations which enable Jose to 'feel' parts of the house. For example, her bedroom door has one of Jose's stuffed toy animals attached to it at exactly the height of Jose's arm. Jose can immediately identify her bedroom door in this way, as well as by its distinctive colour and contrasting door frame. Similarly the bathroom has a toothbrush attached to the door and a wooden spoon adorns the kitchen door. These simple adaptations enable Jose to move about her home with greater confidence and independence.

Fast facts 14.5   Sensory impairment web links

Working to support people with complex physical and sensory needs demands appropriate adjustments to suit the environment to each individual. You can find further guidance and support from organisations, such as:

- Deafblind UK: available at: http://deafblind.org.uk/what-we-do/.
- Sense: available at: www.sense.org.uk/content/communicating-deafblind-people.
- The World Association Promoting Services for Deafblind People: available at: www.deafblindinternational.org/.
- The UK Council on Deafness: available at: http://www.deafcouncil.org.uk/.
- Royal National Institute for the Blind (RNIB): available at: http://rnib.org.uk/aboutus/contactdetails/Pages/contactdetails.aspx.

Conclusion

This chapter draws on two case studies relating to Neil and Jose respectively, in order to explore the nature of cerebral palsy and the support requirements and adjustments necessary to enable people with physical and sensory impairments to live healthy lives. It emphasises the importance of personal, individualised support approaches backed up by skilled therapy and health support, based upon collaboration between all the parties involved from cradle, throughout adulthood.

By engaging with this chapter the reader should be better informed about how to play their own part in supporting people who have physical and sensory impairments and gain a clearer appreciation and awareness of the very wide-ranging and significant health issues that may arise. It is not the aim of this chapter to medicalise disability (treat it as an individual's illness/problem) but rather to ensure that important health issues are not overlooked, misunderstood or ignored, which could easily prove catastrophic. From a position of optimal health and development, we are all in a better position to participate fully in all that life and citizenship have to offer, throughout life.

Points to remember

- Cerebral palsy is a very individual condition and affects all people differently.
- People have many varied needs.
- Ongoing assessment of needs will ensure that changing needs are met.

References

Aird, R. (2012) *The Education and Care of Children with Severe, Profound and Multiple Learning Difficulties.* London: Routledge.

Beresford, B. and Rhodes, D. (2008) *Housing and Disabled Children.* York: Joseph Rowntree Foundation.

Bower, E. (2009) *Finnie's Handling the Young Child with Cerebral Palsy at Home.* Edinburgh: Butterworth-Heinemann Elsevier.

Costigan, F.A. and Light, J. (2011) Functional seating for school aged children with cerebral palsy, *Language, Speech and Hearing Services in Schools*, 42: 223–236.

CPA (Cerebral Palsy Alliance) (2103) ParentWise Podcast Series, Making the Most of Your Child's Mealtimes. Available at: www.cpresearch.org.au/pdfs/pw_tr_Making_the_Most_of_Your_Child's_Mealtimes_2.pdf (accessed 11 April 2013).

CWDC (2009) Department for Education 2012, Children and Young People: Team Around the Child (TAC). Available at: www.education.gov.uk/childrenandyoungpeople/strategy/integratedworking/a0068944/team-around-the-child-tac (accessed 11 April 2013).

Department of Education (2012) *Children and Young People, SEND*. Available at: www.education.gov.uk/childrenandyoungpeople/send/b0075291/green-paper/vision (accessed 16 May 2013).

Dodd, K.J., Imms, C. and Taylor, N.F. (eds) (2010) *Physiotherapy and Occupational Therapy for People with Cerebral Palsy. A Problem-Based Approach to Assessment and Management*, London: MacKeith Press.

Emerson, E. and Baines, S. (2010) *Health Inequalities and People with Learning Disabilities in the UK: 2010, Improving Health and Lives*, Durham: Learning Disabilities Observatory, University of Durham.

Emerson, E. and Hatton, C. (2007). The mental health of children and adolescents with intellectual disabilities in Britain, *British Journal of Psychiatry*, 191: 493–499.

Gerricke, T. (2006) Postural management for children with cerebral palsy: consensus statement, *Developmental Medicine and Child Neurology*, 48(4): 2–44.

Hill, S. and Goldsmith, L. (2009) Mobility, posture and comfort, in J. Pawlyn and S. Carnaby (eds) *Profound Intellectual and Multiple Disabilities*. Chichester: Wiley-Blackwell.

Krageloh-Mann, I. and Cans, C. (2009) Cerebral palsy update, *Brain Development*, 31: 537–544.

McDonald, R., Surtees, R. and Wirz, S. (2004) The International Classification of Functioning, Disability and Health provides a model for adaptive seating interventions for children with cerebral palsy, *British Journal of Occupational Therapy*, 67(7): 293–302.

Medline Plus (2013) Epilepsy. Available at: www.nlm.nih.gov/medlineplus/ency/article/000694.htm (accessed 11 April 2013).

Michael, J. (2008) *Healthcare for All: Report of the Independent Inquiry into Access to Healthcare for People with Learning Disabilities*. London: Department of Health.

NICE (National Institute for Health and Care Excellence) (2012) *Spasticity in Children and Young People with Non-Progressive Brain Disorders: Management of Spasticity and Co-Existing Motor Disorders and their Early Musculoskeletal Complications*, CG 145. Available at: http://publications.nice.org.uk/spasticity-in-children-and-young-people-with-non-progressive-brain-disorders-cg145 (accessed 11 April 2013).

Physiotherapy Treatment (2010) *Postural Drainage Therapy*. Available at www.physiotherapy-treatment.com/postural-drainage.html (accessed 11 April 2014).

Pope, P. (2007) *Severe and Complex Neurological Disability: Management of the Physical Condition*. Edinburgh: Butterworth-Heinemann Elsevier.

Robertson, J., Roberts, H. and Emerson, E. (2010) *Health Checks for People with Learning Disabilities: A Systematic Review*. Durham: Improving Health and Lives, Learning Disability Observatory. Available at: www.improvinghealthandlives.org.uk/uploads/doc/vid_7646_IHAL2010-04HealthChecksSystemticReview.pdf.

Scope (2013a) *Scope to Help and Information: Introduction to Cerebral Palsy*. Available at: www.scope.org.uk/help-and-information/cerebral-palsy/introduction-cerebral-palsy (accessed 11 April 2013).

Scope (2013b) *Scope to Help and Information: Intrathecal Baclofen Therapy (ITB) for Spasticity*. Available at: www.scope.org.uk/help-and-information/z-therapies/intrathecal-baclofen (accessed 11 April 2013).

Scope (2013c) *Scope to Help and Information: Botox™*. Available at: www.scope.org.uk/botox (accessed 11 April 2013).

Scope (2013d) *Scope to Help and Information: Selective Dorsal Rhizotomy*. Available at: www.scope.org.uk/help-and-information/therapies/selective-dorsal-rhizotomy (accessed 11 April 2013).

Scope (2014) *Cerebral Palsy: What Is Cerebral Palsy or CP?* Available at: http://www.scope.org.uk/support/families/diagnosis/cerebral-palsy (accessed 11 April 2014).

15 Supporting people with an autistic spectrum disorder

Stacey Atkinson and Malcolm Richardson

Learning outcomes

After reading this chapter you will be able to:

- understand the nature of autism and the spectrum of biological, psychological and social factors by which it is characterised
- consider the skills that are most appropriate and that you may develop in order to support people who have autism so that they may cope with all aspects of their lives.

Introduction: living within the autistic spectrum

> If you've got a camel which is finding it hard to walk under the weight of all the straws on its back, the easiest way to make it easier for the camel to walk is to take as many straws off as possible. Management is about training the camel to walk or appear to walk while carrying the straws. Cure is about taking the straws off the camel's back. The two can work together.
>
> (Williams 1996)

You will be forgiven for wondering what the above quote can possibly have to do with the autistic spectrum, to put it simplistically the paragraph is about unburdening people and allowing them to be themselves, while helping them to manage the expectations placed upon them. That essentially, is what this chapter is concerned with. Giving health and social care professionals the knowledge to understand what an autistic spectrum disorder (ASD) is and to equip them with the skills to meet the needs of someone with an ASD or to help the person him/herself to manage the needs connected to their condition. There is an outline of the needs of individuals with ASD, including behaviours and mental health needs, and advice given on how to ensure meeting their needs within the health and social care setting. To assist with this, the chapter uses a series of case studies provided by Jon, Jodie and Graham, who are all adults with diagnoses of autism. The scenarios outline some personal experiences which help us to understand some of the differences that an ASD presents.

Table 15.1 The communication and sensory needs of someone who has an autistic spectrum disorder

Someone with autism or Asperger's disease may present in the following ways:

- Difficulty understanding gestures, facial expressions or tone of voice
- Difficulty knowing when to start or end a conversation
- Difficulty choosing topics to talk about
- May use complex words and phrases but may not fully understand what they mean
- May be very literal in their speech and have difficulty understanding jokes, metaphor or sarcasm. For example, may be confused by the phrase 'That's cool' when used to say something is good.
- May have sensory hypersensitivity with regards to touch, sight, auditory, olfactory and taste.

Source: NAS (2010).

Defining autistic spectrum disorders (ASDs)

It is difficult to find an all-encompassing explanation of what ASDs are, as each diagnosis under the umbrella spectrum has so many dimensions. One sentence definitions do not do justice to the complexity of the ASD. Happe's (1994) definition alludes to this fact. Happe described autism as having many different levels: the biological, the cognitive and the behavioural. Among the biological reasons for 'Autistic Conditions,' genetics are sometimes a contributory factor (Rutter, 2000). The symptoms of ASDs, as will be shown, have a biological or physiological impact on the person. For example, ASDs and their effects encroach upon cognitive functioning, while in terms of the behavioural focus, individuals with ASDs may display behavioural needs due to the difficulties caused by their symptoms. Practitioners may find positive outcomes to help the person with ASD when addressing their needs through behavioural interventions (see Chapter 19). Some of the communication and sensory features that a person with ASD may exhibit are presented in Table 15.1.

Williams (2001) describes autism as a 'complex interplay between the identity, personality, environment and experience of an individual. An internal human normality.' This definition nicely illustrates the intertwining relationships that occur for someone with ASD when trying to marry up the forces that exist, i.e. their own personalities and individuality and how they can be themselves in each changing environment and with each experience they encounter and the interplay these challenges present. The ASDs are lifelong conditions; they encapsulate a spectrum or range of conditions, behaviours and characteristics (Figure 15.1). It is essential that those working with people with ASDs

The conditions along the autistic spectrum are also known as
pervasive developmental disorders

Different levels of intellect

Autism ⟵————————————————⟶ Asperger's

Semantic pragmatic disorder
Childhood disintegrative disorder

Figure 15.1 The spectrum of ASD

consider the personal experience of individuals with ASDs, empathise with them and aim to meet their needs. In the UK, about 1 in 100 people have autism, which is more than half a million (NAS, 2010, online). So it is clear that at some point in your health or social care career you will encounter or work with someone with has an ASD, so consideration of their needs is vital.

Reader activity 15.1   ASD

Think about someone with an ASD you have met. What needs did they have?

Along the spectrum illustrated in Figure 15.1, individuals differ in how their particular disorder affects them. About 70 per cent of people with an ASD also have a learning disability (Ghaziuddin *et al.*, 2002; DH, 2012), but vary markedly in their level of learning disability just as they differ as individuals. All this influences how individuals and their autism present. Figure 15.2 shows the specific areas of impact felt by people with ASD.

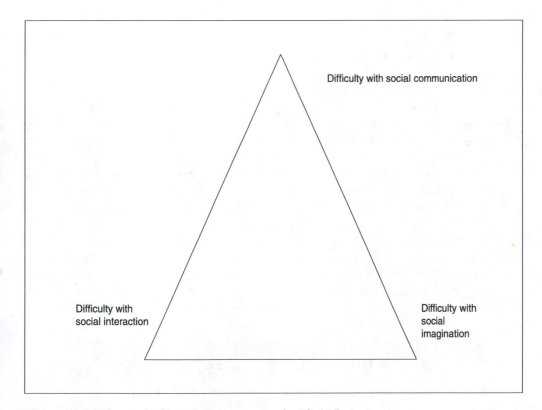

Figure 15.2 The triad of impairments associated with ASD

Source: NAS (2010), and adapted from Wing and Gould (1979).

Case study 15.1   Understanding facial expressions

I couldn't get it at first [facial expressions] even before I got the diagnosis of Asperger's. I struggled really, but am getting there now. I'd say, it's not like 100%. Like, I know if someone is angry and I know when someone is angry with me for no reason, but it still confuses me, if you know what I mean. I think, why are you angry? I think I have done nothing wrong.

Graham talking about his difficulties in recognising facial expressions and how, even it confuses him. Graham is a very able person but still struggles with some aspects of social communication.

Reader activity 15.2   Facial expressions list

List all the facial expressions you can think of that people use. Can you understand the frustration that Graham has in not recognising this aspect of social communication (see Case study 15.1)?

Social communication difficulties

There are many aspects of social communication in daily life that people with ASD have difficulties with. Some individuals may not recognise the need for communicating socially with another person, if something is needed, then pointing or leading the person will enable the child to obtain the object of their desires, using the person as a means to an end. As described by Williams (1999), other people are often not viewed as social beings, just as a means of obtaining what is needed. Once desires are fulfilled, communication, as a means of being sociable, is pointless. Some individuals may not be able to use verbal communication, or if they have it, may for the above reasons not use it. Like Graham, they may not recognise non-verbal cues, including tone of voice, gestures and facial expressions. If they have words, they may have difficulty in making 'appropriate' conversation, often lacking the knowledge of how to act in different social situations; situations when they are the focus, such as birthdays or when attention is paid to them, may be particularly uncomfortable. Individuals may not apply the correct social rules, so, for example, may stand too close to another person or not take turns in conversation. Some people may have the cognitive awareness and ability to learn social rules, but awkwardness or limitations in this area can be a barrier to forging and maintaining relationships.

Reader activity 15.3   Social settings

How do you feel going into social settings that are new to you? These feelings may be exacerbated in someone with an ASD.

Case study 15.2 Social imagination

Jodie, commenting on an aspect of being socially imaginative that is difficult for her says, 'I was diagnosed with autism about two or three years ago [at 17]. I have difficulties coping with new situations. Well, I did, but have got a lot better. Speak-Up [a self-advocacy group] helps me to practise my communication and to meet new people.'

Reader activity 15.4 Late diagnosis

Jodie's diagnosis of autism was not made until she was 17. How do you think not having a diagnosis might have affected her childhood?

Social imagination difficulties

An individual may have difficulties in predicting events especially within social situations or may have trouble transferring skills learnt from one environment to another. Social environments and the people within them may appear unpredictable and confusing. Some people with ASDs detach themselves as far as possible from the social world, and a fear in social situations may lead other individuals to become withdrawn or at least to appear disinterested or distant. Some, like Jodie, can learn the skills they need to adapt to differing situations. In infancy, children with ASD often lack the interest and enthusiasm to react when a parent enters a room or when they speak. Due to this issue and other similar instances, their disinterest is often mistaken for deafness. Doctors often take measures to rule out the possibility of deafness prior to pursuing a diagnosis of autism.

People with autism often have strong interests in predictable events and activities. An autistic child may, for example, line up toys and play with them in repetitive ways, may enjoy bouncing on trampolines or find spinning objects therapeutic ways of finding comfort and pleasure in an unpredictable world. An enjoyment and aptitude for computer work is not uncommon and hardly surprising; most of the time a computer does what you expect it to do, whereas social interactions do not! Some adults with ASD like to organise or catalogue things of interest. They may be attracted by the receptiveness of timetables, or reliability of mathematics or playing rule-led games where the outcomes are 'black or white', with no 'grey areas' to cause confusion.

Understandably, therefore, familiar places or rooms that do not alter much from day to day help to maintain a sense of predictability and comfort. Changes to these familiar environments may precipitate significant alarm or discomfort. Routines help to maintain a sense of control and calm. Breaks in routine can cause distress and may result in great rigidity in adhering to the routines in future. For example, one young person's routine involved being dropped off by taxi at a day service. On one such journey, as the young person arrived and knocked at the door of the day service, instead of being let in as usual, someone came out of the door when it opened. This broke the young person's routine so he got back in the taxi, went home and then repeated the journey again (NAS, 2010, online).

Practice alert 15.1

One person with ASD uses a timetable to help follow the daily routine: 'If I get anxious, I get in a tizz. I have a timetable; it helps me to see what I have to do next, otherwise I get confused' (NAS, 2010, online).

Reader activity 15.5   Stress buster

- For someone with ASD, a lack of predictability can be a major source of stress (Table 15.2).
- What do you do when feeling stressed or distressed, that helps you to feel better again? We all do something to help ourselves to feel better in difficult situations.

Table 15.2 Areas of stress for people with ASD

Area of stress	Example situations
Changes and threats	Having a cold
	Change in task and new directions
	Going shopping
	Change in environment
	Transition in locations
	Transitions from preferred to non-preferred activity
	Engaging in an activity not liked
	Being unable to communicate
	Needing to ask for help
	Participation in a group activity
Anticipation and uncertainty	Having plans changed
	Waiting for an activity
	Having unstructured time
	Waiting generally
Unpleasant events	Waiting to talk about a desired topic
	Having personal objects missing; following a diet
	Receiving criticism and being told no
	Having something marked as incorrect
	A change of teacher/carer
	Losing at a game
Pleasant events	Receiving a present
	Playing with others
	Receiving reinforcement
	Having something marked correct
	Having a quality conversation
	Receiving praise

Sensory/personal	Being in the vicinity or noise or disruption by others
	Being touched
	Receiving hugs and affection
	Feeling crowded
Food-related activities	Waiting in a restaurant
	Waiting for food
Social/environmental interactions	Being in the vicinity of bright lights
	Being unable to assert oneself with others
	Someone else making a mistake
Ritual-related stress	Having personal objects or materials out of order
	Being prevented from completing or carrying out a ritual
	Being interrupted while engaging in a ritual

Source: Grogen *et al.* (2001), cited in RCN (2011).

Difficulties with social imagination can also be the reason why an individual with ASD takes things very literally. They may be unable to comprehend that one word can have several meanings or may not see the humour attached to words in some social dialogue, having very set structures in their minds about the use of language.

Case study 15.3   Social interactions

Graham, talking about problems with social interaction he has experienced, says:

> I struggle explaining a lot of different things, but I am learning, constantly practising. I was once talking to some students and I struggled a bit at first and then I talked about something I knew about and got into the routine, and I was fine and it just flowed. People can learn by experience and often by the time they are out of their teens and into their 20s or 30s, you know, they are building up skills that they used to struggle with.

Difficulties with social interaction

People with ASD often have specific needs which hinder social interaction. A preoccupation with their own agendas, such as toys spinning or an apparent obsession with a particular interest, can cause social interactions to veer towards the subject that the individuals is absorbed with and be a barrier to the sharing of mutual conversation. Anxiety in social situations can, as with Graham's situation, cause people to struggle with the flow of conversation and a lack of insight into the other person's communication needs, exacerbated by a lack of empathy (Attwood, 2006), causes some people with ASD to fail to see the need for turn-taking in conversation. Difficulty in reading facial expressions and cues can all be problematic during conversation. People with ASD may shy away from eye contact, find the intensity of one-to-one situations too intrusive and may find physical contact such as touch or hugs unbearable.

Case study 15.4 illustrates how difficulties with social interaction hinder people with an ASD and the hurt that can be caused by others' lack of adjustment to their needs.

Case study 15.4   Interview with Jon

Malcolm: Jon, thanks for agreeing to help the readers understand and learn a little about autism, where would you like to start?

Jon: When I was a kid, people said I was naughty because they couldn't see my autism, I look just like anyone else. Nowadays I tell people I have autism so that they know I am a bit different. I want them to ask me how they can assist me, like, if I use their services, so I tell them.

Malcolm: Does that always work?

Jon: No, it doesn't always have the effect I want. I moved to a new area and had to register with the GP. I went to the surgery and told the receptionist that I have autism and want to register with the GP. She told me they don't treat people like me. This made me very upset. I went away and told the advocacy group about it and they encouraged me to complain. So I phoned up the doctor's (surgery). A different lady answered and I told her what had happened when I visited. She said she was sorry it had happened and that she would take my details and register me with the GP.

Reader activity 15.6
Helping people with ASD

In relation to Case study 15.4:

*   How would you feel about the situation that Jon has experienced?
*   In your workplace, if Jon, who has autism, came to use the services you provide, how could you adjust your communication so that Jon is not put off or goes away anxious and dissatisfied?

Sensory needs

A chandelier would become a collective of interacting, seemingly playful sparks of colour, the image of which would trigger the associated senses of the chink, chink sound that would be made if the smooth hard glass pieces from which the colours emanated were touched together . . . It caused a drug-like addictive effect such as like 'merging with God' because I would resonate with the sensory nature of the object with such an absolute purity and loss of self that it was like an overwhelming passion into which you emerge and become part of the beauty itself.

(Williams, 2001)

The quotation above illustrates the intensity of the sensory experience felt by many people with an ASD. Smith-Myles *et al.* (2005) found that more than 50 per cent of people with ASD have sensory hypersensitivity or a sensitivity of the senses such as sight, hearing, touch, smell (olfactory) and taste. Their skin, for example, might be so sensitive that the person is unable to tolerate some garments close to their skin or may be intolerant to touch. Sounds may be extremely loud to the point of being painful, with olfactory hypersensitivity, making some smells overwhelming, and visual sensitivity may result, for example, in colours and patterns of great intensity emerging within someone's visual field. Such hypersensitivity may at times result in 'sensory overload' (Williams, 1996) with the concentration of the heightened senses becoming too great so that the individual has to 'switch off' input in order to manage in the situation.

Fast facts 15.1   Sensory overload

Sensory overload is common to individuals with ASD and may be caused by, for example:

- too much noise;
- too many distractions all at once;
- too many instructions at one time;
- too much intense attention/involvement from another person.

Reader activity 15.7   Anxiety creation

A mother contacts your work area to book an appointment for her daughter who is 18 years of age. She explains that her daughter has autism and a severe learning disability and that she cannot sit for long periods of time.

- The appointment will probably represent a break in her daughter's normal daily routine, how might this affect the young lady?
- The young lady may be anxious about attending the appointment, what reasonable adjustments to the booking system can be made to ensure that she does not need to sit waiting for very long?
- Assuming that some waiting may be inevitable, what information would you need to obtain from the young woman or her mother in order to make her waiting time as comfortable and stress-free as possible?
- Are there any further actions you could take to help prepare your department/ workplace and appropriate colleagues so that on the day of this young lady's appointment someone is informed about her needs and ready to support her with her mother?

Behavioural and mental health needs

The specific needs of someone with an ASD, as outlined, can cause the individual to feel anxious, frustrated and distressed, therefore, for this reason both behavioural and mental health needs are prevalent in this client group.

Case study 15.5   Interview with Graham

Graham talks about his anger and how he manages it.

Malcolm: You've talked to students about how you have learned to manage [your anger].
Graham: To manage it, yes, I manage it better now.
Malcolm: So you manage changes in routine better now though, than when you were a young lad?
Graham: Changes in my routine, yes. It can be bad, but I say I manage but it can still get to me even today. I have anger management which helps. I have to. I just try and think about something the anger management counsellor has said and usually it gets me thinking. I think something like 'slow down' 'It doesn't matter, it's not 100% perfect.' I'm a real stickler for perfection. Everything has got to be done right and if it's not done right, it upsets me.
Barry   (Graham's friend): He's just a perfectionist, he knows if I move something, sometimes it makes him awful!

In Case study 15.5 it is evident that some aspects of Graham's anger have links with some aspects of his ASD. As discussed in Chapter 19, the challenges in behaviour sometimes displayed by people with a learning disability are often a form of communication; someone perhaps without speech may have learnt that certain behaviours are responded to by those around them and so they continue to use this behaviour to highlight their needs. Whether seen socially as being 'acceptable' or not, the behaviour gains a positive response that the person needs. Graham's situation shows that behaviours can be indicators of distress felt by someone due perhaps to their sensory, communication or social difficulties, due to his need for control over his environment being challenged.

Groden *et al.* (2001), cited in RCN (2011), highlighted eight areas of stress (see Table 15.2) for individuals who have an ASD in their Stress Survey Schedule. The survey gives practitioners key situations that health and social care practitioners should be aware of. Once aware, adjustments can be made for the management of stress, thus reducing episodes of behavioural or mental distress.

Reader activity 15.8   Stress adjustment

Look at Table 15.2 again, consider each of eight areas of potential stress and why a person with an ASD might find it stressful. Also consider what reasonable adjustments can be made. Two examples have been given already in Table 15.3.

Table 15.3 Stress adjustment techniques

Stressful event	Why it might be stressful	What adjustments can be made?
Receiving a present	It may be stressful as someone will receive intense social reinforcement that they find overwhelming	Tell the person they are going to receive a gift Explain how to respond Do not labour the social side of the gift building
	May lack confidence and may not know how to respond to receiving the gift. It may be unexpected and therefore unplanned for and unpredictable	Do not keep the person in the social situations for longer than they choose to be there
Waiting in a restaurant	The person may be unsure of how to behave in the different environment. They do not know how long they have to wait. They may feel sensory over-stimulated or under-stimulated. The place may feel unpredictable	Explain what to expect in this situation prior to going You may need to use visual aids to ensure a full understanding Keep encouraging their awareness of what is happening throughout the visit Use strategies to manage sensory overload, see section to follow

Now continue yourself!

People with ASDs also suffer more from mental illness needs than other people in general. People with ASDs are, as discussed, often socially withdrawn and isolated. The more intellectually-able are often fully aware of their own differences (Attwood, 2006), while less able people struggle with the condition and its effects, often with limited means of communicating its impact. Due to the needs of people with ASDs the symptoms are often difficult to detect and mental illness may go undetected, particularly in people with more profound autism or greater levels of learning disability who cannot so readily describe what they are experiencing (Stewart *et al.*, 2006). Table 15.4 shows some prevalence rates of mental illness among people with ASDs but it can only be used as a guide due to the difficulties in detection and issues such as diagnostic overshadowing (see Chapter 20).

Reader activity 15.9   ADS diagnosis

You may need to refer to Chapter 20 when considering this question. Why do you think it might be difficult to diagnose a mental illness in someone with an ASD?

Table 15.4 Prevalence rates of mental illness among people with ASD

Researchers	Sample group and results
Gillott and Standen (2007)	Adults with ASD. • Anxiety levels in adults. I.e. the amount of anxiety felt was found to be three times higher than in other people. • Higher levels of panic found • Higher levels of agoraphobia • Higher levels of obsessive compulsive disorder (OCD)
White *et al.* (2009)	Children and adolescents with ASD • 11–84% of children and adolescents had some degree of impairing anxiety.
Stewart *et al.* (2006)	Adults with ASD • Depression is very common but specific rates are difficult to detect due to the symptoms of ASD
Wing (1996), cited in NAS (2004)	Schizophrenia no more likely to occur in people with ASD than any other group

Reasonable adjustments

People with ASDs have a right to fully access and benefit from the environments they utilise. Depending on their needs, it is important to remember that their ability to adapt in different environments may be compromised and when providing care it is the duty of care of service providers, employers, leisure service and other services to make suitable adaptations rather than the person with ASD making them (NHS and Social Care Act, 2008; Equality Act, 2010). Disabling barriers, such as lack of respect towards people with ASD, or failure to make reasonable adjustments so that individuals may access and participate, must be tackled so that a workplace, leisure area, service or care provision become as accessible as possible. The following are examples of reasonable adjustments in support of people with ASDs:

- Knowing about the needs of people with ASD and how the condition itself presents. Where possible, try to obtain some training. This will increase your awareness in meeting the needs of people who have a diagnosis of ASD.
- Get to know people as individuals. In addition to the above recommendation, there is a need to become familiar with people as individuals. If your acquaintance with them is brief, for example, through hospital appointments, ask the person with ASD or a person supporting the individual, how their ASD impacts on them and perhaps more importantly, find out what makes them 'tick' as individuals, such as likes/dislikes, do's/don't's, so enabling you to better enter their world and to form appropriate relationships.
- Be aware of the environment. Assess the environment and question, given the information available in this chapter, is the environment autism-friendly? Rid the environment of distractions such as noise and clutter, keep rooms and routines as predictable as possible. If changes are going

to occur, prepare the person for them. If someone is staying in hospital, the use of side rooms might be considered, however, as Smith and Atkinson (2012) point out, people with communication needs are often very socially isolated, so consideration must be made not to compound that isolation. Therefore, explaining routines through the use of visual timetables can aid the person's orientation into unfamiliar routines and encourage a sense of security.

- Longer appointment times or the chance to explore the environment and equipment are advantageous, allowing someone the opportunity to feel more settled, while communications don't then have to be rushed. Further information about making environments more accessible to people with ASDs can be gained through local hospital learning disability liaison nurses or Community Learning Disability Teams.

- Make communications accessible. Be aware of your own tone of voice, is it potentially painful for someone with an ASD? Are too many instructions being given to someone with an ASD at any one time? Do you tend to use metaphors such as 'butterflies in the stomach' and so forth when talking? These might be difficult for someone to interpret. Are you specific about time spans, for example, do you say 'I will be with you in 5 minutes' and then take 20? Do you readily use touch when talking in a one-to-one? Someone with an ASD may find this intrusive and unpredictable. Being aware of and adjusting any of the above will enable better verbal interactions with someone with an ASD. The use of photographs or objects utilised as reference points or visual cues (Smith and Atkinson, 2012) will also aid someone's understanding of speech.

- Make adjustments for sensory needs. The pain of oversensitivity and unpredictability of sensory stimuli can hinder someone's ability to access health and social care. Many points have been explored already in relation to this but the issue of touch is particularly important and therefore merits reiteration. Health and social care procedures do involve touch. Dental examinations, providing intimate care, brushing hair or physical examination, all involve touch.

As highlighted in previous chapters, the need to gain consent from service users is paramount and has to be obtained prior to the commencement of any procedure. Some people with ASD struggle intensely with touch and for those individuals, therapy obtained through learning disability nursing services or occupational therapy, for example, may be appropriate to desensitise them. For all people, however, a good pattern of communication which includes a detailed explanation of any touch about to occur is vital. It gives the person time to mentally and physically prepare for the procedure, whether that 'procedure' is having hair combed or an intimate examination, it is essential.

Written communications also need attention to ensure accessibility. People with learning disabilities may be unable to read so communicating care plans, procedures, health information and all other health and social care documents pictorially will help. There is a website called Change (2013) that has produced information on how to make information accessible and also has many pictorially accessible health and social care resources available.

New staff could be introduced through the use of pictorial CVs (Figure 15.3). This is an initiative introduced by Lay (unpublished) but described by Atkinson and Williams (2011) whereby new staff may be introduced to service users. There are obvious merits to its use as it familiarises service users with people who are important in their care.

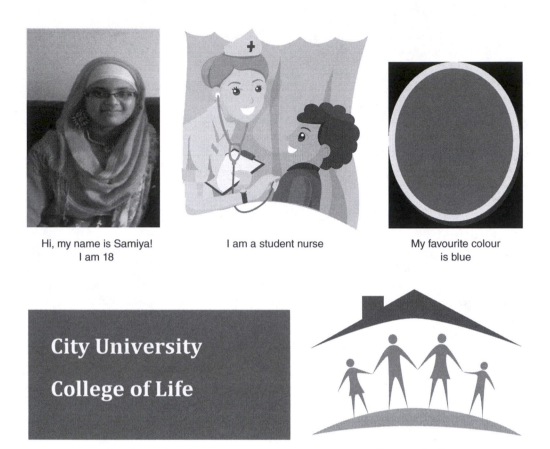

Hi, my name is Samiya!
I am 18

I am a student nurse

My favourite colour
is blue

City University

College of Life

I study at university

I love my family

Figure 15.3 An example of a pictorial CV

Conclusion

In this chapter you have been invited to consider some of the ways in which having an ASD may affect a person's behaviour, including cognitive thinking, perception, sensory and social aspects. Eight broad areas of potential stress to people who have ASD were identified from the literature. You were then invited to identifying examples of reasonable adjustments that you may make in your work area and behaviour in order to support a person who has an ASD to access and benefit appropriately from the services offered. The very activity of attending and using your service may present both a change and therefore a threat to someone with ASD. So it is important for a service user who has ASD to be supported as much as possible prior to visiting your service. That support may, for example, come from someone who knows them well and who will explain to that person what the purpose of the visit is and what will happen. You may have an opportunity to help the person relax and feel more comfortable by remaining calm, respecting their personal space and asking if there are any environmental adjustments you can make, such as making the place quieter, less busy, less waiting around, and so on. Ideally some of these things will need preparing before the person arrives, but that may not always be possible. In that case, take your lead from the person, who may be able to tell you, and sometimes also from someone who has come with them to give that support. This will contribute towards making their experience pleasanter because it will make the environment pleasanter for them. If the visit/appointment conforms to their expectations of what is to happen, this will also help reduce anxiety. If the person with ASD has attended before, then following a similar routine each time will help to reduce anxiety by confirming that sense of familiarity, predictability and, if possible, following a familiar routine. People with ASD are as individual and unique as everyone else, so any one approach that succeeded with one person who has ASD may not necessarily be as relevant or successful for the next person you encounter. Generally, however, the strategies outlined in this chapter are a good place to start making those very reasonable adjustments.

Points to remember

- Autism is individual to each person.
- People with an ASD may have difficulties with social imagination, social interaction or social integration, also sensory hypersensitivity.
- Aspects of the condition may cause the person to develop behavioural or mental health needs.

Resources

The National Autistic Society. www.autism.org.uk.
NHS Choices Autistic Spectrum disorder www.nhs.uk/conditions/autistic-spectrum-disorder
Research Autism. www.researchautism.net.
Local Community Learning Disability Teams.
Local Autism Diagnostic Services.

References

Atkinson, S. and Williams, P. (2011) The involvement of service users in nurse education, *Learning Disability Practice*, 14(3): 18–20.
Attwood, T. (2006) *Why Does Chris Do That?* London: The National Autistic Society.
Change (2013) *How to Make Information Accessible: A Guide to Producing Easy Read Documents*. www.changepeople.co.uk (accessed 23 Jan. 2013).
DH (Department of Health) (2012) *Public Health, Adult Social Care, and the NHS: Estimating the Prevalence of Autism Spectrum Conditions in Adults*, 7 Feb. 2012. Available at: www.dh.gov.uk/health/2012/02/estimating-the-prevalence-of-autism-spectrum-conditions-in-adults/ (accessed 23 Jan. 2013).
Ghaziuddin, M., Ghaziuddin, N. and Groden, J. (2002) Depression in persons with autism: implications for research and clinical care, *Journal of Autism and Developmental Disorders*, 32(4): 299–306.
Gillott, A. and Standen, P. (2007) Levels of anxiety and sources of stress in adults with autism, *Journal of Intellectual Disabilities*, 11: 359–370.

Groden, J., Diller, A. and Bausman, M. (2001) The development of a stress survey schedule for persons with autism and other development disabilities, *Journal of Autism and Development Disabilities*, 312: 207–271.

Happe, F. (1994) *Autism: An Introduction to Psychological Theory*, London: ULC Press.

NAS (National Autistic Society) (2004) *Mental Health in People with Autism and Asperger's: A Guide for Health Professionals*. London: NAS.

NAS (National Autistic Society) (2010) *About Autism*. Available at: www.autism.org.uk (accessed 23 Jan. 2013).

RCN (2011) *The Autism Act 2000: Developing Specialist Skills in Autism Practice*. Middlesex: Royal College of Nursing Publishing Company.

Rutter, M. (2000) Genetic studies of autism from the 1970s into the millennium, *Journal of Abnormal Child Psychiatry*, 28: 3–4.

Smith, J. and Atkinson, S. (2012) Children who have difficulty in communicating, in V. Lambert *et al.* (eds) *Communication Skills for Children's Nurses*. Maidenhead: Open University Press.

Smith-Myles, B., Tapscott Cook, K., Miller, N., Rinner, L. and Robbins, L. (2005) *Asperger Syndrome and Sensory Issues*. Kansas: AA Publishing Company.

Stewart, M., Barnard, L., Pearson, J., Hasan, J. and O'Brien, G. (2006) *Presentation for Depression in Autism and Asperger Syndrome: A Review*. London: Sage.

White, S., Oswald, D., Ollendick, T. and Scahill, L. (2009) Anxiety in children and adolescents with autistic spectrum disorders, *Clinical Psychology Review*, 29(3): 216–229.

Williams, D. (1996) *Autism: An Insight-Out Approach*. London: Jessica Kingsley.

Williams, D. (1999) *Nobody Nowhere: The Remarkable Autobiography of an Autistic Girl*. London: Jessica Kingsley.

Williams, D. (2001) *Autism and Sensing: The Unlost Instincts*. London: Jessica Kingsley.

Wing, L. and Gould, P. (1979) Severe impairments of social interactions of associated abnormalities in children: epidemiology and classification, *Journal of Autism and Developmental Disorders*, 9: 11–29.

16 Specific health needs and conditions

Lesley Montesci and Malcolm Richardson

Learning outcomes

After reading this chapter you will be able to:

- understand the range of health needs and health conditions commonly experienced by people with a learning disability
- be aware of the underpinning principles to support the health of people with learning disabilities.

Introduction

> A wise man should consider that health is the greatest of human blessings.
>
> Hippocrates (date unknown).

This chapter considers some of the many specific health needs and conditions relating to people with learning disabilities. Three guiding principles are recommended to be applied in all circumstances, whether the person has a common syndrome or a rare genetic disorder.

Each case study presented here allows the reader to explore a particular syndrome in depth and can be read as a singular text or collectively to provide insight into specific health needs and conditions. Each scenario is interspersed with activities and reflection points to aid the reader's thinking about how they may address particular health needs, promote health and well-being and reduce the risk of diagnostic overshadowing, such as when a learning disability influences the thinking about and subsequent diagnosis of an underlying health problem (Mencap, 2007).

The four case studies are:

1. Case study 16.1 Living with Prader Willi Syndrome: a service user's account. Prader Willi Syndrome is a genetic condition characterised by obesity and related co-morbidity issues. Affected people have an insatiable appetite for food.

2. Case study 16.2: Jamie explains what it is like to have a condition which causes life-threatening behaviours and how his obsession with food is being managed effectively by staff supporting him. This case study will also discuss other health issues such as cardio-pulmonary effects and respiratory problems, including breathlessness and sleep apnoea.
3. Case study 16.3: Double jeopardy. This case study endeavours to describe the health needs of service users from black and ethnic minority groups and how these can be effectively addressed to promote well-being, reiterating the need to make reasonable adjustments to minimise the risk of ill health. The link between sensory impairments will be a key feature of this case study.
4. Case study 16.4: Living with Turner's Syndrome. This exploratory study will describe some of the many health issues affecting women with this condition and how these might be mitigated to ensure a good quality of life.

Fast facts 16.1   Depressing statistics

People with learning disability

*   are four times more likely to die of preventable causes;
*   are 58 times more likely to die before 50;
*   do not have the same access to health support;
*   have higher levels of unmet need;
*   are discriminated against.

(Michael, 2008)

Three principles

The same three principles apply in all circumstances, whether the person has a common syndrome or a rare genetic disorder (see case studies).

*   Don't let familiarity breed complacency.
*   Do keep a detailed family history.
*   Always consider how a disease or health condition affects a person without a learning disability.

Working with people who have a learning disability involves working with individuals who have a diverse range of health and support needs. These may stem from events that may have occurred before birth (pre-natal), around the time of birth (peri-natal) or some time after the birth of the infant (post-natal). For example, the resulting health and support needs may arise from a genetic or chromosomal condition, resulting in physical, neurological and/or metabolic disorders or from trauma resulting in damage to sensory and/or motor neurones (Table 16.1).

Each of these conditions associated with learning disabilities have their respective co-morbidity factors. While it is not possible to explore each of these in great detail, Table 16.2 provides the reader with an overview of some of the more common disorders and gives a reference point for sources of further information. This will complement the three case stories, providing a more detailed perspective, linking to the current public health agenda; healthy long lives, well-being, health behaviours and health inequalities (DH, 2010a, 2010b).

Table 16.1 Causes of impairments associated with learning disabilities

Pre-natal	Peri-natal	Post-natal
Single gene inheritance	Trauma	Trauma, especially to head Anoxia (lack of oxygen)
Chromosomal, such as Down's Syndrome	Precipitate at labour (too rapid birth may damage infant's skull and underlying neurological tissues)	Infections: meningitis, encephalitis
Ionising radiation	Prolonged labour (too long being born risk of trauma such as lack of oxygen)	Extremely rare effect from vaccination – last occurrence in 1960s due to a single batch of vaccine (Lane et al. 1968)
Maternal ill health or malnutrition	Brain damage due to use of forceps (rare)	Retrolental fibroplasia
Placental insufficiency (lack of nourishment/oxygen to the foetus)	Retrolental fibroplasia (incubated infant receiving too much oxygen resulting in brain damage)	Hypocalcaemia (especially light for dates and low birth weight babies)
Light for dates and premature babies (very underweight or very premature at birth)	Highest peri-natal mortality rates are associated with light for dates and very premature infants	Malnutrition
Drugs, toxins, alcohol, smoking	Kernicterus/hyperbilirubinemia (severe jaundice can result in damage to neurological tissues)	Poisons, e.g. heavy metals – mercury, copper, manganese, strontium cadmium, lead
Infections: Rubella, Cytomegalovirus Virus, Toxoplasmosis, Herpes, Treponema (syphilis)	Respiratory distress syndrome, e.g. immature lungs in very premature babies	Sensory and social deprivation, such as an infant being hidden away in a cellar for months

Table 16.2 Specific conditions and associated health needs affecting people with learning disabilities

Chromosomal abnormalities	Syndrome	Co-morbidity issues	Link to website
	Cri du Chat Syndrome	Congenital heart defects, microcephaly, hypertelorism, hernias, respiratory problems, hypotonia	www.criduchat.org.uk
	Down's Syndrome (see Chapter 8)	Congenital heart disease, cataracts, ear problems, glaucoma, seizures, leukaemia, hypothyroidism, respiratory tract infections, Alzheimer's	www.downs-syndrome.org.uk

(continued)

Table 16.2 (Continued)

Chromosomal abnormalities	Syndrome	Co-morbidity issues	Link to website
	Fragile X Syndrome	Joint abnormalities, cardiac problems	www.fragilex.org.uk
	Klinefelter Syndrome	Low testosterone, diabetes mellitus, scoliosis, osteoporosis and vascular problems	www.klinefelter.org.uk
	Prader–Willi Syndrome	Compulsive eating, hypotonia, obsessive compulsive disorder, sleep apnoea, osteoporosis, diabetes mellitus, orthopaedic problems, endocrine problems	www.pwsa.co.uk
	Turner syndrome	Infertility, lymphodema, skeletal difficulties, heart defects, kidney problems, recurrent ear infections, scoliosis, hypertension, heart problems, diabetes, osteoporosis	www.tss.org.uk
	Angelman syndrome	Microcephaly, ataxia, hypotonia, seizures, scoliosis, feeding difficulties	www.angelmanuk.org
	Rett syndrome	Tremors, scoliosis, muscle wasting, joint contractures, increased spasticity, hyperventilation, seizures, feeding difficulties	www.rettuk.org
	Tuberous Sclerosis	Epilepsy, kidney problems, lung disease	www.tuberous–sclerosis.org
Metabolic disorders	Phenylketonuria	Microcephaly, abnormal gait, seizures, cataracts, skin disorders	www.nspku.org
	Hurler's syndrome	Progressive deterioration, hearing loss, ear infections, bowel problems, respiratory infections, cardiac problems	www.patient.co.uk
		Frequent ear infections, respiratory infections, cardiac disease, sleep apnoea, lung problems, joint stiffness	www.patient.co.uk
Pre- and post-natal factors	Congenital rubella syndrome	Glaucoma, cataracts, blindness, deafness, diabetes mellitus, blood problems	www.deafblinduk.org.uk
	Foetal alcohol syndrome	Kidney problems, cardiac problems, eye defects, hearing difficulties, dental problems.	www.fasaware.co.uk
	Toxoplasmosis	Hydrocephalus, cataracts, blindness, deafness	www.deafblinduk.org.uk

Source: Russell (1997); Hogg and Langa (2005).

The science of genetics

The Human Genome Project has generated lots of media interest and excitement in recent years. The deciphering of genes along each chromosome means that predictive medicine will become part of our future and doctors will be able to better treat or prevent diseases such as cancer, strokes and diabetes (Hirst and Metcalfe, 2009). One could be forgiven for thinking that genetics is a relatively new science but in actual fact, information regarding chromosomal abnormalities and learning disabilities has been known for a number of years. Hence, for example, it is possible for health and social care professionals to relate a syndrome to predisposing health conditions. However, that very familiarity with a syndrome may sometimes lead to a 'blasé' approach to the person's physical health and well-being. For example, when Claire, a lady in her thirties who has Down's Syndrome, began showing signs of mental confusion, her carers and GP assumed that Claire was showing the initial signs of dementia, which is a well-documented health predisposition in older people with Down's Syndrome (NHS Choices, 2012). However, it was subsequently discovered that an underactive thyroid (hypothyroidism) was causing Claire's symptoms. Hypothyroidism is fully treatable, but had it remained misdiagnosed, the consequences for Claire's health would have been serious. In Claire's case, the correct diagnosis of her symptoms arose because a learning disability nurse, with an in-depth knowledge of the health conditions associated with Down's Syndrome, suggested that an underactive thyroid might also explain Claire's symptoms (see also Chapter 8). Hypothyroidism is another health condition more prevalent in people with Down's Syndrome (ibid.). Claire's case demonstrates how having knowledge of predisposing health conditions can potentially lead to misdiagnosis and that other possibilities must also be considered. The potential consequences of not doing so can be dire, with increased risk of premature death and poorer health outcomes; however, such risks can be reduced considerably if the following three principles are applied.

Principle 1: Don't let familiarity breed complacency

It is all too easy to think we know everything about the person we are caring for, particularly if we have been supporting them for some considerable time. Such familiarity may lead to complacency with certain aspects of a condition being forgotten or overlooked, as with Claire above. It is good practice to revisit a text book or use the internet to refresh our memories about a particular condition (including any associated co-morbidity issues) and familiarise ourselves with recent research and developments. Not only will this promote evidence-based practice but more importantly it will promote best practice and care for each individual.

Principle 2: Keep a detailed family history

Family history gives valuable insight into a person's susceptibility to certain medical conditions such as diabetes, breast and bowel cancers and thrombosis. Therefore, it is imperative that staff supporting service users with learning disabilities take a detailed medical history, recording familial traits to ensure this information is not 'lost' in transit or the through passage of time. This is an important and extensive area of practice.

The reader may wish to utilise the following website to support them when taking a family history: www.geneticseducation.nhs.uk/about-us/resources.aspx.

The reasons for taking a family history are threefold:

- Family members can receive genetic counselling to allay their fears or be enabled to make informed choices about having children in future.
- Those with a predisposition to certain conditions can take preventative measures to minimise the risk of developing the condition in later years.
- In families where there is evidence of single gene disorders such as breast or colorectal cancer, individuals can receive targeted surveillance.

Reader activity 16.1   Family history

Michael (born 30 March 1975) has learning disabilities and exhibits behaviours that are described as 'challenging'. He has been referred to your service for support. His mother talks to you about his siblings and from the conversation it is quite clear that other family members are also similarly affected. You manage to ascertain the following information:

- Angela (born 14 April 1949) is married to Richard (12 March 1947) and they have four children: Joshua, Michael, Christopher and Hayley.
- Joshua (born 16 August 1973) has mild learning disabilities and attends a local day service.
- Christopher and Hayley are twins (born 15 Feb. 1978) and though they both attended mainstream school, Christopher struggled with numeracy and literacy and has not been able to hold down a job.
- Hayley and her partner, John, have two children, Sam (born 24 Dec. 1998) and Carly (born 6 Sept. 2000). Sam has been excluded from school on several occasions due to his difficult behaviour.
- Angela's sister, Elizabeth has two daughters (Vicki and Eden).
- Angela recalls that a maternal uncle had learning disabilities and died some years previously.

Using the symbols in Figure 16.1, draw a family tree and then consider the positives and negatives of referring the family for genetic counselling.

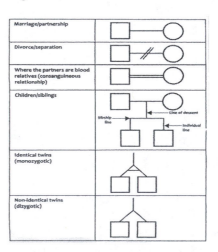

Figure 16.1 Symbols for drawing a family tree

(The NHS National Genetics Education and Development Centre, 2010)

Principle 3: Always consider how a disease or health condition affects a person without a learning disability

People with learning disabilities are often unable to articulate how they feel and this can lead to inequalities in healthcare and poor treatment options (Emerson and Baines, 2010). For example, a person with learning disability might not be able to say they have a headache before or after seizure activity even though we know that people with epilepsy often report migraine-type symptoms and require pain relief. General comparisons with people who do not have a learning disability can give valuable insight into how a person with learning disabilities might be feeling when they cannot self-report and this can minimise the risk of untreated health conditions and diagnostic over-shadowing.

Reader activity 16.2   Sufficient information

The next time you look at a care plan or support plan of someone you are working with, ask yourself:

- Does this contain sufficient information with regards to the person's primary condition, related health issues and family medical history?

Table 16.2 lists some common conditions together with additional information that you might need to consider when supporting the health or social needs of an individual who has the condition. You will see from Table 16.2 that each syndrome or condition has associated health issues and any one of these has the potential to cause additional problems if overlooked or not properly treated. There will now be an opportunity to explore some of these issues in more detail linked to the principles outlined above, beginning with Case study 6.1.

Case study 16.1   Living with Prader Willi Syndrome: a service user's account

Prader Willi Syndrome is a genetic condition characterised by obesity and related co-morbidity issues. Affected people have an insatiable appetite for food and therefore obesity is a major health concern.

Jamie is a 57-year-old gentleman with learning disabilities living in a supported living arrangement with his own tenancy, sharing accommodation with three other people. He attends a day service once a week delivering supplies to various homes within the organisation, making bird boxes and restoring garden furniture.

He cannot remember when he was first diagnosed with Prader Willi Syndrome and is unable to recall what was actually said at the time. While he has some appreciation of what the diagnosis means, he only has a limited understanding of the associated health issues and possible impact on his quality of life. He is justifiably proud of the fact that he has lost a considerable amount of weight (previously he was 25st, now he is 13st 6lbs); improving his mobility and

(continued)

(continued)

skin integrity. However, he is still breathless on exertion and nearly died last year when he developed a serious chest infection. Sleep apnoea is a significant problem and a contributory factor to his tiredness during the day and despite advice to the contrary, Jamie still continues to smoke, although considerably less than he used to. He has a history of deep vein thrombosis and is also being treated for osteoporosis.

Jamie is supported to undertake gentle exercise to promote his health and well-being and enjoys walking.

Reader activity 16.3   Jamie's assessment

Imagine that Jamie has just been referred to your service for assessment:

- How confident are you that the assessment process would capture the complexity of Jamie's needs?
- What information would you need to collate in respect of his family history?
- How would one of Jamie's associated health conditions affect a member of the general population, physically and cognitively?

Assessment formats aim to provide a holistic view of the person but a model is only as good as the assessor using it and all too often the final product is lacking in detail. Not only does this compromise the person involved, but it can have major implications in terms of funding particularly when people are being re-assessed at a lower level of support. In the case of Jamie, it would be imperative that the resulting support plan is person-centred and sufficiently detailed to address all his health concerns; ensuring key information is not lost in 'transit' between one service provider and another.

In terms of family history, it would be important to ascertain what conditions are prevalent in order to prevent something untoward being missed. For example, it would be easy to attribute Jamie's tiredness to sleep apnoea even though there might be a family history of hypothyroidism which, if he is similarly affected, would also make him lethargic. Likewise it would be advantageous to consider the effects of having a specific condition such as diabetes or breathlessness, so that Jamie is appropriately supported. Diabetes is known to cause peripheral neuropathy and people often complain of 'pins and needles' in their extremities which can be extremely uncomfortable and painful. Despite knowing this, one would question how often this has been explained to people with learning disabilities who are diabetic or whether the information provided has been in a format they understand.

Obesity and illness prevention

England has one of the highest rates of obesity in Europe (DH, 2011) with more than half the population now overweight or clinically obese (Hindle and Mills, 2012). The risks associated with obesity are well documented and include: an increased risk of Type 2 diabetes, cancer of the colon, coronary heart disease and osteoporosis (NICE, 2006). The physical and emotional impact on the individual cannot be underestimated and the financial implications of obesity are phenomenal, costing the NHS £4.2 billion every year (National Audit Office, 2014). Consequently there is growing impetus to address this issue, both at a micro and macro level; empowering the individual; promoting preventative and early intervention strategies and taking a community approach to address a multi-faceted problem.

The health gains associated with sustained weight loss are equally well documented (SIGN, 2010) and there are emerging care pathways designed to address obesity (Hindle and Mills, 2012). The main emphasis is on prevention and self-directed support, enabling the person to make healthier lifestyle choices, lose weight and prevent weight gain in future. This might include the person joining a self-help group, increasing physical activity or making a decision to eat a more nutritious diet. A targeted weight management programme is often triggered by a medical diagnosis or a body mass index (BMI) of 30 or above. Such a programme typically involves a combination of dietary advice and physical activity. Sometimes specialist weight management programmes may include intensive support to address the psychological causes of obesity and remedial action such as bariatric surgery. There is a high incidence of obesity among people with learning disabilities (Doody and Doody, 2012) and it is imperative that they are not excluded from such intervention programmes and opportunities to improve their health and well-being. (See also Chapter 26 on promoting the health needs of people with learning disabilities.)

Reader activity 16.4   Weight problems

Look at Case study 16.1. What strategies could you use to help Jamie manage his over-eating and maintain his current weight? See Case study 16.2 for some ideas.

Case study 16.2   Helping Jamie

Jamie realises that he needs help with his diet and admits that he feels much healthier now he has lost a considerable amount of weight. He used to see a dietician but now has the continued support of his staff team and other tenants. The fridge and freezer are kept locked at all times and everyone agrees, including Jamie and the other tenants, that this should happen. However, the other tenants have their own key so are not personally denied access to food.

Jamie is offered smaller quantities of food which includes lots of fruit, low fat yoghurts and jellies and his drinks are restricted; otherwise he would drink excessive cups of tea which could ultimately damage his kidneys. Jamie chooses to monitor his own weight which he records on a daily basis.

Jamie's love for pastries has never wavered and he looks forward to having a vanilla slice once a fortnight on a Friday and he enjoys cooking, an activity that his staff team encourage and support.

Jamie's weight loss is maintained by encouraging him to do gentle exercise and he uses his Wii Sport to play tennis, bowling and golf at home.

Autonomy, choice and the Mental Capacity Act (2005)

It would be all too easy to make decisions on behalf of Jamie in his best interests and exclude him from the decision-making process. However, the Mental Capacity Act (2005) requires all those who work in health and social care to have a good understanding of how the Act applies and how we should respond to those who may lack capacity. As such, we should be familiar with the Mental Capacity Code of Practice (2007) and provide evidence that we have complied with our obligations under the Act. See Chapter 10 (Figure 10.2) for the principles of the Mental Capacity Act (2005).

If we apply the principles of the act to Jamie's case, we would probably conclude that while he has a learning disability, it does not necessarily mean he is unable to make a particular decision at the relevant time. Provided Jamie can understand, retain and weigh up information regarding the decision to be made and communicate his decision verbally or using alternative methods of communication, we must presume he has capacity to consent to the eating regime which is in place. However, it could be argued that the compulsion associated with Prader Willi Syndrome is such that Jamie is unable to make informed decisions and staff are acting in his best interests (Goldstone *et al.*, 2008).

In summary, Prader Willi Syndrome is a genetic condition characterised by obesity and related co-morbidity issues. Although Jamie is actively involved in his weight management regime, he will need support to maintain his health and well-being. His situation is not unique and many people with learning disabilities are reliant on others to support them or take on a caring role. This is particularly evident in the second case study which offers a Black and Ethnic Minority (BEM) perspective, highlighting barriers to communication and difficulties in accessing mainstream services.

Case study 16.3   Double jeopardy

Mr and Mrs Asif emigrated from Pakistan in the 1960s and had five children, two of whom have cerebral palsy and profound learning disabilities. Mother recently died and now Imran (47 years) and Nasreen (36 years) are cared for by their sister Shameen, with additional support from their two brothers and sister-in-law.

Imran has restricted mobility and uses a wheelchair. He is doubly incontinent and has renal problems which will ultimately result in catheterisation. Nasreen also uses a wheelchair and has complex health needs including epilepsy, bowel and bladder problems and a history of deep vein thrombosis, all of which require daily medication. Imran and Nasreen currently attend a day service, five days per week.

Mr Asif is 80 years of age and does not enjoy good health. He had heart bypass surgery two years ago; a stroke affecting his balance, making him prone to falls and has been diagnosed with dementia. He required antibiotics for a urinary tract infection and recently developed bed sores due to his immobilisation and confinement to bed.

The family did not have an allocated social worker when Imran and Nasreen were children because their parents did not know how to access support and they were never offered any respite from their caring obligations.

Shameen constantly 'juggles' the needs of her immediate family and the requirements of her brother, sister and father. She is often near the point of exhaustion and would love some additional support.

Case study 16.3 highlights the need to address two of the principles outlined above, to *obtain a detailed family history* and *consider how a disease or health condition affects a person without a learning disability*.

Evidence suggests that black and ethnic minority groups (BEM) have more health problems than the overall population and that ill-health begins at a much younger age (Parliamentary Office of Science and Technology, 2007). South Asian men are particularly susceptible to heart attacks and angina and there is a high incidence of obesity and diabetes in the BEM population generally. In this particular case it would be useful for staff to know that Mr Asif has a history of coronary heart disease and whether other family members have been similarly affected. Likewise it would be advantageous to know the circumstances surrounding the death of Mrs Asif and if this has implications for their siblings so that Imran and Nasreen can be properly monitored and preventative measures can be instigated if needed.

Good health surveillance is required for people with profound learning disabilities and complex needs who may not be able to communicate verbally (Emerson and Baines, 2010), in order to prevent delayed diagnosis of medical conditions and poorer outcomes. The fact that both Imran and Nasreen have a history of renal problems requires monitoring of their fluid intake and output and early medical intervention if a urinary tract infection is suspected or confirmed. Health care support such as medical or nursing should also consider how renal problems, epilepsy or muscular-skeletal problems associated with cerebral palsy affect people from the general population to ensure parity in treatment. For example, both Imran and Nasreen may benefit from a muscle relaxant which is used to treat painful contractures of the muscles. Such pain may be overlooked in people with severe learning disabilities whose communication difficulties may prevent them from describing their pain.

Shameen's situation is not unique and evidence suggests that there are many black and ethnic minority carers in a similar position. Some of the key themes in the literature relating to the specific needs of people with learning disabilities from BEM communities are presented in Fast facts 16.2.

Fast facts 16.2   Key health themes relating to people with learning disabilities from BME communities

According to Mir *et al.* (2001, p. 9), people with learning disabilities from BME communities suffer from:

- A higher incidence of impairment in a number of areas.
- Low levels of knowledge of services available for the disabled person or carers.
- Poor standards of communication.
- Delays in diagnosis and treatment.
- Isolation, lack of support and high levels of carer stress.
- Low take-up and poor access to services.
- High levels of unmet need.
- Low levels of access to benefits/receipt of lower amounts of benefits.

As a consequence of the above factors, carer health is often poor (even in comparison to other carers) and there is a significant risk of mental illness due to prolonged stress (Parliamentary Office of Science and Technology, 2007). Indeed one Asian carer told me recently that she is 'sometimes happy and sometimes sad' and it was almost if she was resigned to the situation; that there was no alternative but to look after her disabled son, whatever the circumstances. It is not uncommon for carers to neglect their own health needs in favour of continuing their caring commitments (DH, 2008) but the danger is that services only become involved when the situation reaches crisis point. It is therefore imperative that service provision and support are equally accessible to people with learning disabilities and carers from black and ethnic minority communities

Barriers to service provision

There is evidence to suggest that people with learning disabilities from black and ethnic minority (BEM) communities face discrimination on a regular basis and those services offered are either inappropriate or insufficient to meet their needs (DH, 2009). This ultimately means there is a 'hidden' population requiring help and support; and carers struggle to cope with day-to-day activities resulting in a detrimental effect on their own health and emotional well-being.

There are several reasons why this might be the case:

- *Cultural insensitivity*: In our eagerness to treat everyone the same, we do not take into account the specific requirements of a particular culture. This may include dietary requirements, the need for same gender accommodation, the provision of bilingual carers and the use of culturally sensitive information (Mir, 2001).
- *Wrong assumptions*: There is often a mistaken belief that carers from BEM communities have support from extended family networks and that some groups have a more or less favourable attitude towards disability because of their religious or cultural beliefs (Royal College of Psychiatrists, 2011).
- *Language barriers*: This is often cited as a major issue because for many female carers, English is not their first language and they are reliant on relatives or interpreters to convey information. This makes it very difficult for carers to voice their concerns, request additional support and ultimately access services.

> ### Reader activity 16.5   Inter-professional working

- How would inter-professional working benefit the family?
- Which professionals or agencies should be involved and what contribution would they make towards improving the situation?

Support groups such as the Pakistani Asian Carers Group in Sheffield can be a very effective means of addressing difficulties and providing information in an informal environment. Opportunities to share experiences and provide mutual support can be invaluable, and having a chance to meet carers in a similar situation can prevent feelings of helplessness and isolation. Advocacy services can also support individuals and their carers to access culturally sensitive services and bi-lingual carers can provide additional support in terms of translating information to and from family members, as well as raising awareness amongst other staff groups. Organisations will only be truly inclusive if they understand the barriers that exist and involve BEM communities directly in the development of services; otherwise we will continue to perpetuate inequalities and difficulties in accessing support.

The Office for National Statistics (2009) predicts that the BEM population will rise from 16.2 per cent to 20 per cent of the population by the year 2051 and there is an increased sense of urgency for health and social care practitioners to be culturally aware and sensitive to the needs of these groups. People with learning disabilities from BEM groups are often 'hidden' and excluded from services and Mir *et al.* (2001) report that currently 19 per cent of South Asian families have more than one person with a learning disability in the household. The situation described in Case study 16.3 is not uncommon. Services must be responsive and seek ways to minimise the risk of further isolation as a matter of urgency. Similarly, much more needs to be done to prevent health inequalities and ensure that people with learning disabilities have the same opportunities to seek expert advice for medical conditions as the general population. Such is the focus of Case study 16.4.

Case study 16.4   Living with Turner's Syndrome

Jessica is a 48-year-old lady who has a condition called Turner's Syndrome, a chromosomal abnormality associated with complex medical problems (see Table 16.3). She has a super-imposed mental health condition on top of an existing learning disability and requires medication to treat her on-going depression.

Jessica currently lives in a supported living environment after spending considerable time in a secure hospital, detained under the Mental Health Act. It is reported that Jessica's behaviour changed in adolescence, at a time when her parents separated. Making friends has always been problematic causing jealousy and inappropriate behaviour.

In addition to her depression and lack of motivation, Jessica self-harms (anorexia) and has a number of medical conditions, including muscular skeletal problems, amenorrhoea, a congenital heart defect and osteoporosis.

Table 16.3 Recommended health checks for women with Turner's syndrome

Medical condition	Type of screening	Frequency
Obesity	Weight, BMI	Routine
Diabetes	Glucose tolerance test	As required
	Fasting blood sugar test	Annually
Osteoporosis	Bone density	5 yearly
	Fracture history	Routinely
Hearing loss	Hearing test	5 yearly
Hypothyroidism	Thyroid function test	1–2 yearly
	Thyroid antibodies	1–2 yearly

(continued)

Table 16.3 (Continued)

Medical condition	Type of screening	Frequency
Renal system	Ultrasound	Time of diagnosis
	Urine testing to exclude urinary tract infection	As required
	Renal function	Annually
Eye defects	Eye sight checks	1–2 yearly
Reproductive problems	Hormone replacement therapy	Advised every visit
	Mammography	Routinely from 45 years of age
Cardiology problems	Echocardiogram	Time of diagnosis 3–5 yearly
Hypertension	Blood pressure checks	Advised every visit
Coeliac disease	Coeliac antibodies test	1–2 yearly

Turner's Syndrome is an abnormality of the X chromosome affecting 1 in 2000 women in the UK (TSSS, 2012) and those affected by it are often of normal intelligence. It is a complex condition which gives rise to a 'challenging array of genetic, developmental, endocrine, cardiovascular, psychological and reproductive issues' (Bondy, 2007, p. 10); requiring on-going health screening and medical intervention, if needed. There may be an absence of an X chromosome in all the body's cells; an absence of an X chromosome in some of the cells (referred to as mosaicism) or a structural mutation of the X chromosome affecting development before and after birth (Sybert and McCauley, 2004). Turner's Syndrome is rarely inherited and is only passed from one generation to the next if there is a partial deletion of the X chromosome. In this circumstance genetic counselling may be appropriate.

Although women with Turner's Syndrome can enjoy a long and active life, cardiovascular problems such as coarctation of aorta (a narrowing of the main artery from the heart) and other structural heart defects can cause premature death (Sybert, 1998). It is therefore imperative that such abnormalities are detected as early as possible and children are referred to specialist cardiology services for evaluation and intervention; thus minimising the risk of poor health outcomes in later years. Likewise it is important to screen women with Turner's Syndrome throughout their lifetime for common disorders such as hypertension, osteoporosis, diabetes, hypothyroidism and kidney disease. These are preventable conditions and can be identified using simple health checks (see Table 16.3) (TSS, 2012).

The health surveillance checks outlined in Table 16.3 are important for women with Turner's Syndrome to maintain good health, prevent associated conditions and enable early intervention if needed. Given that these checks are evidence-based, it is somewhat alarming that Jessica has never been routinely monitored with regards to her congenital heart defect and possible related problems or offered hormone replacement therapy (HRT) as a preventative strategy for osteoporosis. Neither has she had routine blood tests to exclude hypothyroidism or glucose intolerance. All her mood swings have been attributed to her previous psychiatric history without due diligence being given to other possible causal factors. This is not uncommon and, as previously suggested, diagnostic overshadowing is a contributory factor to people with learning disabilities having a shorter life expectancy or experiencing greater health problems compared to the general population. Hence the third principle: Always consider how a disease or health condition affects a person without a learning disability, if applied in this context, should help to mitigate against diagnostic over-shadowing and improve health and well-being.

Annual health checks for adults with learning disabilities were introduced in England in 2009, following a recommendation made by the Department of Health in its report *Healthcare for All* (Michael, 2008). This constitutes a 'reasonable adjustment' as it recognises that people with learning disabilities are at greater risk of health inequality and that annual checks can, therefore, help to reduce those inequalities and ensure that health services are responsive to the needs of adults with learning disabilities (ibid.). The Commission concluded that GPs should be incentivised to undertake specific health checks in relation to people with learning disabilities, in addition to those identified in the Quality Outcome Framework (QOF) scheme. The response to this has been variable and evidentially there are still concerns that people with learning disabilities have not received an Annual Health Check (Turner and Michell, 2012). Health and social care practitioners have an important role in supporting this process, either advocating on behalf of an individual and ensuring a health check is done or contributing to the development of a Health Action Plan (DH, 2009). This is when actual or potential health needs are identified in collaboration with a person; actions are prioritised and followed up to improve the health of the individual. There may be on-going issues which need to be addressed, such as those identified in the aforementioned case studies or further actions might be needed in terms of health promotion and developing a healthy lifestyle, both of which are equally important.

Conclusion

The sad truth is that people with learning disabilities are 58 times more likely to die compared to the general population and 4 times more likely to have a preventable cause of death in the UK (Emerson and Baines, 2010). There are a significant number of genetic and chromosomal conditions associated with learning disability, ranging from rare syndromes to more common disorders. However, irrespective of the condition, the same three principles cited in this chapter apply. Health and social care professionals need to be mindful of these to ensure that a person with a learning disability remains healthy and enjoys a good quality of life and that tragedies such as those outlined in *Death by Indifference: 74 and Counting* (Mencap, 2012) become a thing of the past.

Points to remember

- The biological, social and cultural psychological issues impacting on individuals with learning disabilities cause specific health needs to arise.
- Genetic influences may also be present.
- Health assessments such as health action plans are necessary for maintaining good health.

References

Bondy, C.A. (2007) Care of girls and women with Turner Syndrome: a guideline of the Turner Syndrome Study Group, *The Journal of Clinical Endocrinology and Metabolism*, 92(1): 10–25.

DH (Department of Health) (2008) *Carers at the Heart of 21st-Century Families and Communities*. London: Department of Health.

DH (Department of Health) (2009) *Valuing People Now: A New Three Year Strategy for People with Learning Disabilities*. London: Department of Health.

DH (Department of Health) (2010a) *Healthy Lives, Healthy People: Our Strategy for Public Health in England*. London: The Stationery Office.

DH (Department of Health) (2010b) *Our Health and Wellbeing Today*. London: The Stationery Office.

DH (Department of Health) (2011) *Healthy Lives, Healthy People: A Call to Action on Obesity in England*. London: The Stationery Office.

Doody, C.M. and Doody, O. (2012) Health promotion for people with intellectual disability and obesity, *British Journal of Nursing*, 21(8): 460–465.

Emerson, E. and Baines, S. (2010) *Health Inequalities and People with Learning Disabilities in the UK, 2010*. Durham: Improving Health and Lives Learning Disabilities Observatory.

Goldstone, A.P., Holland, A.J., Hauffa, B.P., Hokken-Koelaga, A.C. and Tauber, M. (2008) Recommendations for the diagnosis and management of Prader-Willi Syndrome, *Journal of Clinical Endocrinol Metabolism*, 93(11): 4183–4197.

Hindle, L. and Mills, S. (2012) Obesity: self care and illness prevention, *Practice Nursing*, 23(3): 130–134.

Hirst, M. and Metcalfe, J. (2009) *Human Genetics and Health Issues*. Milton Keynes: The Open University Press.

Mencap (2007) *Death by Indifference*. London. Mencap

Mencap (2012) *Death by Indifference: 74 Deaths and Counting. A Progress Report 5 Years On*. London. Mencap.

Mental Capacity Act 2005 *Code of Practice (2007)*. London: The Stationery Office.

Michael, J. (2008) *Healthcare for All: Report of the Independent Inquiry into Access to Healthcare for People with Learning Disabilities*. London: Department of Health.

Mir, G., Nocon, A., Ahmed, W. and Jones, L. (2001) *Learning Difficulties and Ethnicity*. London: Department of Health.

National Audit Office (2014). *Tackling Obesity in England*. Available at www.nao.org.uk/report/tackling-obesity-in-england/(accessed 11 April 2014).

NHS Choices (2012) *Complications of Down's Syndrome*. Available at: www.nhs.uk/Conditions/Downs-syndrome/Pages/Complications.aspx (accessed 29 Oct. 2012).

NICE (2006) *Obesity Guidance on the Prevention, Identification, Assessment and Management of Overweight and Obesity in Adults and Children*. London: Department of Health.

Office of National Statistics (2009) *Population Trends*, No. 138. Winter 2009.

Parliamentary Office of Science and Technology (2007) *Postnote Ethnicity and Health January 2007*, Number 276. London: The Stationery Office.

Royal College of Psychiatrists (2011) *Minority Ethnic Communities and Specialist Learning Disability Services*. Report of the Faculty of the Psychiatry of Learning Disability Working Group Faculty report FR/LD/2. RC PSYCH Publications. London: Faculty of the Psychiatry of Learning Disability of the Royal College of Psychiatrists

SIGN (2010) *Management of Obesity: Quick Reference Guide*. Edinburgh: Scottish Intercollegiate Guidelines Network.

Sybert, V.P. (1998) Cardiovascular malformations and complications in Turner Syndrome, *Pediatrics*, 101(1).

Sybert, V.P. and McCauley, E. (2004) Turner's Syndrome, *The New England Journal of Medicine*, 134: 1227–1238.

TSSS (2012) Turner Syndrome Support Society. Available at: wwwtss.org.uk/index.php/publication-sandinformatio/generalheathcare.

Turner, S. and Michell, B. (2012) Making sure service users receive health checks, *Learning Disability Practice*, 5(5):16–20

17 Emotional difficulties

Malcolm Richardson

Learning outcomes

After reading this chapter you will be able to:

- understand the importance of emotional experience throughout the lifespan
- discover some of the negative emotional experiences more commonly experienced by people with learning disabilities
- recognise practical ways and means by which the emotional well-being of people with learning disabilities may be supported and promoted and outcomes evaluated.

Introduction

> No aspect of our mental life is more important to the quality and meaning of our existence than emotions. They are what make life worth living, or sometimes ending.
>
> (de Sousa, 2010, online)

This chapter explores some elements of the emotional experiences of people with learning disabilities throughout the human life span. Insights are drawn from parts of the lives of people with learning disabilities including David, Leon, Ahmed, Claire, Kevin, Connor and Arthur. These insights will be employed to assist the readers to think about how they may support people with learning disabilities to benefit from life-affirming emotional experiences and some ways of evaluating outcomes.

A review by Arthur (2003) of the research and therapy literature around the emotional lives of people with learning disabilities revealed how little was known about this compared with similar literature on the general population. However, our understanding of emotional aspects in the lives of people with learning disabilities has been increasing gradually over recent decades, drawing on a diverse literature that includes the poetry, prose, art work and verbal accounts of people with learning disabilities, self-advocacy groups and from the clinical work of therapists(e.g. Deacon, 1974; Fido and Potts, 1989; Atkinson and Williams, 1990; Beail and Warden, 1996; Read *et al.*, 1999; Hollins and Sinason, 2000; Arthur, 2003; Simpson and Miller, 2004; LD Pride, 2013).

Abuse

At the start of the new millennium, Nadirshaw (2000) expressed hope that the new century would witness the agenda of inclusion overtaking that of the systems approaches which have dominated learning disability services for more than a century. Many of the emotional difficulties reported by people with learning disabilities are rooted within the systems approach, such as their sense of loss of a personal identity, negative emotions arising from labelling and stereotyping, the emotional traumas consequent upon the self-knowledge that death and annihilation might still be their fate within a society that rejects difference to the extent that the eugenic abortion and euthanasia of people who are different remain pervasive within health, social and other service systems.

Consequently, an inclusive society must, by definition, accept difference and in so accepting come to understand better the emotional lives of people with learning disabilities, how their emotional lives may be enriched, enhanced and find healing.

Fast facts 17.1   Shame and fear

Shame and fear are among the commonest emotions experienced by people with learning disabilities (see also Table 17.1).

Table 17.1 Emotional difficulties commonly experienced by people with learning disabilities (five common examples identified by LD Pride)

Shame – a distorting of self concept e.g. from an emotional history of labelling, stereotyping, negative values attaching to some aspects of 'difference,' rejection by society e.g. eugenics, amniocentesis, abortion.

Examples of Modes of Expression – sense of loss of personal identity; the anguish and distress of labelling; poor self esteem; mentally reliving experiences of being humiliated; fear, knowledge that others like you, if detected in the womb, have been and can still be aborted; hiding one's own difficulties.

Fear – closely associated with shame as above, fear often as a consequence of traumatic life experiences and/or the anticipation of potential repetition thereof, eugenics, amniocentesis, abortion, euthanasia.

Examples of Modes of Expression – often masked by anger or anxiety, fear of one's difference being 'found out'; fear of ridicule, failure, judgment, criticism or rejection; intrusive recollection of traumatic experiences experienced as flashbacks/post traumatic stress disorder, poor sleep patterns, nightmares, reduced mental concentration, re-enactment e.g. in child play, or 'reliving' the experience in adulthood, dissociative reactions, memory distractions or omissions, heightened central nervous system arousal, heightened startle reflex, hyper vigilance, not being able to trust in others, a sense that one might have been and might still be discarded, shyness.

Environmental and emotional sensitivity – a sense of being overwhelmed by too much environmental stimuli (e.g. background noise, more than one person talking, side conversations, reading and listening at the same time).

Examples of Modes of Expression – many people with learning disabilities have associated conditions such as autism (see chapter 15) with a need for familiar routines that bring a sense of security and predictability;

(continued)

(continued)

attention deficit hyperactive disorder (ADHD); some people have specific sensitivities to their environment such as particular foods they cannot tolerate or fabrics they cannot wear, heightened sensory experiences (see chapter 15).

Emotional Regulation – sometimes ordinary emotional expressions, such as being cross, may be misinterpreted by non-disabled people as a symptom of the person's learning disability and requiring a psychiatrist or other specialist psychological intervention.

Examples of Modes of Expression – secondary emotional impairments (sometimes arising from the trauma that caused the original learning disability) such as seeming to under-react to stimuli or conversely displaying a heightened emotional response, sometimes these interfere with emotional adjustment, for example needing longer to calm down, and also with day to day enjoyment.

Difficulty Adjusting To Change – commonly a trait associated with people who fall within the autistic spectrum (see chapter 15), but may also feature in some people where routine and familiarity of day to day life situations enables them to cope better and optimise their sense of personal identity, safety and autonomy.

Examples of Modes of Expression – insistence upon familiar and set routines and patterns of daily life; anxiety triggered by changes to familiar environments and routines.

Emotional experience

Although people with learning disabilities experience the same range of emotions as everyone else, the web-based learning disability organisation LD Pride identifies five emotional difficulties that particularly affect people with learning disabilities (LD Pride, 2013). In no particular order of priority, these include shame, fear, environmental and emotional sensitivity, emotional regulation and difficulty adjusting to change (Table 17.1).

Shame and fear

Shame, fear and related emotions are no strangers to people with learning disabilities, but their shame is seldom due to any wrongdoing on their part, and the fears they may hold spring from many routes, not least fear of abuse.

> Someone calling me, er, nasty names and what have you. And, er, it's not very nice . . . calling me names like BaBa David . . . That was scary.
>
> (David, commenting upon one example of how he was verbally abused)

Fast facts 17.2   Abuse

Regrettably, some 22 per cent of adult abuse reported to local authorities relates to people with learning disabilities and abuse of children with learning disabilities probably exceeds 36 per cent of all child abuse cases (Emerson *et al.*, 2012). The range of abuse includes physical, emotional/psychological, neglect, financial, sexual, and combinations of these.

Of course, human rights are founded on respect for the dignity and worth of each individual adult or child, regardless of race, ethnicity, gender, language, religion, opinions, wealth, ability or impairment (United Nations, 1948, 1971, 1975, 1989, 2005). These rights stem from what all children and adults need to survive, grow, participate and fulfil their potential; they include civil, political, economic, social and cultural rights. For example, English law states that people who work with children must keep them safe (Children Act 1989; 2004; DFE, 2010). Similarly, the Department of Health provides guidance on the protection of vulnerable adults (DH, 2000, 2009, 2010).

Unfortunately the abuse of children and vulnerable adults, including people with learning disabilities, remains such a common occurrence as to feature repeatedly in media headlines. Fairly recent evidence concerning the training of National Health Service staff about protecting children points to a lack of consistency and rigour in training about abuse (CQC, 2009). At the time of writing, proposals to create a vast national database for all children have re-emerged in government thinking on child protection. However, history teaches that databases and related systems and processes seldom protect vulnerable adults and children from abuse. It is people who protect the vulnerable, not databases. So, in the NHS and elsewhere, competent, well-supervised, and well-resourced professionals in frontline posts are best placed to detect and act upon signs of actual or potential abuse. No less importantly, however, taking action to safeguard the welfare of children and vulnerable adults is, potentially, something that both you and I may have to do at some time in our workplaces and, perhaps sometimes, in our capacity as ordinary members of the public.

Reader activity 17.1   Suspecting abuse

- What should you do if you suspect any form of abuse to a child or adult with learning disabilities?
- What might prevent someone from acting upon their suspicion of abuse?
- To whom should suspicions of or abuse and actual abuse be reported? Make a list of potential sources of help.

Table 17.2 contains guidance on how to deal with reporting abuse. All social and healthcare agencies have 'speaking out' or whistle-blowing procedures which you may follow. If you cannot locate them, or if you would prefer, then you may telephone the Local Authority about your concerns or the NSPCC (National Society of the Prevention of Cruelty to Children) or the Care Quality Commission.

The impact of abuse upon an individual is always distressing and the effects can be profound. People with learning disabilities may therefore benefit from therapeutic support in dealing with psychological trauma in a similar way to other non-disabled people (e.g. Simpson and Miller, 2004). Table 17.3 considers some examples of more common causes of emotions in children with disabilities that are not specifically associated with forms of abuse and Table 17.4 outlines some therapeutic interventions.

Our most positive emotional experiences are sometimes referred to as peak experiences; an event that captures a moment of profound joy/peace/transcendence; moments of self-actualisation (Maslow, [1962] 1968). These kinds of experiences often form strong emotional and sensory memories that remain with the person for life. When an individual recollects such an experience, the recollection will tend to rekindle the original emotion that was experienced.

Table 17.2 Acting to stop abuse

- The worst thing you can do is nothing
- Where the person is in immediate danger phone 999 to obtain emergency medical assistance and/or the police
- Do not put yourself at risk
- Preserve evidence if possible
- Where the danger is less immediate, call the Local Authorities Adult Services or Child Services about your concerns. They will listen carefully and take very seriously what you say, even if you wish to remain anonymous.
- They will inform you about what will happen next and if appropriate give advice about how you can help keep the vulnerable person safe until immediate assistance from the police and/or social services arrive.
- If you are an employee, student on placement or volunteer, then you should immediately report your concerns to your line manager, who should call the relevant Child or Adult Services on that same day
- If you think your manager may be implicated or if the manager fails to act on your concerns, you should ring the Adult Services or the Child Services at your Local Authority even at weekends when they will normally have a cover service
- If you know or suspect another worker, student or volunteer has harmed a child or vulnerable adult, or failed to provide the proper care and support, you must report this
- You can find further advice on child protection and report abuse at: NSPCC (2013), available at: http://www.nspcc.org.uk/help-and-advice/help_and_advice_hub_wdh71748.html.

The emotional needs of children

Table 17.3 Examples of some causes of emotions in children with learning disabilities

Anger: Frustration arising from demands or experiences they find difficult may lead to emotional outbursts

Anxiety: Fear of failure e.g. at school, with school work and /or, in various social situations

Depression: Not being able to keep pace with non-disabled peers or achieve at the same rates as other children may cause the child to experience sadness and even depression. The child may develop a low self-esteem and may even turn their anger about their disability inwards at themselves.

Self image: May feel a sense of being inferior to others, feel powerless and incompetent because of the failures they have experienced or through not being allowed to do some of the things that other, non-disabled children are permitted. Some children will also have associated physical and sensory impairments such as hearing, visual or mobility, which may also affect their self image negatively, especially if they have experienced taunting or bullying.

Social skill difficulties: Children with learning disabilities are more likely to have associated physical or sensory impairments (see self image above). These may impede social skills. Children with learning disabilities may be less mature than their non-disabled peers, making them feel awkward in some social situations. Many will have difficulties reading social cues (or body language), for some this will be due to autistic spectrum characteristics, they may have trouble with oral language (e.g. tone and volume of voice, stammering, pauses while speaking).

Source: Spedsupport4parents (2011 online).

Table 17.4 Examples of types of therapy and training techniques

Type of therapy and training technique	Examples of application to emotional needs
Psychotherapy	insecure childhood attachment to parent; separation
Cognitive Behavioural Therapy	from significant others, e.g. parent, siblings; bereave-
Family Therapy	ment; grief; low self-esteem; experiences of rejection,
Assertiveness Training	being bullied, tormented; experiences of abuse, building
Cognitive Analytical Therapy	self-confidence; expressing sexuality; expressing intimacy;
Non-Directive Counselling	personal identity; depleted motivational skills; making
Clinical Psychology	transition from childhood to adulthood; phobias; coping
Clinical Psychiatry	with change; self-harming; managing difficult emotions;
	psychological problems; mental health; post-traumatic
	stress disorder; distorted self-image; shyness, aggression;
	problematic family dynamics.

Reader activity 17.2   Positive emotions

Try to recall five positive emotions that you have experienced in your life. They need not be peak experiences but you will probably find that for each positive emotional memory, you can also vividly recall what precipitated them.

Hidden emotions

People with learning disabilities are equally capable of experiencing positive emotions and peak experiences; as many of their stories, recollections and art works reveal (e.g. Deacon, 1974; Fido and Potts, 1989; Atkinson and Williams, 1990). However, they are also more likely to suffer adverse, unpleasant experiences with consequent negative emotions and recollections which can be vividly rekindled whenever they are brought to mind. Sometimes these negative memories may become deeply embedded in their psychology and become expressed in disassociated ways, some of which are indicated in Tables 17.1 and 17.3.

So while people with learning disabilities have attributes that enable them to lead fulfilling emotional lives, the categories represented in Table 17.1 and 17.3, which are neither exhaustive nor definitive, remind us of the negative emotional experiences to which people with learning disabilities are more likely to be susceptible. Our understanding of the range and complexity of such negative experiences and their potential effects has been increasing, drawing on a developing literature base of the emotional experiences of people with learning disabilities, covering aspects such as temperament, levels of activity and excitability; degrees of emotionality; attention span and distractibility; inhibitory controls by which individuals moderate their emotional responses; soothability or the time it takes to reach a state of equilibrium after experiencing something exciting, novel or challenging and approach avoidance, where new or novel situations may be either avoided or sought to differing extents according to the individual's general disposition to change and new experiences (Hollins and Sinason, 2000; Nadirshaw, 2000; Arthur, 2003; Teglasi et al., 2004). Of course, all of these facets of emotionality can and do vary significantly between individuals, whether or not a learning disability is present. They will, to a degree, reflect an individual's nature, experiences and environment. They are of major concern when their presence prevents us getting on with leading a fulfilling life. When that emotional impediment is present, people with learning disabilities, like most other people, can and often do, benefit from having friends and acquaintances who will offer support, sympathy, a listening ear, maybe some wise counsel, but when these are not available or insufficient, then therapy may also be worthwhile. Table 17.4 identifies a range of therapeutic approaches that have been used with success in supporting the emotional needs of people with learning disabilities. These are no different to the range of therapies available to the rest of the population, but there is an increasing literature that demonstrates their potential to assist people with learning disabilities (Beail and Warden, 1996; Hollins and Sinason, 2000; Arthur, 2003).

As seen in Chapters 7 and 8 even the most devoted and loving parents of a child with learning disabilities or an associated physical or mental impairment do not, typically, anticipate their soon-to-be baby will be anything different from the standard model, i.e. perfect, fingers, toes – the works. So when a child arrives who is noticeably different, those comfortable expectations will be challenged significantly. The reason why a child is born with a physical or mental impairment, such as a learning disability, is not always immediately known and sometime takes time to emerge and be recognised. Table 17.5 contains some indications of the kinds of reactions and emotions that parents may experience. Parents may, for example, go through a period of denying their child's disability; they may express anger and grief about the impairment.

Table 17.5 Some common parental reactions to the news that their child has a learning disability

Parents in denial of their child's learning disability
A deep-rooted reaction, usually a temporary stage in the process of acceptance of the child's learning disability, but it can sometimes persist and can be justified, for example, in the attempt to protect the child from labelling and negative stereotyping.
May include:

- making excuses for a child's school failure;
- blaming school failure on teachers or a spouse;
- accusing the child of being lazy or refusing to allow special education to be provided.

Anger – sometimes some parents become angry when a child has a disability
Like denial, anger is based in fear for the child's future well-being. The parent may seek someone or something to blame for their child's disability. This may be expressed at various stages of the child's life, for example, at school by being difficult in parent-teacher meetings, in delivering both warranted or unwarranted criticisms about the availability and adequacy of help and supports.

Grief – some parents feel grief over a child's disability
Many parent feel a powerful sense of loss when they learn that their child has a disability. May include: worries about the future; the grief may reoccur throughout the child's life especially when the key milestones and social rites of passage arrive that other children typically achieve.

Relief – some parents are relieved to obtain a diagnosis
Sometimes the relief of obtaining a formal diagnosis of a disability provides an explanation for many of the difficulties that face the family.

Source: Lodgson (2011).

A diagnosis can sometimes bring a sense of relief, for example, at last knowing some causative agent, or at least giving it a name. It may also serve to stigmatise and create a sense of shame and fear. Of course, the great majority of parents, regardless of the swell and mix of contrasting emotions they both experience and encounter, come to accept and value their child. As we will consider below, a major part of how we all learn about ourselves and what we *feel* about ourselves and others, stems from how other people react to us and treat us, especially during our formative childhood years. For example, Maslow's hierarchy of needs (Maslow, 1943, [1954], 1970, [1962] 1968, as illustrated in Chapter 1) expresses the growth of a human being in terms of the person's early socialisation into the world where, being accepted, kept safe and nurtured are the foundations by which each individual begins to engage with the world, develop a sense of belonging, self-confidence and a desire to know and explore life more generally (Figure 17.1).

Reader activity 17.3   Maslow's hierarchy of needs

- Consider each stage in Maslow's hierarchy of needs.
- What positive outcomes might a person gain at each stage of the hierarchy when born with or without a learning disability?
- What kinds of negative experiences might make progression through the hierarchy more difficult for a child or adult with learning disabilities? Make some notes and compare these with the contents of Tables 17.1 and 17.3 which contain examples of contributory factors.

Impacting on negative emotions

People with learning disabilities often have one or more associated difficulties, with things such as telling the time, basic literacy, attention difficulties, slow processing of information, motor coordination, genuine forgetfulness and/or difficulties organising things generally. These are things that can sometimes make them stand out as 'different' in some way and therefore influence other people's reactions and treatment of people with learning disabilities, not always for the better. Naturally, people with learning disabilities respond emotionally, like anybody else, to how other people treat them. Negative emotions tend to stem from negative experiences. Table 17.3 gives some examples of the kinds of responses that may be triggered during childhood, some of which may spill over into adult contexts. Not surprisingly, therefore, people with learning disabilities will sometimes choose to defend themselves from stigmatising labels and their frightful consequences by trying to hide their difficulties and deny their learning disability.

To help explore this a little further I would like to introduce you to some people with learning disabilities, beginning with Leon, whom I first met many years ago when I was a student and Leon was in his forties.

Case study 17.1   Leon's story

The system approach to disability, mentioned earlier in this chapter, had a significant impact upon Leon, from at least his youth onwards, by ascribing to him a diagnosis that condemned him to a stigmatised institutional life for a large part of his life. However, rather than deny his stigmatising institutional label, Leon appeared to do the opposite. Perhaps he felt it pointless to deny his disability after decades of being told by the institution that he was 'mentally subnormal' and later in the 1980s that he was 'a person with a mental handicap'. So in the 1970s, Leon introduced himself to me thus, 'Hello, my name's Leon, I'm mentally subnormal and EP, that means epileptic fit case!' By internalising the labels that institutionalisation had attached to him, Leon appeared at one and the same time to both accept the label of incapability (Gerber *et al.*, 1992), yet also to mock it by cleverly jesting the part he had been ascribed. Today Leon lives in supported accommodation and usually introduces himself as Leon.

So Leon has moved on and now defines himself in more diverse ways. We will think some more in this chapter about supporting people to move on and to define themselves in more diverse ways. For example, consider Ahmed's case study.

Case study 17.2   Ahmed's story

Ahmed is 19 and has social skills difficulties. He tends to miss some social cues and worries about being rejected, though he wants to get on well with his peers, he makes out that he is shy in order to hide his social difficulty. His support worker has been supporting Ahmed by helping him to rehearse social situations such as meeting new people and taking turns in conversation. The result is that Ahmed now understands better how to take turns, to have a conversation without interrupting quite so often when others are talking.

Reader activity 17.4   Social skills

- List some emotional strengths that you anticipate Ahmed will gain from becoming more adept at social interactions.
- What reasonable adjustments can you make if you meet someone like Ahmed who wishes to socialise and be accepted, but has not quite mastered all of the social skills necessary to take turns in conversation?

Case study 17.3   Claire

Claire sometimes hides her disability. She finds humour a little bit baffling at times and she will pretend to laugh at a joke she does not really understand in order to hide her learning disability.

Reader activity 17.5   Hiding a learning disability

- Can you suggest some ways that you may support someone like Claire to feel more at ease in such social situations? Adults like Ahmed and Claire may also need support to deal with ordinary things such as budgeting, shopping, reading a recipe or filling out an application form.
- In your line of work, what support (reasonable adjustments, see Chapter 3) might Ahmed and Claire need from you in order to use your services effectively, without shame or fear that they will be less well treated because of their learning disability?
- What potentially positive emotional outcomes might adults like Claire and Ahmed experience if you can successfully support them when using your service?
- How might you evaluate that their experience has been positive? Make some suggestions of ways that you could obtain feedback from Claire or Ahmed and or people who are supporting them to use that service.

Fear of failing is one of the major disincentives to motivation in people with learning disabilities. Having failed at something in the past may only serve to convince oneself that failure is inevitable. We all make mistakes and hopefully learn from them. So to support people like Claire and Ahmed to develop skills and competences in some of the ordinary activities mentioned above, it is important to develop an accepting yet supportive relationship with them and look at their strengths *with them*. In other words, to find out what they can already do well and what they like to do. It then becomes possible to build on those strengths. For example, by breaking down more complex activities and skills into a series of small achievable steps, it becomes possible for people with learning disabilities, like Ahmed and Claire, to practise those steps successfully. Take making a bed, for example, sometimes learning the last step in a sequence, such as smoothing the bed duvet, helps a person achieve the last task in a skill, like bed making, first. Teaching a complex skill like making the bed or dressing oneself may be made more immediately successful by teaching the last step in the sequence first and giving praise and encouragement. Once that last step has been successful a few times, teaching the step immediately before it can follow. In this way, before very long Claire and Ahmed can learn many complex self-help skills and do them completely by themselves when appropriate.

Reader activity 17.6   Ahmed's Goal Plan

An example of Ahmed making his bed is given in Table 17.6 (see also Swaggart *et al.*, 1995; Silver, 1998; Baker and Brightman, 2003; Browder and Spooner, 2011; ehow mom, 2012). What do you think step 3 will be? What instructions will you give John?

Using a stepped approach and, sometimes, reversing the order in which it is taught can help make success really immediate and rewarding. Otherwise, making the bed, learning to cook a meal, and so on from beginning to end might seem too difficult to Claire or Ahmed. We all enjoy being confident and capable. Each of us loves a sense of achievement.

Reader activity 17.7   Emotional strengths

- What do you imagine will be the emotional consequences for Ahmed upon completing each step and receiving praise in the sample goal plan in Table 17.6?
- When a person with a learning disability learns a new skill, what emotional strengths do you anticipate might be enhanced?
- Why is it important that Ahmed should be involved in choosing what he wishes to learn?

If you know someone with a learning disability who wishes to learn new skills, this gentle, supportive and positive approach using clear goals and positive encouragement is highly effective.

Table 17.6 An example from Ahmed's Goal Plans of a skill Ahmed has chosen to learn

Some of Ahmed's strengths that are used to help Ahmed achieve his plan	Some of Ahmed's aspirations/hopes
Ahmed likes John Ahmed likes to learn new skills Ahmed responds to encouragement and verbal praise	Ahmed wants to be more independent – do more things for himself such as: • dressing • making breakfast • making his bed
One of Ahmed's goals for this week: By the end of day five Ahmed will make his bed with minimal support from John.	1. John makes Ahmed's bed to the point where only the pillow needs placing on the bed.
Day one, step 1: Ahmed will put his pillows on his bed	2. John shows Ahmed how to put one pillow on the bed and asks Ahmed to place the second pillow on top. John praises Ahmed for placing the pillow.
Day 2, Step 2: Ahmed smoothes the duvet and adds the pillows to his bed	1. John makes the bed, adding and straightening the duvet. 2. John smoothes half the duvet and asks Ahmed to smooth the rest and add the pillows, praising Ahmed for his efforts and giving guidance if necessary.

You can find out more about how to facilitate this type of approach from the people who practise this regularly such as physiotherapists, occupational therapists, behavioural skills teachers and behavioural psychologists. There are further examples in the following references (Baker and Brightman, 2003; Browder and Spooner, 2011; ehow mom, 2012).

Some final words on issues of fear and shame come from Kevin and David. First, Kevin talks about being harassed in a shopping precinct: ' I've never been a fearful person, . . . there were these, er, lads they were peashooting at me and the support worker so we dashed round to [supermarket] and we were disgusted with them.'

Fortunately Kevin, with assistance from his support worker, was able to enlist the support of the local supermarket security people, who now know Kevin and told him, 'If you get any trouble, Kevin, you come down to us and we will sort it out for you.'

Fast facts 17.3   Safety in Doncaster

In the town of Doncaster in South Yorkshire, a local scheme called Safety in Doncaster (SID 2013) was developed by a self-advocacy group of people with learning disabilities who secured support from the local council and shops to display the SID logo on their windows. The SID logo signifies that the shop will assist anyone with a learning disability who feels unsafe for any reason, including the kind of harassment Kevin described above. The success of the scheme has spurred some other towns in South Yorkshire to develop similar schemes.

David has also experienced harassment, for example, during some visits to his local market, he explains:

> Someone calling me, er, nasty names and what have you. And, er, it's not very nice . . . calling me names like BaBa David . . . That was scary. One minute he's not there, then he is straight in t'back of you, yeah.

Kevin and David are both members of local learning disability self-advocacy groups. They are involved in a wide range of educational activities, including teaching university students and people in commerce, the public sectors and industry about disability issues. If you met them today, you would see two quite confident people. But they have not always been so confident. They both describe examples of how their self-confidence and self-esteem have improved greatly through their involvement with the advocacy groups.

> I used to go around town a lot, doing nowt, getting bored stiff. People used to come and target me, like I used to be a target for bullying . . . it got worse as I got older . . . One day we went to Gateway [a club for people with learning disabilities] . . .we had this launch to get this group going . . . Speaking Up For Action (SUFA, 2013) . . . we started sticking up for our rights, in a good way . . . that we could stick up for ourselves.
>
> (David)

The next example demonstrates how Kevin uses his self-confidence and the support from his advocacy group.

Malcolm: Did something happen that made it so you wanted to speak out . . . as a voice for people with learning disabilities?

Kevin: Hmm, it were all from the self-advocacy group with me, 'cos I do, like, volunteer work with them and all that.

Jacqui: This morning when we first met, one of the first things you said to me was that you'd heard that story about those people being abused in that care home.

Kevin: That's right, yeah.

Jacqui: Yeah, and that, that made you angry or

Kevin: Ooh, it has!

So Kevin channels the upset he feels about the mistreatment of people with learning disabilities into educating the wider public about learning disabilities. Here is an example of Kevin's work:

> I went into hospital and . . . I got a load of jargon and stuff [thrown] at me and I had to slow this here doctor down and consultant down, and it weren't very nice of hearing it when he were talking a load of jargon, so I were able to say, 'Look, can you draw pictures, and can you put a lot more easier language in for me, because I'll not be able to tell your jargon?' And he has done.
>
> (Kevin)

Kevin went on to help design information leaflets for use in the local hospital: Kevin says:

> This year we've had, like, the open day with the nurses and the big chief who come round, he says to me, he says, 'We, know we've got to listen at you now and not listen at what we want to do. We got to listen at you in future.'

Reader activity 17.8   Accessible information

- In your area of work are there easy read leaflets and information accessible to people like David and Kevin, written in ordinary words with helpful pictures and photos?
- If you were to develop or update such leaflets, how might you find and engage local people with learning disabilities to demonstrate that your organisation and you are listening?

Environmental and emotional sensitivity

People within the autistic spectrum are particularly prone to environmental sensitivity (see Chapter 15). In order to regulate and control this sensitivity, they will adopt regular daily routines and stick to familiar places, preferring their surroundings and routines to remain the same and unchanging. For some individuals, changes in their familiar environments can be overwhelming to their sense of order and control, provoking extreme anxiety and distress.

Some adults with learning disabilities have a heightened emotional sensitivity (e.g. Williams, 1996; Walker, 2000). This trait can enable them to intuitively understand both their own and other people's emotions and so form meaningful relationships. However, some people with learning disabilities have significant difficulties coping with strong emotions. An example would be feeling moved to tears quite easily by one's own or other people's distress. Conversely, it is quite usual for people who have autism to experience greater difficulty recognising emotions in other people and empathising. Yet people with autism will often have strong emotional experiences themselves, especially anxieties in response to changes in their familiar environment and daily routines.

Heightened emotional sensitivity, if it is expressed as aggression, may understandably lead to social rejection. Yet the person expressing that aggression may simply be trying to communicate their sense of emotional overload and be unaware of the effect this is provoking in others. The expressed behaviour stems from an urgent need to communicate, so in order to communicate more appropriately and obtain the desired result, the person may benefit from skilled support to enable them to recognise strong emotions and express them more acceptably.

Reader activity 17.9   Coping with strong emotions

- How do you cope with your own strong emotions and or an urgent need to communicate?
- Imagine you work on a reception desk. Today you are expecting a visit from one of your regular service users, Erica. Erica has a strong and vocal personality. She has lots of energy and doesn't like waiting, so if she has a long wait she may start pacing about and talking out loudly. You know that you need to think about how you can help to calm the environment so that Erica doesn't get over-stimulated.
- What else can you do to make Erica's experience and use of that service an all-round success?

Emotional regulation

Everyone sometimes needs to control strong emotions, and impulses. Young children often have difficulty coping with emotions (Table 17.3). Some people with learning disabilities struggle to control stronger emotions or impulsive thoughts and actions (Walker, 2000). Many of these strong emotions will have links to negative experiences in the past which have left the person highly sensitive to some kinds of emotions and experience which echo that past. These may even lead to anxiety and depression.

- A person with a learning disability is likely to have experienced less schooling, or segregated schooling, possibly integrated schooling and bullying. Later inability to obtain paid employment and social success may follow.
- How do you think these experiences, collectively, may contribute to the person's emotional well-being? Tables 17.1 and 17.3 contain indicative examples.

If you have been ridiculed by people close to you, perhaps by teachers, peers, perhaps by some professionals you have encountered, these experiences may understandably leave some psychological and emotional scars. Consequently heightened emotional responses to rejection, social anxiety and even a phobia of social events may exert powerful influences upon your behaviour and the activities and experiences with which you feel comfortable.

Difficulty adjusting to change

Both adults and children with learning disabilities may prefer familiar routines and environments, this becomes especially more likely where the individual has some behavioural features that fall within the autistic spectrum (see Chapter 15). The neurological underpinning for this behaviour may stem from the condition or trauma that caused the learning disability. However, the ability to cope with change can be nurtured. Consequently as children mature and pass through adulthood, many of these aspects become much less marked, provided that this supportive nurturing is present consistently and, where necessary counselling and therapy are available (see Table 17.4).

However, difficulty adjusting to change is often something with which adults with learning disabilities struggle. For example, some adults, especially if there is some degree of autism, will always want to stick to routines such as travelling by the same route to work, enter always by the same door, and so on (see Chapter 15). Even a slight change in this routine may cause acute distress, perhaps even the need to start the routine again from the very beginning. This sometimes gives people with this attribute a reputation for being inflexible when more accurately it is a device by which they try to avoid the unexpected for which they are less well equipped. Therefore some individuals feel 'safer' by staying with the known and familiar, by exerting some firm control over the complex world of sensory and emotional experiences.

Many people with learning disabilities do therefore benefit from opportunities to improve their ability to cope with change. As Ahmed (above) found, practice with social skills leads to more positive results because the social skills he learns actually succeed in affirming his desire for social acceptance, which otherwise might have resulted in him retreating to avoid social hurt. Ahmed has therefore improved his ability to tolerate social change.

Reader activity 17.11   Increasing confidence

Make some notes on how you in your role may support adults with learning disabilities to feel more confident, safe and in control in the environments where they encounter you and your colleagues.

Emotions throughout the life span

In the next part of this chapter we will explore emotional life throughout the life span by drawing on the writings of Eric Erikson (1950, 1968) who developed a theory of Psycho-social Life Stages (Table 17.7).

Table 17.7 Erikson's theory of Life Stages

Each life stage holds the potential for a positive or a negative outcome. A negative outcome in any of the stages may have the potential to be resolved later, under more favourable conditions.

Stage 1. Infancy – Birth to 18 months
Ego Development Outcome: Trust vs. Mistrust
Basic strength: Drive and Hope

Stage 2. Early Childhood – 18 Months to 3 years
Ego Development Outcome: Autonomy vs. Shame
Basic Strengths: Self-control, Courage, and Will

Stage 3. Play Age – 3 to 5 years
Ego Development Outcome: Initiative vs. Guilt
Basic Strength: Purpose

Stage 4. School Age – 6 to 12 years
Ego Development Outcome: Industry vs. Inferiority
Basic Strengths: Method and Competence

Stage 5. Adolescence – 12 to 18 years
Ego Development Outcome: Identity vs. Role Confusion
Basic Strengths: Devotion and Fidelity

Stage 6. Young adulthood – 18 to 35
Ego Development Outcome: Intimacy and Solidarity vs. Isolation
Basic Strengths: Affiliation and Love

Stage 7. Middle Adulthood – 35 to mid-60s
Ego Development Outcome: Generativity vs. Self absorption or Stagnation
Basic Strengths: Production and Care

Stage 8. Late Adulthood – approximately 55 or 65 to death
Ego Development Outcome: Integrity vs. Despair
Basic Strengths: Wisdom

With regard to Erikson's (1950) life stages (Table 17.7), potentially, if an individual was unfortunate to be landed only with the negative outcomes at each life stage, this would resemble the following characteristics of that person's life experience and emotions:

Mistrust + Shame + Guilt + Inferiority + Role Confusion + Isolation + Stagnation + Despair

Reader activity 17.12 Physical and mental exercise

Find a quiet place where you can do this physical and mental exercise:

- Begin by sitting down, then adopt a body posture and expression that conveys to other people MISTRUST.
- Hold on to that mistrust and add to it SHAME and GUILT.
- Hold on to the above and add a good helping of INFERIORITY to your expression and body language.
- Spice it up with some ROLE CONFUSION.
- Now imagine there are people nearby, Hold on to all of the above and ISOLATE yourself from them.
- Do not change anything, hold on to all of the above, stay as you are: STAGNATE.
- Now, DESPAIR!

I have used Reader activity 17.12 with small groups of students. By the time some of them reach ISOLATION, the students have backed away from everyone else, some of them have pulled furniture between them and other people and crouched low behind it! As you read on, I will introduce you to Connor. For those of us who have completed the exercise above, then just perhaps we may gain some sense of how Connor was feeling.

If Erikson's psycho-social life stages are anything to go by, then as people with learning disabilities live through the same life stages, the outcomes at each stage may have a significant bearing upon their quality of life and emotions, just as much as anyone else's. However, for a variety of reasons people with learning disabilities are more at risk of suffering the negative outcomes. Reader activities 17.13 to 17.20 will assist you to explore some of the factors that may impinge upon some powerful emotions at each stage of life for a person with a learning disability; you may also like to look again at Tables 17.1 and 17.3. We will work our way through Erikson's Life Stages.

Reader activity 17.13 Erikson's Life Stage 1

Erikson's Life Stage 1: Infancy: Birth to 18 Months; Ego Development Outcome: Trust vs. Mistrust. Basic strength: Drive and Hope. Most significant relationship – maternal parent.

In the early months after birth the most significant relationships are typically those between the infant and the maternal parent, or whoever is the most significant and constant caregiver. All infants need positive, loving care. When this occurs, the infant will learn that s/he has a right to be here and will develop trust that life is basically alright and confidence in the future. If, however, the infant is constantly thwarted in relation to that positive and loving care, then trust in others becomes difficult to establish because the infant's needs are not adequately satisfied. The infant may be left with deep-seated feeling of worthlessness and a mistrust of the world in general.

- What kinds of experiences during this stage of life might lead a person with a learning disability to develop a sense of trust in others? What kinds of experiences might counter this and lead towards a sense of mistrust?
- How do you imagine feeling mistrust towards other people might be expressed by the person in infancy, childhood, adolescence and adulthood respectively?
- In thinking about the above, it may help to remember that in our society the tacit belief that it is better to be dead than disabled has by no means vanished. For example, we still have eugenic abortion of foetuses with, for example, Down's Syndrome, and the rising count of deaths by indifference such as *74 Deaths and Counting* (Davies, 1987; Mencap, 2007, 2012; DH, 2010a).

Reader activity 17.14   Erikson's Life Stage 2

Erikson's Stage 2: Early Childhood: 18 Months to 3 Years, Ego Development Outcome: Autonomy vs. Shame/Basic Strengths: Self-control, Courage, and Will. Most significant relationships – parents.

During this stage children start to accomplish some skills such as fine motor skills, learning to walk, talking, feeding themselves and becoming toilet trained. The acquisition of these new skills holds many opportunities to develop self-esteem and autonomy. During the so-called 'Terrible Twos' children love to use the word 'NO!' which contributes to their formation of a sense of autonomy.

- At this stage children are vulnerable if they are made to feel ashamed when learning important skills such as toilet training. Feeling shame or doubt about their abilities may diminish their self-esteem.
- What kinds of experiences during this stage might lead a person with a learning disability to develop a sense of autonomy?
- What kinds of experiences might counter that sense of autonomy and perhaps lead to feelings of shame or doubt about oneself?
- How do you imagine feelings of shame and self-doubt might be enacted by the person in infancy, childhood, adolescence and adulthood respectively?

Reader activity 17.15   Erikson's Life Stage 3

Erikson's Life Stage 3: Play Age: 3 to 5 Years; Ego Development Outcome: Initiative vs. Guilt. Basic Strength: Purpose. Most significant relationship – basic family.

During this period children take the initiative in making creative and imitative play. For example, imitating what they see adults doing such as pretend cooking, wearing a parent's shoes, putting teddy to bed, using toy phones/cars, role playing at what the child thinks it means to be a grown-up. Children also begin to explore their environment more widely and to ask, 'WHY?' Because Erikson was influenced by Freud, he also argued the importance of the child identifying with a suitable same sex role model. Without this identification, the child could be left to feel guilt and frustration at having not formed that role identification.

- What kinds of experiences during this stage do you think would be suitable to enable a person with a learning disability to develop a sense of initiative, strength and purpose?
- What kinds of experiences might counter this and lead towards feelings of guilt?
- Imagine a young adult person with a learning disability wishing to try her hand at, for example, boiling the kettle to make a cup of tea. Her sense of guilt might lead her to try this in secret, perhaps in a hurry before anyone notices, hesitantly and so on. How might you support a person with a learning disability to develop a sense of initiative and purpose (i.e. to feel it is OK for me to try this for myself)?
- You might consider here how some of the skills teaching approaches mentioned above may be useful, for example, the effects they had on Claire and Ahmed (see above).

Reader activity 17.16   Erikson's Life Stage 4

Erikson's Life Stage 4: School Age: 6 to 12 Years; Ego Development Outcome: Industry vs. Inferiority/ Basic Strengths: Method and Competence. Most significant relationships – school, neighbourhood; parents no longer hold complete authority, though they are still important.

During this stage children continue to expand their learning and creativity, accomplishing many new intellectual, social and other life skills which develops in them a sense of industry. Children who experience unresolved feelings of inadequacy and inferiority in comparison to their peers can be left with significant problems in terms of competence and self-esteem.

- What kinds of experiences during this stage might lead a person with a learning disability to develop a sense of industry and capability?
- What kinds of experiences might counter this and lead towards feelings of inferiority?
- How might you support a person with a learning disability to expand their learning and creativity, widen their social networks and relationships so they feel increasingly confident and capable about life and their participation?

Reader activity 17.17 Erikson's Life Stage 5

Erikson's Life Stage 5: Adolescence: 12 to 18 Years; Ego Development Outcome: Identity vs. Role Confusion/Basic Strengths: Devotion and Fidelity. Most significant relationships – peer groups.

During previous stages, Erikson argued that personal development was dependent upon what is done to us. From this stage what we do socially is of more importance. During adolescence we struggle away from our childhood identity toward that of finding our own adult identity. Adolescents will experiment with social interactions, different identities and wrestle with moral issues. Discovering their own identity, beyond that of the narrower family, causes many adolescents to resist general responsibilities. This can be a trying period for families, but, once resolved, leads the adolescent to become more adept at adult self-expression. However, an unsuccessful outcome will result in role confusion. Adolescents seek to develop their philosophy of life, but life is seldom without conflicting values and beliefs. Adolescents tend therefore to think idealistically. Nevertheless, they are capable of forming strong attachments to friends and causes.

- What kinds of experiences and activities during this stage might lead a person with a learning disability to develop a positive sense of identity?
- What kinds of experiences might counter this and make the person feel confused about his or her identity?

Recall Leon, whom I introduced above, sometimes described himself to other people as 'mentally handicapped and EP – that means epileptic fit case'. People in authority had told Leon that he was this person many times, for example, his medical diagnosis when he was admitted to the institution stated as much and would be repeated at each case conference he attended over many years.

- How might you support Leon, or someone like him, to broaden his sense of who he is and what he can be?

Reader activity 17.18 Erikson's Life Stage 6

Erikson's Life Stage 6: Young adulthood ages 18 to 35; Ego Development Outcome: Intimacy and Solidarity vs. Isolation/Basic Strengths: Affiliation and Love. Significant relationships – marital partners and friends.

In the initial stage of being an adult we seek one or more companions and love. We try to find mutually satisfying relationships, primarily through marriage and friends, and generally begin to start a family. A successful journey through this stage can produce intimacy on a deep level. Lack of success may result in isolation and distance from others, causing one's world to shrink, yet in defence of our ego, one may develop a feeling of superiority over others.

(continued)

(continued)

- Think about the people who have shaped your emotional life, people with whom you became close; people with whom you shared your most intimate thought, feelings, sense and sense of self.
- Take some of these away, can you imagine the effects upon you? Now read the case study about Connor.

Case study 17.4   Connor's story

I mentioned above that I would introduce you to Connor. This case study is taken from a part of Connor's life when this author knew Connor personally for a number of years (Richardson, 1994). Connor spent about 40 years, from his childhood onwards, in an institution. When I first met Connor, he kept himself well apart from other people in the residential unit where he lived. He refused to wear any clothing. He used no speech. During the daytime he would barricade himself into a corner of a room or the outside yard with pieces of furniture, rugs and cushions that he commandeered. Connor might suddenly lurch forward to push away anyone who approached too near to his barricade.

Did you complete the exercise above (Reader activity 17.12) where you were asked to compound all of the negative outcomes in Erikson's life stages and observe the effects upon yourself? Connor's behaviour and body language appeared in many respects to signal these same negative outcomes (Richardson, 1994): mistrust, shame, guilt, inferiority, role confusion and isolation. In other words, Connor appeared to have accrued mainly the negative outcomes depicted in each of Erikson's (1968) psycho-social stages of development.

Many factors will have contributed to Connor's view of himself, the world and people generally and we can never know for sure. Most probable are lack of consistent, loving parent figures in infancy and childhood, compounded by his experiences of institutionalisation, which did not permit Connor to do many of the things that children, young people and adults should come to experience naturally, like being with people who value your company, identifying with other appropriate role models, role playing, acting autonomously, taking some risks, learning how to socialise in a supportive environment and forming friendships and intimate relationships. Such things as these, that most of us can experience and take more or less for granted as we grow and develop, were typically repressed within the institutions that Connor experienced during his formative years.

Reader activity 17.19   Trust

Clearly people with a learning disability need to be able to trust those closest to them, you may sometimes be that person.

- How can you demonstrate in your behaviour and actions towards a person like Connor that you merit that trust?
- Once you have established some trust, how important would it be to maintain it and how can you do that?

Richardson (1994) described how Connor's carers eventually established mutual trust with Connor. After establishing that initial trust, Connor was gradually introduced to other people whom he also came to trust, all of whom supported him to try out new experiences and activities over a period of weeks and months. During this time Connor was also taught new skills (or to re-acquire some that he had abandoned), using the positive goal-focused methods outlined earlier in this chapter. As Connor's trust in other people grew and some of his basic life skills expanded, so his self-confidence and self-esteem appeared to flourish. For example, Connor learnt to cooperate in putting on his clothes, he participated in activities such as taking a beach holiday and sitting with other people listening to music.

Reader activity 17.20   Erikson's Life Stage 7

Erikson's Life Stage 7: Middle Adulthood, ages 35 to 55 or 65; Ego Development Outcome: Generativity vs. Self-absorption or Stagnation/Basic Strengths: Production and Care. Significant relationships – in the workplace, community and the family.

Erikson observed that in middle age the important things we enjoy include creative, meaningful work and engaging with the family. At this time in life we can expect to 'be in charge'. Perpetuating and transmitting cultural values through the family (taming the youngsters) and working to establish a stable environment. Strength comes from care about others and from others and contributing to the common good of society, Erikson calls this generativity, and during this stage we tend to loath inactivity and meaninglessness. Relationships and goals in life may face us with major changes, for example, the children leaving home. We struggle to find new meaning and purposes – the mid-life crisis. If we do not negotiate this stage fortuitously, we can become self-absorbed and stagnate.

Creative and meaningful relationships, activities and work are all important to people with learning disabilities but such activities will often have been less accessible, often non–existent in the case of paid employment. How can you support a person with learning disabilities to find and maintain relationships, friends, creative work and activities (paid or otherwise)?

People with learning disabilities like to be in charge too, not just in terms of personal autonomy, but also contributing to wider agendas. Self-advocacy groups, social enterprises where people with learning disabilities employ other people are examples of how people can find fulfilment as they make their way through middle life, as David and Kevin testify above, and such activities and related training and support where necessary can promote the kind of outcomes sought in the reader activity above.

Fast facts 17.4   Personal integrity

Statistically, people with learning disabilities are less likely to live into late adulthood due to a variety of factors. Nevertheless, those who do experience and feel a sense of inclusion and participation in their lives are more likely to feel a sense of personal integrity and fulfilment (see Case study 17.5 Arthur).

Case study 17.5   Arthur

Arthur, now in his tenth decade, shares a home with a group of men and women like him who, many years ago, were institutionalised. But Arthur expresses no bitterness. When asked about the institution, he said, 'that was a long time ago . . . I made friends . . . there's happy memories too.' And of his current home, Arthur says, 'I like my telly, I like to get out once or twice in t' week. Sometimes I bet on the horses.' And if you are willing to listen, Arthur will tell you stories all about when he was a lad, or what he did yesterday! So Arthur seems to have a positive view of his life.

Reader activity 17.21   Erikson's Life Stage 8

Erikson's Life Stage 8. Late Adulthood: 55 or 65 to Death; Ego Development Outcome: Integrity vs. Despair/Basic Strengths: Wisdom. The significant relationship is with all of mankind, 'my-kind'.

Erikson felt that much of life is preparing for middle adulthood, and the last stage is recovering from it. Perhaps that is because as older adults we have often developed or found meaning in life and can look back on our lives with happiness, contentment and a feeling of fulfilment, that we have contributed to life; very like the case study of Arthur above. Erikson calls this a feeling of integrity. Wisdom from understanding the vastness of our world gives us the strength to hold a detached concern for the whole of life, accepting death as life's completion.

Conversely, some people upon reaching this stage despair at their life experiences and perceived failures. Still struggling to find a purpose or worthwhile meaning in their lives, they may fear death, questioning the value of their journey through life. Some come to feel that they alone possess the 'right' knowledge (similar in some respects to adolescence) dogmatically expounding their 'correct' views.

Having read Arthur's case study, think about these questions:

- What do you think will be important to supporting Arthur and other elderly people with whom he lives to feel fulfilled?
- Can you identify some activities that will help Arthur and his peers remember and celebrate past times?
- Some memories may be painful, sad or full of emotional hurt, how can you support someone to deal with such memories?

Thus far, we have used some of the theories developed by Maslow and Erikson respectively to explore emotional development and to relate this specifically to people with learning disabilities. What comes through forcefully in both of these approaches is that how we all come to know and understand and feel about ourselves and other people, is largely a reflection of how the world 'feels and reacts' to us.

Reader activity 17.22   Achievement

Thinking about where you work and may encounter people with a learning disability, make some notes about general principles and reasonable adjustments that you can apply that may assist people with learning disabilities that you encounter to feel safe and to express:

- their sense of personal worth;
- self-confidence;
- trust;
- the optimism to explore new experiences;
- a sense of achievement and personal fulfilment.

Conclusion

In conclusion, the emotional experiences and emotional lives of people with learning disabilities derive from much the same roots as those experienced by the rest of society. However, differences do arise in terms of how these emotional experiences are mediated by discrimination, prejudice and eugenics. While some significant differences have neuro-biological routes, such as being within the autistic spectrum or having Down's Syndrome, the positivity or negativity of the emotions people with learning disabilities experience are more accurately and more generally down to the differing reactions of those around them: parents, siblings, other relatives, neighbours, other children, professionals, and so forth. All of these people are subject to the same values and beliefs about people with learning disabilities as the rest of society.

Therefore, how well we as a society value difference, and learning disabilities are a form of difference, will determine the extent to which people with learning disabilities feel shame and fear or the extent to which they self-actualise. People with learning disabilities respond in flourishing ways to experiencing acceptance, inclusion and even celebration of some of the differences they possess. In your working environment, if you are able to promote these kinds of experiences, then you are probably already doing some of the right kinds of things to support positive emotional lives and outcomes. All of us benefit from education and skills teaching, but we must remember how important these are to supporting the emotional lives of people with learning disabilities, for example, to support and enhance the ability to cope with environmental and emotional sensitivities, emotional self-regulation and the difficulties of adjusting to change.

Thinking back to the story of Connor, above: trust, autonomy, initiative, industriousness, identity, intimacy, generativity and integrity are founded upon positive emotional experiences as we travel life's path. These were just as much Connor's birth right as they are yours and mine. In studying this chapter you should now be in a better position to support people with learning disabilities to find rewarding and positive emotional experiences. We have seen that those kinds of experiences come from many avenues such as respect, inclusion, education and developing skills (e.g. Claire, Ahmed and Connor), peer support and educating other people about learning disabilities (David and Kevin), being autonomous and defining oneself (Leon), and finding inclusivity, citizenship and some sense of fulfilment (Arthur). This chapter began by pointing out that emotions make life worth living, so we must be aware that additional therapeutic support will sometimes be necessary to help traumatised individuals find greater emotional well-being.

Points to remember

- People with learning disabilities experience the same emotional needs as other people.
- Life experience including disability and its impact can effect people.
- Human therapeutic and caring approaches are needed to discourage negative emotions and encourage more positive ones.
- It is important to reflect upon the needs of people with learning disabilities to ensure their needs are being met.

References

Arthur, A.R. (2003) The emotional lives of people with learning disability, *British Journal of Learning Disabilities*, 31: 25–30.

Atkinson, D. and Williams, F. (eds) (1990) *Know Me As I Am: An Anthology of Prose, Poetry and Art by People with Learning Difficulties*. London: Hodder and Stoughton.

Baker, B.L. and Brightman, A.J. (2003) *Teaching Everyday Skills to Children with Special Needs*, 4th edn. Baltimore, MD: Brookes Publications Co.

Beail, N. and Warden, S. (1996) Evaluation of a psychodynamic psychotherapy service for adults with intellectual disabilities: rationale, design and preliminary outcome data, *Journal of Applied Research in Intellectual Disabilities*, 9(3): 223–228.

Browder, D. M. and Spooner, F. (2011) *Teaching Students with Moderate and Severe Disabilities*. New York: Guilford Press.

Children Act (1989) Available at: www.legislation.gov.uk/ukpga/1989/41/contents (accessed 15 Nov. 2012).

Children Act (2004) Available at: http://www.legislation.gov.uk/ukpga/2004/31/contents (accessed 15 Nov. 2012).

CQC (Care Quality Commission) (2009) *Review Safeguarding Children: A Review of Arrangements in the NHS for Safeguarding Children*. Available at: www.cqc.org.uk/sites/default/files/media/documents/safeguarding_children_review.pdf (accessed 3 Jan. 2013).

Davies, A. (1987) Women with disabilities: abortion or liberation? *Disability Handicap and Society*, 2(3): 275–284.

Deacon, J. (1974) *Tongue Tied: Fifty Years of Friendship in a Subnormality Hospital*. London: National Society for Mentally Handicapped Children.

De Sousa, R. (2010) Emotion, in E.N. Zalta (ed.) *The Stanford Encyclopedia of Philosophy* (Spring 2010 Edition). Available at: http://plato.stanford.edu/archives/spr2010/entries/emotion/ (accessed 28 Nov. 2011).

DFE (Department for Education) (2010) *Working Together to Safeguard Children: A Guide to Inter-Agency Working to Safeguard and Promote the Welfare of Children 2010*. Available at: www.education.gov.uk/publications/standard/publicationdetail/page1/DCSF-00305-2010 (accessed 15 Nov. 2012).

DH (Department of Health) (2000) *No Secrets: Guidance on Developing and Implementing Multi-Agency Policies and Procedures to Protect Vulnerable Adults from Abuse*. Available at: www.dh.gov.uk/en/Publicationsandstatistics/Publications/PublicationsPolicyAndGuidance/DH_4008486 (accessed 15 Nov. 2012).

DH (Department of Health) (2009) *Responses to Consultations. Safeguarding Adults: Report on the Consultation on theRreview of No Secrets*. Available at: http://webarchive.nationalarchives.gov.uk/+/www.dh.gov.uk/en/Consultations/Responsestoconsultations/DH_102764 (accessed 15 Nov. 2012).

DH (Department of Health) (2010a) *Clinical Governance and Adult Safeguarding: An Integrated Process*. Available at: www.dh.gov.uk/en/Publicationsandstatistics/Publications/PublicationsPolicyAnd Guidance/DH_112361 (accessed 15 Nov. 2012).

DH (Department of Health) (2010b) *'Six Lives' Progress Report*. London: Department of Health.

ehow mom (2012) *How to Teach Life Skills for Developmentally Delayed Teenagers*. Available at: www.ehow.com/how_6374043_teach-skills-developmentally-delayed-teenagers.html (accessed 1 Nov. 2012).

Emerson, E., Hatton, C., Robertson, H., Roberts, P., Baines, S., Evison, F. and Glover, G. (2012) *Improving Health and Lives*. Durham: Learning Disabilities Observatory: People with Learning Disabilities in England 2011, Services and Supports. Available at: www.improvinghealthandlives.org.uk/publications/1063/People_with_Learning_Disabilities_in_England_2011 (accessed 15 Jan. 2013).

Erikson, E.H. (1950) *Childhood and Society*. New York: Norton.

Erikson, E.H. (1968) *Identity: Youth and Crisis*. New York: Norton.

Fido, R. and Potts, M. (1989) 'It's not true what was written down!': experiences of life in a mental handicap institution, *Oral History*, 17(2): 31–34.

Gerber, P.J., Ginsberg, R. and Reiff, H.B. (1992) Identifying alterable patterns in employment success for highly successful adults with learning disabilities, *Journal of Learning Disabilities*, 25(8): 475–487.

Hollins, S. and Sinason, V. (2000) Psychotherapy, learning disabilities and trauma: new perspectives, *British Journal of Psychiatry*, 176: 23–36.

LD Pride (2013) *Top Five Emotional Difficulties of People with Learning Disabilities*. Available at: http://ldpride.net/emotions.htm (accessed 3 Jan. 2013).

Lodgson, A. (2011) *Parent Reactions to a Child's Disability: Learn How Many Parents Respond to a Child's Disability*. Available at: http://learningdisabilities.about.com/od/parentsandfamilyissues/tp/Parent-Reactions-To-A-Childs-Disability-Reactions-To-A-Childs-Disability.htm (accessed 15 Jan. 2013).

Maslow, A.H. (1943) A theory of human motivation, *Psychological Review*, 50: 370–396.

Maslow, A.H. ([1954] 1970) *Motivation and Personality*. New York: Harper and Row.

Maslow, A.H. ([1962] 1968) *Towards a Psychology of Being*. Princeton, NJ: Van Nostrand Company.

Mencap (2007) *Death by Indifference: Following up the Treat Me Right! Report*. London: Mencap.

Mencap (2012) *Death by Indifference: 74 Deaths and Counting. A Progress Report 5 Years On*. London: Mencap.

Nadirshaw, Z. (2000) Expert or experience? Public or private? A personal view of a psychologist within the health care system, *Journal of Learning Disabilities*, 4(3): 187–191.

NICHCY (National Information Centre for Children and Youth with Disabilities) (2002) *General Information about Learning Disabilities*, Fact sheet #7. Available at: www.ldonline.org/ld_indepth/general_info/nichcy_fs7.pdf (accessed 2 Nov. 2002).

Read, S., Frost, I., Messenger, N. and Oats, S. (1999) Bereavement counselling and support for people with a learning disability: identifying issues and exploring possibilities, *British Journal of Learning Disabilities*, 27(3): 99–104.

Richardson, M. (1994) Erikson's model as a nursing tool, *Nursing Standard*, 8(17): 29–31.

SID (2013) Doncaster Council: Safety in Doncaster. Available at: www.doncaster.gov.uk/sections/socialcareforadults/adviceandsupport/learningdisabilitiesadults/S_I_D__Safety_In_Doncaster_.aspx (accessed 15 Jan. 2013).

Silver, L.B. (1998) *The Misunderstood Child: Understanding and Coping with Your Child's Learning Disabilities*, 3rd edn. New York: Random House Books.

Simpson, D. and Miller, L. (eds) (2004) *Unexpected Gains: Psychotherapy with People with Learning Disabilities*. London: The Tavistock Clinic Series.

Spedsupport4parents (2011) *How to Advocate for Your Child from the Outside In*. Available at: http://spedsupport4parents.wordpress.com/2011/07/31/learning-disabilities-and-socialemotional-difficulties/ (accessed 15 Jan. 2013).

SUFA (2013) *Speaking Up for Advocacy*. Available at: http://www.sheffieldmentalhealth.org.uk/providers/display?providerId=166 (accessed 15 Jan. 2013).

Swaggart, B.L., Gagnon, E., Bock, S.J., Earles, T.L., Quinn, C., Myles, B.S. and Simpson, R.L. (1995) Using social stories to teach social and behavioral skills to children with autism, *Focus on Autism and Other Developmental Disabilities*, April(10): 1–16.

Teglasi, H., Cohn, A. and Meshbesher, N. (2004) Social–emotional side of learning disabilities: temperament and learning disability, *Learning Disability Quarterly*, 27(1), (Winter).

United Nations (1948) United Nations General Assembly, Universal Declaration of Human Rights, 10 December 1948, 217 A (III). Available at: www.unhcr.org/refworld/docid/3ae6b3712c.html (accessed 19 January 2010).

United Nations (1971) UN General Assembly, Declaration on the Rights of Mentally Retarded Persons, 20 December 1971, A/RES/2856. Available at: www.unhcr.org/refworld/docid/3b00f04e5c.html (accessed 15 November 2012).

United Nations (1975) Office of the United Nations High Commissioner for Human Rights. Declaration on the Rights of Disabled Persons 1975. Available at: www2.ohchr.org/english/law/res3447.htm (accessed 15 Nov. 2012).

United Nations (1989) United Nations Cyber Schoolbus (2012) Children's Rights. Convention on the Rights of the Child (1989). Available at: www.un.org/cyberschoolbus/treaties/child.asp (accessed 15 Nov. 2012).

United Nations (2005) UN Convention (2005) UN Committee on the Rights of the Child (CRC), Report of the UN Committee on the Rights of the Child, Thirty-Ninth Session (Geneva, 17 May–3 June 2005), 21 December 2005, CRC/C/150. Available at: www.unhcr.org/refworld/docid/44182d714.html (accessed 15 Nov. 2012).

Walker, K. (2000) *Self Regulation and Sensory Processing for Learning, Attention and Attachment*. Gainsville, FL: Occupational Therapy Department, University of Florida.

Williams, D. (1996) *Autism: An Insight-out Approach*. London: Jessica Kingsley Publications.

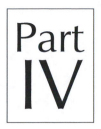

Part IV

Psychological and psychotherapeutic interventions

Introduction

My world is a world of confusion. I don't understand lots going on around me and that makes me mad! Things have happened in my life that have been bad, people have told me they were bad. I have been hurt by them. I get so angry sometimes and so upset as well. I need someone to listen and tell me everything will be OK!

Part IV will explore the needs of someone with a learning disability who also presents with psychological, behavioural and mental health needs. Such a person is complex and challenging to work with. It may be unclear as to how best to meet their needs. Once again, the topics will be explored through the use of a case study and the reader will be encouraged to use exercises to explore the needs of the person with a learning disability. There will be an investigation of the issues that are important to people with learning disabilities with suggestions of how best to address the person's psychological conditions and possible approaches outlined in detail. Ultimately the aim is for the reader to gain greater confidence in working with such an individual within the health and social care area, recognising the need for psychological interventions, to better understand the service users' condition and to more effectively meet needs.

The chapters which make up Part IV are:

Chapter 18 Sexuality and people with a learning disability
Chapter 19 The behavioural needs of people who have a learning disability
Chapter 20 The mental health needs of people with a learning disability
Chapter 21 Addressing the needs of people with learning disabilities who have offended
Chapter 22 Bereavement and loss
Chapter 23 Ethical issues when meeting the psychotherapeutic needs of people with a learning disability

18 Sexuality and people with a learning disability

Stacey Atkinson

Learning outcomes

After reading this chapter you will be able to:

- allow the reader to consider the importance of sexuality generally and to highlight the need for addressing sexuality when meeting the holistic needs of an individual.
- identify potential barriers in enabling someone with a learning disability to reach their full sexual potential and to acknowledge the ways in which barriers may be overcome.
- emphasise the need for people with a learning disability to become more aware of matters of a sexual nature. Such awareness is important in increasing their knowledge and insight, reducing vulnerability and increasing sexually responsible behaviours.
- provide guidance regarding how people with a learning disability may have their sexuality needs met through informal and formal support mechanisms and teaching strategies.

Introduction

I have a learning disability. Sex is a word I have heard. People giggle or go red when they say it. Lots of people talk about it. My carers mention it with secret voices and laugh! People on telly go on about it all the time but no one talks about it to me. Why not? What is this thing that I am left out of? I want to have shiny hair and red lips, I want to look like those women in magazines. I want people to look at me and think 'she is beautiful.' I want to kiss someone and see how it feels and for someone to touch me down below, that feels nice. Arrrggggghhhh I want to know about this sex thing!

This chapter will, through the use of Lawrence's case study and reader activities, address the sexuality needs of people with a learning disability. It will highlight what the important issues are for people with a learning disability, giving students historical and contemporary sociological perspectives regarding why many people with a learning disability still have unmet sexuality needs. It will suggest ways in which these sensitive needs can be developed, acknowledging the rights of people with a learning disability as sexual beings and increasing the reader's skills in this area.

Case study 18.1 Lawrence's story

Lawrence, aged 28, has a moderate/mild learning disability and he has been admitted to a medium secure unit for people with a learning disability and mental health needs who have offended. Lawrence has several times exposed his genitalia in public recently, generally targeting children. In the most recent incident he exposed himself and asked a child to 'touch it' and was reported to run after the children until they got away. Lawrence's account of the event is that they were teasing him and encouraging him to expose himself. The incident resulted in public outrage and Lawrence was arrested for indecent exposure under section 66 of the Sexual Offenses Act (2003). He was felt to be a threat to the public.

Lawrence's history is that following abandonment in infancy, he spent many years in and out of foster care, where it was later suspected he may have suffered episodes of sexual abuse. He eventually was given permanent accommodation at the age of 8 in a Local Authority children's home but was vulnerable to sexual, physical and psychological abuse (bullying) from older children and despite staffs' attempts to protect Lawrence, he would place himself in positions whereby he was vulnerable to exploitation and some further incidents of abuse occurred. Lawrence attended special schooling for children with learning disabilities and required extensive supervision as he had a tendency to approach younger children for sexual purposes.

In adulthood, due to his sexualised behaviour, it was felt that Lawrence would be better supported within a hostel for people with a learning disability. It was in the hostel that Lawrence began a loving, sexual relationship with a much older man of 65 called Bill, who had a mild learning disability. Their relationship appeared consensual and lasted for three years before Bill suddenly died. During their relationship Lawrence's sexualised behaviour towards others stopped and he appeared much happier and more settled than he had previously been. However, following Bill's death, the behaviour became much more determined and despite staff attempting to constantly supervise Lawrence, something he found extremely intrusive, he would invent ways of leaving the home unnoticed and readily approach unaccompanied children asking them to touch his exposed genitalia. At home Lawrence became increasingly more aggressive and had generally changed from the carefree person he had become with Bill to someone who was short-tempered, who would throw furniture and shout if disturbed or challenged. He had become increasingly afraid of being left alone, particularly at night, when he often asked staff to stay with him until he fell asleep.

Lawrence was assessed on admission to the unit and it was felt that in addition to his learning disability, he also was depressed and had an anxiety disorder. He appeared confused about sexuality issues, while he readily sought sexual gratification from males, he stated that he 'fancied' women and thought they were beautiful. Lawrence was placed on medication to reduce his depression and anxiety and to control his libido.

Each of Lawrence's psychological needs will be explored in the sections to follow.

Lawrence has many areas of confusion with regards to his sexuality. Consider the reasons why this confusion has occurred. Circle the relevant reasons.

A high libido	Due to his learning disability
Ignorance about the law	Lack of knowledge of how to behave in public places
Lack of good sexual education	Childhood instability
Communication problems	His learning needs
Not knowing how children should be treated	Exposure to sexual abuse.

What is sexuality and why is it important?

It is important to gain an understanding of the importance of sexuality and sexual health within all our lives, to realise the breadth of these areas and to gain an appreciation of how it might be for someone to be denied the opportunity to know about, to explore or be able to address such issues. In order to do this, it is important to define sexuality and sexual health.

In this day and age sexuality is a word so much more readily discussed but it is often linked to what sexual orientation someone has, with many people considering sexuality to be whether someone is 'gay or straight'. Sexuality is much more than this. The World Health Organisation (WHO, 2008) define sexuality as

> A central aspect of being human throughout life which encompasses sex, gender identities and roles, sexual orientation, eroticism, pleasure, intimacy and reproduction . . . Sexuality is influenced by the interaction of biological, psychological, social, economic, political, cultural, ethical, legal, historical, religious and spiritual factors.

Sexuality is all-encompassing; it includes gender issues, not just with regards to what sex someone is, or what sexual orientation they have; it is so more than this. If you were not female, perhaps you would be someone else completely. Not just a man, you perhaps would have a whole different outlook on life. Perhaps you would aim to achieve things in different ways, you might have different goals, different opportunities. You might be as far removed from the person you are today as you could be. Sexuality affects how someone relates to the world. It, at times, affects the job someone has and, it can affect the wage someone earns. It affects a person's perceptions of life and of what that life holds for them. It is relevant to the ability to bear children. A person uses their sexuality as a source of fun and enjoyment or they might gain employment through their sexuality such as if involved in prostitution or pornography. All people are affected by sexuality, by virtue of being human and having a gender; it is important for us all. In view of this, sexuality is something that perhaps health and social care professionals who work with people within care settings need to be especially aware of. They have to understand the impact not only of their own sexuality but also the sexuality of the people with whom they work and generally the impact of sexuality on everyday life.

In nursing, Roper, Logan and Tierney (1996), well respected nursing theorists who compiled a model for nursing; outlined the activities of human living. They identified the importance of meeting the fundamental needs of the holistic person and highlighted sexuality as one of the activities of living as shown in Chapter 9 (Figure 9.6).

Reader activity 18.2   Importance of sexuality

Lawrence's case illustrates the importance of sexuality as an issue in someone's life.

Lawrence was sexually exploited from an early age and went on to behave sexually inappropriately himself. He began to be protected because of his sexuality. Later he had a sexual partner and was happy and contented. He lost his partner and was saddened. Following this he sexually offended. Sexuality has played a large part in Lawrence's life.

Is it the case that sexuality is important in one way or another in all our lives? Perhaps our lives have not followed the same pattern as Lawrence's, but isn't sexuality still important?

Seeing sexuality as an essential part of the whole person is vital. If a health practitioner was to neglect any of the elements of the human person, for example, the activity of breathing, by not opening an airway when necessary, the person would suffer and may die. Similarly, if sexuality were not addressed, severe suffering might also occur. Sexuality is as important to the person as breathing is. Soble (1998, p. 22) saw sexuality as being not only natural, but due to our need to reproduce, sexuality and sex, as an element of our sexuality, is an innate part of a human being, a 'hormone-driven instinct implanted by nature'. He highlighted the natural, 'hormone-driven' nature of our sexuality and as such it is something that we cannot but help but get involved in. It could therefore be argued that the desire for sex and the nature of one's sexuality are autonomic or instinctive and therefore not dependent on a person's level of intellect.

For people with a learning disability as well as those without learning disabilities, sex, sexuality and sexual health are important matters. How important they are at a given time may depend on the individual needs at any point in a person's life. Someone's sexuality needs may come more to the fore when someone is worrying about sexuality issues, for example, during adolescence, when they may be becoming sexually active; if someone is in need of a smear test or perhaps when wanting to attract a partner. Throughout life the role that sexuality plays in the life of people with a learning disability should never be underestimated. It is important to be treated as a female or male, to have a sexual identity, to be respected and treated with dignity with regards to your sexuality and know that your sexuality is being acknowledged by those around on a continual basis. At the specific times mentioned above, someone with a learning disability may require heightened support.

Reader activity 18.3   Mammogram

You may know someone you can think about for the following exercise or you may have to use your imagination.

Think about the needs of a woman with a severe learning disability who is attending a clinic for a mammogram. What information/support/advice might she need before the appointment?

Sexual health and sexuality

Sexual health was defined by the WHO (2008) as:

> A state of physical, mental and social well being in relation to sexuality; it is not merely the absence of disease, dysfunction or infirmity. Sexual health requires a positive and respectful approach to sexuality and sexual relationships, as well as the possibility of having pleasurable and safe sexual experiences, free from coercion, discrimination and violence.

When an individual becomes aware of their sexuality, then some type of sexual behaviour might occur. Teenagers, with or without learning disabilities, on becoming more aware of their sexuality often engage in increased sexual behaviours at different levels such as flirting, exploring fashions or having a first girl/boy friend. It is important therefore to address sexual health, so that if the sexuality is expressed in more intimate ways such as within relationships, then sexual health is recognised and maintained. Or if sexual health is lost, through, for example, developing a venereal infection, or through the potential psychological torment of an unwanted pregnancy, at such times sexual health is a goal to be reached. If someone is taught about their sexuality, then they must also be taught how to remain sexually healthy. If someone is sexually unhealthy, then this might impact on the person's sexuality.

Reader activity 18.4   Expressing sexuality

Sexuality is important to all of us. How do you express your sexuality? List the ways.

Case study 18.2   Lawrence's ideal sexuality scenario

Lawrence is a sexual being, just like everyone else. But perhaps due to the nature of his previous sexual experiences, specifically the previous sexual abuse, some of the ways he expresses his sexuality, for example, exposing his genitalia to children in public places, are inappropriate. He has become confused about sexuality issues and is now actually committing sexual offences. This might have been actually avoided and if his sexuality had been addressed, the pattern of Lawrence's life would perhaps have altered.

   The ideal case scenario would be if, in his earlier life, Lawrence had received accessible information about sexuality in pictorial forms from a learning disability nurse. Lawrence can trust this person, he has formed a good relationship with her and she has the skills to develop the programme which meets his specific needs. She liaises with the multi-disciplinary/multi-agency team involved with Lawrence such as his carers, his social worker and medical practitioners and all contribute to the education he receives by being consistent in their approaches and treating him with respect and acknowledging him as a sexual person. Through his nurse Lawrence learns that children are not sexual beings and learns how he should behave sexually. He falls for Bill and learns to love. On Bill's death he grieves but he has no previously sexually

(continued)

(continued)

inappropriate behaviour to revert back through his bereavement. He talks to those around him about how he feels at the loss of his partner. He may go on to love again. If this ideal case scenario had occurred, the outcome for Lawrence might have been very different.

Reader activity 18.5   Sexuality scale

How would you feel on a scale of 1–10 if someone stopped you expressing your sexuality in one of the ways you have identified?

Not concerned 1   2   3   4   5   6   7   8   9   10 Angry/Upset

---

The barriers to addressing the sexuality needs of people with a learning disability

Societal views

As illustrated, people with a learning disability have the sexual needs, desires, hopes and dreams like other people but many face barriers which prevent them expressing their sexuality. Due to such barriers within learning disability services and indeed within society, people with learning disability may be denied the opportunity to engage with their sexuality in ways that other people do. They may be prevented, for example, from talking about issues to do with sex and sexuality or in having privacy with regards to intimate matters. In extreme cases people may feel that they are not being seen as or treated as a man or a woman or people with learning disabilities are denied the opportunity to have intimate relationships (Henault, 2006). Previous care regimes for people with a learning disability, i.e. the institutionalisation of people with a learning disability, coupled with strongly held views about the 'nature of learning disabilities' have led some to believe strongly that individuals with learning disabilities should not be taught about sexuality matters; deep fears have prevailed and perhaps still do with regards to sexuality and people with a learning disability.

On one hand, as highlighted by Craft (1987), many people in society believed that people with learning disabilities were like children and thus would have no need for knowledge about matters of a sexual nature. In the Victorian era at the other extreme, they were seen often to be sexual deviants. They were seen as a group of individuals who 'bred like rabbits', had limited morality and reproduced more sexual and intellectual deviant offspring, who due to the high numbers they were expected to produce, would be responsible for the intellectual and moral decline of society. Allen (1997) reports how these thoughts heralded the eugenic period.

This was a significant time in the history of learning disability care. Geneticists, led by Sir Francis Galton (c.1865), were powerful and influential people, who having done some exploratory work on genetics and the hereditary nature of talent and character traits, reported on the hereditary nature of undesirable traits such as reduced intelligence or ugliness (Stubblefield, 2007). The influence of these geneticists coupled with the already swelling distaste for 'undesirables' in society led to the introduction of laws which supported the sterilisation of thousands of people with learning disabilities across

Europe from circa the 1920s until the 1950s. The thought of sterilising would perhaps be humane. As mentioned, people with learning disabilities were seen as childlike imps and what would such creatures need with reproductive organs. 'Children' do not give birth. Sterilising the 'moral defective', a definition provided by the 1913 Mental Health Act, would be a highly effective way of curbing their reproductive patterns. Sterilisation was coupled with the mass admission of people with learning disabilities into large prison-like institutions where the mixing of sexes was highly regulated; such practices restrained the sex lives of people with learning disabilities. In such an environment, the only type of sex education was the strong message about the wrongness of sex and sexual expression. The presumptions of promiscuity led to the sterilisation of hundreds of people with a learning disability in Britain also. This continued until the middle of the twentieth century with institutional care being the preferred mode of care until the Community Care Act (1990) (Grant *et al.*, 2005).

Reader activity 18.6   Providing sex education

When thinking about Lawrence, what reasons might there be for those around him to perhaps be afraid of providing sex education/information to him?

Carers' views

Despite moving away from mass care for people in institutions and introducing legislation which promotes person-centred approaches, individualised care and consideration of the mental capacity needs of people with a learning disability, many still see the learning disability and make assumptions about their inabilities as a group of people. This is especially the case when working around sensitive topics such as sexuality and there are many reasons why addressing the sexuality needs of people with a learning disability is deemed a tricky, if not a risky thing to do. This is one reason why many professionals and carers including family members, shy away from addressing the sexuality needs of those people they care for. Sexuality is shaped by social forces; social contexts define what is legitimate (Ross and Rapp, 2009). How someone is able to express their sexuality often depends on environmental influences, for example, if a carer does not believe sexuality should be addressed, then it most probably won't be. There are many reasons why carers shy away from addressing the issue, leaving many people with a learning disability in the dark about such matters.

Reasons include:

- Seeing people with a learning disability as not needing information about sexuality and sexual health due to misunderstandings about their need for information or about their level of capacity to learn from the information (McCarthy, 2001).
- Carers may feel that that people with a learning disability may be vulnerable to abuse or exploitation, so may react by limiting the information or advice given. To somehow protect them and keep them safe from a world they do not yet have awareness of. This is almost like, don't tell them about it and they will never know. Such actions could be likened to the 'Pandora's box' principle. Pandora was, according to Greek mythology, the first woman. She owned a box which she was told to never open, then one day, out of curiosity she opened it and out of it spilt

all the evils of mankind – greed, slander, vanity, envy and pity, leaving only hope in the box (Lindeman, 1997). The story of Pandora may be applied when considering sexuality issues as it warns that if one opens the sexuality box needlessly, then nothing but negative outcomes will occur. If one agrees with the premise that people with learning disabilities should be kept ignorant with regards to sexual matters, then one might worry about a professional teaching them about sexuality, maybe putting ideas into innocent heads that can lead to them exploring things they would never have previously contemplated; in this case leading perhaps to them getting into sexual situations they did not bargain for.

- Concerns about the level of one's own skill as a practitioner in addressing sexuality when someone perhaps has communication needs/deficits. The person's communication needs may prevent the assessor fully ensuring the person's understanding and they may not be able to show effectively what their sexual choices are (Garbutt, 2008).

- Fears about a lack of support from others, for example, within an organisation if a person acting as a member of staff addresses someone's sexuality (Davies *et al.*, 2005). Will others support me? Will others agree with my actions? It might be feared by some that if you teach people with learning disabilities about sexual matters, it is giving them the green light to be sexual. Sex education may be something that perhaps not everyone will agree with.

- The religious or moral beliefs of those caring for people with a learning disability may prevent them from promoting the sexuality of those they care for. If sex if occurring outside marriage or sexuality is being expressed in a manner they do not agree with, such as through same-sex relationships, this can be an issue of contention for carers, causing them to hesitate to promote sexual behaviour (Craft, 1987).

- Being employed by/for the person with a learning disability can cause difficulties when addressing their best interests, particularly around something as sensitive as sexuality. Murphy (2001) discussed the difficulties in allowing people with a learning disability some freedom and autonomy with sexuality issues while still protecting them. There is a balance required when meeting the needs of people with a learning disability which requires practitioners to encourage an individual's autonomy while actively promoting their independence and rights; also ensuring that the practitioner works within their duty of care. This is extremely complex and difficult to get right! All of these issues have perhaps contributed to the fact that Lawrence has, of yet, not had education on sexual issues.

Reader activity 18.7   Helping Lawrence

Circle the areas that it might be helpful for Lawrence to know and learn about, thus enabling him to develop more sexually and socially appropriate behaviour.

1. Naming body parts
2. What is abuse
3. How to protect oneself from abuse
4. Identifying private body parts
5. The law and sex
6. How to form relationships

7. Ways of being intimate
8. Sexual intercourse
9. Different types of relationships
10. Methods of contraception
11. Safe sex.

Continue the list with anything else you feel needs to be included.

Reader activity 18.8   Sex education

If you were considering delivering a programme of sex education to someone with a learning disability, what do you think you might be concerned about at this present stage of your career?

The sexual knowledge of people with a learning disability

As already outlined in this book, the term learning disability refers to a group of people with sometimes very different needs. Someone can be labelled as having a profound, severe, mild moderate or mild learning disability, the scale advancing as their level of intellect increases. People who have a diagnosis of profound learning disability may have very different needs to those said to have a mild learning disability. The former group may be unable to communicate verbally, may have profound physical disabilities and also have specific sensory needs, while those at the milder end of the spectrum may be able to articulate well, be fully mobile and have no sensory differences to others in society, but may be slower at developing literacy and numeracy skills than other people. Clearly, as a group, this diversity is both in relation to their needs generally and also in their awareness of all matters sexual. While it is difficult to say what many individuals with learning disabilities know about such issues, as outlined above, some may be unable to communicate verbally. Research by Zdravka and Mihoković (2007) explored the level of sexual knowledge of people with a mild and moderate learning disability and found that their knowledge of sexual matters is very much dependent on their level of intellect, so, for example, someone with a more severe level of learning disability would have less knowledge on sexuality matters than someone with a milder learning disability. Zdravka and Mihoković found that as a group, when compared to others of a similar age without a learning disability, their knowledge was lacking in many areas with regards to sex and sexuality, but most concerning was their lack of knowledge in relation to protecting themselves from sexual exploitation, sexually transmitted infections and knowing how to avoid them, also how pregnancy occurs and its prevention. Many members of the group Zdravka and Mihoković studied, however, were sexually active. It could be argued therefore that people with learning disabilities, if unaware of sexual matters while being sexually active, may be vulnerable to abuse, sexual ill health and unwanted pregnancies. Zdravka and Mihoković's (2007) research was undertaken with the most able of the client group but for those with a lesser level of intellect, though they may perhaps be less sexuality active due to mobility needs or higher levels of support, they, however, are no less in need of sexual knowledge. They are often reliant on others to provide intimate care and due to their subsequent vulnerability, they may be more at risk of sexual abuse or unwanted pregnancy. Garbutt (2008) outlined the need for sex education aimed at a level cognitively accessible to the person with a learning disability. In view of this, the support given would need to be planned following a holistic assessment of individual need which will be provided by a learning disability nurse or psychologist.

Reader activity 18.9 Resources

If you were to provide some education for Lawrence about his sexuality, what sorts of equipment/aids/teaching resources might you use to make the information more accessible to him?

Addressing the sexuality of people with a learning disability: techniques and the reasons for doing so

Having intimate and/or sexual relationships is important. Morrall (2001) states that being sexual is biologically, evolutionally and socially normal, it can bring immense enjoyment and satisfaction. Having sexual relationships can make people feel desirable and attractive; they can build the general sense of well-being and confidence. Lowenthal and Haven (1968) and Horwitz et al. (1998) revealed that good mental health is linked to the value of one's intimate relationships. Generally, people with better close relationships, including sexual ones, have raised self-esteem and enjoy better mental health. McConkey (2007) found that generally people with learning disabilities have much fewer social relationships of any kind than other people. As highlighted, poor mental health can be the result of poor/limited social and sexual relationships (Priest and Gibbs, 2004). It is vital therefore that those supporting people with learning disabilities encourage them to form and maintain relationships, especially more intimate ones. It is interesting to note also that where sexuality is addressed with individuals like Lawrence, the issue of same-sex relationships is even more rarely discussed (Burns and Davies, 2011). Being able to express your sexuality is a fundamental part of being human. The sexuality needs of people with a learning disability should be addressed as readily as other needs.

Reader activity 18.10 Relationship

You may have a partner now, or had one previously. Think of the times you have had a partner in your life. What positive impacts are there or were there when you were involved in that relationship?

Why shouldn't someone with a learning disability also be able to feel this way?

Sexual abuse and people with a learning disability

Sexual abuse is defined by DH (2002, 2.7) as the involvement in 'sexual acts to which the vulnerable person has not consented, or could not consent to or was pressured into consenting to'. There are often imbalances of power between the perpetrator and victim and, in the case of child sexual abuse, there may be large age differences and it is a crime. People with a learning disability are highly vulnerable to sexual abuse. There are many points which must be considered here.

- The term sexual abuse covers a variety of sexual acts against the victim. Some, such as rape or sexual assaults, involve direct physical contact and others such as voyeurism can be without direct contact. There may be violence involved.
- Abuse can affect both adults and children.
- Hall and Innes (2011) report that in the general population, between 2009 and 2010, 2 per cent of women and just less than 1 per cent of men had experienced a sexual assault. The prevalence in learning disabilities is not fully known and different studies report different findings but Brown (1993), cited in Jenkins and Davies (2004), suggests that up to 50 per cent of adults with learning disabilities may have experienced sexual abuse, while Sullivan and Knutson (2000) in a very large epidemiological study identified that children with disabilities were 3.1 times more likely to be sexually abused. Of the 40,000 children researched, it was found that 31 per cent of children with disabilities had suffered some form of abuse.
- Both Hall and Innes (2011) and McCarthy (2001) point out that sexual abuse is vastly under-reported among people with a learning disability, so its true incidence is unknown.
- In reported cases perpetrators are in two-thirds of cases already known to victims.
- Mencap (2001) reports that the prevalence of abuse is up to four times higher among people with a learning disability than in the general population. Not to address sexuality leaves people like Lawrence vulnerable to sexual abuse, as highlighted by Peckham (2007), Davies *et al.* (2005) and DH (2002).
- People with learning disabilities are vulnerable to sexual abuse, through for example, the nature of the care environment. It may be actually disabling rather than enabling, through them not knowing about abuse and not being provided with the skills to recognise or report it.
- By virtue of the fact that people are often not taught what abuse is, they may not know about issues such as rights, consent, and choices. This is a concern not only for their well-being but for others with whom they may come into contact. This is a worrying situation, as like Lawrence, it may make them unwittingly become perpetrators of abuse.
- Due to cognitive disability and communication needs, people with a learning disability can have difficulty in reporting crime. The consequence of this is that for many victims, if assaults are reported, they often do not result in the conviction of the alleged perpetrator (Wheeler, 2004). (See Chapter 21.)

People with a learning disability are often not taught about abuse or taught how to protect themselves. Ignorance is not bliss, it is a very worrying state of affairs (Brown, 1993, cited in Jenkins and Davies (2004).

Reader activity 18.11   Vulnerability

Consider the following: why might people with a learning disability may be vulnerable to sexual abuse? You might find some reasons above and you may be able to consider other reasons.

Reader activity 18.12   Safety

What might be done to promote the sexuality of people with a learning disability while also ensuring they are safe?

Informal steps to promote the sexuality of people with a learning disability

While aiming to meet individual needs, carers and family members should be encouraged to foster approaches to support the sexuality needs of people with a learning disability. For family members, emotionally and psychologically this might be a very difficult thing to do. It is difficult to perceive one's offspring as being sexual, particularly if he/she has a learning disability. Professional support and advice can therefore be gained perhaps through learning disability nursing services (or CLDN services). Informal steps to address sexuality might include:

Managing sexual behaviours from an early age: people with learning disabilities learn about appropriate behaviours through being exposed to them, through behavioural reinforcement and through consistent management of sexual behaviours. Sexually inappropriate behaviours can be difficult to manage due to their sensitive nature and the embarrassment they cause. All behaviours, however, serve a purpose otherwise they would not continue. In order to manage behaviour effectively its cause must be found. Sexual behaviours occur in children and adults with a learning disability for several reasons:

1. Due to ignorance and the fact that the person does not know/has not been taught how to behave socially/sexually.
2. The reaction gained from exhibiting the behaviour fulfils a need for the person, for example, it may be occupying their time or a positive reaction may be gained from others when the person acts in that way.
3. No alternative ways of behaving have been taught.
4. It might be a means of communicating pain, distress, boredom or excitement.

Appropriate patterns of behaviour need to be developed and reinforced throughout childhood and into adulthood, so that someone is aware of socially/sexually acceptable behaviours. Behaviours, particularly of a sexual nature can limit the use of ordinary facilities such as shops, general medical services, schools, and so forth. It is essential therefore that they are addressed. See Chapter 19 also on the management of behavioural needs.

Fast facts 18.1   Why behaviours continue

The reasons behaviours continue are varied:

- The acts are enjoyable and personally rewarding.
- No one is addressing the behaviours and correcting them.

- People with a learning disability may have a lack of insight into what is right and may need to be specifically told.
- Socially reinforced by attention being given to the action.
- Mixed messages received from multiple carers.

The media portrayal of sexuality may reinforce behaviours.

Case study 18.3   Inappropriate behaviour

For Lawrence, inappropriate sexual behaviours were reinforced as he experienced sexual abuse from an early age and learnt that this inappropriate behaviour was perhaps acceptable as he had no positive behaviours to compare it to. He had had various carers from early life; this can create inconsistencies in what messages are given regarding the acceptability of behaviours. No sex education was given. Sex is reinforced in itself; it is as discussed, enjoyable and self-gratifying. It is one of Maslow's basic needs, see Chapter 1.

Treating age appropriately

This is a difficult concept for many people working with people with a learning disability. Children grow up quickly and to adapt the way one treats a child as they develop is difficult. Added to this is the fact that when a child has a learning disability, their chronological or real age can often be very different from their cognitive age. Despite this, however, as a child with a learning disability develops, it is essential that the way they are treated changes, so that they are seen as and see themselves as maturing individuals. This can help to develop the child's sense of identity, having an impact on their level of maturity, independence, confidence and assertiveness. A developing child may be treated more maturely in relation to the names they are called. They are no longer given shortened versions of their names or pet names. This impacts on how they are treated within the family. Rough and tumble play becomes something less boisterous and sitting on dad's knee evolves to sitting beside dad. The door is closed or locked when taking a bath or when on the toilet. Those with complex intimate care needs may be cared for with more privacy and general reinforcement of the person as a young man/woman with more grown-up behaviours and all this entails.

Encouraging situations where sexuality can be celebrated!

McCarthy (2001) discussed the fact that people with learning disabilities do not learn about sexuality through the informal routes through which others gain insight. For example, they do not socialise with their peers as much, so they fail to benefit from playground banter or heart-to-hearts during sleepovers. If not addressed, this again can cause them to have a reduced awareness of sexual matters.

Though a difficult time for any child, Atkinson (2002) highlighted how many parents/carers fear the emerging sexuality of people with a learning disability and adolescence can be seen as a time of dread and concern. This can be perhaps counteracted, however, through actively seeking situations whereby someone with a learning disability can illustrate their sexuality in an appropriate manner. This might be through attendance at local integrated social clubs, being actively encouraged to dress in a fashionable manner, engaging in sleepovers, or generally doing things where appropriate social and sexual behaviours can be learnt. Mistakes may be made, but by making mistakes, more responsible behaviours are learnt and carers then respond in a timely manner and in a consistent way to the learning needs of those they care for. Ultimately encouraging the person to take pride in being a sexually/socially responsible self!

Encouraging assertiveness and rights

Phrases such as 'Be good' and 'Behave' are often the last things said to a child before they leave for school; what we are effectively saying is ' toe the line', 'don't rock the boat', 'don't stand out as being different'. Barber (1992, cited in Beckett and Taylor, 2010) suggests that it is right to develop individual needs and psychological autonomy, on the one hand, and know behavioural boundaries, on the other. Assertiveness is the ability to be confident in declaring one's own rights or views and is something that people generally need in modern-day societies. It maintains our individuality and keeps us from being oppressed. People with a learning disability, it could be argued, need assertive skills for the same reasons. Due to the recognised fine line between aggression and assertiveness or the concerns about people already perhaps appearing different, they are not often taught to be assertive. In fact, they are often taught the opposite, to do as they are told. As a result of this reinforcement 'not to make waves', also due to being part of a society that somewhat devalues disability (Beckett and Taylor, 2010) and due to the subsequent failure of that society to listen to people with a learning disability, many people with a learning disability lack assertiveness skills.

Fast facts 18.2   Assertive skills

Assertiveness skills are needed so that people with a learning disability can state what they want in life generally and what they want/do not want with regards to matters of a social/sexual nature. Having such skills will help to prevent submissiveness and vulnerability, even in some cases, preventing abuse.

Actively encourage assertiveness by listening and responding to the views of someone with a learning disability. DH (2001) advocates for the rights of autonomy and choice for people with a learning disability. If the person has the mental capacity to make autonomous decisions, then they have the right to have their decisions upheld (DH, 2005). An assertive individual can influence household or organisational plans, their assertiveness should be seen as a positive thing and services should be person-centred where the needs of the service user are paramount (DH, 2001). The Department of Health advocated four main principles for "valuing people", no matter who they are (Figure 18.1).

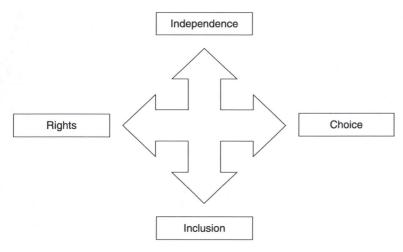

Figure 18.1 The four principles of valuing people
Source: DH (2001).

Reader activity 18.13 Assertiveness skills

When thinking about Lawrence, what steps might be taken to help him to develop assertiveness skills?

Communicate to others so that all are aware of the plan

Ensure those working with the person with a learning disability, including relatives and all staff members, are aware of the approaches made to promote the sexuality of the person with a learning disability, thus encouraging continuity of approach and avoiding mixed messages being given.

Formal steps to address the sexuality of people with a learning disability

The Department of Further Education Enterprises (DFEE) (2000) guidance promotes the provision of sex and relationship education in schools tailored to the age and cognitive levels of children. The guidance states that such education should address:

- attitudes and values
- personal and social skills
- knowledge and understanding.

Children with special needs are included in the guidance, but in practice perhaps for the reasons already discussed, the reality is that many children with learning disabilities are not included in this kind of education. Sex education should occur ideally as it does for other children, with peers learning together in mixed sex groups. Such groups provide individuals with support. Discourage the singling out of anyone who might be having particular sexuality issues/problems. The nature of mixed sex groups reinforces the naturalness of the subject, reinforcing it as something which one need not be embarrassed about. It is a topic to be spoken about freely within the group. Male and female facilitators complement the mixture of the groups and act as role models for the two sexes. Children and adults with a learning disability can and do benefit from formal sexuality education.

Where group involvement is not possible or necessary, sex education can be given individually or perhaps where couples are involved in a relationship, they may be educated together. However the education occurs, a lot of preparation should be made before and during sex education work to ensure the process is as successful as possible.

- Before sex education begins, check what the participants already know. This can be done using a sexual knowledge tool such as those outlined in NHS (2009) or by Bustard and Stewart (2011). In doing an assessment before the intervention, an individual's baseline knowledge is discovered, and repeating the assessment after the lesson will aid the evaluation of the overall process, giving insight into what students have learnt.

- If working in groups, ensure you are aware of their possible dynamics or consider how compatible the individuals within the group might be. Thinking about this beforehand will assist you in managing dynamics; it might involve seating people in particular positions within the groups, whereby they may be more comfortable or encouraging quieter individuals, and so forth. By assisting better communication, you will be aiming for a more successful experience. The dynamics of the groups should be something that is continuously assessed; dynamics can change as relationships are made and broken. Be aware of this and make time for its continuous evaluation as the process continues.

- Consider the different cognitive levels of the people within the group and how their disability affects their ability to understand and access information. It may be that some information has to be service-user accessible, therefore supported by symbols, sign language such as Makaton or British Sign Language. Some individuals require the attention of a 1:1 supporter within the group to explain issues in ways that are more accessible to that person (Smith and Atkinson, 2012). Consider the different ways that people learn; the behaviourist theories and the need to reinforce issues, the social learning theory and the need for people to have role models. The learning styles such as theorist, activists, pragmatist and reflector, as suggested by Honey (Honey and Mumford, 1982), will all have a bearing on the teaching styles adopted to encourage learning. A successful programme of education could, for example, incorporate the use of role play, discussion, question and answer, art work, singing, moving to music, blackboard work and book work.

- Education of this nature can provide an arena where people disclose sexual abuse. If sexuality issues are addressed in a natural and relaxed way, disclosures might more readily occur. Individuals may realise through the course of a programme that what they have seen or experienced was actually sexual abuse. Abuse might be disclosed for a first time, or it might have been previously known about. The possible occurrence of disclosures needs to be acknowledged prior to the commencement of a programme, therefore minimising the element of surprise, and a plan should be made for the appropriate management of any disclosures. Necessary authorities should be informed in a timely manner.

- Group rules should be established by participants on their first meeting. The premise should be to encourage a sense of group ownership, a feeling of belonging and comfort within the group. Confidentiality should be one of the group rules, thus encouraging individuals to speak more freely, but regarding potential disclosures of abuse, it should be said that if facilitators feel someone is being hurt, then it might be necessary to talk to someone else about what is going on.
- It would be useful if those caring for individuals were made aware that the formal education is being undertaken. If working with a child, DFEE (2000) states that parents should be made aware of the content of sexual education programmes. If working with an adult, parental involvement is a courtesy rather than a requirement. It might be useful for them to be informed of the nature of the education. Parental involvement has the aim of encouraging parents/carers to adopt approaches such as those highlighted previously. Encouragement of a holistic approach to the person's sexuality is important. This encourages the person's development as a sexually responsible individual.
- Finally, all the resources need to be available for sessions prior to the commencement. Attention should be given to individuals with regards to their learning needs and facilitators should not be distracted due to poor planning.

Reader activity 18.14 Group rules

Group rules are important if doing group work. What possible group rules do you think might be decided upon by a group at their first meeting?

Reader activity 18.15 Improving formal sex education

Think about the formal sex education you had at school, make two lists and decide:

- What was positive about it?
- What needed to be improved?

By considering this you might also think about how the needs of people with a learning disability might be met. In many respects, it is not so different.

A programme of sexuality work

NHS (2009) provides a comprehensive guide to teaching people with a learning disability about sexuality issues and includes ideas for facilitation and resource tools. The pack details the following topics:

- knowledge of self and group membership;
- life cycle;
- hand washing;
- attractiveness, self-esteem and body parts;
- public and private places and behaviours;
- puberty and personal hygiene;
- menstruation and wet dreams (including the management of);
- arousal, masturbation and dignity;
- consent and assertiveness (including abuse);
- sexual intercourse and contraception;
- testicular and breast care.

The items should be covered in an all-inclusive way. People with a learning disability who are gay or lesbian face discrimination and find it harder to find acceptance of their sexuality than heterosexual people (Abbott and Howarth, 2003). Education on any topic should be inclusive of sexual diversity, ethnicity, age and disability issues so that no group member is segregated. Education should be flexible, further items should be included if individuals would benefit from them. Different relationship types (i.e. friendships/lover, etc.), how relationships differ, greeting behaviours, parenting and many more items can be included, greater emphasis may also be paid to one particular issue depending on individual need. The above-mentioned programme certainly forms a starting point to sex education work.

Reader activity 18.16   Educational content

What educational content do you think might be useful for Lawrence within a sexual education programme?

Conclusion

People are sexual by their very nature, and having a learning disability does not detract from this. Someone like Lawrence, however, who has had limited sex education can, at best, be confused about sexuality issues and, at worst, may be vulnerable to abuse. He may through confusion about consent issues or the law, also do things which are sexually irresponsible or illegal. It is not easy to provide sex education, particularly if one is unsure if the information is being understood or if it is going to result in a positive outcome. Many practitioners shy away from providing information to service users and this reinforces the cycle of ignorance with its negative outcomes. This chapter has aimed to promote the need to provide formal and informal support to people with a learning disability around sexuality issues, with the goal of raising their awareness, promoting sexually responsible behaviours and decreasing vulnerability. People with a learning disability can be taught about sexuality with very positive outcomes.

Fast facts 18.3   Multi-disciplinary working

Both the NMC Nursing and Midwifery Standards for Pre-Registration Nurse Education (2010) and Professional Capabilities Framework for Social Workers (2010) advocate multi-agency and inter-professional partnerships within the care of service users. The following individuals might be involved in meeting the sexuality needs of someone with a learning disability. Depending on individual needs, other professionals may also be involved:

- The person with a learning disability should have choice, independence, rights and inclusion (DH, 2001). They therefore should where possible, be involved in any discussions about them or for them.
- The carers of people with a learning disability can give advice on the person's level of development, communication and educational needs. They will also provide informal support to a formal programme.
- A learning disability nurse would develop an assessment of sexual knowledge and carry out a sexual health programme, also would evaluate the programme and advice on further input.
- A social worker could give advice on the dynamics within care environment, for family issues or child/adult protection concerns.
- A psychologist will assess and intervene regarding more complex sexuality needs.
- A speech therapist will advise on communication with someone with complex communication needs.

Reader activity 18.17   Reflection on practice

What have you learnt? Reflect on your own practice. Tick the correct answer to the following questions in Table 18.1, making notes of any thoughts you have.

Table 18.1 Reflection on practice

Question	Yes	No
Sexuality and how it impacts on someone with a learning disability is something I need to think about and talk to my supervisor about	Plan how this can occur and what you might say	Consider why you have answered no to these questions and the reason for this. You may feel embarrassed about the issues or may be still need clarification of some points. Discussions with other professionals in the field might help, for example, a learning disability nurse or talking to someone with a learning disability.

(continued)

Table 18.1 Continued

Question	Yes	No
There should be a considered/planned approach which meets needs and protects people.	What sorts of things should be considered?	
If sexuality is not addressed, there can be dire consequences for someone with a learning disability	What consequences?	
Services for people with a learning disability should have policies in place to address the sexuality needs of individuals. Do I know these policies and how to access them?	What are the policies, both local (the organisational ones) and national?	
Being open to talk about sexuality is an important first step for my client group. Am I able to do this with confidence?	What can I do to help the people I work with you to express their sexuality?	

Points to remember

- Sexuality is natural and normal.
- People with learning disabilities should be taught about sex and sexuality.
- Not educating people with learning disabilities about sex leaves them vulnerable.

Resources

The following resources are also recommended when working with people with a learning disability around sexuality issues. They may give you more insight into the topic or provide you with valuable support and guidance.

Bustard, S. and Stewart, D. (2011) *Living Your Life: The Sex Education and Personal Development Resource for People with Learning Difficulties and Disabilities*, 3rd edn. London: Brook Publishers. Available at: www.brook.org.uk.

Family Planning Association (FPA) literature available on sex, learning disabilities and the law. Available at: www.fpa.org.uk.

Your local organisational policy on working with people with a learning disability around sexuality and relationships.

Local Sexual Health Centres for good practice ideas and advice on sexual health.

References

Abbott, D. and Howarth, J. (2003) A secret love; a hidden life, *Learning Disability Practice*, 6(1): 14–17.

Allen, G. (1997) The social and economic origins of the genetic determinism: a case history of the American eugenics movement, 1900–1940 and its lessons for today, *Genetica*, 99: 77–88.

Atkinson, S. (2002) It's great to grow up, *Learning Disability Practice*, 5(10): 28–32.

Beckett, C. and Taylor, J. (2010) *Human Growth and Development*. London: Sage.

Burns, J. and Davies, D. (2011) Same-sex relationships and women with intellectual disabilities, *Journal of Applied Research in Intellectual Disability*, 24(4): 351–360.

Bustard, S. and Stewart, D. (2011) *Living Your Life: The Sex Education and Personal Development Resource for People with Learning Difficulties and Disabilities*, 3rd edn. London: Brook Publishers. Available at: www. brook.org.uk.

Chapman, A. (2001) Maslow's hierarchy of needs. Available at: www.businessballs.com.

Craft, A. (1987) Mental handicap and sexuality; issues for individuals with a mental handicap, their parents and professionals, in A. Craft (ed.) *Mental Handicap and Sexuality: Issues and Perspectives*. Tunbridge Wells: Costello.

Davies, R., Northway, R., Jenkins, R. and Mansell, J. (2005) *Abuse of People with Learning Disabilities: Everyone's Responsibility*. Available at: www.learningdisabilitywales.org.uk.

DFEE (Department for Education and Employment) (2000) *Sex and Relationship Guidance*. Nottingham: DFEE Publications.

DH (Department of Health) (2001) *Valuing People: A New Strategy for the 21st Century*. London: HMSO.

DH (Department of Health) (2002) *No Secrets: Guidance on Developing and Implementing Multi-Agency Policies and Procedures to Protect Vulnerable Adults from Abuse*. London: HMSO.

DH (Department of Health) (2005) Mental Capacity Act. London: HMSO.

Dimond, B. (2008) *Legal Aspects of Mental Capacity*. Oxford: Blackwell.

Dixon, H. (2006) *Beyond Biology*. Available at: www.sexeducationforum.org.uk.

Garbutt, R. (2008) Sex and relationships for people with learning disabilities: challenges for parents and professionals, *Mental Health and Learning Disability Research and Practice*, 5: 266–277.

Grant, G., Goward, P., Richardson, M. and Ramcharan, P. (2005) *Learning Disability: A Life Cycle Approach to Valuing People*. Maidenhead: Open University Press.

Hall, P. and Innes, J. (2011) Violence and sexual crime, in *Crime in England and Wales 2009/10: Findings from the British Crime Survey and Police Reported Crime*. Available at: www.homeoffice.gov.uk.

Henault, I. (2006) *Asperger's Syndrome and Sexuality*. London: Jessica Kingsley Publications.

Honey, P. and Mumford, A. (1982) *The Manual of Learning Styles*. Maidenhead: Honey Publications.

Horwitz, A., McLaughlin, J. and White, H. (1998) How the negative and positive aspects of partner relationships affect the mental health of young married people, *Journal of Health and Social Behaviour*, 39(2): 124–136. Available at: http:www.jstor.org/stable/26766395.

Jenkins, R. and Davies, R. (2004) The abuse of adults with learning disabilities and the role of the learning disability nurse, *Learning Disability Practice*, 7(2): 30–37.

Lindeman, M. (1997) Pandora's box, in *Encyclopedia Mythica*. Available at: www.pantheon.org/articles/p. pandora.html.

Lowenthal, M. and Haven, C. (1968) Interaction and adaptation: intimacy as a critical variable, *American Sociological Review*, 33(1): 20–30.

McCarthy, M. (2001) *Sexuality and Women with Learning Disabilities*. London: Jessica Kingsley Publications.

McConkey, R. (2007) Variations in the social inclusion of people with intellectual disabilities in supported living and residential settings, *Journal of Intellectual Disability Research*, 51(3): 207–217.

Mencap (2001) *Behind Closed Doors: Preventing Sexual Abuse against Adults with a Learning Disability*. London: Mencap.

Morrall, P. (2001) *Sociology and Nursing*. London: Routledge.

Murphy, G. (2001) The capacity to consent to sexual relationships in people with learning disabilities, *British Journal of Learning Disabilities*, 29(1): 35.

NHS (2009) *Puberty and Sexuality for Children and Young People with a Learning Disability* (A supporting document for National Curriculum Objectives). Leeds: The Children's Learning Disability Team. Available at: www.leeds.communityhealthcare.nhs.uk/document.php?o=328.

Nursing and Midwifery Council (2010) *Standards for Pre-registration Nursing Education*. London: NMC. Available at: http:standards.nmc-uk.org.

Peckham, N. (2007) The vulnerability and sexual abuse of people with learning disabilities, *British Journal of Learning Disabilities*, 35: 131–137.

Priest, H. and Gibbs, M. (2004) *Mental Health Care for People with Learning Disabilities*. London: Churchill Livingstone.

Roper, N., Logan, W. and Tierney, A. (1996) A model for nursing based on a model for living, in A. Tomey and M. Alligood (eds) *Nursing Theorists and Their Work*. Mosby, MO: Elsevier.

Ross, E. and Rapp, R. (2009) Sex and society: a research note from social history and anthropology, *Society for Comparative Study of Society and History*, 23: 51–72.

Sexual Offenses Act (2003) www.legislation.gov.uk (accessed June 2011).

Smith, J. and Atkinson, S. (2012) Children who have communications difficulties, in V. Lambert, T. Long and D. Kelleher (eds) *Communication Skills for Nurses*, Maidenhead: Open University Press.

Soble, A. (1998) *Philosophy, Sex, Love*. Michigan: Paragon Publishers.

Social Work Task Force (2010) *Proposed Professional Capabilities Framework for Social Workers*. London: Department for Education.

Stubblefield, A. (2007) 'Beyond the pale', tainted whiteness, cognitive disability and eugenic sterilisation. *Hypatia*, 22(2): 163–188.

Sullivan, P. and Knutson, J. (2000) Maltreatment and disabilities: a population-based epidemiological study, *Child Abuse and Neglect*, 24: 1237–1274.

Wheeler, P. (2004) Sex, the person with a learning disability and the changing legal framework, *Learning Disability Practice*, 7(3): 32–38.

WHO (World Health Organisation) (2008) Sexual health. Available at: www.who.int/reproductive-health/gender/sexualhealth.html.

Zdravka, L. and Mihoković, M. (2007) Level of knowledge about sexuality of people with mental disability, *Sex Disability*, 25: 93–109.

19

The behavioural needs of people who have a learning disability

Mick Wolverson

Learning outcomes

After reading this chapter you will be able to:

- allow the reader to explore how being labelled as having challenging behaviour can affect the lives of people with a learning disability
- encourage the reader to consider the reasons why some people with a learning disability display challenging behaviour
- provide an understanding of how health and social care practitioners can be involved in the assessment of people who have challenging behaviour
- offer an outline of a range of appropriate interventions that health and social care staff may be involved in when supporting people who have behavioural needs
- enable staff to identify and understand the role of key professionals within a multi-professional/multi-agency context
- help carers understand why sometimes there are barriers in place that prevent appropriate ways of supporting people who have challenging behaviour from working as well as they should.

Introduction

> When you always do what you always did, you always get what you always got.
> (Attributed to Mark Twain and adapted in Gates *et al.*, 2004)

This chapter will explore the needs of people with a learning disability who also present with challenging behaviour. This will be achieved by use of Lawrence's case study already outlined in Chapter 18. Reader activities will also be used to help develop an understanding of this complex area of care.

Case study 19.1   Labelling

Although this chapter primarily focuses on Lawrence's behavioural needs, it should be noted that many other complex factors need to be considered in order to support Lawrence. At this stage in the case study it is evident that labelling and diagnosis add to the complexity of understanding the situation that Lawrence is in. He has been variously labelled as being:

- a sexual offender;
- mentally disordered;
- a person with challenging behaviour;
- a person with a learning disability.

All of these labels have negative connotations. The likelihood is that if an individual had just one of these labels, they would require skilled support. Lawrence's case is far more complex because he has more than one label. Because of this, any support/nursing care plan put in place for him would need to thoroughly assess his needs in relation to all four labels and the interaction between them. Key considerations that should be taken into account are:

- how to prioritise needs and support interventions;
- the need to develop an understanding of how each of Lawrence's 'labels' interacts with other labels;
- which member of the multi-disciplinary/multi-agency team should take responsibility for specific assessments and interventions;
- how to implement person-centred care within a secure setting;
- the need to identify the causation of Lawrence's behaviour so that appropriate interventions can be implemented.

What is challenging behaviour?

It is vitally important that this chapter begins by exploring the meaning of the term challenging behaviour and the possible impact of this on the lives of those so labelled. Atkinson *et al.* (1990) suggest that 'behaviour' is any activity exhibited by a person that can be observed by another person. If this is the case, then every person, with or without a learning disability, displays 'behaviour' at all times. This chapter will enable the reader to develop an understanding of how society judges and categorises behaviour with the result that some behaviours are perceived to be 'challenging'. Use Reader activity 19.1 to develop some ideas about the subjective and objective nature of challenging behaviour.

Reader activity 19.1 What is challenging behaviour?

Think about what challenging behaviour means and write down your thoughts:

- Make a list of your own behaviours that you think are challenging.
- Make a list of the challenging behaviours you have witnessed displayed by people with a learning disability.
- Are there any differences between the list of your own challenging behaviours and that of people with a learning disability? If there are, try to explain why this might be so.
- Some people think that 'challenging behaviour' is a negative label, can you think of a better and more person-centred way of defining it?

Defining and understanding challenging behaviour involve some discussion of how objective and subjective interpretations of behaviour influence the labelling process. Objectivity involves interpreting a situation in a balanced and unbiased way with judgement based on as much provable fact as is possible. Subjectivity involves offering judgements that are often based on an individual's opinions that have been influenced by partial information or expressions of feelings. Slee (1996) explained how language leads to assumptions, creates an individual's history and ultimately results in how a person is treated by others.

Lawrence's case study contains some key indications that, from a subjective viewpoint, he might be labelled as having challenging behaviour. This is because of some of the terminology used in the case study and the way that society reacts to some of Lawrence's behaviours. Examples from the case study include 'exposed his genitals', 'targeting children', 'public outrage' and 'Sexual Offences Act'. All of these examples are likely to engender an immediate subjective negative response from the majority of people reading this case study, resulting in Lawrence being labelled as having challenging behaviour. Care staff should carefully consider their initial subjective responses to information presented in such a way because it may jeopardise any future person-centred interventions.

The lives of people like Lawrence are often defined by case notes, assessments, and referral letters which, by their very nature, tend to use terminology that creates a negative perception of the individual and defines them as being permanently challenging. This process can result in someone like Lawrence enduring a lifetime within specialist services which fail to understand the reasons why Lawrence displays challenging behaviour or offer holistic and person-centred interventions.

Wolverson (2011) has discussed how challenging behaviour has become a convenient 'catch-all' umbrella term that is inconsistently applied and over-used in relation to people with a learning disability. It is therefore extremely important that some objective consideration is given before people are labelled as having challenging behaviour. Some attempts have been made to define challenging behaviour in a broad sense. The first of these was by Blunden and Allen who stated:

> We have decided to adopt the term challenging behaviour rather than problem behaviour or severe problem behaviour since it emphasises that such behaviours represent challenges to services rather than problems which individuals with learning difficulties in some way carry around with them. If services could rise to the 'challenge' of dealing with these behaviours, they would cease to be problems.
>
> (1987, p. 14)

This definition encourages health and social care practitioners to view behaviour as a challenge to them and to find ways of supporting a person with behavioural issues as opposed to perceiving the individual as the problem. This is a very important shift in emphasis, particularly as many people with a learning disability and challenging behaviour do not perceive or understand that their behaviour is judged by others as being difficult. To some extent, Lawrence's case study illustrates how his presenting behaviours are a 'challenge' to others rather than himself. As already touched on in Chapter 18, this may be because of Lawrence's level of cognitive ability, sexual knowledge and emotional congruence with younger people.

A second widely used broad definition of challenging behaviour is that of Emerson *et al.*, who in 1988 suggested that:

> Severe challenging behaviour refers to behaviour of such an intensity, frequency or duration that the physical safety of the person or others is likely to be placed in serious jeopardy, or behaviour that is likely to seriously limit or deny access to the use of ordinary community facilities.
>
> (1988, p. 16)

This, or derivatives of it, is likely to be the most widely used definition of challenging behaviour. Lawrence's case study objectively indicates that it could be applied to him. This is because some of his sexual behaviour has been 'intense', quite 'frequent' and it has persisted over time (duration). In addition to this 'the safety of others is likely to be placed in serious jeopardy' by him approaching children for sexual gratification. His behaviour has also resulted in him being admitted to a medium secure unit, thus his behaviour was 'likely to seriously limit or deny access to the use of ordinary community facilities'.

A third broad definition of challenging behaviour was provided in the Mansell Report for the Department of Health in 1992:

> People with learning disabilities who have challenging behaviour form an extremely diverse group; including individuals with all levels of learning disability, many sensory or physical impairments and presenting quite different kinds of challenges. The group includes, for example, people with mild or borderline learning disability who have been diagnosed as mentally ill and who enter the criminal justice system for crimes such as arson or sexual offences: as well as people with profound learning disability, often with sensory handicaps and other physical problems who injure themselves, for example, by repeated head banging or eye poking.
>
> (DH, 1992, p. 3)

Once again, to some extent, this definition can apply to Lawrence's case study because it extends to 'people with mild or borderline learning disability who have been diagnosed as mentally ill and who enter the criminal justice system for crimes such as arson or sexual offences'. Quite clearly, this part of Mansell's definition can be applied to Lawrence. Use Case study 19.2 to help you develop your understanding of definitions of challenging behaviour.

Case study 19.2   Focus on the individual, not the label

Lawrence's case illustrates that a number of broad definitions of challenging behaviour can be applied objectively to people with a learning disability; however, in the case of Lawrence and of all other cases, it is of the upmost importance that care staff focus on the needs of the individual rather than the expected behavioural outcomes of the label.

Definitions, labels and diagnoses can be useful because they are part of a common language that is shared by care staff and to some extent this can be convenient; however, care staff should question the accuracy of labels and attempt to see the person and not the label.

Things to consider are:

- If a person is admitted to a unit specifically designed for people with challenging behaviour and does not display any behavioural distress, do they have challenging behaviour?
- Does a person have challenging behaviour if they hit someone who has been trying to dictate how they should behave?
- Does a person who is acting out of character in an 'abnormal' environment have challenging behaviour?

Challenging behaviour and social constructionism

The discussion so far has explained that the label challenging behaviour can lack precision in defining an individual's behaviours. This can be extremely problematic for an individual such as Lawrence as it can lead to potentially negative outcomes. There is a great deal of literature that suggests that the use of language and labelling results in a socially constructed perception of individuals and groups within society. Social constructionism is an academic term that means that people are 'pigeon-holed', often as a result of the labels they have been given. Wolverson (2004) has explained that it is often the case that terminology is often applied to people with a learning disability, which results in them being perceived negatively by society. You can see how negative labelling has affected a group of people with learning disability by the comments they have contributed in Reader activity 19.2.

Reader activity 19.2   Negative labels

York People First are a self-advocacy group. They kindly offered to share how the label of challenging behaviour has affected them. Try to imagine how you would feel if this had happened to you, and consider how this might affect the people whom you work with. They said: 'These are some of the names people have called us and things people have said about how we behave':

- naughty
- challenging
- difficult
- demanding
- attention-seeking
- disruptive
- mongy
- don't obey rules.

Staff saying things like, 'I'll be glad when it's 2 o'clock so that I can go home and get away from you lot.'

This has made us feel:

- depressed;
- suicidal;
- angry with myself;
- angry with others;
- scared;
- not listened to;
- physically sick;
- shaking with temper;
- tearful.

These are some things that have happened to us when people used negative labels:

- physically punished for throwing teddy bears to each other at residential school;
- being punished for trying to be 'normal';
- made to do things that we didn't want to do;
- people put condoms in the letter box;
- not being allowed to develop and be independent.

Wolverson (2004) has also discussed how once a label has been applied to an individual, it is very difficult for an individual to escape the assumptions that society associates with that label. In the case of challenging behaviour, it can be the case that a person may have one episode of distressed behaviour and be labelled as having challenging behaviour forever. Subsequently the individual may exhibit behaviour that is not challenging but the label remains and is carried around by that individual in case notes, referral letters and in general communication between health and social care staff. This will certainly be the case with Lawrence. It is undeniable that some of his behaviours have been challenging, but even if there have been times when he has not displayed challenging behaviour, and there are likely to be times in the future when he doesn't, he will still be labelled negatively. Pilgrim and Rogers (1999) have discussed the concept of primary and secondary labelling. By this, they mean that once a label has been given, then the individual with the label will sometimes 'act out' the behaviours associated with the label and care staff will expect these behaviours to be inevitable. Another way of interpreting this is that a person with a label becomes a 'self-fulfilled' prophecy. This concept has been described by Bicknell and Conboy-Hill (1992) as a 'deviancy career' that often results in significant negative outcomes for the individual. Similarly, Wolfensberger (1975, p. 2) stated:

> It is a well established fact that a person's behaviour tends to be profoundly affected by the role expectations that are placed upon him. Generally, people will play the roles that they have been assigned. This permits those who define social roles to make self-fulfilling prophecies by predicting that someone cast into a certain role will emit behaviour consistent with that role. Unfortunately, role appropriate behaviour will then often be interpreted to be a person's 'natural' rather than elicited mode of acting.

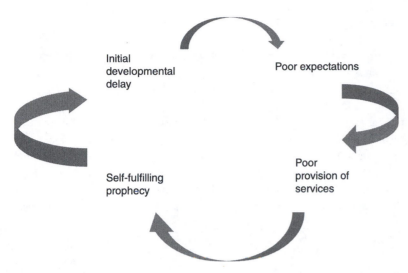

Figure 19.1 The deviancy cycle

It can clearly be seen from Lawrence's care study that this concept can be applied to the circumstances he has experienced (Figure 19.1).

Since his youth, Lawrence has had a variety of potentially negative labels applied to him and has indeed become a self-fulfilled prophecy as he has been admitted to the medium secure unit and he is labelled as a 'sex offender'. Arguably, in contemporary British culture, there is a no more pejorative or negative label than being a 'sex offender'. It can be the case that people with this label such as Lawrence will be both viewed and treated negatively with care staff focusing on the label and its connotations without seeing the person behind the label or understanding the significant factors that caused him to behave in such way. People who are negatively labelled become stigmatised as a result and are often treated in controlling ways. Goffman (1961, 1963) commented on how labelling can lead to stigma and discrimination. Goffman (1963) described stigma as being a personal characteristic that 'discredits' a person in the view of mainstream society which considers stigmatised groups and individuals as being 'of a less desirable kind in the extreme, a person who is quite thoroughly bad or dangerous' (ibid., p. 12). Lawrence's case study evidently indicates that he is very likely to be stigmatised as a result of him being labelled negatively. Reader activity 19.3 will help you to explore stigmatisation in more depth.

Reader activity 19.3   Stigmatisation

Learning disabilities and challenging behaviour are both labels that can result in stigmatisation:

- Differences between people such as skin colour, hair colour, age, weight and even having freckles can result in labelling and stigmatisation. Have you ever experienced, or felt that you have been labelled in a negative way? If so, write down how this made you feel.

- Now think about and write down how you would feel if you were labelled as having a learning disability and challenging behaviour.
- Think about and write down what might happen to somebody who has been labelled as having a learning disability and challenging behaviour.

This process can result in people with a learning disability and challenging behaviour spending much of their lives in specialist services which often tend to control an individual's behaviour rather than use person-centred interventions that can effectively be used to manage challenging behaviour. Such services tend to maintain rather than ameliorate challenging behaviour and they often result in institutionalisation. Institutionalisation is the pernicious process that results from people with a certain label being isolated from mainstream society in controlling environments. The characteristics of institutionalisation include:

- disempowerment;
- devaluation of individuals;
- learned dependency;
- the encouragement of inappropriate attention-seeking behaviours;
- dehumanisation;
- impersonal service provision;
- the development of inappropriate behaviours;
- little attention to individuality;
- control of individuals by the care regime.

Goffman first identified these characteristics in 1961 and a broad consensus emerged that the large institutions in which many people with learning disabilities and challenging behaviour were accommodated should be shut down. In their place it was envisaged that community-based services and the process of normalisation would improve the lives of people with a learning disability. In essence, the contemporary philosophy of care for people with a learning disability is encapsulated by the four key principles of *Valuing People*: rights, inclusion, independence and choice (DH, 2001). It was anticipated that these four key principles would result in a reduction in the challenging behaviour. However, Mansell, for the Department of Health (2007), reported that in general the closure of long-stay institutions has not resulted in a decrease in challenging behaviour and that increases can be expected. Mansell also reported that the development of specialist services for people with challenging behaviour has resulted in the re-institutionalisation of people with challenging behaviour. Mansell outlined the environmental factors associated with contemporary specialist challenging behaviour which are likely to increase rather than decrease the use of challenging behaviour services as follows:

- increased risk of abuse;
- poor care practices;
- lack of control and choice;
- unskilled 'caring' and 'minding';
- the 'silting up' of specialised services;
- limited access to psychotherapeutic interventions;

- high turnover of staff, resulting in poor continuity of care;
- limited interaction between staff and clients (around 9 minutes per hour);
- poorly trained and organised staff;
- demoralised staff;
- crisis intervention, placement breakdowns and out of area placements.

Case study 19.3   Institutionalisation

It is evident from Lawrence's case study that some of the factors relating to institutionalisation have had an impact on his behaviour and that others may do so in the future. Examples of this include the institutional abuse he experienced as a child and his history of being involved with a range of services. He is now held under a section of the Sexual Offences Act in a medium secure unit which may well to some extent involve Lawrence experiencing some of the factors outlined by Mansell and listed above. If this is the case, then it is likely to result in an increase rather than a decrease in his challenging behaviour.

Unfortunately there are many examples of poor services that exhibit the factors outlined by Mansell (2007), the most notorious of which was brought to public attention by the BBC *Panorama* documentary and subsequent police investigation relating to Winterbourne View (BBC, 31 May 2011) (as discussed in Chapter 6). It is self-evident that the systematic abuse of the people at Winterbourne was directly contrary to the principles of *Valuing People* and that it would be likely to increase rather than decrease the occurrence of challenging behaviour. Lawrence's case study illustrates to some extent how environmental factors have contributed to the causation, maintenance and interpretation of his challenging behaviour.

So far this chapter has discussed the problematic aspects of defining challenging behaviour and how this label can impact on an individual such as Lawrence. From this discussion it is apparent that health and social care practitioners should give careful consideration to the use of this label and attempt to use it as accurately as possible. Therefore, the next section of this chapter will outline various assessments that can be used to ascertain the nature of an individual's challenging behaviour.

The cause of challenging behaviour

It is vitally important that care staff can accurately identify the reason for a person's challenging behaviour. Often care-givers and services can be reactive to the presenting behaviour and fail to identify the complex causative factors that have contributed to the development of it. To some extent this is understandable as sometimes challenging behaviour can endanger both the person displaying it and others, and as such care staff need to respond quickly in such situations; however, only dealing with challenging behaviour in a reactive way will not address the deep-seated causative factors that have led to its development. In the case of Lawrence, it is evident that some of his presenting behaviours have caused alarm and presented a danger to others. It is also evident that these behaviours have been responded to reactively and in ways that maintain the deviancy cycle. Care staff and services need to develop proactive rather than reactive strategies. These strategies should be carefully chosen so that they can have a beneficial effect on specific causations. The following section of this chapter will outline good practice in relation to the assessment of challenging behaviour. The discussion of the assessment process will reinforce the importance of accurately identifying the reasons for that behaviour. It will do so by categorising causation into three interlinking categories as discussed by Wolverson (2011): organic/biological, environmental and psychological domains, each of which will be outlined in turn.

Organic/biological causation

It is the case that some manifestations of challenging behaviour can be attributed to an organic causation. An organic causation is an innate component of an individual's biological make up. Organic causations include chromosomal abnormalities and certain medical conditions. It is important to note that though sometimes challenging behaviour can be attributed to an organic or biological causation, direct specific links are uncommon. Murphy (1994) has suggested that there are only two identified conditions which inevitably lead to specific challenging behaviours. These are Lesch-Nyhan Syndrome and Prader-Willi Syndrome. Both of these conditions are extremely rare. Wolverson (2011) discussed how there are some conditions that are sometimes more associated with learning disability than in the general population and which can lead to challenging behaviour. These associated conditions include epilepsy, autistic spectrum disorder and diabetes. Unlike Lesh-Nyhan and Prader-Willi Syndromes, challenging behaviour will not inevitably occur as a result of a person having the condition. Challenging behaviour may result if the condition remains undiagnosed or if it is inadequately treated and managed. The fact that there are only two conditions known to cause specific challenging behaviours, and that the challenging behaviour that results from an associated condition can be treated and managed, indicates that these are not usually the specific cause of the challenging behaviour. Certainly in the case of Lawrence, it is unlikely that there is an organic or biological cause of his challenging behaviour as he has not been diagnosed with an associated condition. Although this is likely to be the case, it is still important to consider organic factors in Lawrence's case because people with a learning disability and challenging behaviour are often treated in response to the 'medical model'.

There are several ways and models of interpreting disease, illness and challenging behaviour. A prevalent model in Western industrial countries such as Britain is the medical model. Many theorists, such as Swain et al. (2004), maintain that even if a person has not been diagnosed with a specific condition, they might still be treated under the medical model because they are associated with a devalued client group, such as learning disability. As a result of Lawrence having a mild to moderate learning disability, it is entirely plausible to suggest that some aspects of the medical model may be applied to him in an attempt to manage his challenging behaviour. Bilton et al. (2002) have discussed how the medical model which is also discussed in Chapter 3, is based on the following assumptions:

- The disease is organic: and the non-organic factors are considered unimportant or ignored.
- Disease is a temporary organic state that can be eradicated/cured by medical intervention.
- Disease is experienced by the sick individual who becomes the object of treatment.

- Disease is treated after the symptoms/behaviour appear; the application of medicine and treatment is reactive.
- Disease is treated in a specialist/medical environment, away from where the symptoms appeared.

Case study 19.4 offers an explanation of how the medical model can be applied to Lawrence.

Case study 19.4   The medical model

It is quite clear from Lawrence's case study that to a large extent these assumptions have been applied to Lawrence. So, though no organic causation has been identified, he is currently being treated in a specialist medical environment away from where his behaviours occurred in a reactive way. As a 'sick' individual, it is Lawrence who is being treated rather than any action being taken to act on the potential environmental causal factors. In a general sense, it is plausible to suggest that Lawrence's learning disability has to some extent been interpreted as a condition under the medical model and that this has resulted in complex emotional factors being ignored. Lawrence's case study illustrates that though it is unlikely that there are organic causations of his challenging behaviour, this can still have an impact on the lives of people with a learning disability due to the power of the medical model.

Behavioural interpretations

The range of human behaviour is extremely diverse. Sometimes it can seem quite simple to explain why people behave in certain ways whereas other behaviours seem to be inexplicable. It is also the case that some behaviours result from a variety of motivations and that they can serve more than one purpose for the person displaying them. Use Reader activity 19.4 to explore the reasons for some behaviours that people in the general population might engage in.

Reader activity 19.4   Explaining behaviour

The development of human behaviour can be difficult to explain. Attempt to offer some explanations for the following behaviours:

- People write poetry.
- You go to work.
- You have a partner.
- You drink alcohol.
- You go shopping.
- To give is better than to receive.
- Less is more.
- You work with people with learning disability.
- People gamble.
- People enjoy sport.

- You get angry.
- You sulk.
- People paint pictures.
- People mourned the death of Princess Diana.
- People go to church.
- People climb mountains.

The behavioural interpretation of challenging behaviour is based on the assumption that behaviour is learned and maintained as a response to reinforcing responses to the behaviour. That behaviour can be learned has been proven by early behavioural psychologists such as Pavlov (1927) and Skinner (1953). In order to explain how behaviour can be learned, theorists have developed and use what has become known as the antecedent, behaviour, consequence (ABC) sequential triad or functional analysis. How this can work is demonstrated by the following example:

1. *Antecedent*: A person with a learning disability living in an institutional setting has made appropriate attempts to gain the attention of care staff. These attempts have either been ignored or responded to inadequately.
2. *Behaviour*: The individual picks at scabs until they become open wounds.
3. *Consequence*: Care staff give attention to the individual by attempting to stop the behaviour and by administering first aid that the individual finds soothing. (See also Chapter 9.)

The likelihood is that this behaviour will be repeated because it was reinforced or 'rewarded' by the 'soothing' intervention of care staff and the attention associated with it. This scenario demonstrates how challenging behaviour can develop in an attempt to gain attention. Every human being requires attention, however, it is often the case that some people with a learning disability have been compelled to seek attention in challenging ways as this is possibly the only way that attention has been given. Wolverson (2003) has also discussed how even if the response to challenging behaviour appears to have a negative outcome for the individual, it is still reinforcing, as any attention is more reinforcing than none. The term 'attention-seeking behaviour' can pathologise those so labelled and suggests that it is a form of challenging behaviour to seek attention. It is the case that most people seek attention and social contact and they have developed appropriate strategies in order to gain these. Health and social care practitioners should develop an alternative frame of meaning in relation to how they interpret and the attempts made by some people to gain social contact and appropriate attention. Examples of this could be:

- Rather than being described as 'manipulative' this could be reframed as 'finding creative ways of having their genuine needs met'.
- Lawrence is a victim of sexual abuse and as such he might describe himself as 'not being normal'. This could be reframed by staff as 'you are a normal person coping with an abnormal situation'.
- Being described as 'attention seeking' could be reframed as 'needing acknowledgement'.

Reader activity 19.5 provides an opportunity to explore the development of socially acceptable behaviours. It can be used to help you consider the development of some commonly observed challenging behaviours associated with learning disability.

Attempt to offer some explanations for the following challenging behaviours:

- self-mutilation;
- projectile vomiting;
- head banging;
- constantly stripping off their clothes;
- throwing furniture around;
- stealing from peers;
- hoarding belongings and carrying them about;
- refusing to eat;
- attacking family members;
- walking around in circles;
- masturbating in public;
- constantly being incontinent;
- repeatedly telling fantastic lies;
- feigning seizures;
- constantly 'whirling' about;
- jumping at the feet of passers-by;
- making extremely loud and strange noises.

There is also an assumption that behaviour can be learned vicariously. Bandura (1977) postulated that individuals can learn to behave in certain ways by observing the behaviour of others. Bandura called this social learning theory. It is entirely feasible that individuals such as Lawrence who are being cared for in specialist units can develop a repertoire of challenging behaviours developed as a consequence of observing others.

Environmental and psychological causation

When exploring the environmental causations of challenging behaviour in relation to Lawrence, it is worth considering the famous Jesuit adage 'give me the child for the first seven years and I'll give you the man'. There is much evidence to suggest that the formative experiences of childhood have a huge impact on the development of challenging behaviours. It is clear from Lawrence's case study that his challenging behaviour may be attributable to his childhood experiences. Sinason (2010) has explored how children with a learning disability are perceived differently from others. It is this perceived difference which to some extent can account for the development of subsequent challenging behaviours.

This perception of difference can lead to 'faulty' parenting that often results in behaviour that is perceived to be challenging. Rolland (1993) has discussed the concept of centripetal forces (those that push family members together) and centrifugal forces (those that force family members apart). This does seem to be the case with Lawrence as he was abandoned in childhood.

In relation to caring for a child with long-term needs. McConachie (1986) has suggested that centripetal forces can result in challenging behaviour as a result of children with learning disabilities being over-protected, 'infantilised' and not being expected to reach developmental milestones. If this is the case, then behaviours associated with early stages of child development can endure into adulthood when they are viewed as challenging. Thus, in Lawrence's case, the sexual experimentation that is expected as part of usual child development may have become an enduring pattern of behaviour for him and explain his sexual 'congruence' with children. Vetere (1993) explored how children with learning disabilities can be 'infantilised'. Infantilisation is the process in which people with a learning disability are perceived to be 'eternal children' who are expected to display some of the problematic behaviours associated with childhood. Centrifugal forces can also result in the child with a learning disability being blamed for family disharmony and ultimate disintegration. From Lawrence's case study it does seem that significant contributory factors for his challenging behaviour are related to attachment issues such as emotional abandonment and psychological abuse.

Lawrence's case study indicates that he has experienced abuse periodically throughout his life. Cambridge (1999) has discussed how people with learning disabilities are more vulnerable to abuse than the general population. Hepworth and Wolverson (2006) explain how challenging behaviour can be a manifestation of socially learned behaviour that can develop as a result of consistent exposure to environments in which abuse and aggression are accepted behaviours. Hames (1993) and Campbell *et al.* (2001) proposed that people who have been the victims of abuse can themselves become abusers as a result of experiencing inappropriate sexual behaviour. Once again, Lawrence's case study indicates that these environmental factors may have contributed to his challenging behaviour.

Case study 19.5   The assessment process

Lawrence's case study is in many ways indicative of the life stories of many people with a learning disability who develop challenging behaviour. Lawrence's case study presents a complex picture that involves many potential reasons that may indicate why he has developed challenging behaviour. It is therefore imperative that the assessment process in relation to Lawrence and people with challenging behaviour in general includes an extensive contextual assessment of his challenging behaviour that includes his past history.

Sometimes it has been the case that the assessment of challenging behaviour has had a narrow focus on presenting behaviour and other important broader factors have been ignored. Therefore, the assessment of challenging behaviour should be holistic and assess all aspects of a person's life and seek as much involvement from interested parties as possible. It is therefore important to include both direct and indirect care givers within a multi-disciplinary and multi-agency context. Lawrence's case study indicates that this 'global' holistic assessment should include aspects of his personal history. Important aspects of this include his abandonment in infancy, his time in foster care, his experiences in local authority care and special education and his time spent in the hostel. In Lawrence's case multi-disciplinary and multi-agency involvement could include the social services, police, psychology/ psychotherapy, occupational therapy and learning disability nurse specialists.

Assessment should be person-centred and involve the individual being assessed as much as possible. Although it might not be feasible or desirable in this case, Lawrence's parents or other family members should be included as much as possible. Although some assessment formats might not be appropriate for use with Lawrence, there are specific assessment tools that focus on each of these three areas of the causation of challenging behaviour as discussed earlier in this chapter.

Assessment of organic causation

It can be the case that diagnostic overshadowing (which has been discussed in several places in the book) influences assumptions and the assessment of challenging behaviour. Diagnostic overshadowing is the process whereby an original diagnosis, condition or label can lead to any behaviours or symptoms a person may have being attributed to the original diagnosis, irrespective of whether there are any provable links. An example of this which may well apply to Lawrence is the diagnosis of learning disabilities. Care-givers may perceive challenging behaviour to be an inevitable outcome of having a learning disability and expect people with a label of learning disability to display it. It is equally problematic to account for challenging by describing it as 'attention seeking'. The assessment of challenging behaviour should therefore attempt to ascertain demonstrable causal links between possible reasons for a person's behaviour and the behaviours displayed.

In order to begin the assessment process it is recognised good practice to ascertain if there may be an organic causation of a person's challenging behaviour. This is unlikely in the case of Lawrence but even though this is the case, it would be dangerous to assume that there may not be an organic causation. A 'global' assessment of an individual's health should be undertaken to ascertain if there are any previously unknown or underlying conditions that might explain the development of challenging behaviour. An example of this is the well-regarded 'OK' Health Check (Matthews, 2004). A global assessment can be used to identify conditions such as epilepsy, conditions which might lead to undiagnosed pain and sensory deficits that may account for or contribute to the challenging behaviour. If specific conditions are identified, then more specific and detailed assessments should be undertaken. An example of this is the Dementia Scale for Down's Syndrome (Gedye, 1995). An assessment tool such as this can be used to verify the causation of the behaviour so that appropriate care planning can take place.

Behavioural checklists and rating scales

There are a wide variety of behavioural checklists that can help identify, target and prioritise specific behaviour. These are often used at the beginning of the assessment process. They can be used in all situations though they are used most frequently if it is suspected the challenging behaviour has an environmental causation and that the behaviour has developed in response to environmental triggers. One that is frequently used is the Aberrant Behaviour Checklist (ABC) (Aman and Singh, 1986). This is a generalised rating scale that categorises behaviours into the subscales of hyperactivity, irritability, stereotypy, lethargy and inappropriate speech. Originally developed for the assessment of self-injurious behaviour and stereotypical behaviour, the Behaviour Problems Inventory (BPI) is another frequently used checklist that has been further developed to also assess for aggressive/destructive behaviour (Rojahn et al., 2001). Hill et al. (2008) have suggested that both of these are reliable and valid assessment tools. In the case of Lawrence, a checklist such as the ABC could be used to identify his problem behaviours and prioritise those which require the most attention. Findings from these assessment tools should underpin care plans designed to target the specific behaviours identified.

Assessment of mental ill health

Lawrence's case study indicates that he has been admitted to a medium secure unit for people with a learning disability and mental health needs. The focus of this chapter is on challenging behaviour; however, it is crucial to emphasise that mental ill health and challenging behaviour are often conflated. Moreover, it can be hugely problematic attempting to identify whether the behaviour a person displays is as a result of experiencing mental ill health or has a functional purpose.

Priest and Gibbs (2004) have identified that people with a learning disability experience mental ill health and can do so more frequently than other groups of people. Studies have demonstrated that a wide range of challenging behaviours displayed by people with learning disability, including destructiveness and self-harm, can be an atypical feature of mental ill health within this client group (Emerson *et al.*, 1999; Taggart and Slevin, 2006). Assessment tools have been developed to screen for the existence of psychiatric disorders in people with a learning disability. These should be used to ascertain if an individual with challenging behaviour also has a mental health disorder. Assessment should also allow for an exploration of the inter-relationship between challenging behaviour and psychiatric disorder and whether they exist independently of each other. In the case of Lawrence, it does seem that he may well have a psychiatric disorder or challenging behaviour. Chapter 20 provides a comprehensive overview of the links between learning disability and mental illness and it offers guidance on the use of specific assessment tools.

Interventions

The discussion of the causation and assessment of challenging behaviour has indicated that there are many complexities in understanding and accurately identifying the origins of challenging behaviour. It has also been made clear that there is a spectrum of causations that can influence the development and maintenance of challenging behaviour. Because of this complexity and spectrum of causation it is vitally important that the most appropriate intervention or range of interventions is carefully selected to have the maximum benefit for the individual. This section of the chapter will outline a range of interventions that can be used in supporting people with challenging behaviour. As with the discussion of causations, not all of these would be the most appropriate in the case of Lawrence, however, readers will benefit by being aware of them so that they could consider using them with other individuals.

Wolverson (2006) has discussed how historically the management of challenging behaviour has often involved an element of control and 'aversion'. The approaches to working with people with challenging behaviour that will now be outlined have been grouped into aversive and non-aversive interventions. Aversive approaches have been discredited and deemed to be ineffective because they are controlling, not person-centred and are seen to be a form of punishment. Conversely, non-aversive approaches are person-centred and seek to modify behaviour by utilising the therapeutic relationship. The approaches outlined below represent this spectrum and move from those with an element of potential aversion to the non-aversive.

Chemotherapeutic and physical interventions

There is a likelihood that some care staff will have little direct involvement with this type of interventions; however, it is important that care staff gain some knowledge of these factors as they will have an impact on the individuals receiving these treatments and an awareness of them is desirable as part of the multi-disciplinary role. The section of this chapter which discussed causations outlined how there are some organic conditions that have the potential to cause an individual to display challenging behaviour. Some of these conditions can be treated by the use of medication. An example of this is the use of Naltrexone in the treatment of self-injurious behaviour (Murphy, 1999); however, it is often the case that a mainstay of clinical intervention in challenging behaviour is the prescription of anti-psychotic or psychotropic drugs. As touched on earlier when discussing the medical model, it is highly likely that Lawrence may well have received a variety of anti-psychotic or psychotropic drugs in an attempt to manage his behaviour. It is also probable that he will continue to be prescribed medication, as doing so is often the primary response to managing challenging behaviour within a medium secure unit. The likelihood of Lawrence being prescribed medication is also increased by him being under a section of the Sexual Offences Act. It should be noted that though Lawrence's case study does not indicate that he has been sectioned under the Mental Health Act 1983 (amended 2007), people detained under some sections of this Act can compulsorily be given medication even if they do not give their consent to this. Lawrence's case study is indicative of some people with a learning disability and offending or challenging behaviours who are often prescribed medication in an attempt to manage these behaviours, whether or not as a result of being sectioned under the Mental Health Act. It can happen in such cases as represented by Lawrence, anti-psychotic or psychotropic drugs are prescribed even when there is not a diagnosis of a psychiatric disorder in attempt to suppress challenging behaviour. Whereas these drugs can be effective if there is an underlying psychiatric disorder, there are concerns that they can be used instead of adequate staffing (DH, 2001, 8.43) and more appropriate behavioural support (Emerson *et al.*, 2000). Chapter 20 discusses best practice in relation to the use of medication in more depth.

Medium secure units also sometimes use other aversive interventions, including physical restraint and time out from positive reinforcement. It is widely acknowledged that these are examples of undesirable but occasionally unavoidable practice. These are generally used in specialist in-patient units such as the one where Lawrence has been admitted. Physical restraint should only be used as a last resort by staff trained to use it. As alluded to earlier in this section, the terrible abuse of people at Winterbourne View included the wilful misuse of restraint. If restraint is a technique used in a care setting, then staff should be guided in how to use it by the Revised Mental Health Act Code of Practice 2008 as it provides comprehensive guidance on the legality and use of restraint. These interventions can have a hugely negative effect on clients, such as poor self-esteem and it is important that care staff are aware of this when working in practice. In the case of Lawrence, it is entirely likely that major life events such as his abandonment in childhood and being a victim of abuse will have led to him experiencing emotional distress and low self-esteem. Health and social care staff would need to give careful consideration to Lawrence's emotional needs if he was subject to restraint in the medium secure unit. All those involved in Lawrence's care should also be involved in the monitoring of the side effects of medication and the implementation and review of care plans that include the use of physical interventions.

Behavioural approaches and functional analysis

The discussion of the causations of challenging behaviour offered an explanation of how challenging behaviour can be learned. Indeed, Hames (1993) has outlined how sexual abuse can be a learned behaviour. Although it may not be the most appropriate intervention for Lawrence, behaviour modification is an approach that is based on the premise that if behaviour can be learned, equally it can be 'unlearned', and people with challenging behaviour can learn to behave more appropriately. A further key tenet of the behavioural approach is that all behaviour has a meaning and a communicative function regardless of how challenging and meaningless it may appear. This approach is firmly based on the antecedent, behaviour, consequence triad, and functional analysis is the process by which attempts are made to identify the potential reasons why a person may display challenging behaviour and which factors serve to reinforce the behaviour (thus making it more likely to be repeated).

Functional analysis is conducted by using charts that accurately record the three stages of the antecedent, behaviour, consequence triad. Once these charts have been completed, hypotheses are made as to what purpose the behaviour serves for the individual and what may reinforce it. Care plans can then be devised that alter the reinforcement of the challenging behaviour. Lawrence's complex offending behaviour may be unresponsive to behaviour modification due to the following criticisms of this intervention. Note that these criticisms can be generalised across the spectrum of challenging behaviour:

- The recording of the antecedent, behaviour, consequence triad can be extremely inaccurate.
- Rewards and reinforcements aimed at altering behaviours may be meaningless to the individual.
- It is too simplistic and can ignore emotional and cognitive causations of behaviour.
- Care-givers lack the knowledge and skills to apply it adequately.
- It is controlling and mechanical and therefore potentially ethically questionable.
- It can be inconsistently applied.
- The process is heavily focused on the individual and environmental factors can be overlooked.

Practice alert 19.1

Because of these criticisms of behaviour modification, McCue (2000) has argued that behaviour modification can be effective if a more person-centred approach is incorporated into the implementation and the following concepts are considered:

- Interventions should be designed to alter systems and not individuals.
- Behavioural approaches should seek to improve the quality of life of individuals and not merely attempt to eradicate challenging behaviour.
- Some behaviours may have more than one function and they may operate differently in different contexts.
- Detailed functional assessment must be conducted prior to intervention.

This more holistic and person-centred approach to applying behaviour modification has become known as Positive Behavioural Support (PBS). It has been demonstrated that PBS can be effective in the management of challenging behaviour across a wide range of service settings (McClean et al., 2005).

Gentle teaching

Gentle teaching developed as a rejection of the physical and behavioural approaches due to their potentially 'aversive' nature and the criticisms of them outlined above. Both behaviour modification and physical approaches can be criticised because of the perception that they are controlling and that they are not person-centred. The proponents of gentle teaching assert that the primary objective is not only to eradicate the symptoms of challenging behaviour but also to encourage valued and meaningful life changes. The components of gentle teaching that are designed to improve the lives of people with challenging behaviour are:

- unconditional positive regard – even when the individual is displaying challenging behaviour;
- equity – the development of an equal relationship between carer(s) and the individual with challenging behaviour;
- mutual change – care giver(s) and client develop mutual coping strategies.

It is clear that the central premise of gentle teaching is based on person-centred approaches and is an attempt to view the person displaying the challenging behaviour in a humanistic way. This is a commendable approach that could enable Lawrence to increase his self-esteem and reduce his emotional distress; however, gentle teaching does have its limitations. In the case of Lawrence, it can be very difficult to adopt a person-centred gentle teaching approach within a medium secure unit, which by its very nature will have some elements of control that mitigate against this approach. It is also the case that Lawrence's offences are of an emotive nature and some care-givers may find it difficult to support him in ways that encourage 'unconditional positive regard'. As well as these issues, other criticisms of gentle teaching include:

- The suggested ways of engaging in gentle teaching are poorly defined and difficult to implement.
- It is merely a variation of the behavioural approach because it is an attempt to control and alter behaviour.
- It lacks an evidence base – all interventions should be proven to be effective by research studies. There is very little research available that proves that gentle teaching in itself is an effective intervention.
- It can 'trigger' challenging behaviour as the function of some challenging behaviours are to 'escape' from proximity to care staff who may be attempting to engage the client in gentle teaching.

The term 'teaching' implies that there must be a didactic element to gentle teaching and some professionals and care staff make the mistake of implementing this approach on a sessional basis, as one would for teaching. It is the author's contention that the central principles of gentle teaching should be an underpinning philosophy of any human service or care regime and as such will contribute to a person-centred ethos.

Cognitive behavioural therapy or 'talking therapies'

Priest and Gibbs (2004) have identified that people with learning disabilities experience significantly more mental ill health across most diagnostic categories than the general population and that this is often associated with challenging behaviour. Lawrence's case study reveals that he has been diagnosed with a mental disorder. It is highly likely that this disorder is inextricably linked to environmental factors from his past that have resulted in a significant amount of emotional distress. If this is the case, then an appropriate intervention to support Lawrence and people with a mild or moderate learning disability could be the use of 'talking therapies'.

In Chapter 18, Atkinson outlined how some aspects of the 'talking therapies' can be applied specifically to Lawrence's thinking in relation to sexuality. It is also worth considering how the 'talking therapies' can be applied in a more generalised way to people with a mental disorder and challenging behaviour. Some theorists (Wilberforce, 2003; Turnbull, 2007) postulate that many manifestations of challenging behaviour associated with a mental disorder are the consequence of errors in thinking and 'faulty' cognition. It is also plausible to suggest that these, often unconscious, negative cognitions are attributable to the life experiences, environmental and social 'setting' conditions discussed by Wolverson (2003). Reader activity 19.6 provides an opportunity to explore how negative labelling and stigma can lead errors in thinking and low self-esteem.

Reader activity 19.6   Self-esteem

Here is a list of the ways people who have been labelled as disabled think that the general public feel about them. Write down which of these apply most to Lawrence and try to explain how these perceptions might influence his behaviour.

- We feel ugly, ashamed of our disability and inadequate.
- Our lives are a burden to us and barely worth living and that we crave to be normal.
- Whatever we do or think or work we undertake is done as a therapy to take our minds off our disability.
- We can never really accept our condition and it seems that we are putting on a brave face.
- We need taking out of ourselves with diversions provided by the non–disabled.
- We desire to emulate and achieve normal behaviour and appearance in all things.
- We go through the daily necessities or pursue an interest merely to provide a challenge and so prove ourselves.
- We are envious and resentful of the able-bodied normal population.
- Any emotion or distress we feel is inevitably linked to our disability.
- Our disability has affected us psychologically, making us bitter and neurotic.
- We are ashamed of our inabilities.
- We are asexual or sexually inadequate.
- If we are single, it is because nobody wants us and not through choice. Any able-bodied person married to us must have done so for suspicious reasons, such as desire to hide their own inadequacies, a saintly desire to be a caring rescuer, gold digging or neurosis.
- If we have a disabled partner then it is for no other reason than to be with our own kind.
- It is irresponsible of us to have children.
- We should put up with indignity, inconvenience and discomfort in order to participate in normal activities.
- Our right to privacy and dignity is not as important as other people's because often our lives are seen to be in need of monitoring.
- If we are lesbians or gay, it can only be because we cannot find a heterosexual partner.

(Adapted from Morris, 1991)

In recent years there has been an increase in the use of cognitive approaches in alleviating challenging behaviour. Cognitive behavioural therapy, rational emotive therapy and cognitive analytical therapy are now employed by psychotherapists in learning disability services. The use of these non-aversive approaches has been met with a degree of scepticism because of the following points:

- There is a presupposition that the client must have adequate cognitive ability and expressive language skills to benefit.
- The client must be willing to engage in the process.
- They require conformity to a 'normal' world view rather than an acceptance that some people with a learning disability may interpret their existence in different ways.

In spite of these criticisms there are some universal benefits of therapy that can help to lessen challenging behaviour as follows:

- a relationship based on trust, mutual respect and genuineness;
- support and reassurance;
- a working alliance in which client and therapist work in partnership;
- the client develops insight into their patterns of behaviour;
- healthy and positive responses are reinforced by the therapist;
- the client feels empowered and listened to.

Wilberforce (2003) concludes that in many ways it is the process of therapeutic interventions that can be as important as the content. It should also be noted that attempts have been made to adapt cognitive behavioural therapy (CBT) to suit the requirements of people with learning disabilities, and that these should be considered when attempting to engage someone like Lawrence by the use of the 'talking therapies'. It can be the case that people like Lawrence have difficulty in understanding some of the language used by professionals and they may find it difficult to use expressive language. Hurley *et al.* (1998) have explained that CBT can be made more accessible to people such as Lawrence by simplifying language and ideas and by the use of materials such as plasticine and dolls to develop representations of emotions.

Case study 19.6   A person-centred ethos

It seems evident that the challenging behaviour displayed by Lawrence may have resulted from a combination of complex and interlinking causative factors. Because of this, service providers and care staff should attempt to apply a combination of appropriate interventions within an overarching person-centred philosophy of care. It is acknowledged that it can be difficult to encourage a person-centred ethos within some settings such as the medium secure unit in which Lawrence is currently being treated; however, attempts must be made to support people like Lawrence in person-centred ways.

Other therapeutic approaches

This chapter does not allow for an in-depth discussion of all the potentially useful interventions that could be used to support a person with a mental disorder and challenging behaviour; however, readers should be aware that some other approaches could be used to support other people with a learning disability and challenging behaviour as follows:

- family therapy (Wolverson, 2003);
- structured teaching (Barr *et al.*, 2000);
- the arts therapies (see Liebmann, 2000);
- complementary therapies (Wray and Paton, 2003);
- intensive interaction (Caldwell, 1999);
- functional communication training (Murphy, 1999).

As with the 'talking therapies', the individual needs and abilities of the person concerned should be considered before any of these interventions are implemented. It is often the case that it is a person's degree of learning disability that influences both the choice and efficacy of the intervention. Lawrence's case study indicates that he has a mild learning disability and therefore functional communication training, intensive interaction and structured teaching might not be helpful. This is because these interventions are more often used to help people with more profound and complex needs than Lawrence. Wolverson (2003) outlined how family therapy could be a useful intervention, depending on individual circumstances. In Lawrence's case, very careful consideration would need to be given to its use as it is apparent that Lawrence's emotional distress could be directly linked to his abandonment as a child. The likelihood is that it would be impossible to engage Lawrence and his family in this process. If family therapy is a possibility, it would be have to be implemented very skilfully due to Lawrence's abandonment and abuse. Lawrence's case study would indicate that he might well benefit from the use of both art and complementary therapies. It can be the case that professional care-givers can over-theorise and over-professionalise ways of helping people with a learning disability and challenging behaviour. In order to help people, health and social care practitioners should empathise and attempt to 'walk in the shoes' of those they care for who have challenging behaviour.

Challenging behaviour can be interpreted as a coping mechanism. Most people have developed a variety of socially acceptable and appropriate ways of coping with emotional and psychological stresses These coping mechanisms are known as a 'self-help tool kit' and can include generally accessible activities that a person can absorb themselves in such as gardening, exercise, listening to music, eating chocolate, and taking a soothing bath (Sonnet and Taylor, 2009). Reader activity 19.7 can help you develop your understanding of self-help tool kit coping mechanisms.

Reader activity 19.7   Self-help tool kit

We all have a self-help tool kit.

- Consider the strategies that you have developed to help you cope if you feel stressed and make a list of these.
- Write down a list of your hobbies and consider what purpose these serve for you.

- Now compare your self-help tool kit list and the list of your hobbies with people you know who have a learning disability and challenging behaviour.
- Consider ways in which you could enable people with a learning disability and a challenging behaviour to develop a self-help tool kit.

It is important that within the constraints of the medium secure unit that Lawrence is given access to his individual self-help tool kit. In general, services and care-givers need to develop an understanding that therapeutic interventions can help people with a learning disability and care plans should be developed that give people access to a self-help tool kit.

Points to remember

- Labels hurt and can be damaging.
- So-called challenging is socially constructed and learnt.
- Challenging behaviour is a subjective term. We all see things differently.
- Assessments are vital in meeting behaviour distress.
- There are many varied interventions that may be used to meet the behavioural needs of people with leaving disabilities.

References

Aman, M.G. and Singh, N.N. (1986) *Aberrant Behaviour Checklist Manual*. New York: Slossom Publications.

Atkinson, R., Atkinson, C., Smith, E., Bem, D. and Hilgard, E. (1990) *Introduction to Psychology*, 10th edn. London: Harcourt Brace Jovanovich.

Bandura, A. (1977) *Social Learning Theory*. Englewood Cliffs, NJ: Prentice Hall.

Barr, O., Sines, D., Moore, K. and Boyd, J. (2000) Structured teaching, in B. Gates, J. Gear and J. Wray (eds) *Behavioural Distress: Concepts and Strategies*. London: Balliere Tindall.

Bicknell, J. and Conboy-Hill, S. (1992) The deviancy career and people with mental handicap, in A. Waitman and S. Conboy-Hill (eds) *Psychotherapy and Mental Handicap*. London: Sage.

Bilton, T., Bonnett, K., Jones, P., Lawson, T., Skinner, D., Stanworth, H. and Webster, A. (2002) *Introductory Sociology*, 4th edn. Basingstoke: Palgrave Macmillan.

Blunden, R. and Allen, D. (1987) *Facing the Challenge: An Ordinary Life for People with Learning Disabilities and Challenging Behaviour*. Kings Fund Paper No.74, London: Kings Fund Centre.

Caldwell, P. (1999) *Person to Person: Establishing Contact and Communication with People with Profound Learning Disabilities and Extra Special Needs*. Brighton: Pavilion.

Cambridge, P. (1999) The first hit: a case study of the physical abuse of people with learning disabilities and challenging behaviours in a residential service, *Disability and Society*, 14(3): 285–308.

Campbell, D., Glasser, A., Leitch, I. and Farrelly, S. (2001) Cycle of child sexual abuse: links between being a victim and becoming a perpetrator, *The British Journal of Psychiatry*, 179: 482–494.

DH (Department of Health) (1992) *Mansell Report on Services for People with Learning Disabilities and Challenging Behaviour or Mental Health Needs*. London: HMSO.

DH (Department of Health) (2001) *Valuing People: A Strategy for Learning Disability*. London: TSO.

DH (Department of Health) (2007) *Services for People with Learning Disabilities and Challenging Behaviour or Mental Health Needs*, rev. edn. London: TSO.

DH (Department of Health) (2008) *Revised Mental Health Act Code of Practice*. London: TSO.

Emerson, E., Cummings. R., Barret, S. *et al.* (1988) Challenging behaviour and community services, 2: Who are the people who challenge services? *Mental Handicap*, 16: 16–19.

Emerson, E., Moss, S. and Kiernan, C. (1999) The relationship between challenging behaviours and psychiatric disorders in people with severe developmental disabilities, in N. Bouras (ed.) *Psychiatric and Behavioural Disorders in People with Severe Developmental Delay and Mental Retardation*. Cambridge: Cambridge University Press.

Emerson, E., Robertson, N., Gregory, N., Hatton, C. and Kessissoglou, S. (2000) Treatment and management of challenging behaviours in residential settings, *Journal of Applied Research in Intellectual Disabilities*, 13: 197–215.

Gates, B., Wolverson, M. and Wray, J. (2004) Accountability and clinical governance in learning disability nursing, in S. Tilley and R. Watson (eds) *Accountability in Nursing and Midwifery*. Oxford: Blackwell.

Gedye, A. (1995) *Dementia Scale for Down Syndrome*. Vancouver, Canada: Gedye Research and Consulting.

Goffman, E. (1961) *Asylums: Essays on the Social Situations of Mental Patients and Other Patients*. Harmondsworth: Pelican.

Goffman, E. (1963) *Stigma: Notes on the Management of Spoiled Identity*. Englewood Cliffs, NJ: Prentice Hall.

Hames, A. (1993) People with learning disabilities who commit sexual offences: assessment and treatment, *NAPSAC Newsletter*, 6: 3–6.

Hepworth, K. and Wolverson, M. (2006) Care planning and delivery in forensic settings for people with intellectual disabilities, in B. Gates (ed.) *Care Planning and Delivery in Intellectual Disability Nursing*. Oxford: Blackwell.

Hill, J., Powlitch, S. and Furniss, F. (2008) Convergent validity of the aberrant behaviour checklist and behaviour problems inventory with people with complex needs, *Research in Developmental Disabilities*, 29(1): 45–60.

Hurley, A., Tomasulu, D.J. and Pfadt, A.G. (1998) Individual and group psychotherapy approaches for persons with intellectual disabilities and developmental disabilities, *Journal of Developmental and Physical Disabilities*, 10: 365–386.

Liebmann, M. (2000) The arts therapies strategies, in B. Gates, J. Gear and J. Wray (eds) *Behavioural Distress: Concepts and Strategies*. London: Ballière Tindall.

Matthews, D.R. (2004) *The 'OK' Health Check: Health Facilitation and Health Action Planning*, 3rd edn. Preston: Fairfield Publications.

McClean, B., Dench, C., Grey, I., Shanahan, S., Fitzsimons, E., Hendler, J. and Corrigan, M. (2005) Person focused training: a model for delivering positive behavioural supports to people with challenging behaviours, *Journal of Intellectual Disability Research*, 49, part 5: 340–352.

McConachie, H. (1986) *Parents and Young Mentally Handicapped Children: A Review of Research Issues*. Beckenham: Croom Helm.

McCue, M. (2000) Behavioural interventions, in B. Gates, J. Gear and J. Wray (eds) *Behavioural Distress, Concepts and Strategies*. London: Ballière Tindall.

Morris, J. (1991) *Pride Against Prejudice: Transforming Attitudes to Disability*. London: The Women's Press.

Murphy, G. (1994) Understanding challenging behaviour, in E. Emerson, P. McGill and J. Mansell (eds) *Severe Learning Disabilities and Challenging Behaviour: Designing High Quality Services*. London: Chapman and Hall.

Murphy, G. (1999) Self- injurious behaviour: what do we know and where are we going? *Tizard Learning Disability Review*, 4(1): 5–12.

Pavlov, I.P. (1927) *Conditional Reflexes*. Oxford: Oxford University Press.

Pilgrim, D. and Rogers, A. (1999) *A Sociology of Mental Health and Illness*. Oxford: Oxford University Press.

Priest, H. and Gibbs, M. (2004) *Mental Health Care for People with Learning Disabilities*. London: Churchill Livingston.

Rojahn, J., Matson, J.L., Lott, D., Esbensen, A.J. and Smalls, Y. (2001) The behavior problems inventory: an instrument for the assessment of self-injury, streotyped behavior and aggression/destruction in individuals with developmental disabilities, *Journal of Autism and Developmental Disorders*, 31: 577–588.

Rolland, J.S. (1993) Helping couples live with illness, *Family Therapy News*, December: 15–26.

Sinason, V. (2010) *Mental Handicap and the Human Condition: An Analytic Approach to Intellectual Disability*. New York: Free Association Books.

Skinner, B.F. (1953) *Science and Human Behaviour*. New York: Macmillan.

Slee, R. (1996) Clauses and of conditionality: the reasonable accommodation of language, in *Disability and Society: Emerging Issues and Insights*. London: Longman.

Sonnet, H. and Taylor, A. (2009) *Activities for Adults with Learning Disabilities; Having Fun, Meeting Needs*. London: Jessica Kingsley.

Swain, J., French, S., Barnes, C. and Thomas, C. (eds) (2004) *Disabling Barriers: Enabling Environments*. London: Sage.

Taggart, L. and Slevin, E. (2006) Care planning in mental health settings, in B. Gates (ed.) *Care Planning and Delivery in Intellectual Disability Nursing*. Oxford: Blackwell.

Turnbull, J. (2007) Psychological approaches, in B. Gates (ed.) *Learning Disabilities: Toward Inclusion*, 5th edn. London: Churchill Livingstone.

Vetere, A. (1993) Using family therapy in services for people with learning disabilities, in J. Carpenter and A. Treacher (eds) *Using Family Therapy in the 90's*. Oxford: Blackwell.

Wilberforce, D. (2003) Psychological approaches, in B. Gates (ed.) *Learning Disabilities: Toward Inclusion*, 4th edn. London: Ballière Tindall.

Wolfensberger, W. (1975) *The Origin and Nature of Institutional Models*. Syracuse, NY: Human Policy Press.

Wolverson, M. (2003) Challenging behaviour, in B. Gates (ed.) *Learning Disabilities: Toward Inclusion*, 4th edn. London: Ballière Tindall.

Wolverson, M. (2004) Language and the social construction of disability, *Therapy Weekly*, 15 April.

Wolverson, M. (2006) Appropriate methods of intervention for those with challenging behaviour, *Therapy Weekly*, 12 January.

Wolverson, M. (2011) Challenging behaviour, in H.L. Atherton and D.J. Crickmore (eds) *Learning Disability: Toward Inclusion*, 6th edn. London: Churchill Livingstone.

Wray, J. and Paton, K. (2007) Complementary therapies, in B. Gates (ed.) *Learning Disabilities: Toward Inclusion*, 5th edn. London: Ballière Tindall.

20 The mental health needs of people with a learning disability

Stacey Atkinson, Dan Dearden and Catherine Dunne

Learning outcomes

After reading this chapter you will be able to:

- show what a mental illness is and illustrate how it might manifest in someone with a learning disability.
- detail specific conditions which have a neurotic or psychotic basis and the presentation of such conditions.
- highlight how psychiatric disorders are more common among people with learning disabilities and attempt to explore the possible prevalence rates of mental illness among this client group.
- identify why people with a learning disability might be more prone to having a mental illness than other individuals and therefore why it is essential that those working in the field are aware of the issues and are alert to possible mental health conditions among the people they care for.
- show that for many people with a learning disability a mental illness is very difficult to detect, so extra vigilance is essential.
- highlight how psychiatric assessment can be made and clarify the role of the different professionals involved.
- illustrate what practitioners in health and social care services might do to help someone with a learning disability to achieve better mental health.

Introduction

They called me mad and I called them mad, and, damn, they outvoted me!

(Nathaniel Lee, cited in Meggit, 2007)

This chapter will again use Lawrence's case study, reader activities and supporting text to highlight the mental health needs of children and adults, with a learning disability. The chapter will explore how factors within present–day society can impact on the mental health needs of people with a learning disability. Mental illness is common in our society. Generally professionals are better at recognising it than ever before, it is better understood and diagnoses are made in shorter time spans, making for a better prognosis. For people with a learning disability, however, this is not always the case, they are also more prone to mental illnesses than others in the general population. Our society is fast moving; where social isolation can exist for those unable to 'fit in'. It is a society motivated by output, those with useful skills or talents are perhaps the most valued. Beauty and perfection are praised and many say selfishness prevails. These and many more contemporary issues affect people with a learning disability and can have an impact on their mental health; modern–day influences on mental health will be explored.

Case study 20.1 Love and affection and loss

For as long as he could remember, Lawrence had felt that he was different. Children in his neighbourhood would not play with him when he was younger and he became introverted. He had experienced episodes of victimisation and abuse. This added to his feelings of self-loathing. When he entered the children's home at last he found a way of obtaining some physical 'comfort'; when older individuals approached him for sex, he accepted their advances, seeing this form of attention as something near to what he wanted – affection. He learnt as he grew bigger that he could target weaker individuals and try to get contact in the same way from them. Lawrence was deeply hurt; deep down he felt unlovable.

This changed all of a sudden when he met Bill, he was elated and someone wanted him and valued him. Their relationship filled him with joy and the feelings of self-doubt and self-loathing disappeared.

Following Bill's death, Lawrence withdrew into himself again. He obtained no joy in what had previously made him happy, he reverted to old ways of behaving. He cried easily and the things that had previously frightened him such as being left alone and sleeping alone panicked him more than ever. He now began to remember vividly how he had been sexually abused the very first time and how he had felt. He regularly woke up sweating and screaming.

He was diagnosed as having mental illness, specifically depression, and an anxiety disorder. It was questioned if he was also experiencing post-traumatic stress, but due to his learning disability it was difficult to fully ascertain this.

What is mental health and what is mental illness?

What is mental health? Is it something everyone has unless they have a specifically diagnosed mental illness? It is not something readily talked about in society. We tend to talk more about physical well–being rather than mental well–being. We say, 'Are you well?', we don't say, 'Are you mentally well?' People experience different moods but when does feeling mentally low or deflated become a recognised mental illness, such as depression or extreme happiness become mania? What is mental illness? Is a mental illness only present when it has been diagnosed as a mental illness or is it just mental illness when it becomes debilitating? How much impact does a mental illness have? These are all relevant questions when defining what mental illness is. Mental health and then subsequently mental illness will be explored in this chapter with specific reference to the mental health needs of someone with a learning disability.

The World Health Organisation (WHO) (2013) defines mental health as:

> A state of well-being in which every individual realises their potential and can cope with the normal stresses of life, can work productively and fruitfully and is able to make a contribution to his/her community.

Taking this official definition, one might ask, does anyone actually ever achieve mental health? It is a very broad and some might argue idealistic definition. 'A state of well-being'? Does this mean consistently a state of well-being every day or over a period of time or intermittently? There are days when I feel stressed and in a panic, so am I mentally ill then? There are days when I don't have a sense of well-being because I am not physically well or maybe have suffered a bereavement or loss. I might not realise my potential until I have reached the pinnacle of my chosen profession, so am I mentally unwell until that point? In the present economic/political climate, many graduates do not gain employment in their chosen field, so are unable to realise their potential. Are they then mentally unhealthy? This is not ideal; it may be a worry or something which is distressing but may perhaps not be the cause of mental illness. Having a learning disability can compromise the ability of someone to 'work' as productively as other people and they may not contribute fully to their community. This again might be a contributory factor but perhaps not a reason in itself for any mental ill health.

The WHO (2013) definition was perhaps more about the influences on mental health/ill health than how it actually impacts on individuals. Mind (2011) prefers to define mental health in the following way:

> You care about yourself and you care for yourself. You love yourself, not hate yourself. You look after your physical health – eat well, sleep well, exercise and enjoy yourself. You see yourself as being a valuable person in your own right. You don't have to earn the right to exist; you exist so you have the right to exist. You judge yourself to reasonable standards. You don't set yourself impossible goals, such as 'I have to be perfect in everything I do' and then you don't punish yourself when you don't reach those goals.

A long definition; which perhaps sounds more achievable for everyone and indeed especially someone with a learning disability but it also needs some consideration. Let's explore it more in Reader activity 20.1.

Reader activity 20.1   The Mind definition

Personal Development exercise *box*

Explore the Mind (2011) definition whilst doing the following exercise on different days (preferably not in the same week). Use different colours to highlight the scores on different days.

Day 1

Day 2

Day 3

| 1 | 2 | 3 | 4 | 5 | 6 | 7 | 8 | 9 | 10 |

Not very well   Very well indeed

How would you rate the following on each of the days covered.

- How much do you love yourself today?
- How much you care for/look after yourself today?
- How well are you eating today?
- How well did you sleep last night?
- How much exercise have you had today?
- Are you enjoying yourself today?

It is expected that over the course of the different days, the rate of functioning is variable; you might love yourself, sleep and exercise more or less on different days. Mental health is variable. It could be argued that mental health is on a continuum and depends on internal and external influences. Internal influences are factors such as physical health, cognitive and emotional ability to cope with life events, problem-solving skills, resilience and personality traits such as optimism, and so forth. External influences may, for example, include the relationships someone has, some may be more supportive than others, job stability or satisfaction, and factors such as social life or financial security. Internal and external factors are often interlinked, for example, if someone is unwell, they may be prevented from enjoying a varied social life, the illness and the isolation caused by their illness may impact on mental health.

Reader activity 20.2
Continuum of well-being

Look at Figure 20.1, it is similar to how you measured your own well-being earlier. Thankfully, for the majority of us, for most of the time, mental health remains within the 1–10 section of the continuum, even if we are 'a bit fed up', 'feeling down in the dumps' or alternatively 'over the moon', we are still able to manage our own needs and we do not need professional support. However, if something occurs in life, an internal stressor such as illness or external influence, such as a bereavement, this may be something which is too great for us to adjust to and it causes our mental health to move from the 1–10 range, into areas we have not previously experienced, in the plus or minus areas, and we may be unable to manage independently. Professional support from specialist mental health services may or may not be needed at this time depending on the severity of the situation.

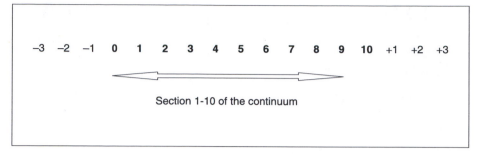

Figure 20.1 The continuum of mental health and well-being

Reader activity 20.3   Lawrence's needs

Consider Lawrence's life and the needs he has presented with:

- childhood sexual abuse, for which he appears to have had no support;
- previous experiences of being bullied;
- approaching children for sexual favours;
- the death of a partner;
- having a learning disability;
- being left alone at night;
- confusion about sexuality issues;
- anything else?

What factors might have contributed to him developing depression and anxiety disorder?

Types of mental illness

Neuroses

Mental health and mental illnesses are defined under two headings: neuroses and psychoses. Neuroses are mental health disorders in which moods or thoughts are disturbed or varied to such a degree that the person's ability to manage their own needs is intermittently disrupted (Norman and Ryrie, 2009). Examples of neuroses are anxiety disorders, post-traumatic stress disorder, obsessive compulsive disorder, phobias, such as agoraphobia (fear of open spaces) or arachnophobia (fear of spiders) and some forms of depression. In neuroses, the person has not usually lost touch with reality, in fact, the neurosis may be a direct reaction or response to something which has occurred. An example of this is a phobic reaction following someone spotting a spider or someone being anxious at an interview. The reactions in neurosis are, however, more extreme than the feelings of fear and anxiety that would ordinarily be felt. Repeated negative experiences can impact on the person's ability to cope and can cause a neurosis to be more severe.

Holmes and Rahe (1967) rated how specific life events can impact on mental health and well-being. Below are some of the most stressful life events:

- death of a loved one;
- break-up of an important relationship;
- sex difficulties;
- change in living situation;
- change in social activities.

Lawrence experienced all of these.

Holmes and Rahe's (1967) list of stressful events is a useful indicator of life's stressors and of course these stressors also affect people with a learning disability. If one of the events occurs, a person may manage, with support, to overcome the situation and adjust to a new routine. However, if, for example, more than one event occurs within a short space of time, this could have a huge impact on the person, causing their mental health to be affected. The person's internal factors such as their ability to cope with change, intellectual understanding of the events or ability to rationalise the event may also determine how well the person adapts. Lawrence has experienced a number of life events which might have impacted on his mental health; these may have contributed to the neurosis he has felt but further stress may make mental health needs more extreme.

Types of neuroses and impacts on people with a learning disability

Anxiety disorders

The group of mental health issues defined under the label of neurosis have great significance for practitioners working within the field of learning disabilities. Anxiety disorders, which include post-traumatic stress disorder and phobias, all occur among people with a learning disability. Studies suggest that anxiety disorders are as common in people with learning disabilities as they are in the general population, if not arguably more so (Cooray and Bakala, 2005). Indeed, it is often the case that whatever an individual's primary mental health diagnosis is, anxiety issues are ever present and, if left untreated, can create a major barrier to quality of life. Once someone with a learning disability has actually presented to services with an anxiety disorder, effective clinical interventions must be devised, as often the condition has become so severe and is impacting significantly on the person.

How someone with a learning disability experiences anxiety does not appear to differ to how other anxious people feel. We may often feel irritable towards others and occasionally agitated or angry. In many situations most people recognise the feelings of anxiety for what they are and are able to cope with them. It is well recognised that due to factors such as intellectual impairment, social isolation and past history of abuse, people with a learning disability have a reduced capacity to cope with distressing feelings. When a behavioural issue has occurred within learning disability services, post-incident reviews occur. These are opportunities to explore the reasons for the incidents, including factors which may be relevant to the environment and to the person him/herself. When discussing with service users, during these reviews, particularly in cases of violence, it is often found that feelings of anxiety were at the heart of critical incidents (Joyce *et al.*, 2005). Due to a reduced ability to articulate their feelings, symptoms of anxiety among people with learning disabilities can manifest in self-harming behaviours, e.g. head banging, self-punching/biting and cutting. Physically also there may be symptoms such as sweating, shaking, nausea and behaviours such as nail biting, 'tics' or even flu-like symptoms may be evident (McMurran *et al.*, 2009). It is important for practitioners to remember that people with learning disabilities often present with unusual behaviours that may seem bizarre. In these cases practitioners must arm themselves with thorough background knowledge of their service users to prevent misdiagnosis.

Post-traumatic stress disorder (PTSD)

Post-traumatic stress disorder (PTSD) presents as a delayed and/or protracted response to a stressful event or situation (Raghavan, 2007). The preceding events are generally of a hugely threatening or catastrophic nature which would in all likelihood cause long-lasting distress for the vast majority of individuals (ibid.). Symptoms usually include the repeated re-living of the experienced trauma in the form of intrusive memories more commonly known as 'flashbacks'. It has been suggested that people with learning disabilities are far more likely to have been the victim of physical/sexual abuse than the rest of the population (Slevin, 2007) so it is perhaps easy to see how PTSD may occur frequently among individuals with learning disabilities.

Obsessive compulsive disorder (OCD)

OCD is characterised by repeated and persistent obsessional thoughts and/or compulsive acts. Obsessional thoughts take the form of ideas, impulses or images that enter into the service user's mind repeatedly in a stereotyped form (Raghavan, 2007). For some, the compulsions create a sense of security and predict-ability, in an otherwise chaotic world. Generally, on the whole, however, the symptoms of OCD are extremely distressing to the sufferer. They may present as violent or repugnant in some way, or seemingly make no sense to the sufferer. Sufferers often try to resist the urges of OCD but generally are unsuccessful, which can cause great distress (ibid.). Unlike psychosis, the thoughts experienced in OCD are recognised as being the individual's own rather than any form of thought insertion (Blankenship, 2012). Compulsive or ritualistic acts are repeated in a stereotypical fashion; no particular joy or satisfaction is derived from them. The individual holds the belief that performing the tasks has the end result of preventing some catastrophic, usually highly unlikely, outcome (ibid.). The prevalence of this disorder among people with learning disabilities appears higher than that of the general population and people with autism, attention deficit hyperactivity disorder (ADHD) or paranoia may be more prone to OCD, and the condition can also have a strong link to depressive illness (Raghavan, 2007).

Phobias

People with learning disabilities experience phobias much more so than the general population (Deb *et al.*, 2001, Gravestock *et al.*, 2005). Phobias elicit high degrees of excessive anxiety in situations that to others would not appear particularly stressful (Raghavan, 2007). Examples are agoraphobia whereby the sufferer fears to be in large crowds or away from home, social phobia whereby the individual fears attention from others in social situations, or specific phobias such as fear of certain animals, using public toilets or fear of illness (Blankenship, 2012). People with a learning disability may have limitations in understanding in a variety of areas. With this in mind, it could be argued that it is relatively easy to see why phobias occur so frequently in people with learning disabilities.

Depression and depressive disorders

The WHO (2012) cites depression as the fourth most common cause of illness worldwide and by far the most common mental health issue in the UK (McMurran *et al.*, 2009). Prasher (1999) suggested that for people with learning disabilities, depression was at least as common as that of the general population and argued that it may, in fact be twice as high. The symptoms of depressions in people with learning disabilities are often the same as that of the general population; emotional flattening, self-neglect and in some cases suicidal ideation (Morrison and Weston, 2012). In mainstream psychiatry it is often the case that service users are able to articulate their feelings of depression which aids diagnosis and treatment. As many people with learning disabilities have major communication impairments, it is often necessary to closely monitor them for marked changes in behaviour that might indicate a depressed mood. Such changes might be in relation to eating habits, sleep patterns and in relation to self-care routines.

Case study 20.2   Lawrence's depression

For Lawrence, following Bill's death and due to his childhood abandonment, victimisation and abuse, it became more acutely obvious that he was suffering from a depressed mood. He experienced withdrawal, emotional bluntness and feelings of acute anxiety.

Reader activity 20.5   Indication of depression

Consider how someone with a learning disability who has limited speech might show how they are depressed.

Types of psychosis and the impact on people who have a learning disability

Psychosis is perhaps a more intense condition than neurosis and is often referred to as a more severe psychiatric disorder (Norman and Ryrie, 2009). It is characterised by the loss of reality. The person may be unable to manage their life, as the disturbance of the mind may be so severe that it results in a change of behaviour, distortion of reality, including changed mood and thought processes (Wrycraft,

2009). Schizophrenia, bipolar disorder, dementia or severe forms of depression are conditions classi-fied under the psychosis heading. Psychotic depression can alter the person's ability to think ration-ally, and hallucinations and delusions can be the extreme result of this. Hallucinations may involve any of the five senses and may be pleasant or unpleasant in nature. If pleasurable, they may be more difficult for carers to notice as signs of distress may not be seen. During delusions the person experi-ences 'mistaken' beliefs, some of which may be based on past events. In dementia, someone perhaps reverts back to previous life events while in schizophrenia someone might perhaps take on a persona they have never had. During delusions thought processes are altered so that the person accepts the situation they are now involved in, though it is not a real situation. It is very real to them (Norman and Ryrie, 2009).

Psychosis was thought of previously not to be possible alongside a learning disability and that any change in behaviour or presentation was a direct result of the learning disability (Smiley, 2005). It is now known and accepted that people with learning disabilities do experience psychosis and in fact that the prevalence of this disorder is higher in this group. In psychosis there are 'positive' symptoms, which are so called as they 'add' something to a person's experience of life, and 'negative' symptoms which limit people's emotional range and are often considered more disabling while generally being less known (Lencz et al., 2004). The following is a, by no means exhaustive, list of positive symptoms, shown in the presentation of psychosis.

- *Bizarre and grandiose ideation*: e.g. believing oneself to be ruler of the world or possessing special powers.
- *Paranoid/delusional beliefs*: this may manifest in a belief that one is being watched or harassed by an external agency or that people are trying to harm you by sending threats through an external source, such as the radio or TV.
- *Thought extraction*: the belief that an outside source is removing thoughts from one's mind, often to great distress.
- *Thought insertion*: the opposite of the above, in this case the belief that someone or something is implanting thoughts into your mind.
- *Hallucinations*: these may take the form of voices, a feeling that something is touching you or causing pain. Alternatively smelling odours that are clearly not present, for example, smelling rotten meat in a field of flowers. To follow on from this, you may also experience 'command' hallucinations that may order a person to carry out unpleasant tasks or even hurt someone.
- *'Pressured' speech*: which is part of the clinical term 'thought disorder'; during which you may have fast and jumbled speech, in severe cases words may be so distorted and lacking meaning. The term 'word salad' is often used for this condition.
- *Flight of ideas*: this is a form of talking where you may switch from one conversation to another, making it difficult for people to follow you. You may babble in an incomprehensible way or just have trouble sticking to one subject.

(Lencz et al., 2004)

The negative symptoms present in psychosis, particularly common in schizophrenia, are severe. They can include enduring apathy, causing a disconnection from the world, a reduction in cognitive ability, with a restriction in emotional expression. These symptoms can also be as the result of factors such as mood disorder or medication side effects (Raghavan, 2007). For Lawrence, there are no features of his presentation that would suggest psychosis to a skilled practitioner. While there is withdrawal, this is in context with his bereavement and the experiences he has endured throughout much of his life. Should Lawrence present to specialist services, however, it is essential that conditions such as psychosis are assessed for. If no evidence of psychosis is found, it can be ruled out and further assessment made regarding the possible presence of other conditions.

For people with a learning disability, while access to greater life experiences has generally improved since the closure of large-scale institutional care, it is often the case that many people with learning disabilities still lead more sedentary and restricted lives than those of the general population. In people without learning disabilities, hallucinations of any sort and delusional beliefs can be extremely complex and grandiose. Often they contain references to sophisticated plots and beliefs in advanced scientific ability. In people with learning disabilities, the concept of 'psychosocial masking' or 'bland' hallucinations is often evident; a good example of this would be the delusional belief that one can drive a car or that they can hear a voice telling them in simple terms that they are bad or shameful (Raghavan, 2007). These examples taken at face value do not appear grandiose or complex as people with milder levels of learning disabilities can learn to drive; this dream may be a hallucination in someone suffering from psychosis, so its presence should not be merely ignored. Psychotic illness can be distressing. While people with learning disabilities often report relatively bland or simple hallucinations, in people who have a reduced capacity to cope with such stressors, it must still be taken seriously and treated the same as it would be in the general population (ibid.).

Bi-polar disorder

Bi-polar affective disorder is historically known as 'manic depression'. A person suffering with this disorder will experience periods of mania characterised by extremely elated mood, grandiose delusions, paranoid beliefs, hallucinations (often auditory or visual), irritability and often an increased interest in sex (Morrison and Weston, 2012). An acutely disturbed sleep pattern is often also evident, in some cases there is also a risk of interpersonal violence. During the depressive phase individuals may feel extremely low and unmotivated, cry without reason, experience feelings of irritability and/or suicidal ideation (ibid.).

Dementia

The most common form of dementia is Alzheimer's disease. (See also Chapter 11.) Among people with learning disabilities, this accounts for a larger proportion of irreversible dementia than is found in the general population. Increasing age is a major risk factor for the development of dementia and, with better health interventions and outcomes, people with learning disabilities are living far longer than previous generations. It is known that people with Down's Syndrome may develop Alzheimer's disease by the age of 40 though may not present with all of the clinical symptoms (Raghavan, 2007). Dementia is characterised by a marked and progressive deterioration in an individual's intellectual, affective and behavioural areas; in people with Down's Syndrome the symptoms may be more diverse and can include seizures, mood changes, cognitive declines and personality changes (ibid.). It is important to remember that, if assessing for dementia in someone with a learning disability, a thorough assessment that includes baseline functioning and day-to-day presentation should be obtained. Due to impaired ability to carry out everyday tasks, symptoms may be missed in the early stages of the illness.

Personality disorders

In people diagnosed with the diagnostic term of personality disorder, their difficulties appear to stem from these characteristic ways of thinking, feeling and acting (McMurran *et al.*, 2009). People with personality disorder typically have difficulties in managing their emotions and relating to others. People with learning disabilities exhibit the full range of personality difficulties, and it must not therefore be assumed that they cannot develop personality disorders (Gravestock *et al.*, 2005), and yet in view of their behavioural and psychiatric needs, it must not be overly presumed that an individual is likely to develop them.

There is a dearth of literature regarding the manifestation of personality disorders in people with learning disabilities, but if present for someone with a learning disability, they are often part of a complex symptomology. There are, for clinical purposes, three groups of personality disorders known as 'clusters', specifically clusters A, B and C (WHO, 2010). Each cluster presents with different symptoms and challenges for sufferers. The clusters are as follows:

1. *Cluster A*: People with cluster A disorders often appear odd or eccentric. This cluster includes the paranoid and schizoid personality disorders. Paranoid personality disorders, in brief, are characterised as excessive sensitivity to setbacks, a tendency to interpret the actions of others as threatening, a highly suspicious nature and an excessive sense of self-importance. Schizoid personality disorders are characterised by an emphatic degree of emotional coldness. Individuals may have an inability to derive pleasure from activities and have a preference for solitary actions. There is also the schizotypal personality disorder; individuals with this condition often present as odd/ bizarre in how they think and speak. They may hold odd beliefs and experience unusual perceptual disturbances and feel anxious in social situations due to irrational fears (WHO, 2010).

2. *Cluster B*: Those with cluster B conditions appear 'dramatic' individuals who may present with a diagnosis of dissocial or anti-social. They may show a callous disregard for the feelings of others and have a pattern of violating the rights of others. Individuals may also be diagnosed with emotionally unstable or borderline personality disorder, in which the individual shows a pervasive pattern of impulsive behaviour. They can experience intense outbursts of anger, may have an unclear or distorted self-image. They often experience repeated thoughts and may self-harm. Some people have strong feelings of emptiness and a tendency to involve themselves in damaging and unstable relationships. There is also the narcissistic form of personality disorder in which an individual has a grandiose sense of self-importance, an exaggerated sense of entitlement and requires constant admiration from others (Psych.org 2013).

3. *Cluster C*: Those with cluster C disorders present as anxious or fearful types. An individual may present with the obsessive, compulsive personalities in which they hoard seemingly worthless items and experience feelings of excessive self-doubt and caution. They may also present with the anxious or avoidant traits in which a person shows a preoccupation with being rejected in social situations, has constant and pervasive feelings of self-doubt and apprehension or avoids new activities due to a strong fear of being embarrassed. Lastly, there is the dependent type in which a person experiences extreme discomfort or fear when left alone due to fear of being unable to self-care. This person may have intense difficulty in making normal daily decisions without reassurance from others and subordinates their care to others whom they feel dependent upon.

(McMurran *et al.*, 2009)

People with cluster B type disorders generally present to services, particularly forensic services. Lawrence has not been formally diagnosed with any personality disorder; no diagnosis of this type is ever made lightly by clinicians. There are certain factors of Lawrence's case, however, that warrant attention in this vein. Lawrence has been the victim of abuse and victimisation as well as social isolation from an early age. Raghavan (2007) highlighted how borderline personality disorders have strongly indicated the aforementioned abuse and trauma experiences as significant factors in their development. It is also worth noting that Lawrence has feelings of deep self-loathing and, it could be argued, a feeling of emptiness and need for affection, even if it is inappropriate and exploitative in nature. Many people with borderline personality disorder report such feelings (Mind, 2011). As a presentation of the condition, people with personality disorders may violate the rights of and exploit others; Lawrence has used his size in the intimidation of others into sexual activity with him. It appears in his situation to be a learned behaviour; however, it is important to consider a personality disorder as a diagnosis in such a case. This is a dissocial trait that would need serious intervention to prevent a potentially dangerous escalation.

The impact of mental illness on people with a learning disability

Psychiatric conditions affect individuals in different ways. The effect is dependent on the severity of the condition and the physical, emotional and mental resources of the person concerned (RCN, 2010). It could be argued that due to the specific biological, psychological and developmental factors inherent in people with a learning disability that not only is the prevalence of mental illness greater in this client group (Cooper *et al.*, 2007), but perhaps due to these same factors, they are perhaps more severely affected by mental illness once they have acquired it. The individuality of people with a learning disability is unquestionable. Not only are the natures of people determined by the causes of their disability, but like all of us, nature versus nurture, specifically our genetic make-up, our upbringing and learning, play a part. Mental illness can affect someone with a learning disability in the traditional ways; a 'textbook case', they may present with all the features you would expect when they have a particular psychiatric condition (RCP, 2006) but there may be some people who do not display their mental illness in traditional ways due to the nature of their pre-existing learning disability and due to other genetic and learnt behaviours.

Fast facts 20.1   ASD and depression

Stewart *et al.* (2006) reviewed various research studies of depression in intellectual disability and found that the following were described as the major symptoms of depression found in people with a learning disability who also had an Autistic Spectrum Disorder (ASD):

- depressed mood;
- increase in aggression;
- alteration in obsession behaviours (either an increase or decrease);
- increase in self-injurious behaviours.

The above symptoms may have already been present, to some degree, in someone with ASD due to the nature of the spectrum of conditions (see Chapter 15). The person with ASD may use aggression, self-injurious behaviours or obsessional behaviours, for example, as coping mechanisms for managing an unpredictable world. They may present with what appears to be a 'depressed mood' due to the social presentation of ASD and behaviours also may have been reinforced, so they are learnt prior to the onset of their mental illness; nature plus nurture has played a part. The key to recognising the impact of the mental illness in someone with a learning disability, therefore, is to know the person or assess the person with regards to their previous patterns of behaviours and how they presented under 'normal' conditions, so an awareness of their deviation from the norm can be recognised.

> **Reader activity 20.6   Does Lawrence have a psychiatric condition?**
>
> Look back at Lawrence's case study. List all the behaviours that Lawrence displays which cause you to wonder if he might have a psychiatric condition.

Why mental health needs might be masked in someone with a learning disability

Meeting the needs of someone with a dual diagnosis is challenging. The first challenge is to recognise that someone with a learning disability has a mental health need. Many people with a learning disability have characteristics which create difficulties in recognising when a mental health need is present. In Table 20.1, the ways in which mental health issues are identified in the general population are compared to people with a learning disability. Table 20.1 clearly shows how mental illness can be masked within the learning disability population.

Diagnostic over-shadowing

A major reason why mental health needs may be masked in someone with a learning disability is diagnostic over-shadowing. Defined by Reiss (1994, 2000) and discussed briefly in other areas of the book, diagnostic over-shadowing is the term used to describe the situation whereby someone's needs are not being recognised because they are attributed to a pre-existing condition such as a learning disability itself. A carer or professional may know that someone has a learning disability; perhaps the person is a wheelchair user or has a specific syndrome. On hearing a diagnosis, all other needs may be wrongly attributed to the original diagnosis. A professional told of the presence of hallucinations, for example, may not consider a mental illness and believe the person 'talks to himself' because of his learning disability or a person who self-harms due to emotional distress may be overlooked as carers believe the person self-harms due to having a learning disability. Diagnostic over-shadowing is dangerous and is born out of ignorance and prejudice; it is something that can cause people with a learning disability to have mental health or behavioural needs disregarded and therefore not addressed. It is important that those who care for people with a learning disability recognise diagnostic overshadowing; it might be something that carers and professionals have to challenge in themselves or that you as someone who is interested in addressing the needs of people with a learning disability have to challenge in others.

Causal factors creating a predisposition to mental illness among people with a learning disability

As discussed, until recently the mental health needs of people with a learning disability were unrecognised, as it was felt that due to their limited cognitive skills, people with a learning disability could not experience mental illness (Hardy and Bournas, 2002; Wallace, 2002). Contrary to this, it is, however, now known that people with a learning disability, such as Lawrence, do suffer from mental illnesses and in fact are actually much more likely than others to develop mental health needs (Bournas *et al.*, 2004; Priest and Gibbs, 2004). RCN (2010) suggested that the rate of mental illness among people with a learning disability is 20.1–22.4 per cent compared to 16 per cent in the general population. There are many factors associated with having a learning disability which cause increased

Table 20.1 Identifying mental health needs

Identifying mental health needs in someone without a learning disability	*Mental health needs in someone with a learning disability.*
• Detection is easier because the person is generally able to articulate how they feel and state what their symptoms are • Detection is easier as the person may experience an alteration in their ability to self-care, for example, may not maintain hygiene as well as they previously have, others may notice the difference • The mental health need may be detected due to physical changes such as alterations in sleep or appetite patterns • Speech may become more monotone or slurred during a mental illness such as depression or dementia • Needs are perhaps more detectable as behavioural differences may become apparent with the progression of the mental illness.	• Detection is more difficult because the person may have communication needs which limit their ability to express their needs • They may also have had chronic symptoms for so long that they fail to appreciate that they have a condition (Bournas *et al.*, 2004) • Detection is more difficult because due to their learning disability the person's ability to self-care may already be limited and care needs may be carried out by others, irrespective of mental health status. As care may be dependent on others, there may not be deterioration in the person's presentation. • It might be difficult to detect because sleep patterns may already be erratic, particularly in children with learning disabilities, needing specialist learning disability intervention to correct • Meals may be given by carers who are unaware of appetite changes • Speech may be limited or monotone due to conditions such as autistic spectrum disorder or slurred due perhaps to cerebral palsy or medication • A person with a learning disability may have pre-existing learnt behaviours due to, for example, communication needs, which may be a barrier to recognising mental health needs • Recognition of the illness may be reliant on the observation skills of carers. The full-time care role may limit objectivity skill in recognising needs may not be present.

vulnerability to mental health disorders. The Stress Vulnerability Model (Zubin and Spring, 1977) helps to show how people with a learning disability already have a vulnerability when exposed to extreme life events which ultimately impacts upon their mental health.

Reader activity 20.7 Contributory factors

Think of someone with a learning disability that you know. List the possible factors which might contribute to them experiencing a mental health need.

Emerson and Hatton (2007) researched the mental health needs of children with learning disabilities, many of their findings are also appropriate to adults (RCN, 2010). They highlighted how specific causes of learning disability such as cerebral palsy or genetic disorders such as Fragile X, for example, can impact on the brain structure and/or cerebral chemical balance to such a degree that mental illness can result. They found that people with a learning disability suffer poorer health; some conditions remaining chronic over prolonged periods of time before they are detected. People with more severe learning disabilities have higher levels of sensory problems; these may be unrecognised, particularly in people with more complex needs and can interfere with the person's ability to integrate socially (Emerson and Hatton, 2007; RCN, 2010). Social problems are prevalent too. People with a learning disability are more likely to live in poverty, many carers have mental health needs, perhaps contributing to the fact that many people with learning disabilities lead socially isolated lives and people with a learning disability are exposed to more adverse life events, such as abuse and accidents than other people (RCN, 2010). Predisposing factors such as abuse or neglect can cause psychological distress and possibly depression. In addition to these, learned helplessness (Seligman, 1975), labelling and stigma can add to psychological distress and perhaps create anxiety in social situations (Thomson and McKenzie, 2005). Thomson and McKenzie researched what people with a learning disability felt about having this label and found that people who were aware that they had a learning disability suffered more readily from poor self-esteem and held negative views about having a learning disability, with some of the group linking the negativity they felt to feelings of depression. People with learning disabilities obviously encounter the stresses as described by Holmes and Rahe (1967) that face us all, but due to a reduced cognitive ability and coping mechanisms, they may struggle with life changes. A lack of meaningful relationships or people to turn to for emotional support is also detrimental (Kawachi and Berkman, 2001).

Reader activity 20.8 Circle of support

Look at Figure 20.2. Think about someone with a learning disability you know and consider your own and that person's social circle. If you had a problem, who could you turn to for support? Write the names of all the people you might turn to in shape A. Now consider someone with a learning disability you know. Who might they turn to for support? List all the people in the person's social circle B.

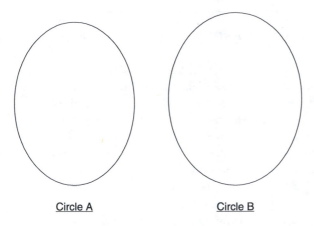

Circle A   Circle B

Figure 20.2 Circles of support

How does your circle of support compare to the person who has a learning disability?

How would you feel if this circle of support didn't exist for you? These feelings are probably very similar to how someone with a learning disability feels without support.

The prevalence of mental illness for someone with a learning disability

Although studies have consistently reported the higher prevalence of mental health disorders among people with a learning disability (Ghaziuddin *et al.*, 2002; Smiley 2005; Hemmings *et al.*, 2006; Kirk *et al.*, 2006), the point was raised by Cooper *et al.* (2007) that generally the studies overall provide conflicting prevalence rates. This is somewhat confusing. Actual prevalence rates are unknown. Cooper *et al.* (2007) suggest that the reasons for the different rates are due to studies often having different sample groups, and different interpretations are given for what constitutes a learning disability and/or a mental health need. Some sample groups are biased with those involved being specifically chosen due to the presentation of their needs. Sample groups chosen in this way are often not representative of the wider learning disability population. Some sample groups are very small and the different studies vary in the extent and breadth of information covered. Some studies, for example, include behavioural needs and hyperactivity when exploring psychiatric disorder, both of which may not be related to a mental disorder (Cooper *et al.*, 2007). Some people with learning disabilities may be unknown to services until a difficulty arises, at which point services may intervene. Other people may consistently be presented to services; their presence can, however, at times be due to the stress felt by carers rather than a reflection of needs of the individual. These issues have an effect on the research findings. As a whole, therefore, the information given in research studies about the prevalence of mental health needs among people with a learning disability is difficult to decipher. Whitaker and Read (2006) also deduced that, in addition to higher prevalence rates of mental illness, people with more severe learning disabilities were more affected by psychiatric disorders than people with milder or no learning disability. The assumption that can be made therefore is that the risk of developing a mental illness and the level of mental illness are greater as the level of learning disability increases, due to the increased impact of the causal factors as previously discussed.

Case study 20.3   Looking for clues

Lawrence has depression, an anxiety disorder and possibly though no diagnosis has formally been made, he may also have post-traumatic stress disorder. Lawrence's many presenting behaviours gave clues to his distress which were noted by his carers. Their alertness and objectivity led to a diagnosis and treatment for Lawrence. Sometimes, however, people with a learning disability live at home and parent/carers may be less able to recognise the signs and symptoms of a psychiatric disorder. They may be busy and lack the insight of trained staff. In view of the needs of carers, it is important that as professionals in health and social care we are vigilant to the ongoing changing needs of the person with a learning disability. Don't always rely on someone else's judgement because it might not always be obvious to someone else that a person with a learning disability needs support and while considering and wondering about the needs of the person with a learning disability consider also if the carers are needing some support too.

Reader activity 20.9
Diagnostic over-shadowing

You take Lawrence to the GP to discuss your suspicions that he may have a mental health need. Together you and Lawrence detail the features of his symptoms. Finally, the GP says 'This is because Lawrence has a learning disability. He is unable to feel depressed. His sexual behaviour is because he is highly sexed and he is too disabled to grieve the loss of a friend.' This is a case of diagnostic over-shadowing.

- How will you feel?
- What impact do you think this may have on Lawrence?
- What do you think you can do in this situation?

Diagnosing mental illness in someone with a learning disability

Practice alert 20.1

Early diagnosis of mental illness is essential in encouraging a timely recovery. The following is necessary:

- Doing an assessment; getting to know someone (and deciding that a problem may be present).
- Making referrals for diagnostic investigations.

- Receiving a diagnosis.
- Making plans to meet the person's needs.
- Implementing treatment.
- Evaluation of needs and recovery.

If you are meeting needs from a nursing perspective, the nursing process cycle (Figure 20.3) will aid in meeting Lawrence's needs. The stages involved are:

- *Holistic nursing assessment*: Also discussed in other areas of the book, assists in obtaining a full picture of the individual, including presenting problem and its history. The outcome of the assessment helps in the development of the further stages of the nursing process.

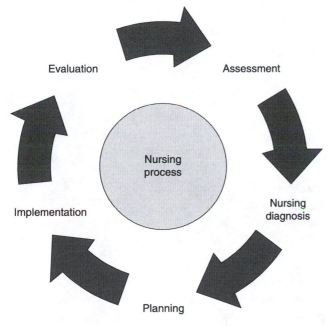

Figure 20.3 The nursing process cycle

- *Nursing diagnosis*: Using professional judgement and evidence to decide upon the diagnosis of a need that merits a referral for a medical diagnosis.
- *Planning*: Setting nursing plans to meet psychiatric needs.
- *Implementation*: Having communicated the person's need for a mental health diagnosis, using a consistent approach during therapeutic approaches which are aimed at meeting the person's needs, as advised in the nursing care plans.

- *Evaluation*: Ongoing, objective evaluation of the person's needs will highlight if mental health needs are improving or if further assessments or care planning are required. It will show if treatment is effective or not.

The first step is a holistic nursing assessment. A holistic nursing assessment takes in many aspects of a person's health. Is the person having regular health checks? If not, their health should be checked. It is essential that people with a learning disability receive regular health checks in order to rule out possible health conditions which may cause deterioration in their mental health or may cause the person to present in a particular way so that a psychiatric condition is suspected. As shown below, some health conditions have symptoms which may cause lethargy or lower mood. If the person is in pain or if they have unwittingly experienced deterioration in their sight or hearing, behavioural change can occur. DH (2001) and DH (2009) recommend that people with a learning disability receive annual health screening, using tools such as the OK Health Checklist (Matthews, 1997) to rule out health conditions which they, as individuals, are unable to report on. Ongoing health needs should be detailed in health action plans (DH, 2001, 2009). The person's health status should be checked particularly if the person is unable to communicate discomfort.

Fast facts 20.2   Symptoms and conditions

Some conditions that affect people with a learning disability can appear, like the symptoms of mental illness:

- Hypothyroidism causing loss of energy and sluggishness.
- Sensory loss, including hearing, sight and sense of smell can cause people to be detached and isolated.
- Sleep apnoea/disturbance can cause daytime lethargy and apathy.
- Hepatitis can cause weakness and confusion.
- Being overweight can cause someone to be sluggish and to lack energy.

During the assessment it is essential to discover how people usually behave. People with a learning disability sometimes present in ways that are not considered usual. They may have stereotypical, self-stimulatory or idiosyncratic ways of presenting that are usual for them as individuals, but perhaps others do not behave that way. It is essential to be aware of how the person presented prior to the onset of the suspected mental illness and to see if this has altered. This is difficult to assess if the suspected psychiatric condition has been present for some length of time. Previous assessments, care plans and progress notes will help to establish previous patterns of presentation and help in making the decisions regarding the requirement for psychiatric assessment. Remember Lawrence's needs, look specifically for changes in the person's self-help skills and their behaviours, for example. An increase in behavioural outbursts which appear to be untriggered or someone becoming more withdrawn or changes in an individual's sleep or appetite. If changes have occurred, this may be an indication of a mental illness being present.

Be aware of the person's lifestyle issues. Consider if the person has experienced one or more significant life changes such as those identified by Holmes and Rahe (1967). There may be questions you can explore in relation to life events. Ask specifically, has the person experienced the death of a loved one or has someone who has had a major role in the person's life suddenly left? You may have not been aware of the important role the person played in the individual's life. Has the person moved home or work? Are they well occupied or perhaps bored? Have there been traumatic experiences, such as abuse or bullying? Maybe you are unaware of them. Has the person unfulfilled hopes or dreams? Does the person enjoy a good social network, is there family involvement? What are relationships like between family members? Does the person have intimate relationships; is there someone the person can confide in? Do they have the ability to say when things are troubling them? The answers you obtain from these questions and other similar ones might help you to decide if the person with a learning disability has experienced a major life change/event which may well have impacted on their psychological well-being. The answers to such questions might determine whether you make a referral to a psychologist or mental health professional for a mental health assessment.

> ### Reader activity 20.11 Stressful life event
>
> Remember if the life event that has affected the person with a learning disability is something that would have an impact on you or other people, it probably also would have had an impact on the person with a learning disability. The level of learning disability often causes people to feel even more stress when life events occur. Think about something stressful/difficult in your life. What psychological impact did it have on you?

This stage of the nursing process cycle involves carrying out a mental health checklist. There are a number of mental health assessments designed for people with a learning disability which can be done to help decide if a deterioration of mental health has occurred and if a referral for more in-depth diagnosis is needed. Doing such assessments is vital as they provide a baseline, providing a picture of the present situation; a measurement point which can be revisited and compared against later, when treatment has begun. Examples of these types of assessments are:

- the Assessment Scale (Krawiecka et al., 1977);
- the Psychiatric Symptom Rating Scale (Haddock et al., 1999);
- the Psychiatric Assessment Schedule for Adults with Developmental Disabilities (PAS-ADD) (Moss, 2002).

The GP or psychiatrist may wish you to be involved in the reassessment of someone as treatment progresses. If they do not request this, perhaps it is something you can suggest.

Making plans to meet the person's needs

Making a referral for a mental health diagnosis can be a difficult decision. If a diagnosis of mental illness is not made, this is not a problem, at least you will know someone is well. If someone has a mental illness that is not detected, then this is a problem. Always make a referral if you feel something may be wrong. It is better to make a referral that shows someone is healthy than not to make a referral and a serious problem is missed. Psychiatric help will be given through the GP, who may treat some individuals and refer more complex cases on to a psychiatrist. The Royal College of Psychiatrists (2007) suggests that most family doctors are experienced in recognising emotional problems in the general population but highlight that they may have limited insight into recognising mental health needs among people with a learning disability. Carers and family members often have a good overall perspective and should be seen as 'experts' in the person's care, therefore their attendance at appointments is vital especially if the person themselves cannot report on their own needs (ibid.). Learning disability or mental health nurses may be involved in assisting with the diagnosis. Both do assessments from their separate professional perspectives and assist at the treatment stage again from their individual viewpoint. These nurses should, where possible, work together in order to meet a person's needs. They should work collaboratively to ensure the best approach is decided upon for that individual, or one nurse may be involved depending on the precise nature of the person's presenting need. A psychologist may assist with delving into specific causes of psychiatric need in more complex cases. A speech therapist may assist with the diagnosis, identifying which communication strategies are needed to support the person and the multi-disciplinary team. An occupational therapist can suggest therapies to aid improved mental well-being.

Diagnosis of a mental health need

The diagnosis of a mental health need may take some time. If a person feels comfortable in the environment where they are being assessed, this will aid diagnosis. The RCN (2010) provides some excellent hints on how to make health appointments more effective for someone with a learning disability. The key points below are vital in ensuring the best outcome:

Those involved in the diagnosis should aim to forge a relationship with a person with a learning disability. The therapeutic relationship as outlined by Peplau (1952) (see Practice alert 20.2) is important, in particular the development of trust, empathy and unconditional positive regard (Rogers, 1951). This is essential when working with someone with a learning disability. A therapeutic relationship will enable the healthcare professional to learn more about the person's condition, gain more understanding and develop a greater level of empathy. The development of the relationship may take some time. The person may have to attend a clinic or see the clinician several times before feeling at ease with the practitioner and with the environment. Building the relationship will be assisted through the removal of items which can create a professional barrier such as white coats, stethoscopes or equipment. For some people with a learning disability, the best place for an assessment would be in the person's own home or at day placements. If this is not possible or not necessary, an atmosphere and professional manner as unclinical as possible will aid a relaxed environment which enables a relationship to develop and a diagnosis to be made.

Practice alert 20.2

According to Peplau (1952), the person with a learning disability should have someone to help them. Below are some roles in the therapeutic relationship.

- *Stranger*: Meets someone and provides an environment in which trust can develop.
- *Resource person*: Someone who has resources available which the other person can utilise in order to meet their needs.
- *Teacher*: Shows understanding in considering the other person's needs and imparts knowledge to the person regarding how their needs might be met.
- *Leader*: Discusses the care with the person, including them leading the way until the person is able to emotionally stand on their own feet again.
- *Surrogate*: Acts as an advocate and emotional supporter for someone in times of need.
- *Counsellor*: Listens and helps the person to gain an understanding of how present circumstances impact on them and helps the person to develop strategies to address their present situation and recover.

The RCN (2010) recommends ensuring predictability. For many people with a learning disability, routine is important. Be aware of this and make appointments as predictable as possible. Explain what the appointment process is going to be, prior to the event. Identify who will be present, what will occur, and where it will be and keep to the plan. Someone who is familiar with the routine of appointments is more likely to engage, be comfortable and cooperative.

Consider the person's individual communication, behavioural, mobility and sensory needs. It is advised that professionals involved in the diagnosis make contact with the rest of the multidisciplinary team beforehand and enquire about such issues prior to appointments. With good insight, an environment conducive to good communication and the use of adapted approaches, appointments can be more successful. Accessibility is vital. Chapter 2 highlights important information about this, the RCN (2010) also advise extensively on communicating with individuals with intellectual disabilities but in short, the following advice adapted from Smith and Atkinson (2012) is useful:

- Make use of the communication methods already employed such as Makaton, PECS, bliss boards.
- Use language that is easier to understand. Check with carers which words the individual already uses regularly and how best to communicate with the person. Avoid jargon, fully explaining the terms you utilise and use shorter sentences.
- Give the person time to respond so they can adapt to what is being said.
- Too often people with a learning disability say what they think they should say instead of what they truly feel/think. Be aware of this and ask questions in different ways and explore the meaning of the answers given.
- Sensory/cognitive needs many hinder the ability of individuals to absorb information. Check their understanding by asking them to repeat key points back to you in the course of the diagnosis and treatment.
- Despite their learning disability and the presentation of their mental health needs, remember the person is a person first! This might sound like a very strange thing to say, but too often person-centred approaches are forgotten and the practitioner treats the person like just another patient or, worse, forgets that they are someone with feelings and needs. Give autonomy and rights and treat with respect; this will make care more successful and satisfactory for everyone!

The treatment options for someone with mental illness who has a learning disability

On receiving a diagnosis of mental illness there are various treatment options available to assist someone like Lawrence (Table 20.2). Each one will be discussed in detail.

Sectioning

The severity of mental illness might determine the necessarily for admission into a mental health unit. Such admissions would provide the opportunity for some of the interventions as follows to occur.

Fast facts 20.3   The sections of the Mental Health Act (1983)

The sections of the Act are:

- Section 2: Compulsory admission for assessment.
- Section 3: Compulsory admission for treatment.
- Section 4: Emergency admission for mental health need.
- Section 5: Detention to prevent for from leaving.
- Section 37: Used by criminal courts to transfer someone to hospital rather than prison.

Learning new skills and coping/problem-solving strategies

Teaching people with learning disabilities new skills, for example, leisure activities, things to keep people occupied or self-help skills can prove to be therapeutic and be an escape for them in times of stress or insecurity. Such skills can include painting, exercise or doing jigsaws. Learning how to use the phone could equip someone with the ability to phone for help in time of need and learning new communication skills could enable someone to indicate the need for help. It could be that there is a particular trigger for someone's mental illness, helping the person to recognise this, manage it and resolve the situation will aid mental well-being. Assessment should be done to highlight what skills someone might learn to enable their growth and empowerment, which will aid mental health.

Table 20.2 Possible treatment options for someone who has a learning disability and a mental illness

Learning new skills	Admission to hospital in-patient unit under the
Desensitising	Mental Health Act (1983)
Alternative therapies	Distraction techniques
Talking therapies	Coping strategies
Manipulation of the environment	Flooding
Use of medication	Problem-solving strategies
Breathing and relaxation	Admission to an in-patient unit under a section of the Mental Health Act (1983)

Many people with learning disabilities can be taught how to cope with their symptoms of mental illness. Distraction techniques such as counting, breathing exercises, listening to music or thought control, as explained in talking therapies, for example, may be ways that people can learn to manage symptoms. Consider ways or ask a mental health or learning disability professional about ways of enabling someone with psychiatric disorders to manage their illness.

Desensitisation and flooding

Both are processes used in the treatment of someone with phobias. Desensitisation is a means of gradually and measurably introducing the object that is feared, thus lessening its intensity. It has been done successfully with people with a learning disability (Dansey and Peshawaria, 2009).

In flooding, the individual is 'flooded' with thoughts and images of the things he/she most fears and their anxiety levels carefully measured to ensure efficacy. Both procedures should be done with extreme care, by trained professionals following a thorough assessment. Both methods cause anxiety and over-exposure can be extremely anxiety-provoking. Measured desensitisation work of either kind, when done in a measured way, can assist in considerably reducing phobic reactions in some individuals.

Alternative therapies

Alternative therapies such as relaxation, massage or aromatherapy, for example, can relax people and provide a therapeutic encounter which calms someone and aids mental well-being. Some care must be taken with the use of touch in someone who has sensory hypersensitivity, such as in people with autism, and essential oils must also be used with care. Nonetheless, this is an area of benefits for people with learning disabilities which is worth further exploring (Lindsay et al., 2007).

Manipulation of the environment

A calm, predictable environment which is not over-stimulating is helpful to people with mental health needs such as dementia or anxiety. Where possible, rid the environment of loud noises and overbearing decor and so forth and encourage calmness.

Talking strategies

Approaches such as cognitive behavioural therapy (CBT) counselling and other talking therapies (Chapter 19) fall within this category of therapeutic approaches, and if geared at the right level by trained professionals, both can be used very effectively with some people who have learning disabilities (Brown and Marshall, 2006; Sams et al., 2006). Talking therapies are both ways of encouraging the person to explore their thoughts and feelings and of managing them. CBT, it could be argued, has a further remit, which is to seek out more damaging thoughts, providing a structured way of addressing them so their damage is lessened (Edelman, 2006).

Medication

Caution must be taken when deciding upon and using medication to treat the mental health needs of someone with a learning disability. Medication is generally used successfully in the treatment of both neurosis and psychosis but there is limited research to show the efficacy of medication in treating people with a learning disability. One assumes, however, that if non-learning disabled people's mental illnesses can improve with medication, then the same must be true of people with a learning disability. Worryingly, however, there have been many concerns raised about the use of medication with this client group, yet, despite such reservations, it is worth noting it is still the most readily used treatment option. McGillivray and McCabe (2004) and Holden and Gitlesen (2004) reported on high levels of prescribing of anti-psychotic medication to people with a learning disability. Anti-psychotic medication can cause severe side effects, but despite this, the above authors also report episodes of more than one medication being given, increasing the possibility of side effects. Many researchers have raised concerns about anti-psychotic medication being used despite the lack of a diagnosis of mental illness (Robertson *et al.*, 2000; Chapman *et al.*, 2006; Dhumad and Markar, 2007). The use of medication to control behaviours in the absence of management plans has also been recounted (Wolverson, 2011). Robertson *et al.* (2000) and McGillivray and McCabe (2004) highlighted that staff shortages and the absence of structured approaches to meet behavioural/psychiatric needs have been known to create situations whereby medication was called upon as a control, rather than used for its therapeutic effects. The same authors also reported on incidents of extended use of medication, raising concerns that the period of medication usage was without reviews or monitoring, therefore, there was little awareness if the perceived need for medication was still present (Chapman *et al.*, 2006). It is essential that there is a multidisciplinary team (MDT) approach to the use of medication and that steps are taken by the MDT to ensure a therapeutic dose is given for specific and relevant needs.

Wolverson (2011) emphasised that medication, if assessed to be required for a specific mental illness, should be used alongside a range of other therapeutic approaches. Deb *et al.* (2006) recommend the following actions are taken by members of the MDT when the administration of medication is recommended to someone with a learning disability.

- Ensure holistic and specific assessments have been done prior to the commencement of the medication in order to ascertain a baseline of behaviours and a benchmark for measurement against, once the medication regime has begun.
- Thoroughly monitor the effect of the medication. Is the situation improving?
- Be clear about the side effects and look out for them.
- Ensure the person consents, where possible, to treatment. Informed consent will mean that information is given in an honest and meaningful way. The person must be informed of the consequences of receiving the treatment, including the possible side effects of the treatment and any alternative treatments available. If the person lacks capacity to consent, then steps should be taken by the MDT to ensure a decision is made in his/her best interests.
- Ensure the views of the family and carers are listened to with regards to the treatment options offered.
- Ensure that service users and carers have a very clear treatment plan, with review dates and reduction of medication dates made explicit.
- Administration of medication should occur as prescribed with no changes unless agreed with the medic.

- Ensure regular reassessments of the person's mental health and follow-up appointments to check ongoing progress.
- Where possible, there should be a reduction or a termination of medication once an improvement in mental health has been established.

(Adapted from Deb *et al.*, 2006)

Evaluation of mental illness

The evaluation of care is an essential part of the nursing and care process. How can one ensure that interventions are applicable to need unless their efficacy is evaluated? Evaluation occurs in two ways: subjectively, involving thoughts and feelings about how things are going, for example, asking, 'How do you feel compared to last week?' Or objectively, which is a more involved, perhaps complicated process as it involves collecting data to look the person's well-being compared to other data collected. Both methods of evaluating care are important. Feelings and thoughts matter. They help us judge if individuals and their carers feel better overall but objective data collection perhaps can provide a more reliable picture of whether the overall situation has improved. The following are examples of information that can be collated in a more objective way:

- how much sleep someone gets;
- how much someone is eating/drinking;
- the number and severity of behavioural outbursts;
- mood: if scaled on a 1–10 or recorded or charted across a timespan or through an event;
- skill base: whether someone is able to perform different skills at different periods of time;
- how often voices are heard.

By recording information, where possible before and throughout an episode of psychiatric disorder, changes in pattern can more clearly be recognised. Such recordings can then be transferred to graphs and charts so the impact of the data is more easily seen by all.

Recovery in mental illness

Increasingly, services for people with mental health problems are adopting a 'recovery' based approach. Recovery must be thought of in a holistic and person-centred framework. 'Clinical' recovery involves the treatment and eventual absence of symptoms, while a person's 'personal' recovery focuses on rebuilding a meaningful and purposeful life as defined by that individual. Many individuals, if treated early, completely recover clinically, return to their homes, jobs and families, never to enter into psychiatric services again. There are challenges in building a recovery based approach for people with learning disabilities but they can be overcome.

Murphy and Brewer (2011) provide compelling evidence that shows that for psychosis, for example, if treated with both pharmacological and with talking therapies in its early stages, then a profound recovery is often observed. With regards to 'personal' recovery, however, many individuals with learning disabilities may have reduced meaningful employment/occupation and frequently live in staffed settings. It is important to consider how life is for them and potentially what it could be like with better mental health. Aim in such cases to ensure also that nurturing environments exist, whereby people with a learning disability can achieve better recovery.

The 'My Shared Pathway' (NHS Networks, 2013) initiative, which is used in many forensic services, aims to involve service users as active partners within their care, charting their progress through services to eventual recovery. As person-centred care is strived for, their views are respected and taken into account, as well as the views of carers and family members. Clinical evidence suggests that the more an individual is involved in their care, the greater the chance for positive outcomes; this may include an individual remaining concordant with medication upon discharge and being more willing to discuss difficult issues in counselling sessions.

It must not be assumed that people with learning disabilities cannot live fulfilling lives, having made a full recovery from a mental illness. Many with a learning disability in fact do. However, for others with a learning disability, recovery may not be a symptom-free ideal in which the person is able to live without interventions from psychiatric services. While it is usual for someone with a learning disability to experience some limitations in social and intellectual functioning, mental health issues will, from their onset, further deteriorate any present skill base and therefore recovery may be the successful reinstatement to the individual's pre-morbid state. Someone may, for example, once again begin to perform self-care tasks without support on recovery or a reduction in challenging behaviours may be seen. Intermittent reviews through psychiatric services and ongoing reassessment should occur to ensure any return of mental illness is recognised again in a timely manner.

Conclusion

People with learning disabilities are more vulnerable to mental health problems than the general population. This chapter has highlighted the difficulties in diagnosing, treating and managing psychiatric problems within this client group. Assessment aids the recognition of mental health needs and while diagnostic tools may need to be adapted for use with people with a learning disability, they are extremely valuable. Gathering a detailed history from the individual is essential as well as gaining information from the primary caregivers so that an accurate picture of the presenting problem can be gained.

The RCN (2010) states that in most cases, it is rarely the solution that a single approach will meet someone's mental health needs. The approaches used must complement each other. The approaches used in this chapter are by no means exhaustive; all possible avenues of treatment should be explored. Unfortunately people with a learning disability are still more likely to receive medication than psychological interventions. This should be addressed. It is essential that approaches used to meet their mental health needs are meaningful, driven by individual needs, promote inclusion and, where possible, aid recovery (DH, 2006).

Points to remember

- People with learning disabilities are susceptible to mental health problems.
- Assessment is needed to find out if someone has a mental health problem.
- There are many approaches which can be used to meet psychiatric need.
- Medication should not be the presumed treatment option. A thorough assessment will help to ascertain the possible benefit of any treatments used.

Resources

Mental Health Foundation: Mental health in people with learning disabilities.
www.mentalhealth.org.uk

Mind for better health
www.mind.org.uk

RCN (1992) Mental health nursing of adults with learning disabilities.
www.rcn.org.uk

References

Blankenship, K.M. (2012) *Anxiety Disorders*. Chichester: John Wiley and Sons Ltd.

Bournas, N., Martin, G., Leese, M., *et al.* (2004) Schizophrenia: spectrum psychosis in people with and without intellectual disability. *Journal of Intellectual Disability Research*, 48(6): 548–555.

Brown, M. and Marshall, K. (2006) Cognitive behavioural therapy and people with learning disabilities: implications for developing nursing practice, *Journal of Psychiatric and Mental Health Nursing*, 13(2): 234–241.

Chapman, M., Gledhill, P., Burton, M. and Soni, S. (2006) The use of psychotropic medication with adults with learning disabilities: survey findings and implications for services, *British Journal of Learning Disabilities*, 34: 28–35.

Cooper, S.A., Smiley, E., Morrison, J., William, A. and Allen, L. (2007) Mental ill health in adults with intellectual disabilities, prevalence and associated factors, *The British Journal of Psychiatry*, 190: 27–35.

Cooray, S. and Bakala, A. (2005) Anxiety disorders in people with learning disabilities, *Advances in Psychiatric Treatment*, 11: 355–361.

Cowan, A.E. (2012) *Psychotic Disorders*. Chichester: John Wiley & Sons Ltd.

Dansey, D. and Peshawaria, R. (2009) Adapting a desensitisation programme to address the dog phobia of an adult on the autism spectrum with a learning disability, *Good Autism Practice*, 10(1): 9–14.

Deb, S., Clarke, D. and Unwin, G. (2006) *Using Medication to Manage Behavioural Problems Among Adults with a Learning Disability*. London: Royal College of Psychiatry. Available at: www.rcpsych.ac.uk.

Deb, S., Thomas, M. and Bright, C. (2001) Mental disability in adults with intellectual disability. 1. Prevalence of functional psychiatric illness among a community based population aged between 16–64 years, *Journal of Intellectual Disability Research*, 45(6): 495–505.

DH (Department of Health) (2001) *A New Strategy for Learning Disabilities in the 21st Century*. London: HMSO.

DH (Department of Health) (2006) *From Values to Action: The Chief Nursing Officer's Review of Mental Health Nursing*. London: HMSO.

DH (Department of Health) (2009) *Valuing People Now: A 3 Year Strategy for People with Learning Disabilities*. London: HMSO.

Dhumad, S. and Markar, P. (2007) Audit of the use of antipsychotic medication in a community sample of people of people with a learning disability, *The British Journal of Developmental Disabilities*, 53(104): 47–51.

Edelman, S. (2006) *Change Your Thinking*. London: Vermillion.

Emerson, E. and Hatton, C. (2007) *The Mental Health of Children and Adolescents with Learning Disabilities in Britain*. Lancaster: Foundation for People with Learning Disabilities, Lancaster University.

Ghaziuddin, M., Ghaziuddin, N. and Greden, J. (2002) Depression in persons with autism: implications for research and clinical care, *Journal of Autism and Developmental Disorders*, 32: 4.

Gravestock, S., Flynn, A. and Hemmings, C. (2005) *Psychiatric Disorders in Adults with Learning Disabilities.* Brighton: Pavilion Publishing.

Haddock, G., McCarron, J., Tarrier, N. and Faragher, E. (1999) Scale to measure dimensions of hallucinations and delusions the psychotic symptom rating scale (PSYRATS), *Psychological Medicine*, 29: 879–889.

Hardy, S. and Bournas, N. (2002) The presentation and assessment of mental health problems in people with learning disabilities, *Learning Disability Practice*, 5(3): 33–38.

Hemmings, C., Gravestock, S., Pickard, M. and Bournas, N. (2006) Psychiatric symptoms and problem behaviours in people with intellectual disability, *Journal of Intellectual Disability Research*, 50: 269–276.

Holden, B. and Gitlesen, J. (2004) Psychotropic medication in adults with mental retardation: prevalence and prescription practices, *Research in Developmental Disabilities*, 25(6): 509–521.

Holmes, T. and Rahe, R. (1967) The social readjustment rating scale, *Journal of Psychosomatic Research*, 11: 213–218.

Joyce, T., Newrick, G., Geer, D. and Molloy, J. (2005) *Challenging Behaviour.* Brighton: Pavilion Publishing.

Kawachi, I. and Berkman, L. (2001) Social ties and mental health, *Journal of Urban Health*, 78(3): 458–467.

Kirk, L., Hick, R. and Laraway, A. (2006) Assessing dementia in people with a learning disability, *Journal of Intellectual Disabilities*, 10(4): 357–364.

Krawiecka, M., Goldberg, D. and Vanghu, M. (1977) A standardised assessment scale for rating chronic psychotic patients, *Acta Psychiatrica Scandinavica*, 55: 299–308.

Lencz, T., Smith, C.W., Auther, A., Correll, C.U. and Cornblatt, B. (2004) Non-specific and attenuated negative symptoms in patients at clinical high risk of schizophrenia, *Schizophrenia Research*, 68(1): 37–48.

Lindsay, W.R. and Morrison, F.M. (2007) A comparison of the effects of four therapy procedures on concentration and responsiveness in people with profound learning disabilities, *Journal of Intellectual Disability Research*, 41(3): 201–207.

Matthews, D. (1997) The OK Health Checklist: a health assessment checklist for people with learning disabilities, *British Journal of Learning Disabilities*, 25(4): 138–143.

McGillivay, J. and McCabe, M. (2004) Pharmacological management of challenging behaviour of individuals with intellectual disability, *Research in Developmental Disabilities*, 25(6): 523–537.

McMurran, M., Khalifa, N. and Gibbons, S. (2009) *Forensic Mental Health.* Cullompton: Willan Publishers.

Meggit, J.J. (2007) The madness of King Jesus: why was Jesus put to death, but his followers were not? *Journal of the Study of the New Testament*, 29: 379.

Mind (2011) www.mind.org.uk (accessed August 2012).

Morrison, A.K. and Weston, C. (2012) *Mood Disorders.* Chichester: John Wiley & Sons Ltd.

Moss, S. (2002) *Psychiatric Assessment Schedule for Adults with Developmental Disabilities: The Mini PAS-ADD Interview Pack.* Brighton: Pavilion Publishing.

Murphy, B. and Brewer, W. (2011) Early interventions in psychosis: clinical aspects of treatment, *Advances in Psychiatric Treatment*, 17: 408–416.

NHS Networks (2013) Available at: www.networks.nhs.uk/my-shared-pathway/background (accessed Dec. 2012).

Norman, I. and Ryrie, I. (eds) (2009) *The Art and Science of Mental Health Nursing*, 2nd edn. Maidenhead: Open University Press.

Peplau, H. (1952) Interpersonal relations in nursing, in A. Marriner Tomey and M. Raile Alligood (eds) (2006) *Nursing Theorists and Their Work*, 6th edn. Philadelphia, PA: Mosby Elsevier.

Prasher, V. (1999) Presentation and management of depression in people with learning disabilities, *Advances in Psychiatric Treatment*, 5: 447–454.

Priest, H. and Gibbs, M. (2004) *Mental Health Care for People with Learning Disabilities.* London: Churchill Livingstone.

Psych.org (2013) Available at: www.psych.org (accessed Jan. 2013).

Raghavan, R. (2007) *Mental Health Disorders in People with Learning Disabilities*. Oxford: Elsevier.

RCN (Royal College of Nursing) (2010) *Mental Health: Nursing Adults with Learning Disabilities*. London: RCN.

Reiss, S. (1994) Psychopathology in mental retardation, in N. Bournas (ed.) *Mental Health in Mental Retardation: Recent Advances in Practice*. Cambridge: Cambridge University Press.

Reiss, S. (2000) A mindful approach to mental retardation, *Journal of Social Issues*, 6: 65–80.

Robertson, J., Emerson, E., Gregory, N., Hatton, C., Kessissoglou, K. and Hallam, P. (2000) Receipt of psychotic medication by people with intellectual disability in residential settings, *Journal of Intellectual Disability Research*, 44(6): 666–676.

Rogers, C. (1951) In *Interprofessional Communication and Psychology for Healthcare Professionals*, 4th edn. Oxford: Butterworth-Heinemann.

Royal College of Psychiatrists (2007) *Depression in People with Learning Disabilities*. Available at: www.rcpsych.ac.uk.

Sams, K., Collins, S. and Reynolds, S. (2006) Cognitive therapy abilities in people with learning disabilities, *Journal of Applied Research in Learning Disabilities*, 19(1): 25–33.

Seligman, M. (1975) *Helplessness*. San Francisco: W. H. Freeman Publishers.

Slevin, E. (2007) in B. Gates (ed.) *Learning Disabilities: Towards Inclusion*, 5th edn. Oxford: Elsevier.

Smiley, E. (2005) Epidemiology of mental health problems in adults with learning disability: an update, *Advances in Psychiatric Treatment*, 11: 214–222.

Smith, J. and Atkinson, S. (2012) Children who have communications difficulties, in V. Lambert, T. Long and D. Kelleher (eds) *Communication Skills for Nurses*, Maidenhead: Open University Press.

Stewart, M., Barnard, L., Pearson, J., Hasan, R. and O'Brien, G. (2006) Presentation of depression in autism and Asperger's syndrome: a review, *Autism*, 10: 103. Available at: wwwsagepub.com/jounals-Reprints.nov.

Thomson, R. and McKenzie, K. (2005) What people with a learning disability understand and feel about having a learning disability, *Learning Disability Practice*, 8(6): 28–32.

Wallace, B. (2002) The challenge of 'dual diagnosis', *Learning Disability Practice*, 5(3): 24–26.

Whitaker, S. and Read, S. (2006) The prevalence of psychiatric disorders amongst people with intellectual disabilities: an analysis of the literature, *Journal of Applied Research in Intellectual Disabilities*, 19: 330–345.

WHO (World Health Organisation) (2010) *International Classification of Diseases, ICD-10*. Available at: www.who.com (accessed Dec. 2012).

WHO (World Health Organisation) (2012) Depression. Available at: http: www.who.int.topics/depression/en v (accessed Dec. 2012).

WHO (World Health Organisation) (2013) Principles. Available at: http://www.who.int/features/99/62/en/index/html (accessed Jan. 2013).

Wolverson, M. (2011) Challenging behaviour, in H.L. Atherton and D.J. Crickmore (eds) *Learning Disability: Towards Inclusion*, 6th edn. Oxford: Elsevier.

Wrycraft, N. (ed.) (2009) *An Introduction to Mental Health Nursing*. Maidenhead: Open University Press.

Zubin, J. and Spring, P. (1977) Vulnerability: a new view on schizophrenia, *Journal of Abnormal Psychiatry*, 86: 103–126.

21 Addressing the needs of people with learning disabilities who have offended

Anne Todd

Learning outcomes

After reading this chapter you will be able to:

- consider what offending behaviour is, including a consideration of Lawrence's behaviour, with some focus on his sexual offending behaviour
- consider the prevalence of offending behaviour in adults with learning disabilities and reflect on the accuracy of suggested prevalence rates
- reflect upon why people with and without learning disabilities offend and briefly outline specific theories about why people commit sexual offences
- recognise how social factors impact upon the development of offending behaviour and consider the characteristics of offenders with learning disabilities
- identify issues involved in reporting offending behaviour
- highlight the multi-disciplinary professionals involved in the processes of the criminal justice system
- outline problems for people with learning disabilities within the criminal justice system and highlight the important role that all health and social care staff can play in supporting adults with learning disabilities through the criminal justice system
- gain a very brief overview of the needs of youths with learning disabilities who offend
- provide an overview of some interventions available within secure care.

Introduction

I have really messed up now, big style, I have been locked up, I could be for years, I might never get out! They teased me and wanted me to do it, so why did I get in trouble? I have been doing this on and off for years. I suppose it is a problem, really, I'm not sure. I just went along with what the police and court said. I haven't got a clue what it all means really. I hope that someone can explain it all and help me get out of. I will do what it takes to get out.

(Lawrence – Case study 21.1).

Using the case study of Lawrence, reader activities, evidence from the literature and clinical experience, this chapter aims to highlight the issues around offending behaviour and people with learning disabilities. People with learning disabilities have historically been criminalised and vilified by some just because they were labelled as having learning disabilities. Being viewed as menaces in society who are more likely to commit crimes resulted in a culture of stigma, deeply entrenched negative public perceptions, marginalisation and exclusion as people were hospitalised and incarcerated to protect the rest of society (Harding *et al.*, 2009). Thankfully, in the last century there have been vast changes in care provision for people with learning disabilities with deinstitutionalisation, the closure of the long-stay institutions and the move to people living back in the community. Stigma does continue but not to the extent it did historically and generally people with learning disabilities are no longer immediately presumed to be associated with criminal activity and behaviour.

Case study 21.1   Lawrence's history

Lawrence has just been admitted to a medium secure unit where he is currently detained on Section 37/41 of the 1983 Mental Health Act (amended 2007). (See Chapter 20). He was convicted of indecent exposure after he exposed his genitals to children and asked the child to touch it. He chased the child until the child managed to get away. There had been an increasing number of these incidents since the death of his partner Bill. Lawrence was charged and convicted of a number of similar offences in his recent court appearance. Lawrence had run away from the hostel on several occasions and had been found by care staff and police in the park.

Historically, Lawrence had approached children while he was at school and exposed his genitals to them and asked them to touch him. He would also ask to see their genitals. Throughout various care placements this behaviour has continued except when he was in the three-year relationship with Bill. He has been a victim of sexual abuse. He has been vulnerable to abuse and has put himself in positions where he has been sexually exploited.

Lawrence has described feeling 'confused' about his sexuality. He has always sought sexual gratification from males and the children he has targeted have been boys but he has spoken of finding females beautiful and attractive. He has been on anti-libidinal medication in the past to try and control these behaviours but he stopped taking this when he was in his relationship with Bill.

Types of offending behaviour

Offending behaviours are any behaviour which breaks the law of the land where it is committed. The vast spectrum of offending behaviours can range from driving offences, theft, drug offences to physical assaults, arson, sexual crimes to homicides and anything else illegal in between. People with learning disabilities can commit a range of offending behaviours along this whole spectrum of offending behaviours, like the rest of the general population. Traditionally, it was thought a higher percentage of people with learning disabilities committed sexual offences and arson but more contemporary research questions this.

Lawrence's offending behaviour: sexual offending

Lawrence has displayed a range of behaviours which are sexual offending behaviours. The term 'sexual offending' encompasses a wide range of different sexually offensive behaviours covering both contact (i.e. where there is physical contact between the perpetrator and the victim, for example, vaginal and anal rape, forced oral sex, touching of sexual body parts) and non-contact offences (i.e. where there is no physical contact between the perpetrator and victim, for example, voyeurism, exhibitionism, making obscene telephone calls and, more recently, downloading obscene images from the internet). This range of behaviours is exhibited without the consent of the victim. Religion, race and culture can impact upon the perception and attributions of whether the behaviour is appropriate or inappropriate behaviour or legal. Read and Read (2009, p. 38), propose a continuum of sexual offending behaviour ranging from exhibitionism, indecent assault to serious sexual assault and rape. There is a greater prevalence of people with learning disabilities at the lower end of the spectrum of sexual offending behaviours.

Some people with learning disabilities can display a number of sexually inappropriate behaviours. These may be seen as a sexually inappropriate challenging behaviour especially where there is a greater degree of learning disabilities. The key difference between challenging and offending behaviour is the underlying intent, challenging behaviour is one form of trying to communicate whereas sexually abusive behaviour is deliberate and may be about abusing others so as to gain power or control (Doyle, 2004).

> ### Reader activity 21.1   Challenging behaviour or sexual offence?

Some people with learning disabilities can display a number of sexually inappropriate behaviours. Think about Lawrence and his history; think about the following behaviours listed in Table 21.1. Do you view these are sexually inappropriate challenging behaviours or sexual offences? Write down your thoughts.

Table 21.1 Defining events

Event	Challenging behaviour or sexual offence?
A child approaching another child at school asking to see their penis	
A child approaching another child at school asking to touch their penis	
A child touching the genitals of another child at school	
Walking around on the ward with their fly open	
Walking around on the ward exposing their penis	
Walking around on the ward masturbating	
Exposing penis to people on the ward	
Walking down the street with their fly open	
Walking down the street exposing their penis	
Walking down the street masturbating	
Exposing penis to a child in the park	

Prevalence of offending behaviour in adults with learning disabilities

Prevalence rates have generally focused on the rates of offending within specific services for people with learning disabilities or the rate of people with learning disabilities within specific offending populations (Rose *et al.*, 2008). Precise figures about the prevalence of offending behaviour in adults with learning disabilities are unclear and unknown.

UK prevalence rates of 5–10 per cent of the offending population as having a formal learning disability are widely acknowledged (Talbot, 2012). Cooper (1995) reported a prevalence of learning disabilities as 9 per cent of the offending population, people with learning disabilities committed 10–15 per cent of sex offences. Lyall *et al.* (1995b) found that 15.2 per cent of suspects at a police station had learning disabilities and the same authors (1995c) stated that 2 per cent of 385 people in a learning disability service were suspects in the previous year. Approximately 10 per cent of people with learning disabilities will have contact with the criminal justice system at some point (McBrien *et al.*, 2003).

In a study by Harrington *et al.* (2005), 23 per cent of juvenile offenders and 20–30 per cent of prisoners had learning difficulties. Research across three prisons in the UK proposed that 6.7 per cent of the population had learning disabilities, 25.4 per cent had borderline learning disabilities (Mottram, 2007). In a 10 per cent sample of a UK prison 140 people were interviewed; 7.1 per cent had learning disabilities and 23.6 per cent had borderline learning disabilities (Hayes *et al.*, 2007).

Lawrence has been detained in a medium secure unit due to his sexual offending behaviour. The hypothesis that men with learning disabilities are more likely to commit sexual offences is not supported (Holland, 2004; Lindsay *et al.*, 2004; Michie *et al.*, 2006). The prevalence rates of sexual offending in people with learning disabilities are again not clear. The percentages of the learning disabilities population committing offences range from 28 per cent (Walker and McCabe, 1973) to 26 per cent (Rose *et al.*, 2008) and 30 per cent (O'Brien *et al.*, 2010). The percentage of a sample of offenders with learning disabilities ranged from 9.5 per cent (Winter *et al.*, 1997) to 7.1–10 per cent (Hayes *et al.*, 2007) depending on measure used. Much of the research around sexual offending and adults with learning disabilities centres on the male population. Summarising, the research findings cannot conclude that the prevalence of offending behaviour is higher or lower for people with learning disabilities when compared to the general population.

The problem with prevalence rates

As with research into the mental health needs of this client group (see Chapter 20) research studies undertaken with this population have not used a clear and consistent definition of learning disabilities. People with learning disabilities do not represent a homogeneous group. Different intelligence tests and cut-off points for learning disabilities have been used. Much research has been based on the prison system which misses people diverted from custody, those found not guilty and offences not reported. There is a lack of a unified identification system for people with learning disabilities, meaning people may be missed (Talbot, 2012). People with learning disabilities are sometimes absorbed into larger population studies (Simpson and Hogg, 2001). The sample groups of people with a learning disability are often small and lack statistical power and significance or transferability to other settings (Craig and Lindsay, 2010). Research areas can hugely influence prevalence, such as secure settings having higher rates than community settings. Care staff may not report offending behaviour (McKenzie *et al.*, 2001). Rates suggested could be the tip of the iceberg. Given these factors, it is expected that the actual prevalence of offending behaviour and sexual offending behaviour in adults with learning disabilities could be higher than what the literature suggests.

Reader activity 21.2   Why do people with and without learning disabilities offend?

Write down some suggested reasons for why the following populations with and without learning disabilities may offend;

1. Why might young people start to display offending behaviours?

2. Why might young people with learning disabilities start to display offending behaviours?

3. Why do adult men commit offences?

4. Why do adult men with learning disabilities commit offences?

5. Why do adult men commit sexual offences?

6. Why do adult men with learning disabilities commit sexual offences?

7. What do you think are the differences between what makes women and men offend?

Why people with learning disabilities might offend

Counterfeit deviance (Hingsburger *et al.*, 1991) proposes that inappropriate sexual behaviour in men with learning disabilities is triggered by poor and limited sexual knowledge, inadequate social skills, and limited interpersonal and communication skills (Craig and Lindsay, 2010). Traditionally, people with learning disabilities live with their parents or in learning disability services. As previously discussed in Chapter 18, some services provide limited opportunity for sexual expression and the development of sexual knowledge. Some people with learning disabilities may lack knowledge of appropriate boundaries so may behave sexually inappropriately. These people lack understanding about the law and societal norms.

Research studies have questioned this hypothesis. Michie *et al.* (2006) found that the sex offender group with learning disabilities had greater sexual knowledge than the non-offender group with learning disabilities. No significant difference between sex offender groups and non-offender groups of people with learning disabilities was found following treatment (Talbot and Langdon, 2006). Other studies have found that deviant and persistent offenders often had greater levels of sexual knowledge, with good knowledge about some aspects of sexuality such as contraception demonstrated.

Children who have been victims of sexual abuse can become perpetrators of abuse when they become adults (Fryson, 2007), but this is not a clear causal relationship and cannot be assumed. In the Thompson (1997) study, 75 out of 120 men with intellectual disabilities referred for a sex education course were allegedly perpetrators of sexual abuse. Out of these 75 men, 17 had experienced sexual abuse and one was suspected of experiencing sexual abuse.

Deviant sexual interests are as likely to be found among people with learning disabilities as in the general population. People with learning disabilities are more likely to commit sexual offences against male children and younger children (Craig and Lindsay, 2010).

As discussed in Chapter 20, mental ill health in people with learning disabilities is hard to accurately establish with prevalence rates estimated between 20–74 per cent of sample populations. Diagnostic overshadowing (Reiss *et al.*, 1982) and mental health issues could be a risk factor for some people and their offending behaviours. Personality disorders are proposed to be present in 1–28 per cent of samples of people with learning disabilities (Haut and Brewster, 2010). Anti-social traits and poor impulse control have been linked to deviant sexual interests and recidivism. Substance misuse of either alcohol or illicit substances can be linked to offending behaviours. Some research suggests links between autism and autistic spectrum disorders, attention deficit hyperactivity disorder, epilepsy, brain damage and offending behaviours.

The offender perspectives of people with learning disabilities regarding their lived experiences around the onset of their offending behaviours were reported in a qualitative study of six men detained in secure units (Isherwood *et al.*, 2007). Social factors contributed to their vulnerability of being exploited and manipulated by more able peers. People tried to fit in but isolation, victimisation and bullying were issues. Individual interpersonal difficulties played a part, for example, anger, revenge and retaliation. People felt the need for safety, security, structure and routine. People stated that if they had a 'normal' life such as having a job and girlfriend that this would have stopped them getting into trouble. External destabilising factors such as drugs and alcohol impacted on their offending behaviour. Internal individual inherent factors were incorporated, such as the impact of bereavement and mental health experiences. Obsessions and fascination with specific offending behaviours were a factor for some people.

Specific theories about why people commit sexual offences

Numerous diverse causal models and multifactorial theories have been proposed which attempt to explain why people sexually offend. These have been proposed when considering the general population so their applicability to people with learning disabilities is questionable as it is unclear if exactly the same underlying principles apply. Finkelhor (1984; Finkelhor and associates, 1986) postulated a four-stage model to explain sex offending against a child. The perpetrator has the motivation to sexually abuse as this meets their emotional needs and they are sexually aroused. Their internal inhibitors are challenged and the desire or urge to resist is overwhelmed. They overcome external inhibitors and the barriers protecting the child and they then overcome any resistance from the child. This key model has underpinned the development of most sex offender treatment programmes. Marshall and Barbaree (1990) suggested an integrated model where negative early attachment and adverse childhood and life experiences impact upon the development of self-esteem, self-worth and coping strategies so people are vulnerable to being exploited (Craig *et al.*, 2008). Hall and Hirschman (1992) developed the quadripartite model where there is a physiological sexual arousal which is deviant in response to children. Problematic personality traits based on negative early life experiences are evident. Ward and Brown (2004) suggested 'the good lives model'. All humans need purpose and meaning in life and strive for 'primary human goods' such as friendship, knowledge and intimate relationships in order to get this. People may use maladaptive ways to meet these needs which is where offending occurs.

> ### Reader activity 21.3   Which social factors impact on why people offend?

- How have people with learning disabilities been socially excluded in society?
- How do these factors impact on why people with learning disabilities offend?
- Which of these social factors could apply to Lawrence?
- Look at the social and individual factors outlined in Figure 21.1. Which factors could have impacted on Lawrence and his offending?

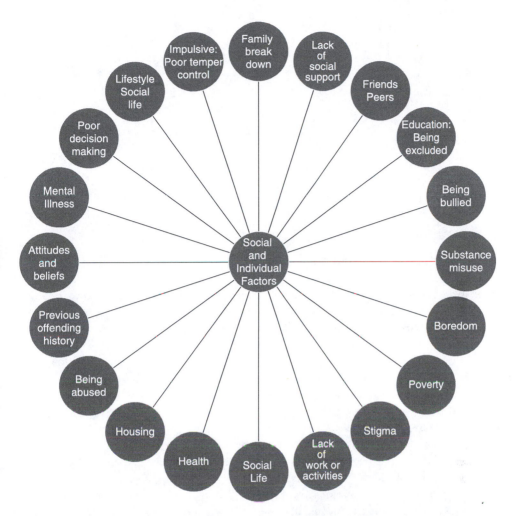

Figure 21.1 Social and individual factors that can impact on offending behaviours

The characteristics of offenders with learning disabilities

Many researchers have outlined the over-representation of young males with learning disabilities and males from ethnic minorities who are convicted of offences. Green *et al.* (2003), suggest that people with learning disabilities are more likely to target younger people. The onset of offending is often at a younger age (Barron *et al.*, 2004). The importance of being able to engage in society is crucial in the rehabilitation of sex offenders. This study found sexual offenders more isolated from parental support with some having no contact with either parent, suffering from poor attachments and emotional detachment. These people were also likely to make less use of leisure time, have fewer relationships and hobbies and be satisfied with lower-level relationships and lower integration into society as a whole. There are a number of social background characteristics that are often reported in research studies which are outlined below. Interventions also need to address these issues as well as using direct CBT interventions. The social background factors are:

- social deprivation/poverty;
- exclusion from school;
- family breakdown;
- relationship problems;
- anti-social behaviour history;
- unemployment;
- child sexual abuse;
- mental illness;
- substance misuse.

Reporting offending behaviour

Care staff often find themselves in a difficult dilemma when deciding whether to report a potential offence to the police. Staff groups often tolerate offending behaviours as they see managing behaviours as being part of their role and many would fear negative repercussions of reporting incidents to the police. In a study by Lyall *et al.* (1995a) only 9 per cent of the sample stated they would report a sexual assault or indecent exposure to the police. Staff may think they will be blamed for these incidents occurring. Staff are unclear about when they should report the behaviour to the police or other external agencies, and there is a dearth of clear policies to guide staff about this. Preference for approaching child welfare and social services was evident in 54 per cent of the sample compared with 23 per cent being reported to the police.

Some staff may think they should not report offending behaviours because the person has learning disabilities. People with learning disabilities could be perceived as being unable to make decisions and hence are not in control of their actions. It could be perceived as being punitive or oppressive to report them as they are not legally culpable (Kearns, 2001). Staff may think that by reporting offences that they are being unfair, unkind and it could have negative consequences and cause distress or upset for the person in their care (Jaydeokar and Barnes, 2009). This could have a detrimental and long-lasting impact upon their therapeutic working relationships. Previous negative experiences of reporting offences and seeing little response from the police could deter people from reporting offences.

If offending behaviour is not reported, this can have a devastating impact on victims and perpetrators. Increased distress can be created for victims as no action could imply that people are not bothered about what has happened to them. A police investigation could demonstrate to victims that they have been listened to. Perpetrators may believe that their behaviour is acceptable or not serious if there are no consequences of it. They may continue the behaviour and will not break the vicious cycle by developing more insight and ways of managing the behaviour. Containment may for some people be the only way that they will be able to access intervention services to address the offending behaviours. Behaviours could escalate so they are more frequent or more severe offending behaviours. Barnes and Robertson (2009) suggest that offenders with learning disabilities should be reported to the police so they can take responsibility for their actions with the appropriate consequences. Staff teams are made up of individuals who have their own sets of attitudes, values and beliefs. People have their own boundaries about what is acceptable and this will impact on when they will report things to the police.

Reader activity 21.4   Reporting behaviour to the police

Lawrence has a long history of sexually inappropriate behaviour towards others. Would you have reported the following behaviour to the police or any other external agency such as social services?

- Approaching children at school when he was a child asking them to touch his genitals?
- When he was exposing himself to younger children at school?
- When he was masturbating in the classroom at school?
- The incidents of abuse in the children's home?
- Lawrence putting himself in vulnerable positions?
- Having a sexual relationship with a peer aged 65 with learning disabilities in the hostel?
- Approaching young children alone in the park asking them to touch his genitals?
- Approaching young children alone in the park exposing his genitals to them and asking them to touch his penis?

The multi-disciplinary professionals and processes involved within the criminal justice system

Reader activity 21.5   Professionals

- What professionals or groups of people could people with learning disabilities like Lawrence come into contact with in the criminal justice system? Make a list.
- List which processes are involved in the criminal justice system.

Figure 21.2 illustrates some of the professionals or groups of people that people with learning disabilities could come into contact within the criminal justice system. Figure 21.3 illustrates some of the processes which are part of the criminal justice system.

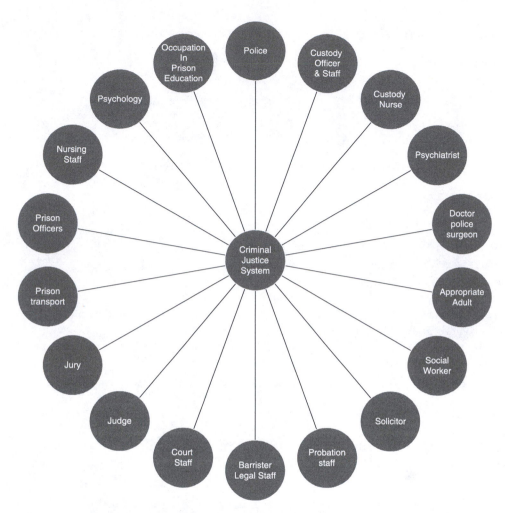

Figure 21.2 Some of the professionals or groups of people that people with learning disabilities could come into contact within the criminal justice system

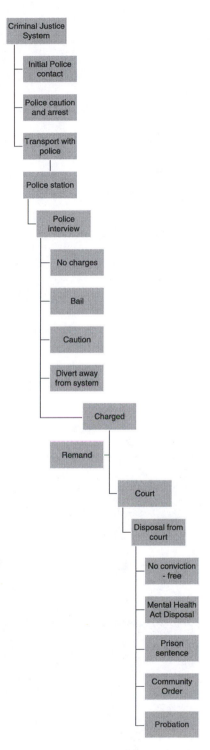

Figure 21.3 Some of the processes which are part of the criminal justice system

Can you think what role each of the following might have in the criminal justice system when working with someone with a learning disability? Complete Table 21.2.

Table 21.2 Role of professional in the criminal justice system

Professional	Role and duties
Police	
Custody Officer and staff	
Custody Nurse	
Psychiatrist	
Doctor/Police Surgeon	
Appropriate Adult	
Social Worker	
Solicitor	
Probation	
Barrister and legal staff	
Court staff	
Judge	
Jury	
Prison transport	
Prison Officers	
Nursing staff	
Psychology	
Prison staff: Occupation/Education	

What difficulties could people with learning disabilities like Lawrence face in the following stages and processes of the criminal justice system? Complete Table 21.3.

Table 21.3 Potential difficulties for people with learning disabilities in the criminal justice system

Stage of system/process	Potential difficulties
Initial Police contact	
Caution and arrest	
Transport	
Police Station	
Police Interview	

Outcome of Interview
Court
Outcome of Court
Prison
Probation Services

Experiences of the criminal justice system

Progressing through any stage of the criminal justice system poses potential difficulties for any adult, let alone adults with learning disabilities. Talbot (2012) identified that there is a lack of any consistent, routine and systematic procedure to identify people with learning disabilities and that not having a learning disability recognised at the start of the process can impact upon the whole experience within the system. Talbot found that some people could deliberately try and hide their learning disabilities while for others, such as people with mental health symptoms or those experiencing the effects of substances, their learning disabilities could be hidden.

When someone's learning disability is unrecognised, they may not have access to an appropriate adult. An appropriate adult should be called to the police station when someone has any mental 'disorder'. The role is to assist the person, protect their rights and to protect them from giving unreliable, incriminating information. They should support the person through the whole criminal proceedings process; insist on legal representation and a psychiatric assessment. They should advise the person being questioned, observe if the interview is conducted properly and help facilitate communication during the interview. Appropriate adults can be family, friends, professionals or trained volunteers. Family may not always be the most appropriate and in terms of confidentially, guidelines were updated in 2006 so the appropriate adult could be someone experienced or trained in their care. There is a National Appropriate Adult Network (NAAN) which sets out national standards for people undertaking this role.

The arrest process will be distressing. The initial police caution may be hard to understand. The police may use jargon and people may not fully understand their rights. People may have issues around sensory perception so having to put handcuffs on and being in close proximity to people could pose a challenge for them. The police interview can be stressful. People could feel intimidated by the uniform or the environment; they could be anxious, scared, worried, confused, excited and stressed and give a false confession just so they could get out of the situation quicker. People with learning disabilities are more likely to be suggestible, so may agree to things they have not done and may not protect themselves or their rights in what they say. A small qualitative research study of the experiences of 15 men with learning disabilities of being interviewed by the police (Leggett *et al.*, 2007) found that 27 per cent of the sample were not allocated an appropriate adult; 18 per cent of the sample did not understand the purpose of the appropriate adult. The feedback was generally negative about the appropriate adult having limited input and saying nothing. It was most important that the appropriate adult should be somebody whom they knew and trusted. The sample group made comments about the negative environment and appeared to underestimate the importance of what had happened. Feelings were mostly negative about feeling anxious, scared and bored due to the waiting time. There was some positive feedback that some people felt understood and listened to.

Court rooms can instil fear in anybody. The accused needs to be able to understand what they have done wrong which may be an issue for some people. The Ministry of Justice (2011) allows vulnerable or intimidated witnesses to be interviewed via a video link from a different room or in a recorded interview but this does not apply to the accused. The court building, processes, language used, waiting around and having to sit and stand when directed could all have issues for offenders with learning disabilities.

Prison will be very stressful for everybody. Mills (2005) stated that despite the NHS taking over prison health services in 2003 there were still a number of issues for offenders with learning disabilities. The deprivation of liberty, rules and regulations, the environment and facilities, long cell lock-ups can lead to isolation, depression, bullying, loneliness and despair in anybody. Due to cognitive deficits, people with learning disabilities often fail to understand and function in such environments.

The work of the Prison Reform Trust though the 'No One Knows' project has been pivotal in understanding the needs of this particular group of offenders and is looking at making changes to ensure that people's needs are met. The needs of offenders with learning disabilities are not clearly identified so support in meeting their needs is lacking. They are vulnerable to manipulation, exploitation and being bullied by other prisoners. There is a lack of systematic screening for learning disabilities. Talbot and Riley (2007) highlighted how conventional treatment programmes are largely inaccessible as an IQ of 80 is needed and people with a learning disability will not benefit from these. They cannot make progress to move on which impacts upon their human rights. The same authors highlighted how prison staff often have some awareness of the issues but lacked the confidence and appropriate skills to manage the issues due to a lack of specialist training. Prisons have a written culture, forms need to be filled to request visits, routines are written down which may be an issue for people with learning disabilities who cannot read and write. Information should be available in formats that people can understand. Some people with learning disabilities would prefer to get a prison sentence as if they are diverted from custody they may stay on a section for a longer time than their sentence.

O'Brien (2008) summarises the key recommendations of the 'No One Know' Projects. He summarised that:

> There should be some information flow about the people being detained. Easy-to-use screening tools should be used routinely and systematically. A multi-disciplinary team approach is crucial. Accessible information about the prison regime should be provided in a format that people can understand. Standards for safe and supportive care should be developed to meet underlying needs. Specific training should be developed for all staff on learning disabilities awareness so as to develop staff understanding, attitudes and values and confidence when working with these people. Good practice should be developed along with a strategic plan and ministerial group. (O'Brien 2008).

Role of health and social care staff

Health and social care staff have a crucial role to play in supporting adults with learning disabilities who offend. Some staff members work directly within the criminal justice system with very specific healthcare roles such as custody nurses, prison healthcare staff, community forensic nursing teams or probation services. Alternatively, anyone working in a variety of different care settings, ranging from local community teams, day services, group homes and residential services to hospital inpatient facilities and secure services may need to support somebody in their care though the criminal justice process at some point.

Care staff could be called upon to act as appropriate adults and to provide the person with support through all stages of the police interview process. They may advocate for the person to ensure the interview process has been fair and offer them support. Custody staff may need to offer emotional support and have an educator role as they help the person to understand what is happening. Care staff could support offenders by taking them to court. Prison staff will ensure appropriate observations are carried out. Healthcare staff in the prison may assess the person and plan appropriate interventions. Prisoners may attend specific treatment groups, education groups or undertake work activities. The care staff in the community forensic team will work with the person to actively manage any risks of reoffending. They will devise appropriate risk management and supervision care plans.

Youth offending

Youth offending teams form part of the youth justice system which is separate from the adult system. Health and social care professionals work together with children aged 10–18 who have been involved in criminal activity where the police and courts have been involved. Teams work to prevent reoffending and to divert people away from the criminal justice system. Teams are made up of the police, probation, health services, children's services, housing, schools and education authorities, substance misuse input, charities and local organisations. They provide support and interventions so young people do not end up in custody. People with learning disabilities should have input from this system the same as anybody else, but unfortunately some fall through the net as they receive input from other services. There are higher rates of mental health issues and socio-economic stressors in young people with learning disabilities.

Meeting Lawrence's needs while in a secure setting

Caring for adults with learning disabilities in a secure units, the interface of the medical and criminal justice systems, involves effective multi-disciplinary working. Figure 21.4 outlines the different members of the team who would work in a secure unit.

Risk assessment and management are a key priority and care staff have an essential role in this process (DH, 2007). Providing a safe and secure environment for staff and patients is essential to allow high quality care to be delivered. Healthcare staff work together as part of the multi-disciplinary team to complete the relevant risk assessments for the specific service such as the HCR–20 risk assessment (Webster *et al.*, 1997).

Security is a key issue on a secure unit and care staff are at the forefront of managing the security of the unit on a daily basis. Security can be physical, procedural and relational (Mason and Phipps, 2010). Physical security incorporates the management of physical violence, the management of the building and the environment. Procedural security involves working within the remit of the policies and procedures that are in place such as observation and search policies. Observation is a time for positive engagement with the patient. It should not just be seen as intrusive surveillance. Lawrence likes to play dominoes. By spending time playing dominoes with Lawrence, the conversation is often lengthy. By being together in this way, it helped the care staff build a relationship with Lawrence but also yielded new information about some of his experiences in the past.

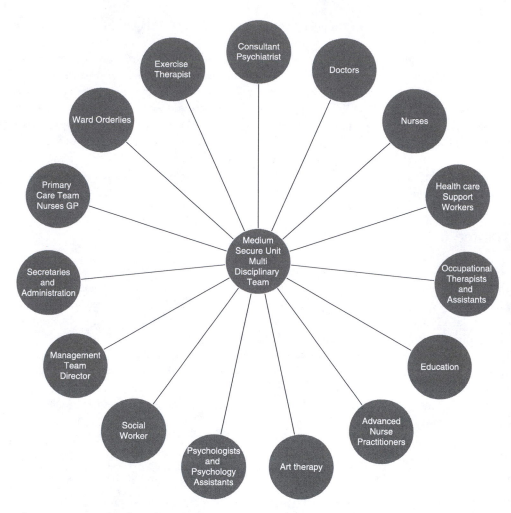

Figure 21.4 Multi-disciplinary team in a medium secure unit

Relational security is about the therapeutic caring relationships that healthcare staff develop within the unit. This aspect is key to quality care delivery working collaboratively toward recovery and progression out of the service. The See, Think, Act policy (DH, 2010) recognises the importance of this and that knowing and understanding the environment and the people in it give a better quality of patient care.

The therapy security paradox debate is one which rumbles on within secure forensic nursing. How can care staff offer therapeutic interventions at the same time as maintaining security? One day staff may have to deny a person's access to community visits, for example because the person's presentation is unsettled, yet the next day they may be approaching the person for an individual therapeutic discussion session. To overcome this, care staff need to have a full awareness of both sides of the coin so they can marry the two. It takes time, skills and experience for staff to be able to balance care in this way. Attitudes and values of the healthcare staff are key.

Nursing tasks are numerous within a secure unit. Risk management and daily shift coordination are essential in sustaining a safe and supportive environment. There are tasks involved in delivering basic nursing care such as promoting physical health, hygiene, diet and healthy living. Legalities of detention create a number of tasks for nurses such as reading of rights at regular intervals, working with the person to understand their rights, ensuring the person has access to advocates, writing reports and attending tribunals with service users. Lawrence was read his rights but did not understand some of the points so the nurse explained this to him. The nurse has also introduced him to the advocacy service who attend the ward and he has now had several discussions with his new advocate. The nurse has a role in administration, involving accurate documentation in notes and reports, writing and reviewing care plans, and effective communication. The nurse supports Lawrence to attend ward rounds and his care planning meetings and provides feedback from, for example, the weekly clinical team meetings that the service users do not attend. Nurses have a role on ongoing monitoring of mental health and the management of any challenging behaviours. When the time is right for the service users, nurses will have a key role in community reintegration by assessing and planning access and facilitating this once it has been agreed by all relevant parties.

Offending behaviour needs are only one aspect of Lawrence's life and he requires input in other areas. Beck, Rawlins and Williams (1993) outline the five dimensions to the person and five care areas: physical, emotional, intellectual, social, spiritual dimensions. All of these interconnect and have an impact on the person as a whole. For example, Lawrence has depression and staff could do some work on behavioural activation and activity scheduling. If Lawrence is occupied, this means he is less likely to have chance to ruminate and plan sexually offending behaviours.

Social interventions will also have a key role to play in Lawrence's rehabilitation. Interventions not directly related to offending can impact on the potential for future reoffending such as anger management and social skills training. If Lawrence develops his skills and understanding, this could impact on how he copes in the future. Psychosocial interventions such as stress vulnerability work, coping strategy enhancement, managing mental health, enhancing strengths, motivation and change work, communication training and staying well relapse prevention work could all have an indirect impact on his offending behaviour. Other interventions such as promoting occupation, developing hobbies, using access to the community, promoting social relationships and promoting physical health also can all have an impact. All members of the health and social care teams have important roles in these interventions. All of these interventions can work together and have a synergetic impact which can also impact on offending behaviours.

Case study 21.2 Anti-libidinal medication

Lawrence was on anti-libidinal medication previously but stopped taking this when he began a consensual sexual relationship. There is inadequate scientific evidence to justify the use of anti-libidinal medication due to the lack of any significant randomised controlled trials. The androgen-depleting drug, cyproterone acetate and the anti-psychotic benperidol are the only drugs licensed for anti-libido usage within the UK and there are huge ethical issues around their use. The side effects of cyproterone acetate included reduced libido, reduced erections and ejaculations, weight gain, low mood, breast development and milk production. One has to wonder whether the therapeutic effects are sufficient to merit its use. Lawrence has stated that he would never take cyproterone acetate again due to the side effects.

Lawrence has depression and the medical team were discussing medication with him for this. Lawrence is happy to take an anti-depressant. This treatment for his depression could potentially impact on his sexually inappropriate behaviour.

Multi-disciplinary professionals follow a therapeutic process so as to build effective therapeutic relationships to meet the needs of individuals. Engagement is the cornerstone of the therapeutic relationship, without engagement the whole therapeutic relationship would collapse. The care team have spent some time in conversation with Lawrence to build up their relationship. A thorough assessment of history, personal background, family, school, occupation, social life, relationships, hobbies and interest, strengths and needs, drug and alcohol use and offending history and behaviours is the next stage. The multi-disciplinary team have worked together to complete a holistic assessment.

Formulation

Traditionally the role of psychologists, many health professionals now see formulation as a core skill. A formulation is 'a hypothesis about the causes, precipitants, and maintaining influences of a person's psychological, interpersonal and behavioural problems' (Eells, 2007, p. 4). The aim is to develop a shared understanding of specific issues which can then be used to guide appropriate interventions. It is important that staff have undertaken some awareness training before undertaking this but it has been shown that staff teams can participate in formulation training and begin to formulate (Ingham et al., 2008). Formulations should be accurate, useful, parsimonious and evidence-based. There are numerous different models of formulation. All care staff should be able to contribute to the formulation process in some way, even if this only means that they can understand what a formulation is and use it to guide their interventions.

Using the five aspects of the 'hot cross bun' formulation (Padesky and Mooney, 1990; Padesky and Greenberger, 1995) (Figure 21.5), the advance nurse practitioner working with Lawrence has

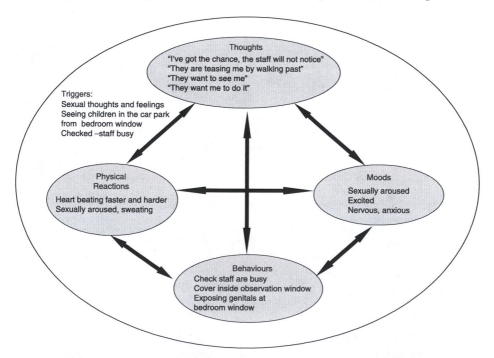

Figure 21.5 Five aspects formulation of Lawrence's recent incident on the ward

completed a formulation of a recent incident where Lawrence had been found exposing his genitals at his bedroom window when there were children in the car park.

Healthcare staff can use this to work with Lawrence at breaking the cycle. The cycle can be broken at any stage. Care staff moved Lawrence to another bedroom after this incident so his new bedroom overlooked an internal courtyard and not the car park. This intervened at the environment stage. It would be possible to work with his thoughts and recognising these and intervening before the behaviour occurred. Lawrence could be asked to seek staff out if he had the feelings so he could be given support and potentially diverted. Care staff should use formulations to underpin their interventions and care plans.

The multi-disciplinary team worked together to develop a '5 P's' formulation for Lawrence (Figure 21.6). This approach uses the case conceptualisation crucible (Kuyken *et al.*, 2009, p. 3) where presenting, predisposing, precipitating, perpetuating and protective factors are identified. This gives an overview of Lawrence's presenting problems that all the different multi-disciplinary professionals can use to guide their interventions.

Needs and goals are identified from the formulation, such as not engaging in sexually inappropriate behaviour and then a plan is formulated. Implementation of the care plan will then be reviewed at regular intervals. The care plan can be amended at any time similar to a formulation, it is dynamic and things change for people. If the plan is working, then it will continue to be implemented as care staff work with Lawrence to maintain well-being, which in this specific example would be not displaying sexually offending behaviours.

My shared pathway

Care staff need to remain innovative and creative. They need to be open to change and to be flexible in their approach to accommodate new ways or working or new interventions in practice. My Shared Pathway (www.networks.nhs.uk/nhs-networks/my-shared-pathway, 2011) is an example of this. This aims to develop an outcomes approach to delivering nursing care using a recovery-focused collaborative approach. This involves the completion of a number of workbooks including shared understandings of how people entered the service, rights, mental health and recovery. The care staff completing this with Lawrence have a good therapeutic relationship with him and will ask questions about his offending behaviours and potential risks as a part of this, as goals are set working towards meeting his agreed outcomes.

Practice alert 21.1

Health and social care staff who work with people with learning disabilities should reflect on and examine their views towards sexuality in this population. Lawrence did experience some hostility from staff in the hostel when he started his relationship with Bill. Some staff on his current ward have commented that he should not have been allowed to have a relationship with a peer, despite the fact that both were consenting. Yool *et al.* (2003) suggest that staff attitudes are now more liberal about the sexuality of people with learning disabilities than they were 30 years ago. They are accepting of holding hands and masturbation but not accepting of other sexual activity. Staff are concerned about risk, capacity to consent, and consent and safeguarding issues preventing exploitation of more vulnerable peers.

Presenting Factors: What is your key problem?

- Approaching children by themselves – when by myself outside such as the park/shops
- Exposing penis to them
- Asking children to "touch it"
- Chasing children
- Did not happen when in 3 year relationship with Bill – loving consensual sexual relationship
- Now, masturbating at bedroom window
- Now, when staff are busy/just done observation checks/visiting times – look out of bedroom window at car park

Predisposing Factors: What caused you to develop this problem? Why do you do it?

- Abandoned as a child
- Number of foster placements
- Lived in a children's home from age of 8
- Sexually abused as a child
- Bullied as a child and adult
- Special school – close supervision – approaching younger children for sexual purposes, asking them to touch him, exposing himself to them
- Vulnerable to exploitation by peers
- Sexual gratification – Thoughts/feelings
- Need a relationship – lack of social network/friends
- No family contact or friends – Nobody cares about me anyway
- The children do not mind, it is part of growing up
- Learning disabilities
- Anxiety and depression
- Living in hostel
- Lack of occupation/hobbies

Precipitating Factors: Why has this become more of an issue now? What are the triggers?

- It gives me a thrill, a nice feeling I enjoy, It is the only sexual thrill I get at the moment
- Sexually aroused by men/boys but think women are beautiful and fancy them – confusion regarding sexuality
- Nobody gets hurt – that was what they used to tell me, they would not look if they did not want to, they talk to me, they like to see me
- Increase in verbal aggression, throwing furniture around if questioned
- Mental Health issues – anxiety and depression
- Getting the chance to run off when in the hostel, seeing children who are alone, planning approach, offering them sweets
- Afraid of being left alone especially at night, asking staff to stay until fall asleep
- Bereavement – loss of relationship and sexual partner
- Being detained – change in behaviour – loss freedom, lifestyle, no access outside, started to look out of bedroom window at car park and saw a child

Perpetuating Factors: Why does this keep happening?

- It gives me a thrill, a nice feeling I enjoy
- It is the only sexual thrill I get at the moment
- Nobody gets hurt – that was what they used to tell me
- They would not look if they did not want to
- They talk to me, they like to see me
- Getting the chance to run off when in the hostel

Protective Factors: Who or what helps you with this problem? What are your strengths?

- Being busy so not thinking about it
- Not being alone – being with people
- Being in a Relationship
- Being in hospital and not being able to go out by myself
- Good at listening to people
- Good at cooking, gym, computers

Figure 21.6 Lawrence: a 5 P's formulation

Source: Kuyken *et al.* (2009).

The needs of staff

Healthcare staff working in forensic secure services can experience stress, burnout and low morale and all staff need adequate support and supervision. Debriefing after incidents should be offered and people should feel supported by both formal systems and informal systems by their peers. Staff should feel supported if they want to report offences to the police. Supervision should be available individually or as groups. McKenzie *et al.* (2001) outline how therapists need support and space to discuss their thoughts and feelings especially when undertaking highly specialised interventions.

Reader activity 21.8   Care planning

Care planning is a key role of health and social care staff. Following a period of assessment on the ward, and with agreement with Lawrence, his team have suggested the following care plans are required:

- Observation/engagement
- Sexualised behaviour
- Management of mental health
- Management of aggression
- Bereavement support
- Social relationships
- Activities/occupation.

Write the care plans for observation/engagement and the sexualised behaviour. For each, you will need to identify the specific problem or need, identify the goals, and specify the interventions and the time when this will be reviewed. You will need to add the evidence base for the interventions. Consider how you will collaboratively discuss this with Lawrence and involve him in the whole process before you both agree and sign the care plan and implement it.

Specialist interventions

Specialist interventions for sexual offending are undertaken by professionals such as psychologists, psychiatrists and specialist nurses who have undertaken specific training in this area. They are not to be attempted by people who have not undertaken this specialist training.

In the 2009 Cochrane Review, Ashman and Duggan highlight how traditional approaches in the management of sex offenders have focused on behavioural interventions. Pharmacological interventions using medication have also been used. There is a growing evidence for the use of cognitive behaviour therapy interventions with this group. Interventions have been developed for a general population so adaptation of these interventions is required so they can be used appropriately with adults with learning disabilities. Their true effectiveness is not known as yet as there has been no randomised control trial conducted in interventions for people with a learning disability who are sex offenders.

Cognitive behavioural interventions represent the most used form of intervention to date. The Adapted Sex Offender Treatment Programme (ASOTP) was adapted in 1997, to treat the needs of learning disabled sex offenders. SOTSEC-ID (2010) reported on 13 CBT treatment groups that ran over nine collaborating sites over one year. Content included: social skills, addressing denial, sex education, consent, and cognitive. The model is used beginning with non-offending examples working up to disclosure of offence using Finkelhor's (1984) four-stage model, which included victim empathy – how they felt when abused, how their victims felt, and relapse prevention. Some 46 men attended, 92 per cent completed the treatment programme and gave good feedback. Their knowledge increased and cognitive distortions decreased which were maintained at 6-month follow-up. Victim empathy did increase but this was not maintained. Three of the men displayed sexually abusive behaviour during treatment which increased to 4 at 6-month follow-up. Autism was observed to be linked to reoffending.

Goodman *et al.* (2008) adapted Finkelhor's (1984) model to use with people with learning disabilities as part of their sex offender treatment programme. The four stages of the model were: thinking about it/wanting to do it, making excuses, getting the chance, and doing it. It followed a graduated approach to full disclosure at 20 weeks into the course. Relapse prevention work was shared with the person's key worker. Progress was noted in terms of increased personal responsibility, reduced victim blaming but there was little evidence to show that the risk of reoffending reduced. It was noted that 'Effective interventions are likely to be multi-faceted and enduring over time' (Goodman *et al.*, 2008, p. 254). A holistic approach is necessary to include such features as housing, employment, activity and relationships, as all of these needs still need to be met and could impact on sexual offending behaviour.

Murphy *et al.*'s (2007) group content included studying body parts, social rules, relationships, what is legal, feelings in stressful situations, consequences of behaviour, disclosure of offences, how hard it is to talk about it and how people cope, experiences of being victims, how others feel when victims, how victims feel, causes of sexual behaviour, understanding their own cycle, choice and consent and relapse prevention.. The CBT was simplified for this population but this study had a limited sample size and no treatment comparison group. People with learning disabilities need the adaptations they had made to the group to cater for people with learning disabilities. This included breaks in sessions, warm-up games, use of symbols, old me/new me, why people offended, who you are now and who you want to work towards becoming. Minimum written tasks were used and a buddy system was used to help with written tasks. Role play and practical activities were also useful. Craig (Craig and Hutchinson, 2005) demonstrated how cognitive behavioural approaches have a greater impact on reoffending, 9.9 per cent compared to 17.4 per cent.

Healthcare professionals have a role in supporting specialist interventions like those mentioned in this chapter. Care staff could be asked to support a person with their homework. They may be an allocated support staff member to speak to if the person has become upset. They may provide feedback to the practitioner about how the person is finding therapy.

Conclusion

This chapter has reviewed aspects of offending behaviour and how this relates to people with learning disabilities. There has been a focus on sexual offending as links have been made throughout with the case of Lawrence, and sexual offending is his offending behaviour. Health and social care staff have a central role to play in the rehabilitation of offenders and sex offenders. Appropriate training is fundamental before offering the specialist interventions outlined but there are other interventions that all health and social care professionals can use as suggested which could have a knock-on effect and help with offending and sexual offending behaviours. Working with people using a holistic, person-centred approach is essential and the therapeutic relationship is crucial to meeting care needs.

Points to remember

- Offenders often have a history of negative life experiences. This includes offenders with learning disabilities.
- Learnt behaviours may be offending behaviours.
- MDT involvement is necessary in meeting needs.
- A measured, risk-assessed plan of care is necessary.

Resources

Table 21.4 presents key relevant legislation and policy.

Table 21.4 Key relevant legislation and policy

Policy/Legislation/Guidance	Year/author	Points of note
No Health Without Mental Health	DH 2011	Good health, recovery, physical health, reduced avoidable harm and reduced stigma and discrimination are the aims, everybody has a role. LD offenders should have same access to services with issues being identified when during first contact with criminal justice system.
See, Think, Act	DH 2010	Knowing and understanding the environment and the people in it gives a better quality of patient care and relational security
Valuing People Now	DH 2009	Promotes inclusion, rights, control and independent living promoting respect and dignity. A right to lead their lives like others and similar opportunities are central. Person-centred approaches are essential to improve outcomes. People with complex needs and offenders should be supported to access mainstream mental health services like anybody else.
The Bradley Report	DH 2009	Diversion of offenders with learning disabilities from prison
Protection of Vulnerable Adults (POVA)	DH 2009	Safeguarding Adults Policies
The Mental Health Act	1983 (amended 2007)	Civil Sections and Hospital Orders for detention and treatment
Best Practice Guidance: Specification for adult medium secure services	DH 2007a	Standards – security – physical, procedural, relational, clinical and cost effectiveness, governance, patient focus, accessible and responsive care, care environment and amenities, public health

(continued)

Table 21.4 (*Continued*)

Policy/Legislation/Guidance	Year/author	Points of note
The Commissioning Specialist Adult Learning Disability Health service Good Practice Guidance	DH 2007b	Quality of care to meet needs, in community where possible or in no greater security than necessary to promote rehabilitation
Policing and Justice Bill	2006	Live Links for vulnerable witnesses to give evidence over video link
The Mental Capacity Act	2005	Framework for making decisions for those over 16 who lack mental capacity to do this – assume capacity unless proven otherwise, try to help make decisions, accept unwise decisions if capacity, do things in best interests where no capacity, least restrictive options. IMCA help support decisions (independent mental capacity advocate)
PACE (Police and Criminal Evidence Act) 1984/2006	1984/2006	Police service, persons with mental disorder or mentally vulnerable – right to appropriate adult, safeguarding procedures
Disability Discrimination Act DDA	1995/2005	Legal responsibility not to discriminate against people with disabilities, aims to eliminate discrimination and harassment
Criminal Justice Act MAPPA Multi Agency Public Protection Arrangements	2000/2003	Police, prison, probation working together to manage dangerous offenders. NOMS – National Offender Management Service
Valuing People	DH 2001	Improve quality of life for people with learning disabilities – rights, inclusion, choice, independence. Person-centred approach.
National Service Framework for Mental Health	DH 1999	Guides decision on level of security an individual needs.
Human Rights Act	1998	Article 5 – right to liberty and security Article 6 – right to a fair trial
The Criminal Procedure (Insanity and Unfitness to Plead) Act	Home Office, 1991	If fit to plead responsible for actions, fitness to plead – ability to plead, understand evidence, understand and participate in court proceedings. Two psychiatrist reports needed to say if fit to plead
Care Programme Approach	DH 1995	Care coordinator, full package care, effective case management

References

Ashman, L.L.M and Duggan, L. (2009) *Interventions for Learning Disabled Sex Offenders*. (Review). The Cochrane Collaboration. Chichester: John Wiley & Sons Ltd.

Barnes, J. and Robertson, D. (2009) in E. Chaplin, J. Henry and S. Hardy (eds) *Working with People with Learning Disabilities and Offending Behaviour: A Handbook*. Brighton: Pavilion.

Barron, P., Hassiotis, A. and Banes, J. (2004) Offenders with intellectual disability: a prospective comparative study, *Journal of Intellectual Disability Research*, 48: 69–76.

Baxter, V. (2002) Nurses' perceptions of their roles and skills in a medium secure unit, *British Journal of Nursing*, 11(20): 1312–1319.

Beck, C.K., Rawlins, R.P. and Williams, S.R. (1993) *Mental Health Psychiatric Nursing: A Holistic Life Cycle Approach*, 3rd edn. St Louis, MO: Mosby Year Book.

Cooper, A.J. (1995) Review of the role of two antilibidinal drugs in the treatment of sex offenders with mental retardation, *Mental Retardation*, 33(1): 42–48.

Craig, L.A., Browne, K.D. and Beech, A.R. (2008) *Assessing Risk in Sex Offenders: A Practitioner's Guide*. Chichester: John Wiley & Sons Ltd.

Craig, L.A. and Hutchinson, R.B. (2005) Sexual offenders with learning disabilities: risk, recidivism and treatment, *Journal of Sexual Aggression*, 11(3): 289–304.

Craig, L.A. and Lindsay, W.R. (2010) Sexual offenders with intellectual disabilities, characteristics and prevalence, in L.A. Craig, W.R. Lindsay and K.D. Browne (eds) *Assessment and Treatment of Sexual Offenders with Intellectual Disabilities: A Handbook*. Chichester: John Wiley & Sons Ltd.

DH (Department of Health) (2007) *Best Practice Guidance: Specification for Adult Medium Secure Services*. London: Department of Health.

DH (Department of Health) (2010) *Relational Security Explorer*. London: Department of Health.

Doyle, D.M. (2004) The differences between sex offending and challenging behaviour in people with an intellectual disability, *Journal of Intellectual and Developmental Disability*, 29(2): 107–118.

Eells, T.D. (ed.) (2007) *Handbook of Psychotherapy Case Formulation*, 2nd edn. New York: Guilford Press.

Eells, T.D. and Lombart, K.G. (2011) in T.D. Eells, K.G. Lombart, P. Sturmey and M. McMurran (eds) *Theoretical and Evidence-Based Approaches to Case Formulation*. Chichester: John Wiley & Sons, Ltd

Finkelhor, D. (1984) *Child Sexual Abuse: New Theory and Research*. New York: Free Press.

Finkelhor, D. and Associates (1986) *A Sourcebook on Child Sexual Abuse*. Beverly Hills, CA: Sage.

Fryson, R. (2007) Young people with learning disabilities who sexually harm others: the role of criminal justice within a multi agency response, *British Journal of Learning Disabilities*, 35: 181–186.

Goodman, W., Leggett, J., Weston, C., Phillips, S. and Steward, J. (2008) Group treatment for men with learning disabilities who are at risk of sexually offending: themes arising from the four stage model to offending, *British Journal of Learning Disabilities*, 36: 249–255.

Green, G., Gray, N.S. and Willner, P. (2003) Management of sexually inappropriate behaviours in men with learning disabilities, *Journal of Forensic Psychiatry and Psychology*, 14(1): 85–110.

Hall, G.C.N. and Hirschman, R. (1992) Sexual aggression against children: a conceptual perspective of etiology, *Criminal Justice and Behaviour*, 19: 8–23.

Harding, D., Deeley, Q. and Robertson, D. (2009) In E. Chaplin, J. Henry and S. Hardy (eds) *Working with People with Learning Disabilities and Offending Behaviour: A Handbook*, Brighton, Pavilion.

Harrington, R., Bailey, S., Chitsebesan, P., Kroll, L. and Macdonald, W. (2005) *Mental Health Needs and Effectiveness of Provision for Young Offenders in Custody and in the Community*. London: Youth Justice Board for England and Wales.

Haut, F. and Brewster, E. (2010) Psychiatric illness, pervasive developmental disorders and risk, in L.A. Craig, W.R. Lindsay and K.D. Browne (eds) *Assessment and Treatment of Sexual Offenders with Intellectual Disabilities: A Handbook*. Chichester: John Wiley & Sons Ltd.

Hayes, S. (2007) Missing out: offenders with learning disabilities and the criminal justice system, *British Journal of Learning Disabilities*, 35: 146–153.

Hayes, S., Shackell, P., Mottram, P. and Lancaster, R. (2007) The prevalence of intellectual disability in a major UK prison, *British Journal of Learning Disabilities*, 35: 162–167.

Hingsburger, D., Griffiths, D. and Quinsey, V. (1991) Detecting counterfeit deviance: differentiating sexual deviance from sexual inappropriateness, *Habilitative Mental Health Care Newsletter*, 10: 51–54.

Holland, A.J. (2004) Criminal behaviour and developmental disability: an epidemiological perspective, in W.R. Lindsay, J.L. Taylor and P. Sturmey (eds) *Offenders with Developmental Disabilities*. Chichester: John Wiley & Sons, Ltd, pp. 23–34.

Ingham, B., Clarke, L. and James, I.A. (2008) Biopsychosocial case formulation for people with intellectual disabilities and mental health problems: a pilot study of a training workshop for direct care staff, *The British Journal of Developmental Disabilities*, 54(106): 41–54.

Isherwood, T., Burns, M., Naylor, M. and Read, S. (2007) 'Getting into trouble': a qualitative account of offending in the accounts of men with learning disabilities, *The Journal of Forensic Psychiatry and Psychology*, 18(2): 221–234.

Jaydeokar, S. and Barnes, J. (2009) In E. Chaplin, J. Henry and S. Hardy (eds) *Working with People with Learning Disabilities and Offending Behaviour: A Handbook*. Brighton: Pavilion.

Jones, G. and Talbot, J. (2010) No One Knows: The bewildering passage of offenders with learning disability and learning difficulty through the criminal justice system, *Criminal Behaviour and Mental Health*, 20: 1–7.

Kearns, A. (2001) Forensic services and people with learning disability: in the shadow of the Reed Report, *Journal of Forensic Psychiatry and Psychology*, 12(1): 8–12.

Kuyken, W., Padesky, C.A. and Dudley, R. (2009) The science and practice of case conceptualisation, *Behavioural and Cognitive Psychotherapy*, 26(6): 757–768.

Leggett J., Goodman, W. and Dinani, S. (2007) People with learning disabilities' experiences of being interviewed by the police, *British Journal of Learning Disabilities*, 35: 168–173.

Lindsay, W.R. (2005) Model underpinning treatment for sex offenders with mild intellectual disability: current theories of sex offending, *Mental Retardation*, 43(6): 428–441.

Lindsay, W.R., Smith, A.H.W., Law, J., Quinn, K. and Anderson, A. (2004) Sexual and nonsexual offenders with intellectual and learning disabilities, *Journal of Interpersonal Violence*, 19: 875–890.

Lyall, I., Holland, A. and Collins, S. (1995a) Offending by adults with learning disabilities and the attitudes of staff to offending behaviour: implications for service development. *Journal of Intellectual Disability Research*, 39(6): 501–508.

Lyall I., Holland A. and Collins S. (1995b) Incidence of persons with a learning disability detained in police custody:aA needs assessment for service development, *Medicine, Science, Law*, 35: 61–71.

Marshall, W.L. and Barbaree, H.E. (1990) An integrated theory of the aetiology of sexual offending, in W.L. Marshall, D.R. Laws and H.E. Barbaree (eds) *Handbook of Sexual Assault: Issues, Theories and Treatment of the Offender*. New York: Plenum.

Mason, T. and Phipps, D. (2010) Forensic learning disability nursing skills and competencies: a study of forensic and non-forensic nurses, *Issues in Mental Health Nursing*, 31(11): 708–715.

McBrien, J., Hodgetts, A. and Gregory, J. (2003) Offending and risky behaviour in community services for people with intellectual disabilities in one local authority, *Journal of Forensic Psychiatry*, 14: 280–297.

McKenzie, K., Matheson, E., McKaskie, K., Patrick, S., Paxton, D., Michie, A. and Murray, G.C. (2001) Health and social care staff responses to working with people with a learning disability who display sexual offending type behaviours, *Journal of Sexual Aggression: An International, Interdisciplinary Forum for Research, Theory and Practice*, 7(1): 56–66.

Michie, A.M., Lindsay, W.R., Martin, V. and Grieve, A. (2006) A test of counterfeit deviance; comparison of sexual knowledge in groups of sex offenders with intellectual disability and controls, *Sexual Abuse: A Journal of Research and Treatment*, 18(3): 271–278.

Mills, A. (2005) In B. Littlechild, and D. Fearns (eds) *Mental Disorder and Criminal Justice, Policy, Provision and Practice*. Lyme Regis: Russell House Publishing.

Ministry of Justice (2011) *Achieving Best Evidence in Criminal Proceedings: Guidance on Interviewing Victims and Witnesses, and Guidance on Using Special Measures*. London: Ministry of Justice.

Mottram, P.G. (2007) *HMP Liverpool, Styal and Hindley Study Report*. Liverpool: University of Liverpool.

Murphy, G., Powell, S., Guzman, A.M. and Hays, S.J. (2007) Cognitive-behavioural treatment for men with intellectual disabilities and sexually abusive behaviour: a pilot study, *Journal of Intellectual Disability Research*, 51(11): 902–912.

My Shared Pathway (2011) *The NHS Quality, Innovation, Productivity and Prevention*. Available at: www. networks.nhs.uk/nhs-networks/my-shared-pathway.

O'Brien, G. (2008) No One Knows: identifying and supporting prisoners with learning difficulties and learning disabilities: the views of prison staff. Jenny Talbot for the Prison Reform Trust. *Advances in Mental Health and Learning Disabilities*, 2(1): 50–53.

O'Brien, G., Taylor, J., Lindsay, W., Holland, A., Carson, D., Steptoe, L., Price, K., Middleton, C. and Wheeler, J. (2010) A multi-centre study of adults with learning disabilities referred to services for antisocial or offending behaviour: demographic, individual, offending and service characteristics, *Journal of Learning Disabilities and Offending Behaviour*, 1(2): 5–15.

Padesky, C.A. and Greenberger, D. (1995) *Mind Over Mood*. New York: Guilford Press.

Padesky, C.A. and Mooney, K.A. (1990) Clinical tip: presenting the cognitive model to clients, *International Cognitive Therapy Newsletter*, 6: 13–14.

Read, F. and Read, E. (2009) Learning disabilities and serious crime: sex offences, *Mental Health and Learning Disabilities Research and Practice*, 6: 37–51.

Reiss, S., Levitan, G. and Syszszko, J. (1982) Emotional disturbance and mental retardation: diagnostic overshadowing, *American Journal of Mental Deficiency*, 86: 567–574.

Riding, T. (2005) Sexual offending in people with learning disabilities, in T. Riding, C. Swann and B. Swann (eds) *The Handbook of Forensic Learning Disabilities*. Oxford: Radcliffe Publishing.

Rose, J., Cutler, C., Tresize, K., Novak, D. and Rose, D. (2008) Individuals with intellectual disability who offend, *The British Journal of Developmental Disabilities*, 54(106): 19–30.

Simpson, M.K. and Hogg, J. (2001) Patterns of offending among people with intellectual disability: a systematic review. Part I: methodology and prevalence data, *Journal of Intellectual Disability Research*, 45(5): 384–396.

SOTSEC-ID (Sex Offender Treatment Services Collaborative) (2010) Effectiveness of group cognitive behavioural treatment for men with intellectual disabilities at risk of sexual offending, *Journal of Applied Research in Intellectual Disabilities*, 23: 537–551.

Talbot, J. (2012) in H.L. Atherton and D.J. Crickmore (eds) *Learning Disabilities: Toward Inclusion*, 6th edn. London: Churchill Livingstone.

Talbot, T.J. and Langdon P.E. (2006) A revised sexual knowledge assessment tool for people with intellectual disabilities: is sexual knowledge related to sexual offending behaviour? *Journal of Intellectual Disability Research*, 50(7): 523–531.

Talbot, J. and Riley, C. (2007) No One Knows: offenders with learning difficulties and learning disabilities, *British Journal of Learning Disabilities*, 35: 154–161.

Thompson, D. (1997) Profiling the sexually abusive behaviour of men with learning disabilities, *Journal of Applied Research in Intellectual Disabilities*, 10(2): 125–139.

Walker, N. and McCabe, S. (1973) *Crime and Insanity in England*. Edinburgh: Edinburgh University Press.

Ward, T. and Brown, M. (2004) The good lives model and conceptual issues in offender rehabilitation, *Psychology, Crime and Law*, 10: 243–257.

Webster, C.D., Douglas, K.S., Eaves, D. and Hart, S.D. (1997) *HCR-20: Assessing Risk for Violence* (version 2). Burnaby, BC, Canada: The Mental Health, Law and Policy Institute of Simon Fraser University.

Winter, N., Holland, A. and Collins, S. (1997) Factors predisposing to suspected offending by adults with self-reported learning disabilities, *Psychological Medicine*, 27: 595–607.

Yool, L., Langdon, P.E. and Garner, K. (2003) The attitudes of medium secure unit staff toward the sexuality of adults with learning disabilities, *Sexuality and Disability*, 21(2): 137–150.

22 Bereavement and loss

Nigel McLoughlin and Paul Armitage

Learning outcomes

After reading this chapter you will be able to:

- facilitate the reader's understanding of bereavement, loss and the grieving process
- provide an overview of the social context within which individuals with learning disability experience bereavement and loss
- identify individual presentations of responses to loss
- provide initial guidance on how to address the needs of newly bereaved individuals with learning disability.

Introduction

The loss of a loved one is one of the most intensely painful experiences any human being can suffer, and not only is it painful to experience, but also painful to witness, if only because we are so impotent to help.

(Bowlby, 1980, p. 7)

Case study 22.1   Grief

Lawrence was abandoned when very young, and erratic care during his childhood affected his ability to form relationships. He enjoyed a close sexual relationship in adulthood but this ended following his partner's death. Grief has shaped much of Lawrence's life, having a bearing on his outlook, his behaviour and psychological and mental health.

The tenet of the above Bowlby quote holds true, witnessing the emotional pain of another human being can indeed be distressing. However, for those of us who are carers, especially those who have a professional duty of care for others, standing impotently by is not an option, neither morally or professionally. Death is the very fabric of life! Managing bereavement issues, however, are still difficult, as such situations can evoke personal feelings for us, causing pain, and they have an impact on the relationships we have with those we care for, causing us to need to readjust our role of caregiver.

Understanding that grief is a normal reaction to a loss is to take the first step towards normalising what can, at times, seem like an abnormal response. This point is very pertinent to people with learning disabilities. Their needs can often be misunderstood and, as a consequence, are unmet. Having a better understanding of bereavement, loss and grieving can help to minimise their impact not only on the individual but also on those around them. It also enables us to provide the right support or, indeed, recognise our own limitations and at times, perhaps in more complex situations, it enables us to recognise the need to refer to others who may be able to help.

Practice alert 22.1

Before considering the content of this chapter we suggest that the reader exercise some degree of self-care with regard to their own bereavement experiences. If you have been recently bereaved or you are finding reading this chapter is proving challenging, we suggest that you return to it later.

What are bereavement and loss?

We experience feelings of bereavement following the loss of a relationship with something or someone we once had. Loss may be felt in relation to many things and may include relationships in their many forms. We might lose personal things such as possessions; we might lose a job or be made redundant or retire and feel a sense of loss. We could become disabled and lose skills or there may be a loss of health. Losses may also be more abstract; some losses may involve things personal to particular individuals. If you lose something of sentimental value, it hurts or you may panic if there is a loss of something you rely upon. All human beings, regardless of their disability, abilities, culture or ethnicity, feel loss. When considering the loss of relationships, some of the relationships we have are also shared by others. Shared loss is also an important aspect of the human condition and though heartache still exists in such situations, when grief is shared, pain is mutually understood.

Although a universal emotion, each individual's journey through grief is unique, in other words, we are all the same but very different. The grief felt by individuals and its intensity depend on different factors. Having an understanding of the concept of grief and our ability to feel losses are important. The latter is exceedingly pertinent in the care of people with learning disabilities; their cognitive needs will often impact on their emotional development. Social circumstances, particularly attitudes, will have a major impact on their experiences of loss, as do the knowledge and skill of those around them.

Fast facts 22.1   Key definitions

- Bereavement is loss caused by the death of someone with whom you had a relationship.
- Loss is no longer having a relationship with someone/something you once had.
- Grief is the psychological and physiological reactions to the loss of a relationship.
- Grieving is how we process and experience our emotional responses related to the loss of a relationship.

Loss has an impact in different ways. Externally, it has its effect. If we have lost our job, moved house or lost a relationship, for example, we experience it externally through the change it has within our lives, internally, our emotions are affected, we may feel a range of different emotions, and thoughts also may flood back to happier times when the person or lost possession was present. We can feel a loss of expectation, maybe there is the need to readjust previous aspiration, aims and goals. Physically too, loss has its impact, we may feel a physical yearning for the object of our grief, have a sense of emptiness inside; it may cause physical symptoms such as headaches, sweating, the immune system can react and we may be more prone to physical ailments while we suffer psychologically. The remaining person from a couple following a long loving relationship can grieve so badly following the loss of their partner, that they do not eat or sleep and block out previous social contacts. Such actions can lead to both physical and psychological deterioration. There is often a behavioural impact; behaviours such as crying, irritability and sadness can be seen in some people while someone with a learning disability might display behavioural outbursts such as hitting out or more challenging behaviours. These behaviours might become more frequent if the person has no other means of highlighting their distress. Other responses to grief may be idiosyncratic, for example, our own individual response to sudden or traumatic loss events.

Fast facts 22.2   Loss

Loss can be felt due to many life events and changes (Table 22.1).

Table 22.1 Kinds of loss

• Loss of relationships due to divorce or separation	• Loss of security, for example, if feeling threatened by someone or insecure within a relationship
• Loss of capacity through becoming disabled or through mental or physical ill-health	• Loss of friendship or relationship
• Loss of self-worth	• Loss of financial stability following job changes or changes to social security benefits
• Loss due to emigration/migration of self or others	• Loss due to feeling different, for example, if you or your children or siblings have special educational needs
• Loss of culture, maybe you have moved from your homeland?	• Loss of dreams or future expectations

- Losing one's sense of belonging, for example, community or group or following a job change
- Losses experienced through starting a new job, new school, college, class. Maybe you miss the old one?
- Losing one's faith or religion
- Loss or perceived loss of freedom

- Loss of attention through the birth of sibling
- Losing one's home
- Loss of one's possessions
- Loss of self-identity

Reader activity 22.1 Effects of loss

The list in Table 22.1 is not exhaustive; use it to consider how many of the above losses shown you have experienced to greater or lesser degree.

- Consider how you responded to the losses.
- Compare your own experiences to those of others.
- Consider what impacted most on the way you coped with your experience of loss.

Past experiences of loss have an impact; if someone has no past experience, then maybe this first experience is felt very strongly. The situation surrounding the felt loss is pertinent. Maybe it was very sudden or followed a tragic event? Death following tragic events may be felt more strongly by those left behind as they maybe feel angry perhaps at the nature of the circumstances.

Outpouring of grief is experienced differently by people from different cultures or by people from varying religious or social backgrounds. People from some cultures, for example, display stiff upper lips when faced with bereavement, while others show public displays of emotion and pain. Religious and social upbringings can have a bearing. Some families may believe that life continues after death and though a mourning of the loss of the loved one on earth may occur, they may feel that the dead person has gone to a better place. Other faiths may advocate a rejoicing of life rather than a mourning of death. All have an impact on the grief felt and the display of that grief. How individuals cope may be due to more personal factors. Maybe the head of a family feels they have to be strong for others. Males and females may be different in how they grieve. Some people may feel unable to grieve openly or may turn to particular family or friends for support or may find solace in religion or taking their mind off things by working or returning to previous routines.

Someone with a learning disability, like Lawrence, may have lived in many varied environments during earlier life, and this has an impact on the ability to form social relationships. They may appear at times therefore not to feel the loss of a close acquaintance, however, they may have learnt to adapt to change quickly. An apparent nonchalance about death can, however, hide a deep sense of hurt and/or confusion, their feelings should not therefore be minimised. Historical factors should be taken into account as they may provide opportunities for understanding and helping people. How much is understood about the loss is important. If it is an expected death, following a long illness, maybe there has been a time for emotional preparation beforehand. If it has been sudden or unexpected, then shock can cause another dimension within the grieving process. Someone with a learning disability may not be aware of the whole picture surrounding the death of a loved one, leaving them feeling unsure about particular aspects of the situation. For all of us, a lack of knowledge can be detrimental, the lack of insight into the full facts may stop normal grieving occurring. A lack of comprehension can be a barrier preventing a normal consolidation of feelings. Young children and people with a learning disability may, due to limited cognitive development, not fully understand certain life events such as death. It is important that events of loss are explained in terms and in ways understood by people with limited cognitive or intellectual development, so enabling understanding in an age-appropriate and intellectually appropriate way.

The contributory factors outlined above highlight the complexities involved in understanding an individual's response to loss and may help us to aid those affected by loss. On the surface a loss may seem uncomplicated, however, it is not until one takes into account all these variables that we are able to understand and respond more fully.

Case study 22.2   Emotional events

Lawrence's early experience of separation may have affected him in many ways. First, there is the actual separation from his family and the nature of this. Even in abusive situations the individual has a relationship with the perpetrator, it may be one fuelled by mistrust and hurt, but nonetheless, a relationship. This is particularly true if the perpetrator is a close family member. On one hand, there may be pain but, on the other, there may be dependence, fear, attachment or loyalty. Lawrence may have felt some comfort in leaving a difficult home but this will have depended on what replaced it and how he was supported with his loss.

We know that Lawrence has a mild learning disability and would have therefore been able to understand some of what was happening to him. How well this was communicated to him, how he adjusted to the loss, if he remained in contact with his family, the type of help he had, if he felt relieved, and so forth, we do not know.

Hollins and Esterhuyzen (1997) illustrated how people with a learning disability respond emotionally to bereavement like other people. It is important that those supporting people with learning disabilities acknowledge this fact. Anxiety is a normal response for everyone and the 'fight or flight' feelings associated with it (Martin et al., 2000) occur as a response to real or perceived threats, individuals with a learning disability who have cognitive of communication deficits may experience more anxiety as their coping mechanisms may be reduced, and anxiety can lead to behavioural problems. Changes in behaviour may be temporary, expressed as a need to readjust, or more long-standing when anxiety, confusion or hurt prevails. Providing an emotionally safe and secure environment at this time is the first step to encouraging healing following bereavement.

Emotional resilience to death and individual experience of grieving often develops through childhood experiences of loss. Reactions to loss may be learnt through experiencing a lost or broken favourite toy; moving house or school or from the direct experience of the death of a family pet, or the more profound loss of a relative. Emotional development depends on the child's age, however, some of the feelings are nevertheless painful. These experiences play a part in the development of the child's perceptions of

Table 22.2 Age of development of awareness of death

0–2 years. Has no cognitive understanding of death. Will experience death as an interrupted attachment. There may be some changes in behaviour.

2–3 years. Sees death as temporary and reversible. It should be noted at this point insecure or interrupted attachment issues should be taken into account as they have the potential to heighten responses.

4–6 years. Will attempt to explain and rationalise death. May experiment through play and acting out with the thought that death might be permanent.

6–9 years. Has the ability to reason; will understand logical explanations of death, including acceptance of mortality. Around 9 years of age the individual will generally have begun to understand the biological basis of death. Their ideas about death are closer to those of an adult.

9 years and above. Will have a more adult-like comprehension of the concept of death. The individual's understanding has the potential to develop depending on their own experiences of death and observed responses of others.

Source: Adapted from the work of South Eastern Connecticut Bereavement programme.

mortality. Knowing about emotional development and the childhood experience of grief is important. Such understanding can help us conceptualise how a child or a person with a learning disability is experiencing or understanding loss. An individual's understanding of death will be largely dependent on their cognitive development coupled with experiences from their socialisation. Table 22.2 shows the suggested ages of the development of awareness of death among people who do not have a learning disability. We suggest, however, that due to the variation of the human norm, it is used as a guide only.

Personality development is another important factor to consider in meeting the psychological needs of the grieving individual. It is a complex area but is one that cannot be ignored, as some personality traits born of difficult or traumatic experiences can impinge on our efforts to therapeutically engage with the individual, and so may require special care. Below are several personality traits which can impact upon the grieving process and on the ability of others to assist the person through this process.

Reader activity 22.2 Traits

Consider these traits and how they may affect talking to someone about their grief.

Untrustingy	Trusting	Defensiveness
Eagerness to please	Anxiety	Relaxed
Over-trusting	Confrontational	Seeking acceptance
Easy-going	Over-active	Confident
Low self-esteem	Seeking reassurance	Self-centred
High self-esteem	Fearful of change	Suspicious
Accepts change readily	Insecure	Affectionate
Invasion of personal space	Eager to please	Stubborn

How do we experience bereavement and loss?

We are all unique individuals, however, there exists some commonality in how we experience loss. It will invariably include a range of responses.

Following a bereavement, professionals are often asked 'How long will it take to get over this?', or 'When will I feel better?' The answer is: it will take as long as it takes. Coming to terms with death is a very gradual process that can take a considerable time to get over and has many determinants. People usually find that over time they are able to get on with their lives. They may think less about the person they have lost and adapt. Most people begin to feel like this within one or two years of the death of someone close to them. It may be difficult to accept the death of a loved one but it is often possible to get on with life in spite of this. On recovering, some people feel guilty if they are beginning to build a life for themselves. They may feel disloyal to the memory of the loved one. The process of grieving can never be underestimated and anyone can feel overwhelmed or that the experience is unbearable.

Many individuals with learning disabilities may be reliant on those close to them and in addition to the sense of loss if that person dies, may feel exceedingly insecure or vulnerable at the thought of a life without them. Conversely, there may be people who appear resilient to life's challenges and they appear to cope exceedingly well. They may use new opportunities to build a different life to the one that they had with the deceased. For others, though the loss may be painful, the experience of starting a new life, can, in fact be quite liberating. Case study 22.3 shows how the loss of his parents impacted on someone with a learning disability. His experiences are very different to those felt by Lawrence.

Case study 22.3   John's story

John had always lived with his parents. They lived an insular lifestyle and he rarely experienced life beyond his local neighbourhood. Aged 50, when his mother died, he moved into sheltered accommodation. It was evident immediately how John threw himself into all the opportunities that were available to him, including joining a hobbies club, learning to dance and visiting the local pub. People who knew him said that he was much more outgoing and seem to be enjoying life.

Theories of grief and loss

Theories of grief and loss offer a perspective on understanding and individual reactions to changes and have existed for thousands of years. Around 2400 years ago Tibetan Buddhists described the life cycle as a constant journey through life and death. Freud (1917), at the height of the First World War, described reactions to death, he described mourning as a natural, albeit painful process but he describes melancholia as a 'pathological' state, in melancholia the reasons for such deep feelings may be forgotten as the unconsciousness becomes involved. Melancholia, which may be likened to depression following the death of a loved one, involves a loss of self-esteem and a sense of the ego being deeply affected. Elizabeth Kübler-Ross (see also Chapter 7) is known for her pioneering work with the terminally ill and for her ideas on the counselling and support of those affected by death and

Table 22.3 The five stages of grief

Stage	Interpretation
1 Denial	Denial is a conscious or unconscious refusal to accept facts, information and reality relating to the situation concerned. It is a defence mechanism and perfectly natural. Some people can remain at this stage for some time, this should not be ignored; the person may need help to move from this stage. Death, however, is not easy to deny indefinitely.
2 Anger	Anger can manifest in different ways. People faced with emotional upset can be angry with themselves and/or with others, especially those close to them. Knowing this helps one to remain detached from the anger to be non-judgemental.
3 Bargaining	Traditionally the bargaining stage for bereaved or dying people can involve attempting to bargain with God. People may seek to negotiate a compromise, for example 'Can it be anything other than cancer?'
4 Depression	There may be different levels of sadness but this stage indicates a sort of acceptance of the reality of the event and an emotional attachment to it. It is natural to feel sadness and regret, fear, uncertainty, and so forth.
5 Acceptance	Again this stage varies according to the person's situation, though broadly speaking, it is an indication that there is some emotional detachment and objectivity. People dying can enter this stage a long time before the people they leave behind, all must pass through to this stage of acceptance as/when they are ready.

Source: Kübler-Ross (1969).

bereavement. Her seminal book, published in 1969, gave an explanation of the 'five stages of grief' or the 'grief cycle' (Table 22.3). Although her work suggests a grief process, it was not intended to be considered as five stages that individuals pass through from start to finish within a given fixed time frame. It is best considered as a cyclical process where the stages of grieving may be repeatedly experienced; the intensity of the feeling felt during the stages, in most cases, diminishing over time until the individual adjusts to the loss and moves to acceptance which then enables the person to cope.

Case study 22.4   Asif's story

Asif has a moderate learning disability and lives with his parents. He leads an active and varied lifestyle outwith the family home but was close to both of his parents. Asif's father died and he was grief-stricken and numbed and later became withdrawn. He was supported, however, to be as involved with the funeral as much as possible. One of his jobs was to work with his brother to put a photo album of dad's life together. Soon after his father's death, he started to pick up on his old routines, which was encouraged. He and his family often talk about dad and they shed a few tears; but they laugh also at all the fun things they all did together. The family always commemorate dad's death and it is at these times that Asif takes out his treasured album and no one ever gets away without listening to the story of how dad taught Asif to ride his bike.

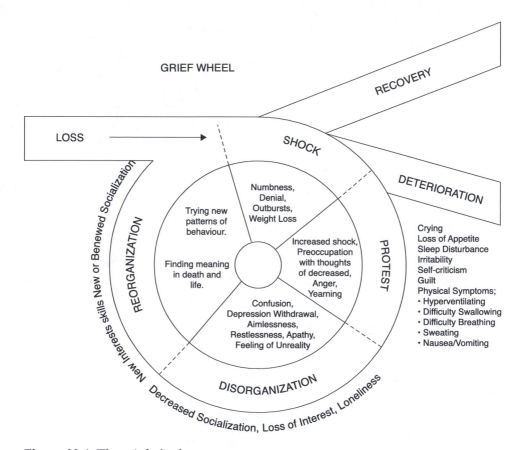

Figure 22.1 The grief wheel

Source: Grace Bible Church of Moorpack; available at: www.gbcmpk.org/site/cpage.asp?sec_id=180008954&cpage _id=180049418.

The grief wheel (Figure 22.1) is an illustration of how we experience loss. At first, our response is one of shock, disbelief, protest, lack of acceptance, followed by disorganisation, eventually moving towards the reorganisation of our lives without the deceased person. There is the potential of deterioration within this process which can serve to lengthen the grieving period. If the deterioration persists, it can indicate that professional help is required. People with a learning disability are particularly sensitive to delayed grief, as the reality of a situation may take some time to become apparent. It is important for carers to understand this and be vigilant to signs of ongoing distress.

The social context within which individuals with a learning disability experience bereavement and loss

Historically people with learning disabilities have been treated as a group, they were not perceived as being capable of having individual needs, including individual thoughts and feelings. More recently people may have been cosseted from the impact of death, by well-meaning carers wishing to minimise their distress. Over-protectiveness often leads to disempowerment and those who do not have the opportunity to grieve and who are not involved in the rituals surrounding death may be described as disenfranchised grievers (Doka, 1989), that is, people who are grieving, but are not permitted openly to do so or are excluded grievers. People with learning disabilities are often reliant upon others to facilitate such grieving opportunities (Read and Elliot, 2003). Some individuals may not be encouraged to say goodbye to their loved ones; may not attend the funeral and are often not informed about the death of their loved ones. Such attitudes may not help bereaved individuals to accommodate their grief.

Fast facts 22.3   Disenfranchised grief

Doka (1989) identified three features of what is termed disenfranchised grief:

- having the grief not recognised;
- having the relationship not recognised;
- having the griever not recognised.

Reader activity 22.3   Lawrence's experience of loss

We do not know exactly what happened to Lawrence when he was received into care at a very young age. We can only try to put ourselves into his shoes and imagine the utter abandonment he felt or indeed the hope he experienced in finding a new home with people who cared for him. What we do know, however, is that as he progressed into adulthood he continued to experience further loss and we need to put this into context in order to try to understand how he may have felt; how he was supported or indeed how a lack of support may have affected his emotional development and particularly his relationships with other individuals.

- How do you think Lawrence's experiences of loss impacted upon him?
- Do you think that Lawrence will have fully appreciated everything that happened to him?

Specifically the following points have been made about people with learning disability, about their involvement in, and their needs during the bereavement process:

- Carers may lack knowledge about the needs of people with a learning disability and be ignorant about death and bereavement and their impact on people with a learning disability, which sometimes resulted in over-protectiveness (Elliot, 1995).
- People with learning disability may exhibit reactions to grief which are labelled as 'challenging behaviour' because of their limited comprehension and ability to express grief (Hollins and Esterhuyzen, 1997; MacHale and Carey, 2002).

- Some individuals are not able to make their needs known and are not involved in the ceremonies surrounding death. This results in grief responses often being delayed (Kitching, 1987).
- There may be additional considerations related to the person's disability and the attitudes of others towards their disability, leading to a 'double taboo' where neither disability nor death is discussed (Oswin, 1991).
- The death of a family member can trigger a need for crisis intervention and cause symptoms of complicated grief for people with learning disabilities (Kloeppel and Hollins, 1989; Emerson, 1997; Bonell–Pascual et al., 1999; MacHale and Carey, 2002; Dodd et al., 2005).
- Bereaved people with learning disabilities may be denied the time and privacy required, causing changes in behaviour to go unnoticed by carers (Oswin, 1991).
- Some 54 per cent of people with learning disabilities do not attend their parent's funeral (Hollins and Esterhuyzen, 1997). Additionally, people who have been excluded from the funeral or who have not been told about the death for some time after the event may need the professional help of a bereavement counsellor (Read, 2000).
- People with learning disabilities are often given confused messages about death or losses, for example, that someone has 'gone to sleep', 'gone to Jesus', 'kicked the bucket', or told someone will not be visiting again with no concrete explanation of why that is (Oswin, 1991).
- Carers may prefer people with learning disabilities to forget about the death of a loved one and to be happy, despite sometimes repeated requests of information being made by individuals themselves (ibid.).

It has become apparent that managing the needs of people with a learning disability who are grieving is difficult. Management of such situations should not, however, be avoided as it is something that carers and professionals working in the learning disability field have a duty to address.

Reader activity 22.4   Coping styles

Parents and carers will have their own individual beliefs and coping styles based on their own experiences of loss which will affect how they respond to grief both among their loved one's or with those with in their care.

- What coping styles have you seen in your personal or professional life?
- Can you identify styles that help or hinder the grieving process?
- What may be the motivation behind styles that hinder the grieving process?

The following issues have an impact upon carers and may influence their ability to discuss grief or loss with the person they care for:

- The carer's emotional intelligence; what they understand about emotions generally and the recognition of those emotions in others.
- Carer personality traits such as openness in talking about sensitive issues and, for example, if someone has a caring nature.
- Their own experiences of death and bereavement.

- The carer's circle of support, this might be either formal, such as through professional supervision, or informal, such as through them having someone close to talk to.
- Having a limited support network can cause carers to limit the support they give to others.
- Their attitudes about disability and the needs of people with a learning disability.
- Their personal beliefs about death and their spiritual beliefs.
- Carers' cultural background and their upbringing all having an impact on belief systems.
- Any fears they may have with regards to talking to people with a learning disability and others generally, about death and bereavement.

Doka (1989) argues that the very nature of disenfranchised grief creates additional problems for grievers. While removing or minimising sources of support, he suggests that for many disenfranchised grievers, such as children and people with learning disabilities, there is no coherent, well-organised or readily available support systems to help them grieve.

Reader activity 22.5   Support

Think about someone you know who has suffered a bereavement and the type of support they had during the grieving process. Is there anyone you perceive to be vulnerable to unresolved loss due to receiving inadequate or poor support?

Childhood bereavement has served to highlight commonly shared experiences with people with a learning disability. They too are often excluded from the process of loss and change, and are reliant on the explanations of parents and carers. Also they may be afforded only limited time to adjust to experiences of loss. Given these facts, it is fair to assume that children with learning disabilities are a particularly vulnerable group.

Oswin (1991) acknowledged that people with a learning disability often experience multiple losses as a result of the death of a partner, carer or parent. The end of such relationships can also result in the following:

- loss of familiar surroundings, as they move to other care environments
- loss of relationships and attachments
- loss of friends
- loss of choices
- loss of dignity
- loss of autonomy
- loss of individuality
- loss of sexuality
- loss of skills as the new carer may not know the person's skill base.

The loss of a significant relationship due to bereavement is often only the beginning of subsequent change; these changes can be challenging to cope with while mourning, individuals with learning disabilities may lose their home; familiarity, independence and sense of identity often due to moving into supervised care either temporarily or permanently (Read, 2005).

Case study 22.5   Past and present loss

Lawrence experienced many changes during his formative years which increased his vulnerability to further loss. We understand that after many years of uncertainty and confusion in his life, he met someone who made him happy. This period only lasted three years as this partner died. Lawrence not only exhibited some of the classical signs of depression at this time but the loss triggered deeper emotional feelings from his distant past, feelings of being abandoned and unloved. Although we would want to concentrate on his immediate needs, we should be mindful of how past and present often have a symbiotic link and any grief work we may undertake would need to take this into account in order to facilitate some closure and enable Lawrence to feel well again.

Case study 22.6   Individual responses to loss

Jane is a 25-year-old woman with moderate learning disabilities with no verbal speech. She lived in a supported group home for several years, however, due to a restructuring in the organisations she had to change home to live with another group of people. Some weeks later she became incontinent and lethargic, which led to some resentment from her carers. On reflection of Jane's experience the care team were helped to understand her emotional position and approach the matter more sensitively. They began to actively support her toilet routine but more importantly began to understand her anxieties about the move. A visual book was produced to help her communicate about her friends and regular contacts with them were re-established. Consequently her well-being improved and she returned very much to her normal self.

Loss identities

Another useful way of determining individual response to loss is through what is Berger (2009) described as grieving identities. These identities may give the clinician or carer clues to how someone is dealing with their loss. Some of them are best described as coping strategies as they serve to displace thoughts and feelings. Defining identities may be dependent on range of psycho-social circumstances, including lifestyle, cognitive ability and adaptive skills.

Berger (2009) identified five ways of grieving, as exemplified by:

- *The nomads*: Nomads have not yet resolved their grief and do not seem to understand the loss that has affected their lives.
- *The memorialists*: This identity is committed to preserving the memory of the loved one they have lost.
- *The normalizers*: This identity is committed to re-creating a sense of family and community.
- *The activists*: This identity focuses on helping other people who are dealing with the same disease or with the same issues that caused their loved one's death.

- *The seekers*: This identity will adopt religious, philosophical, or spiritual beliefs to create/recreate meaning within their lives.

Responses to grief

Grief is shown in many ways. Table 22.4 is a list of possible physical, behavioural and emotional responses to grief. The list is not intended to be exhaustive. It should be noted that if any of the responses become extreme, disproportionate or excessive, resulting in inappropriate behaviour or reactions, as discussed previously, it may suggest that the individual is struggling to come to terms with the loss. If the individual's quality of life is still being adversely affected by the loss in excess of 12 months post bereavement, professional help may be required.

Reader activity 22.6   Responses to loss

Examine the responses to loss in Table 22.4 and identify which aspects you may find easier to assess for in people with a cognitive impairment and limited verbal expressive language.

Bereavement challenges

Recognising the symptoms can be challenging. DH (1995) recognised that life events such as bereavement can cause a person with learning disabilities to experience symptoms of psychological distress more readily than other people, in extreme forms, the symptoms of stress, for example, may manifest in unusual and sometimes bizarre ways that may be difficult to understand or interpret. There

Table 22.4 Responses to grief

Physical sensations	*Behaviours*	*Feelings*
Hollowness in stomach	Sleep	Sadness
Tightness in the chest	Disturbances	Anger
Tightness in the throat	Appetite disturbance	Guilt
Over-sensitivity to noise	Absent-mindedness	Self-reproach
Breathlessness	Social withdrawal	Anxiety
Muscle weakness	Dreaming	Loneliness
Lack of energy	Searching	Fatigue
Dry mouth	Crying	Helplessness
Confusion	Sighing	Shock
Preoccupation	Restless over activity	Yearning
Sense of presence	Visiting old haunts	Relief
Hallucinations	Self-injury	Numbness
	Aggression	

Source: Worden (1991).

Table 22.5 Non-verbal signs of grief

Clinging, not wanting to sleep alone	Reluctance to go out
Uncharacteristic incontinence	Self-injury
Restlessness	Apathy or tiredness
Changes in sleep patterns	Destructive behaviour
Changes in appetite	Clumsiness and accidents

are, however, a number of aspects of behaviour which may be indicators of unresolved grief. These include sudden changes in mood or behaviour. Sometimes the reaction to a loss is delayed, causing feelings to possibly be overlooked or not considered. Multiple losses add to a person's confusion and the carer's assessment of the situation. If unrecognised, the original grief may be compounded and the person is more likely to have difficulties connected to their grief (Blackman, 2003).

Diagnostic overshadowing is discussed elsewhere in this book and it is also important to consider this where grief is concerned. The above is of particular concern for people with severe learning disabilities, as it often difficult to ascertain the true consequence of a loss that has occurred. Communications with people with learning difficulties may be difficult for many reasons. It may be necessary to consider pre-verbal communication patterns or the individual's communication profile in order to establish how they may be experiencing loss. Subtle changes in body language are reasonable determinants of how individuals may feel, however, it may take a keen observational eye and skill to notice them. Unfortunately there is always danger that signs may be attributed to some people's normal pattern of behaviours. Table 22.5 shows some non-verbal signs of grief.

People living in congregate setting are particularly vulnerable to having unrecognised grief as many staff may be employed in such settings. Multiple care staff can affect consistency of care; good communication about an individual's needs is vital in ensuring that those acting as advocates have a thorough knowledge of individuals within their care and that this is supported by adequate documentation. Tools such as Health Action Plans (HAPs) (DOH, 2001) or Anticipatory Care Calendars (WMCCN, 2006) can be exceedingly helpful, assisting in understanding changes in health as a consequence of the effects of grief and loss.

Staff turnover in residential settings may also be high; this can create an erratic environment whereby service users may be unable to form relationships. It is human nature to forge bonds with those around us and for many individuals with learning disabilities carers invariably become or are seen as friends. Changes in staff at short notice can trigger emotional reactions in some individuals, often with underlying reasons for such outburst going unnoticed.

Where expressive language is present, carers also need to be mindful that verbal responses may not always be clear. People with learning disabilities who are grieving, even if vocal, may be unable to speak without intense emotional reactions such as crying or shouting or by showing signs of anger or sadness through verbal or physical aggression. Their loss may be referred to frequently in conversations and seemingly minor events may trigger fresh reactions. Some individuals may cling to possessions of the loved one they have lost and become distressed if such possessions go missing. It can be very difficult to get a full picture of how someone feels, even when they have speech. It is important for carers and professionals to take into account the specific communication needs of an individual when speaking both in an informal and in a more formal therapeutic context such as a counselling situation. Specific difficulties may include:

- *Suggestibility*: 'Yielding to leading questions' and 'shifting' initial response to negative feedback.
- *Acquiescence*: Tendency to say 'yes' whether or not they agree.
- *Automatic 'No' or 'Don't know'*: Often indicates lack of understanding.
- *Learned helplessness or passivity*: Resulting from perceived lack of control.

Having a learning disability can impact upon feeling of choice and control over one's own life and have a bearing on how confident people feel in giving a true account of their feelings, individuals with learning disabilities may find it difficult to be open and honest and indeed some may respond to counselling situations with suspicion, in these instances it may take some time to develop trust. The support of knowledgeable carers is invaluable, as is the use of visual aids, not only in the facilitation of good communication and understanding, but they may also act as a bridge between the carer and those in need. Conversely those with trusting relationships or supportive networks may communicate more readily.

Occasionally anger may also be projected towards others or objects which is typical of a grief reactions. Some 50 per cent of the people with learning disability who presented with sudden emotional and behavioural difficulties had experienced the recent death of a person close to them (Emerson, 1977).

Case study 22.7   Josef's story

Josef lives in residential care and he mostly keeps himself to himself. When other residents receive visitors, however, he often becomes very anxious, agitated and angry. Occasionally he is verbally or physical aggressive towards them. On reflection, the behaviour had been apparent for some years and started after his mother died and ceased visiting him.

How do you think Josef felt when his mother stopped visiting?

Conboy-Hill (1992) cited grief as a major factor for people with learning disabilities who experience behavioural problems, including self-injury, loss of skill, anorexia, and aggression. Bonell-Pascal *et al.* (2000) identified an increase in the measures of aberrant behaviour of 50 people with learning disabilities over a five-year follow-up study. Carers and professionals must be aware of the long-term behavioural consequence of bereavement. Bereavement must be considered when investigating the causes of behavioural deterioration.

Checklists are useful in assessing bereavement issues in people with a learning disability, enabling such needs to be met. Tools, for example, the BNAT tool (Blackman, 2008), guide the therapist, helping to define the potential consequence of loss in areas such as social and emotional responses, cognitive understanding, social impact or changes in identity. Such tools help to navigate through the complexities of grief with vulnerable individuals by providing structure and focusing on the issues at hand.

In care navigation (Blackman, 2008), some example questions are:

- Did the person see the deceased before they died?
- Did the person have access to photos and mementoes of the deceased?
- Is the person able to visit the grave?
- Has this person the ability to communicate with others who have been affected by this loss?
- Has the person lost any skill since this bereavement?

- Does this individual recognise their own emotions?
- What lifestyles changes has this created?
- What significance has this loss had on their social networks?
- Does the individual understand the concept of death?
- Who informed them and how?

Case study 22.8   Overlapping emotional needs

Lawrence has many overlapping emotional needs and it is important to define the true nature of these before one can help him.

The death of his close friend, Bill, was a huge loss not only in terms of friendship but also the loss of a fulfilling sexual relationship. Clearly he experienced the acute symptoms of loss and the inappropriate sexualised behaviour returned. This loss may have precipitated unresolved grief from his early life which would have compounded the whole situation, thus impacting on his mental health and behaviour. What is required at this time is for Lawrence to feel safe; his mental health symptoms need to be ameliorated and any inappropriate behaviour managed, not only to help him but also to protect others who may be vulnerable. The assessment and treatment unit will provide this and once his mental health symptoms start to improve, he will be in a position to engage in a range of therapies. Medication has been introduced to manage acute symptoms, however, we should bear in mind the minimal effect of medication on grieving and keep medication to a minimum, closely monitoring its effect.

As therapy is introduced, a potential link between his sexualised behaviour and loss should be explored; some form of gratifying behaviour may have a dual function, i.e. sexual gratification and emotional comfort. The indicator is that he is seeking sexual contact while clearly grieving. Libido can be increased as a response to loss. It is likely, however, that under these circumstances his libido is low and it is possible that the sexualised acts have become somewhat habitual and have developed as a consequence of loss, searching for loved ones and comfort. This often occurs when an individual does not have the emotional communicative or cognitive skills necessary to meet their needs in an acceptable ways. Our challenge will be to explore all such avenues.

Case study 22.9   Momamba

Momamba is 38 years of age and has been in different forms of care since her late teens. Her present providers try very hard to accommodate her emotional and behavioural needs but they struggle. One-to-one counselling has begun. It creates an arena for understanding Momamba's life, which has been very troubled. She has been exposed to many environmental changes, including losses that have saddened her immensely. The team are forming a picture of Momamba and she is learning increasingly to share her life experience, including the ups and downs. This has been both painful and comforting for her but she seems to be turning a corner and making some emotional adjustments.

Mental health and its link to bereavement

Bimh and Elliott (1982) highlighted how grief can lead to an individual possibly developing mental health disorders. As shown in Chapter 20, people with learning disabilities are particularly sensitive to developing mental illness. The social circumstance in which the loss occurs and the support gained during mourning can determine how the loss will impact on an individual. The lack of a caring environment and nurturing relationships, it could be argued, may predispose some grieving people to the development of some post-traumatic disorders, anxiety or depression. Medication may help to alleviate the symptoms of mental illness, but not of grief. Grief must be fully explored and medication use in situations such as this monitored fully, its therapeutic impact being assessed continually.

Reader activity 22.7 Medication in grief

What are the practical and ethical considerations to take into account when prescribing medication to grieving individuals with a learning disability?

Case study 22.10 Marie

Marie lost her sister at a young age in acute circumstances necessitating ambulance paramedic intervention. Now many years later she becomes very anxious and insecure when she hears an ambulance siren.

Case study 22.11 John's coping strategy

Carers helping John had thought that he had coped well with his mother's death and consequently little was said to him about it for fear that would upset him. Consequently the little changes in him that started creeping in went almost unnoticed. He started spending more time alone and one of his carers found that he had been hoarding a particular chocolate bar in his wardrobe. A visiting relative pointed out that John's mother used to buy the chocolate bar as a treat for him each time she went shopping.

The risks associated with bereavement issues among people with a learning disability

While bereavement is a normal part of life, it carries risks. Severe reactions to grief affect approximately 10–15 per cent of people. Severe reactions mainly occur in people for whom depression was present before the loss event. Parkes (1972) noted that stress-related illnesses are common among bereaved people. His studies in the 1960s and 1970s in England revealed increased doctor visits, with symptoms such as abdominal pain, or breathing difficulties within the first six months following a death. Due to the vulnerabilities that people with learning disabilities experience in identifying their health needs and accessing mainstream health services, it is important that carers are extra vigilant while people are grieving and monitor their health effectively with accessible screening tools. Ward (1995) identified the risk of suicide among teenagers to be five times greater following the death of a parent. Adolescence, by its nature, is a time of emotional turmoil and a time when the support of a parent is perhaps most needed. Carers must be alert to this fact, being vigilant especially with more able people with learning disabilities who show a level of independence or skill.

The impact of complicated grief

The characteristics of complicated grief are:

> Extreme focus on the loss and reminders of the loved one, intense longing or pining for the deceased, problems accepting the death, numbness or detachment, bitterness about the loss and inability to enjoy life, depression or deep sadness, trouble carrying out normal routines, withdrawing from social activities, feeling that life holds no meaning or purpose, irritability or agitation, lack of trust in others.
>
> (MFMER, 2013)

While medication has been shown to have some therapeutic impact upon complicated grief (Rosenzweig et al., 1997), psychotherapy techniques are often useful, and improved access to psychological services is more readily available for those with learning disabilities. Should carers be concerned about a person developing complicated grief, then such services should be sought.

Addressing the needs of individuals with a learning disability following bereavement

The challenges faced by carers in recognising and addressing bereavement issues among people with a learning disability as discussed, though acknowledged, do not detract from the fact that all individuals have the right to know about the death of their loved ones, while ongoing planning and support are crucial in these circumstances (Read, 1998).

The normality of grief should be reinforced before, during and after any death in order to promote emotional preparation and recovery (James, 1995), individuals should be given opportunities to express feelings. When death and bereavement are managed in a supportive, sensitive and consistent way, individuals are encouraged to develop personal coping strategies which enable them also to cope with future losses in a more constructive manner. The majority of bereaved people receive the help and support they need from within their own social network (Worden, 1991). Some individuals, however, may need additional, specialist support to help them accommodate their loss and move on with their lives (Read and Papakosia-Harvey, 2004).

By identifying, acknowledging and addressing such needs in an open, honest and sensitive way, carers can help the person with a learning disability to confront and address their feelings following the death of a loved one. The following must be done in a way that is meaningful and accessible for the individual:

- Provide adequate information.
- Address their fears and needs.
- Give reassurance that they are not to blame.
- Be attentive, watch and listen carefully.
- Give assurance that their feelings are being accepted and understood.
- Support them with overwhelming feelings.
- Include them in rites and rituals.
- Support them engaging in routine activities.
- Allow them to experience the grieving of others.
- Provide opportunities for remembering the relationship they have lost.

The above list is not meant to be exhaustive. Each person will require something slightly different. When sharing the information, it is important to interact at the individual's pace and at a level appropriate to their cognitive development and while communicating in a way that the individual is likely to understand. The person should be provided with the basic facts, using language that is clear, truthful and cannot be misunderstood.

The use of euphemisms

Euphemisms are expressions that we use when whatever we are referring to is considered inappropriate for the circumstances or when we are embarrassed or uncomfortable with the literal version. It is natural to avoid causing emotional upset to others and, consequently, there are many euphemisms related to death. They are often taken literally when received from a trusted carer or parent. The use of euphemisms with bereaved individuals, however, should be avoided as their use can cause confusion, misunderstanding, hinder the grieving process and possibly leave someone searching for their loved one.

Fast facts 22.4 shows a list of commonly used euphemisms, can you think of any others?

Fast facts 22.4   Euphemisms for death

- Snuffed it
- Taken by Jesus
- Kicked the bucket
- Gone to heaven
- Gone to sleep
- Gone to live with the angels
- Passed away/on
- Gone to meet his maker
- Crossed over

- Lost
- Put him/her down
- Pushing up daisies
- At the happy hunting ground

Case study 22.12 Going to sleep

Nigel was told by his carer Ann, 'your Mum went into hospital last night; she went to sleep and passed away'. Shortly after his mum's death, Nigel was admitted to the hospital for a routine procedure. Nigel was extremely anxious and would not go to sleep in the hospital.

Can you understand what caused Nigel's anxiety?

Communicating with people about death and bereavement

Anxiety can be raised when a carer/professional is about to talk to someone with a learning disability about death or bereavement. The following suggestions about how to communicate may therefore be useful. We provide a Do and a Don't list.

The 'DO' list

- Do let your genuine concern and caring show.
- Do be available to listen or to help with whatever seems needed at the time.
- Do say you are sorry about what is happening and for their pain.
- Do ask what they need (but be prepared for 'I don't know').
- Do be able to say 'I don't know' (but you'll find out).
- Do let them cry or be angry.
- Do encourage them to talk about their feelings and their memories of the deceased.

The 'DON'T' list:

- Don't let your own sense of helplessness keep you from helping them.
- Don't say you know how they feel.
- Don't say 'Be brave.'
- Don't say 'It will be all right.'
- Don't say 'You're the man of the house now' or give them responsibility they may not be ready for.
- Don't use euphemisms.
- Don't tell them what they should feel or do.
- Don't change the subject if someone wants to talk.
- Don't point out that at least they have the other people available to them.
- Don't make any comments which in any way suggest that what is happening is their fault.

The Worden (1991) task model of grief counselling is a widely used framework for helping people with learning disabilities to grieve (Elliott, 1975). The Communicating about Loss and Mourning (CALM) curriculum (Yanok and Beifus, 1993) suggests that people with learning disabilities benefit from a formal programme of death education and grief counselling. Working with and recognising memories following a bereavement are fundamental to grief work. Think of it as a way of giving permission to remember which is something that many people with a learning disability really value.

The key to good communication while doing bereavement work is allowing someone to make personal choices and decisions. Some of the choices following bereavement can be difficult and people with a learning disability need to be given the appropriate information at the appropriate time. Decisions might need to be made about whether someone wants to attend the funeral, view the body, and so forth. They are very sensitive issues and it is understandable that often people may want to change their minds about decisions made. People need to be reassured that this is alright. Preparation is vital prior to the person attending a funeral or viewing a body. They need to be informed of how things will look or feel and the process to be followed, for example, if viewing the body they will need to know that the body will not look the same, it will feel cold, the body will not be breathing and will be in a box called a coffin. Here visual information can be invaluable in communicating the procedure but more importantly assist in supporting informed decision-making.

Creative approaches in managing bereavement issues

Carers often need to be creative in using appropriate resources. These include reminiscence work (Stuart, 1999), the use of visual aids, photographs and DVDs. As time passes it can be useful to help the individual to remember anniversaries such as birthdays or the anniversary of the death. It may be helpful for some but not for others. The use of objects may also be helpful; and for the more creative amongst us, art and drama. The digital age has brought photography and computing into creative therapy and indeed into everyday use. Carers may need to be creative in assessing, understanding and meeting the needs of the person with a learning disability. Staff working in other settings such as day services, education or work may also need advice to ensure they support an individual effectively and do not inadvertently create difficulties by communicating or giving advice about the death that may cause confusion. Being able to use resources that the grieving individual is also familiar with can also be extremely helpful and create an element of predictability that is often reassuring. All those supporting individuals should be appropriately trained about loss and bereavement and given adequate policies and procedures to follow so they can safely meet the needs of the people they work with.

| Reader activity 22.8 Bereavement work |

Imagine that you are going to do some bereavement work with someone with a learning disability.

- What might you be concerned about?
- What support might you need?

Case study 22.13   Visual timeline

Somiya was living at home with her parents when her father suddenly died. She attended the funeral and showed many of the signs of normal healthy grieving. She did, however, find it difficult to understand what had happened to him and had many questions to ask carers she came into contact with. The community nurse helping Somiya and her family produced a visual timeline of events. Somiya valued this immensely and took great comfort in sharing this with those close to her.

Reasonable adjustments within mainstream services

Contemporary policy strongly encourages people with learning disabilities to access mainstream services, including counselling and therapeutic services. Services should make reasonable adjustments when providing care or treatment. Reasonable adjustments can range from providing double appointments, in scheduling appointments in a manner that encourages the person to get as much from the appointment as possible or planning care to reduce fears. Adjustments must also be made regarding communication, to ensure the needs of people with a learning disability are met as effectively as possible. These include:

- being prepared to use alternative methods of communication such as signing, charts or books;
- asking if the person has a communication aid;
- providing information or concepts in an easy-to-read or understandable format;
- providing health promotion advice about specific health needs.

This is especially important as the person may not be able to do the following:

- make the connection between something that has happened and how it has made them feel;
- understand the link between an event and their illness;
- understand key concepts of illness, death or mortality because they have been sheltered from them;
- say what has been said in therapy.

Individuals can be disadvantaged unless the above points are considered. However, with skilled support and the use of adjusted therapy techniques, people with a learning disability can benefit immensely and move on from the dark places that grief inhabits to improved well-being and quality of life.

Case study 22.14   Counselling

As Lawrence becomes emotionally settled, he may be offered counselling sessions. Normally these last around one hour; however, initially this may be shorter. Over time it would gradually build up to the therapeutic hour but this would be dependent on how well the early sessions went and how well he coped with them. For counselling or therapy to be effective, the session will need to be weekly and attendance may be required for up to 20 or more weeks. The therapist/counsellor will work on a one-to-one basis with him; however, this may fluctuate depending on the circumstances. It may be appropriate to involve a confidante or carer, especially if Lawrence is fearful or anxious. The counsellor will work towards establishing a safe and trusting therapeutic relationship with Lawrence, establishing effective and appropriate communication to facilitate his engagement in the therapy. The therapy may also include creative ways of meeting his needs and carers may be requested to assist him, for example, in helping him choose and bring certain objects, keepsakes, or photos relevant to the work in hand. Homework activities may also be undertaken between therapy sessions. An example would be some creative work or visiting a grave. The therapist will guide Lawrence throughout the session. However, they may also encourage him to talk about past experiences either as they arise or through sensitive questioning. Grounding or contextualising the work will be an important aspect of the therapy. If there are many issues to take into account, as in Lawrence's case, this may done through the use of objects, pictures or drawing or mapping out experience. One example of this is the above and below timeline. Here the therapist would guide Lawrence along a timeline putting a happy event above the line and a not so happy one below. This not only acts as a record, it can help the therapist see where the blockages are and help Lawrence view his life in some sort of perspective. Sensitive areas may also be parked and picked up again as the sessions progress. We may not see any results for quite some time, so above all we must be prepared to be patient and continue to offer Lawrence sensitive support while simultaneously being prepared to make the most of any opportunity that may arise to help him go forward on the journey to recovery.

Conclusion

Understanding what is happening to us and to others when enduring the trauma of loss is essential. As with other aspects of life, the more understanding we have, the easier it is to cope with it. Theories of grief and loss are best thought of as models of change, transition and adjustment. Experiencing bereavement and loss especially when it relates to the loss of a relationship with another sentient being is life-changing. The process is the transition towards adjustment. Adjusting to the loss of the relationship and acceptance that the physical relationship has ended is a challenging and often painful journey. How an individual experiences the grieving process is dependent on many contributory factors. People with learning disabilities fall into the group of disenfranchised grievers, therefore, they are vulnerable to loss in ways that were previously not well understood. Loss makes them vulnerable to both delayed and chronic grief and many are dependent on those around them to help them.

Meeting the emotional needs of people who have learning disabilities has improved and professional groups such as psychologists, counsellors and learning disability nurses provide a key role. At the moment the mainstream agenda is very strong and we are starting to see some services responding; including acute, primary and mental health services.

Active support and health promotion are vital in enhancing the lives of people with a learning disability. Therapists must use innovative solutions to support people with a learning disability in order to understand and meet their emotional needs. This is an extremely challenging area of work, however, it is essential. Effective bereavement work can ensure that people with learning disabilities go on to live fruitful and meaningful lives following the deaths of their loved ones.

Points to remember

- People with learning disabilities grieve.
- Their grief may manifest in lots of ways including through them displaying behavioural needs.
- There are many ways to support someone with learning disabilites who is grieving.

Resources

Gray, R. (2010) *Bereavement, Loss and Learning Disabilities: A Guide for Professionals and Carers*. London: Jessica Kingsley Publications.

Oswin, M. (1991) *Am I Allowed to Cry?* London: Souvenir Press.

References

Berger, S.A. (2009) The five ways we grieve: finding your personal path to healing after the loss of a loved one, *Bereavement Identities*. Boston: Shambhala Publications.

Bimh, E.M. and Elliot, L.S. (1982) Conceptions of death in mentally retarded persons, *Journal of Psychology: Interdisciplinary and Applied*, 111(2): 205–210.

Blackman, N. (2003) *Loss and Learning Disability*. London: Worth Publishing.

Blackman, N. (2008) Development of an assessment tool for the bereavement needs of people with learning disabilities, *British Journal of Learning Disabilities*, 36: 165–170.

Bonell-Pascal, E., Huline-Dickens, S., Hollins, S., Esterhuyzen, A. and Sedgwick, P. (1999) Bereavement and grief in adults with learning disabilities: a follow-up study, *British Journal of Psychiatry*, 175: 348–350. Available at: www.bereavementanddisability.org.uk/BSLD3/BSLD3_Challenges.htm.

Bowlby, J. (1980). *Attachment and Loss: Loss, Sadness and Depression*, Vol. 3. New York: Basic Books.

Conboy-Hill, S. (1992) Grief, loss and people with learning disabilities, in A. Waitham and S. Conboy-Hill (eds) *Psychology and Mental Handicap*. London: Sage Publications.

Dodd, P., Dowling, S. and Hollins, S. (2005) A review of the emotional psychiatric and behavioural responses to bereavement in people with intellectual disabilities, *Journal of Intellectual Disabilities*, 49: 537–543.

DH (Department of Health) (1995) *The Health of the Nation: A Strategy for People with Learning Disabilities*. London: HMSO.

DH (Department of Health) (2001) *Valuing People: A New Strategy for Learning Disabilities for the 21st Century*. London: HMSO.

Doka, K.J. (1989) *Disenfranchised Grief: Recognising Hidden Sorrow*. Toronto: Lexington Books.

Elliot, D. (1995) Helping people with learning disabilities to handle grief, *Nursing Times*, 91: 27–30.

Emerson, P. (1977) Covert grief reactions in mentally retarded clients, *Mental Retardation*, 15: 46–47.

Freud, S. (1917) Mourning and melancholia, in J. Strachey (ed.) *Standard Edition of the Complete Psychological Works of Sigmund Freud*, Vol. 14. London: Hogarth Press.

Grace Bible Church Moor Pack. Available at: www.gbempk.org.

Hollins, S. and Esterhuyzen, A. (1997) Bereavement and grief in adults with learning disabilities, *British Journal of Psychiatry*, 170: 497–501.

James, A. (1995) Helping people with mental health needs cope with bereavement, *British Journal of Learning Disabilities*, 23: 74–78.

Kitching, N. (1987) Helping people with mental health problems cope with bereavement: a case study with discussion, *Mental Handicap*, 15: 60–63.

Kloeppel, D. and Hollins, S. (1989) Double handicap: mental retardation and death in the family, *Death Studies*, 13: 31.

Kübler-Ross, E. (1969) *On Death and Dying*. New York: Macmillan.

MacHale, R. and Carey, S. (2002) An investigation of the effects of bereavement on mental health and challenging behaviour in adults with learning disability, *British Journal of Learning Disabilities*, 30: 113–117.

Martin, G., Carlson, N. and Buskist, W. (2000) *Psychology*, 3rd edn. Harlow: Pearson.

MFMER (Mayo Foundation for Medical Education and Research) (2013) *Complicated Grief*. Available at: www.symptonmayoclinic.com.

Oswin, M. (1991) *Am I Allowed to Cry?*, 2nd edn. London: Souvenir Press.

Parkes, C.M. (1972) *Bereavement: Studies of Grief in Adult Life*. London: Tavistock.

Read, S. (1998) The palliative care needs of people with learning disabilities, *International Journal of Palliative Nursing*, 4(5): 246–251.

Read, S. (2000) Bereavement and people with learning disabilities, *Nursing and Residential Care*, 2: 230–234.

Read, S. (2005) Loss, bereavement and learning disabilities: providing a continuum of support, *Learning Disability Practice*, 8: 31–37.

Read, S. and Elliot, D. (2003) Death and learning disability: a vulnerability perspective, *Journal of Adult Protection*, 5(1): 5–14.

Read, S. and Papakosia-Harvey, V. (2004) Using workshops on loss for adults with learning disabilities, *Journal of Learning Disabilities*, 8(2): 191–208.

Rosenzweig, A., Progerson, H., Miller, M. and Reynolds, C. (1997) Bereavement and late-life depression: grief and its complications in the elderly, *Annual Rreview of Medicine*, 48: 421–428.

Sinason, V. (1986) Secondary mental handicap and its relationship to trauma, *Psychoanalytic Psychotherapy*, 2: 131–154.

Sinason, V. (1992) *Mental Handicap and the Human Condition*. London: Free Association Books.

South Eastern Connecticut Bereavement Programme. Available at: http://hospicenet.org/html/understand (accessed April 2013).

Stuart, M. (1999) *Looking Back, Looking Forward: Reminiscence with People with Learning Disabilities*. Brighton: Pavilion Publications.

Ward, B. (1995) *Good Grief: Exploring Feelings, Loss and Death with Over Elevens and Adults*, 2nd edn. London: Jessica Kingsley Publications.

White, M. and Epston, D. (1989) *Literature Means to Therapeutic Ends*. Adelaide: Dulwich Centre Publications. (Republished 1990 as *Narrative Means to Therapeutic Ends*.) New York: Norton.

Wirral PCT and Merseyside and Cheshire Cancer network (2006) *Anticipatory Care Plans*. Northwest Project.

Worden, J.W. (1991) *Grief Counselling and Grief Therapy: A Handbook for the Mental Health Practitioner*, 2nd edn. London: Routledge.

White, M. (1989) *Re-authoring Lives*. Adelaide: Dulwich Centre Publications.

Yanok, J. and Beifus, J. (1993) Communication about loss and mourning: death education for individuals with mental retardation, *Mental Retardation*, 31: 144–147.

23 Ethical issues when meeting the psychotherapeutic needs of people with a learning disability

Monica Murphy, Stacey Atkinson and Angela Ridley

Learning outcomes

After reading this chapter you will be able to:

- understand that most decisions made by practitioners which involve people who are being cared for within the health and social care environments evoke ethical dilemmas. Such dilemmas raise the question, 'Should I/we be doing that?' highlighting the fact that as health and social care practitioners we have legal boundaries within which we work. The legal frameworks which guide our care are outlined when analysing the cases of Lawrence and Chrissy
- make difficult and lawful decisions particularly concerning the psychotherapeutic needs of someone with learning disabilities.

Introduction

We do not always know whether we have made the right decisions, but if we have strong values, good knowledge and skills and follow a decision making framework, we at least know our methods in reaching that decision were correct.

(Kraus, a third–year learning disability student, 2010)

The challenges in making decisions about how best to meet the needs of people with a learning disability are the reason why many working in the field of learning disability practice continue to feel stimulated and fulfilled. Issues such as capacity, individuals' presenting needs, resource issues, the law, independence, rights, risks and choices are all considerations which challenge those working within learning disability services. While this chapter will emphasise the challenges that these points create, it will not answer any questions for you! This seems like a very strange thing to see written in a book. But the issues are not straightforward and each scenario is very different to the last. It is difficult to be definitive. The chapter will, with the use of two case studies, highlight the ethical dilemmas when working with individuals who have a learning disability who also present with psychological needs. It will increase your understanding of ethical issues and the law and explore their significance within learning disability practice. Finally, it will promote more ethical decision-making, providing suggestions of how ethical decisions might be made, so that the needs of the person are at the forefront while acknowledging that decisions are made within a context of many influences.

'[Ethics] embraces the range of methods used to critically analyse, interpret and evaluate the variety of ways in which humans interact with each other' (Pinto and Upshur, 2013, p. 19). It is concerned with making decisions about different issues based on moral judgements and beliefs (Burkhardt and Nathaniel, 2008). Following making a judgement, you then act in a certain way because of the decisions you made. Each situation has varied factors pertinent to that situation, the different people involved; where, when, why and how an event happened all have a bearing on the moral beliefs bestowed on the situation. Other intrinsic and extrinsic factors also sway you as the ethical decision-maker, influencing your viewpoint and the moral and ethical decisions you make. The law, for example, places legal obligations upon us, indicating if something is lawful or not. While something may be legal, it may, however, be felt to be morally wrong. It is in fact lawful to terminate a foetus at any stage in a pregnancy on medical grounds. It is legal on grounds of social need to do so up to 24 weeks gestation (The Human Fertilisation and Embryology Act 1990) in the UK (not including Northern Ireland), however, the moral views about this vary widely.

On a personal level there are factors that influence your moral/ethical stance. Your upbringing and the belief systems you were taught as a child may still determine your present value bases. Your educational level or understanding of any given situation will also influence your thoughts. Your religious beliefs may be strong and also sway particular thinking. In relation to people with a learning disability and your role as a health or social care practitioner, there are issues relevant to the client group which will determine particular trains of thought, for example, someone's level of learning disability, their particular needs or their mental capacity will influence thoughts about whether something is right or wrong for that person, how the person is viewed, and sociological issues concerning people with a learning disability will also influence decision-making in relation to meeting their needs. Ethical decision-making is therefore very complex and ethical decision-making with regards to meeting the psychotherapeutic needs of people with a learning disability is multi-faceted and therefore merits considerable thought. The following case studies will help to illustrate these points.

Case study 23.1   Interventions

Lawrence's mental health needs, limited sexual and social awareness, offending behaviour (indecent exposure – an offence under Section 66 of the Sexual Offences Act 2003) and bereavement issues, culminated in him being admitted for treatment under section 37 of the MH Act (2007) onto Marlow Ward, a medium secure unit for offenders with learning disabilities and mental health needs. While on the ward, he received an individualised programme of care with the following nursing and medical interventions given in order to ascertain and subsequently meet his needs:

- An enhanced CPA (Care Programme Approach for people with complex care needs) meeting every six months and monthly care planning meetings during which, with the support of an advocate, Lawrence was able to attend and be involved in the plan to address and meet his ongoing mental health and behavioural needs. Due to the nature of Lawrence's case the following people were involved in the meetings and generally in his care:

  - case manager
  - psychiatrist
  - psychologist
  - occupational therapist
  - primary nurse (learning disability nurse)
  - social worker
  - carers
  - probation officer.

- Weekly wards rounds with the consultant and care coordinator.
- A full nursing assessment using a holistic nursing tool and subsequently more specific assessments:

  - mental health needs assessments using PASS-ADD and HADS (Hospital Anxiety and Depression Scale) depression and anxiety scales and KGV Global Assessment;
  - sexual and social awareness/knowledge assessments using ASK (Assessment of Sexual Knowledge) (CDDHV, 2008) and QACSO (Questionnaire on Attitudes Consistent with Sexual Offending) (William *et al.*, 2007);
  - behavioural analysis interventions following episodes of behavioural distress (see Chapter 19);
  - occupational therapy assessment to assess Lawrence's skill base and to ascertain his future 'occupation' options.

- Medication for Lawrence's anxiety and depression (Lorazepam 1mg TDS and Panoxetine 20mgs OD).
- A sexual and social educational awareness programme delivered by a learning disability nurse aimed at Lawrence's cognitive level to fill the gaps in his sexual and social knowledge.
- Cognitive behavioural therapy to address Lawrence's poor self-image, bereavement issues and lack of confidence. It also has begun to highlight issues in relation to post-traumatic stress.

- A mood chart, led by Lawrence so that he can indicate more clearly to staff how he is feeling on a daily basis.
- Following a HCR–20 risk assessment (Webster *et al.*, 1997), for violent behaviour, done as a precaution, Lawrence engaged in graded/planned, supported access visits to community environments which aimed to support him in the community while assisting with his sexual and social awareness programme.
- It was planned that any possible disclosures about his feelings or further offences made during the access visits would be acted upon within the programme of care and would involve any necessary professional bodies as appropriate.
- A level of supervision of Lawrence to ensure he is not vulnerable to abuse from other patients while encouraging him to form 'legitimate' social and sexual relationships.

The outcome for Lawrence appears positive. He has agreed and signed his care plan. He has a good relationship with staff and ongoing evaluations show he is making excellent progress.

Case study 23.2   Chrissy's story

Chrissy is a lady of African origin who was admitted to Compton Ward; a learning disability/mental health unit in the same hospital as Lawrence. Chrissy has not offended. She has a severe learning disability due to 'global developmental delay' and some 'autistic traits'. Reports are that Chrissy had a deprived childhood. She was the only child of a chronically alcoholic mother. She became known to services when her mother died and she was found hungry and dirty locked in the home. Chrissy doesn't speak. She self-harms, the scars show this is a long-standing behaviour, staff feel this will not improve. She has been on Compton Ward for approximately six months with a Deprivation of Liberty Safeguard (DoL) and is prescribed Risperidone 3mgs BD for self-injurious behaviour. It is felt there has been some reduction in the behaviour of late. Chrissy is expected to stay on Compton Ward for the 'foreseeable future'. Her self-harming is such that during episodes she severely injures herself through self-biting, head banging, scratching, hitting and when possible, if she can access sharp objects or edges, cutting. Due to the high levels of observation needed, level one observation, i.e. constant supervision/observation, there are no services other than Compton Ward that can meet Chrissy's needs.

Some staff are quite negative about Chrissy's needs, they find her difficult to engage with and feel due to the complexity of her situation she will not progress. The nurse in charge has spoken to two members of staff about how they speak to Chrissy. Chrissy presents as being very unkempt and nervous.

There is no one particular approach to addressing potential ethical issues with Lawrence and Chrissy. While requirements for statutory care are supported with appropriate legislation, the difficulties in meeting Lawrence's and Chrissy's needs from an ethical perspective may not, as discussed, produce unequivocal right or wrong answers. In some ways this is probably just as it should be because

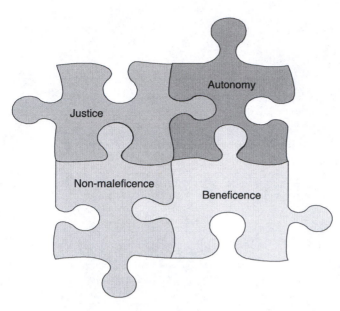

Figure 23.1 Beauchamp and Childress's four principles

living a moral or ethical life is about how to *live a good life* and what constitutes a good life for people is extremely varied! Rarely are ethical issues so polarised as to be *wholly right* (or permissible) or *wholly wrong* (or not permissible). At best, it may be that the role of an ethical approach is to identify which problematic issues are posed and possible ways to address them.

One approach to ethics propounded by Beauchamp and Childress (2008) is that of the four principles (Figure 23.1). These principles are: autonomy, beneficence, non-maleficence and justice. They can be summarised as:

- *Autonomy* – the ability to be self-ruling, make choices and decisions about all aspects of one's life without undue influence.
- *Beneficence* – to do good. Links to advocacy, treating others as you would want to be treated.
- *Non-maleficence* – to avoid harm.
- *Justice* – aspects of equity, fairness, merit, deserving, whether applied to an individual or community.

It can be helpful to view the relationship and interaction between these principles as jigsaw pieces that form a whole rather than viewed as a rigid hierarchical structure. No one principle is regarded as more important than another. They all require equal consideration in ethical decision-making. For example, modern healthcare practice requires that patients give their consent, not merely their assent, to medical procedures and that this requirement derives from a respect for each individual's autonomy – their ability to decide for themselves. To be able to consent requires sufficient information to understand what choices are available and the relative merits of these choices. For example, what a medical procedure is intended to achieve and any associated risks from having the procedure. Treatment options should aim to *do good* and minimise or diminish risk of harm. Justice is also served if the treatment options are available to all who meet the clinical criteria. In a bygone era when medical paternalism was more prevalent, patients were more likely to be told what was going to happen to them, and they were treated as passive recipients who, in the main, went along with decisions that the professionals made. The motivation on the health practitioner's part was probably to do good (act beneficently) and to minimise harm (act with non-maleficence) but in the process an individual's autonomy was ignored or sidelined and a sense of natural justice was not addressed at all. To a certain extent, it is true to say that care for people with learning disabilities in the past was paternalistic in nature. Using the four principles as an approach to ethical decision-making is not unproblematic but it does help in categorising the issues for discussion, so it is with this in mind that the ethical issues with Lawrence's and Chrissy's situations will be explored and some understanding of how to address these are considered.

Reader activity 23.1 Assent and consent

Think about possible ways that Lawrence and other people with learning disabilities might assent to treatment but it is not always clear that they are fully consenting. One example has been given for you.

* Holding an arm out for an injection as it may be felt by the person to be what is expected of them.

Lawrence and confidentiality

The first issue to note is that a team of professionals from health and social care are involved in Lawrence's care. They work together to meet Lawrence's needs and this inevitably involves the flow of information about numerous aspects of his personal life and support. Given his history of inappropriate sexual behaviour, issues to do with Lawrence's sexuality will be discussed. These issues may be felt by Lawrence to be intimate, private and sensitive, however, there is a need in this case for consideration of such issues as they may be relevant to his own and others' well-being. Confidentiality is necessary. But it is not necessarily an absolute prohibiting all disclosure of information. Cooperating with police investigations and preventing harm to the public are instances where professionals are obligated to collaborate with authorities. Confidentiality here at times would be a secondary consideration. But maintaining confidentiality is important in relation to Lawrence's personal dignity and autonomy. Multi-disciplinary team working does not give carte blanche to discussing anything and everything about Lawrence. Careful consideration should take place regarding what the boundaries are for the discussion of Lawrence's disclosures, while also taking into account his decision-making skills, capacity and wishes. This requires assessment of what can be judged as being in his best interests, combined with a consideration of the interests of his own safety and that of others, as well as fostering positive relationships based on trust that Lawrence can have faith in.

Reader activity 23.2   Paternalism

A paternalistic approach to health or social care is one in which practitioners 'treat' people without really involving them in the care. It involves an imbalance of power as the practitioner is invariably seen as being in charge. There is an assumption that the practitioner knows best. As discussed, in the past, the treatment of people with a learning disability was paternalistic.

- Can you think of any examples of what might constitute acting paternalistically towards people with learning disabilities?
- Is there any such thing as 'benevolent paternalism'?
- Can this ever be justified?

If Lawrence is to engage in his care programme in a meaningful way, he needs to feel that he can trust the people who help him, and if this trust were to be undermined through inappropriate disclosure of his expressed thoughts and feelings, it might lead to some degree of self-censure which may inhibit his self-expression. If he believes that he cannot share secrets and have them respected, then trust may be corroded with the potential consequence that he might not fully cooperate with his care programme. In the interests of beneficence, just as Lawrence must be involved in decisions that concern him, he must also be made aware of the boundaries that are meant to protect him. This will help him towards self-fulfilment.

Without trust and honesty, relationships cannot grow. Lawrence needs to be enabled to live a *good life*. His well-being and future depend, in significant measure, on his ability to form relationships based on trust. Trust lies at the core of the Care Programme Approach and is the focus of working with Lawrence. He has the potential to pose a risk to others yet he is also in danger of being subject to coercion from others. This is an area of risk and vulnerability for Lawrence that is double-edged. Ethical thinking is challenging within the field of learning disabilities, because of cognitive impairment, fluctuating capacity and at times the person may make decisions that are deemed unwise to others. Thus, a person with a learning disability may be reliant upon others for support with important decisions. Hence, there is possibility of an imbalance in the therapeutic aspect of the relationship. Coercion is others manipulating Lawrence to do, not what he chooses, but what others want him to do. It does not respect him or foster his developing autonomy nor helps him in his journey towards making decisions independently. In addition, such coercion can involve manipulation and distortion of truth. Lawrence's ability and confidence in being truthful must be reciprocated with truthfulness from those involved in his care. Coercion or deceit could cause someone harm. Without complete transparency there is a danger that openness and honesty are undermined. This in turn can open the door to smaller and greater deceits and further exploitation for Lawrence.

Reader activity 23.3   Without trust

- Imagine that you live in an environment without trust. How would this feel?
- How would you be affected by this situation?

Meeting Chrissy's complex needs

At 18, Chrissy has now entered into a formal care situation. She is completely unfamiliar with it and it is probably quite frightening to her. This situation further compounds her difficulties. Her severe disabilities in many ways shift the onus of care and decision-making on to statutory authorities. Decisions that are deemed to be in her best interests and for her protection will be determined by the application of relevant legislation. Chrissy is clearly owed a duty of care by health and social care professionals. That said, those responsible for her well-being are also obligated to involve Chrissy in as much as she is able to express and fulfil her wishes, preferences and desires so that she might be as independent as she possibly can be. This is quite a task not simply because of Chrissy's communication difficulties but also because it is difficult to determine from her life at home just how much opportunity and experience she has had to exercise choices or be self-determining previously.

What might constitute *doing good* for Chrissy? To answer this, it can be helpful to start by considering what avoids harm for her. Part of the difficulty lies in the apparent stalemate that presently appears to exist with regards to the management of Chrissy's needs. Her self-harming behaviour in itself creates stress because it necessitates such close supervision. In wanting to prevent harm coming to Chrissy, this close observation and containment can fuel her frustrations. This is problematic because this containment may be viewed as neither treatment nor care when what it produces is, in effect, a cycle of restraint. While the only purpose of restraint must be to prevent and protect Chrissy from harm, the degree and frequency with which this is applied must be considered. Containment as part of restraint can involve preventing Chrissy from coming to harm by her staying in Compton Ward and visible to care staff. Containment could include more restrictive measures such as close physical or, where appropriate, medication, as a therapeutic measure. There is a world of difference for Chrissy between a degree of freedom within a safe environment and enforced compliance within a controlled environment. Preventing or minimising the risks to Chrissy may be viewed as non-maleficent action; this is not necessarily the same as acting beneficently. The lowest common denominator for acting beneficently cannot merely be about managing her negative behaviour but must concentrate on fostering all that can constitute a good life for her – such as freedom from abuse, self-determination within her capabilities and the opportunity to develop her full potential.

Verbal chastisement has been given and staff appear to be negative about Chrissy. This suggests that some staff are finding meeting Chrissy's needs challenging. Staff frustration could be understood in relation to justice. Their responsibilities extend to everyone on Compton Ward with equal consideration for individual needs. If any one individual consistently requires greater input, then this can be viewed as potentially detracting from being able to provide therapeutic interventions to other individuals. In other words, Chrissy's needs, and the immediacy of intervention from staff that self harm necessitates, will always trump that of others who require less input. Thus a feeling of injustice or inequity arises in staff simply because Chrissy requires more resources, both in staff and of time. It is important not to act unjustly towards Chrissy or other individuals for whom staff care. Here justice can be interpreted as acting equitably towards Chrissy; her needs simply dictate that more is required. It is assumed that due to the level of her learning disability that she cannot comprehend all the consequences of her behaviour and requires to be both protected and helped to develop less destructive coping strategies. This is going to take time and effort. The focus of a person-centred care approach (DH, 2001) takes into account the uniqueness of the individual with particular regard for their vulnerabilities. Chrissy's challenging behaviour makes her vulnerable to others due to its self-destructive nature and aggressive responses, and she is at risk of receiving a degree of paternalistic care.

For both Lawrence and Chrissy, the same considerations of fundamental human rights, freedom to be self-determining, inclusion in decision-making and living as independently as possible apply. Their differences lie in their relative abilities to be enabled to engage and included in what happens to them and in formulating choices. Both of them are vulnerable from what they might do, to self or to others and also from what others might do to them. Lawrence's and Chrissy's actions may at times be misunderstood, intentions might be lost and the same can be said for staff managing Lawrence and Chrissy's needs. A spectrum of activities that could be interpreted as doing good and/or preventing harm to Lawrence and Chrissy exist but the motivation and intention behind those activities should be carefully examined.

Legal considerations for Lawrence and Chrissy

Detaining anyone against their wishes in the UK can be for criminal reasons – that person has committed an offence against the law punishable by imprisonment (criminal law) or a person is detained under civil law. The latter is for reasons that protect that person from harm (and significant risk of harm) or to protect others from any harm (including risk of harm) that person has already or might yet cause. Legislation that encompasses such detention is provided by the Mental Health Act (MHA) 1983 (amended 2007) (see Chapter 20) and, in some cases, the Mental Capacity Act (2005). Lawrence and Chrissy are likely to come under one or both of these legal frameworks and it is important to understand the care and responsibilities such laws provide when applied to them.

Society recognises that some people, by the very nature of their mental conditions, and learning disabilities is included here, have a lowered threshold of responsibility for their actions which may be temporary or permanent. Some people with a learning disability can do wrong things and break the law, but their degree of understanding and responsibility may be limited or compromised. Punishing that person might be considered harsh, cruel and inappropriate. But justice for any victim of crime would not be served if there was no legal redress. Lawrence is detained on Marlow Ward under Section 37 of the MHA. This is a Hospital and Guardianship Order that detains Lawrence because he has been charged with an imprisonable criminal offence. The purpose of this order is to provide him with the most appropriate care and treatment while also protecting others (and him) from harm, particularly in relation to his offending behaviour. Earlier in this chapter the nature of confidentiality was discussed and Lawrence is owed the same regard for confidentiality as any other person. However, those involved in caring for Lawrence also need to be clear that if his disclosures impacts on or relates to his offending behaviour, then this information is likely to be important in determining his future care and treatment. The obligation to disclose within an appropriate framework overrides other considerations related to confidentiality. The Care Plan Approach, together with the review processes that the MHA provide, mean that communication about Lawrence is transparent.

Reader activity 23.4 Uncomfortable feelings

Caring for people who have committed criminal offences and especially offences of a serious nature, e.g. arson, assault, sexual offences, can give rise to uncomfortable feelings in those responsible for their management within the healthcare setting. What issues, personal and professional might this raise for you?

In time, it may be that Lawrence is shown to pose less of a risk to others because of his previous offending behaviour and the courts will decide on how best to manage his ongoing care and treatment. It is also possible that this risk does not diminish, in which case, the MHA gives provision for his ongoing engagement with services. It should be remembered that though Lawrence does have some insight into his behaviour, he is, nevertheless, a vulnerable person. It is important now to consider the rights and care owed to vulnerable people and the responsibilities this places on those who care for them.

Vulnerable persons

The Mental Capacity Act (MCA) has been touched upon in other areas of this book; however, in view of Lawrence's needs, it is important that it is revised again in this chapter. The Mental Capacity Act (2005) safeguards the interests of adults (persons over the age of 18) who are at risk for reasons of their age, disability, mental condition, illnesses or through their inability to care for themselves. It also applies to persons who are unable to protect themselves from harm or are considered to be at risk of significant harm from others; the latter also includes risk of harm from exploitation. The MCA places a duty to protect those who lack capacity and to make decisions for their welfare that are in their best interests. This does not necessarily mean that decisions are simply imposed, far from it, they should be involved in the process as much as possible. When making decisions under the MCA, five statutory principles apply:

1. Assume a person has capacity unless it is proved otherwise.
2. Take all practicable measures to help a person make their own decision.
3. Just because a person makes an unwise decision, do not assume they lack capacity.
4. Decisions and actions made about a person must always be in that person's best interests.
5. In all decisions and actions, that which is least restrictive on a person is the option that should be taken.

It is worth considering aspects of these principles in a little more detail.

Assessment of capacity

Capacity is not always clear-cut and it is possible that capacity can fluctuate. So it is important to determine whether a person has sufficient capacity to make a particular decision. This is a two stage process that first of all requires a determination of whether a person has a permanent or temporary impairment of the mind or brain. If there is an impairment, then the assessor must then ensure that the person is able to understand the decision that needs to be made and why it needs to be made. To be able to do this, that person must be able to understand the information being given to them, remember or retain this information sufficiently to be able to consider the merits or importance of the information in relation to the decision to be made. This is important because they also need to fully appreciate the possible consequences of their decision. Finally, they must be able to communicate their decision by an appropriate means – this could be verbal, written or by sign. If a person cannot do these measures, they may lack capacity. This process of assessing capacity mirrors exactly

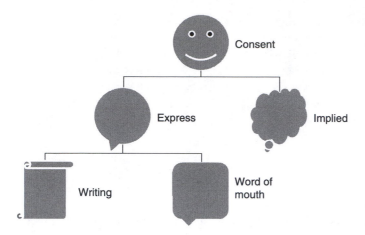

Figure 23.2 Giving consent

Source: Adapted from Dimond (2011).

what is required for anyone to be able to give their consent as, for example, to a medical procedure (Figure 23.2).

Assessing capacity may take time and if the decision to be made is not urgent, then it is a requirement of the MCA that all reasonable and practicable measures are taken to involve the person in the decision-making. It is important to be mindful of that person's values and beliefs, plus any other decisions they may have made previously so that, where possible, decisions reflect that person's value-base.

| Reader activity 23.5 Making decisions |

Lawrence's level of learning disability means that he probably has capacity to make some decisions about his welfare but not others. How could you help him to make decisions? What information is essential in order for him to make the following decisions?

- What time he gets up and goes to bed.
- Declining to take his medication for anxiety and depression.

Best interests

Most Local Authorities provide a checklist to be used in both the assessment of best interests and how to act in someone's best interests. There are also specially trained Best Interests Assessors. Once again it is important when considering a person's best interests to be mindful of the individual's values and beliefs, so they can be involved as much as possible in determining their own care. This has relevance in the situation where a person might have capacity at a future date and then can express their wishes on a particular decision that has been made for them. If a decision can wait until the person can fully engage in the decision-making, then it might be prudent to do so, particularly if the decision made has a permanent impact on an individual (e.g. a surgical procedure). Involving significant others through consultation (e.g. relatives, carers and friends) is also required so that a fuller picture of the individual's previous wishes, attitudes and feelings can be established. Finally, any decision taken in a person's best interests must be that which is least restrictive.

Reader activity 23.6 The Independent Mental Capacity Advocate

Chrissy lacks capacity to make most, if not all, decisions. Under the MCA (Section 36[2]) an Independent Mental Capacity Advocate (IMCA) can be appointed for Chrissy. What do you think the role of the IMCA involves for Chrissy? What do you consider should be taken into account when deciding what is best for her future care and well-being?

The MCA (2005) allows for persons who anticipate that they may lose capacity at a future date to make provision for decisions that respect their wishes, values and beliefs through an Advanced Directive and also for the appointment of a Lasting Power of Attorney (LPA) in proxy decision-making. This is important for anyone whose mental capacity may deteriorate.

Fast facts 23.1 The Mental Capacity Act (MCA) (2005)

The Mental Capacity Act (MCA) (2005) helps staff to consider the capacity of individuals and aims to ensure that people's human rights are not being denied. It is an integral facet in the field of learning disabilities, and came into force following a dearth of case law. It clearly defines mental capacity as cognitive ability to do the following:

- understand information;
- weigh up that information;
- recall that information;
- believe in the information;
- arrive at a decision.

Deprivation of Liberty Safeguard (DoLS)

Chrissy is subject to a Deprivation of Liberty Safeguard (DoLS). This provision was introduced as an amendment to the MCA for adults who lack capacity to make decisions about their welfare. It applies to persons who are not detained under the relevant sections of the MHA and it aims to protect them from harm or risk of harm, allowing for arrangements to be made for their care or medical treatment. A DoLS applies when that person resides in Local Authority care or in NHS care. Depriving anyone of their liberty is serious and sits at the heart of fundamental human rights, so wherever such restrictions can be avoided, they should be. Application for assessment of DoLS may well be triggered if a person is requiring some form of restraint and they lack capacity. If a DoLS is required, then it should be for no longer than necessary (with a review process) and specify restrictions including minimising restraint on the person concerned. The person's care plan should reflect the specific management measures agreed that minimise the degree of restraint used, e.g. sedation, electronic tagging, level of observations.

Adult safeguarding

According to the Department of Health (2011): 'In fulfilling your responsibilities you should follow these five safeguarding principles':

1. *Empowerment*: There should be a presumption of person-led consent and decisions. Where decisions are made for others, there must be a clear justification and the decisions must acknowledge and respect the individual's culture, beliefs, age and lifestyle choices.
2. *Protection*: A primary goal is protection of harm or abuse to the person. This includes reducing risk of neglect or abuse within health services.
3. *Proportionality*: The least restrictive or intrusive response that addresses harm or abuse should be used. Proportionality here also means responding to concerns efficiently and effectively.
4. *Partnership*: Safeguarding requires working collaboratively with colleagues in partner agencies to secure the welfare of vulnerable persons.
5. *Accountability*: Work openly and transparently with agencies to ensure public confidence.

So far, legislation has been considered that applies directly to the care and welfare of Lawrence and Chrissy. Legislation should be proactive and seek to determine the best course of action for their futures. But, as vulnerable adults, Lawrence and Chrissy may be subject to risk of harm from others. Everyone working in health and social care have a responsibility to safeguard the well-being of persons they come into contact with. This responsibility is enshrined in your professional duty of care.

The prosecution of workers from health and social care at the Winterbourne View Hospital (DH, 2012) was a just response to the criminal abuse and neglect of vulnerable adults (see Chapter 6). The death of Steven Hoskin (Flynn, 2007) also highlighted the failure of statutory services to protect this vulnerable man with a learning disability from the abuse and exploitation of people he came into contact with. As an accountable professional, you are responsible for raising an alert within the safeguarding process if there are concerns of actual harm or risk of harm under the relevant categories of abuse, whether this harm occurs in the care environment or outside it. After six months on Compton Ward, Chrissy is described as being unkempt – could this be neglect? The Charge Nurse has spoken to two members of staff about how they address Chrissy – could this be psychological/emotional harm? Communicating your concerns to an appropriate authority, reporting your concerns according to safeguarding policy and recording these concerns are important. Raising concerns is not always easy or comfortable and you may be fearful of reprisals but if the concerns are legitimate, then you have a duty to act and safeguard a vulnerable person.

Being an ethical and law-abiding practitioner

The ethical and legal issues raised in this chapter have illustrated how difficult it is often to know what the right actions are to take and that being a law-abiding, ethical, moral and just practitioner is not straightforward! People have the right to decide what they want for themselves if they are competent to make those decisions. Assisting with the care of someone who may be less able to make choices is more difficult. Sometimes we have to make choices for people and hope that these are the right ones. If someone has a learning disability, choices are not easy; if behavioural challenges, offending behaviours and additional psychological or mental health needs are present, this impacts further and can render care-giving to be even more complex. The difficulties of this are evident when you consider a well-meaning, well-trained multi-disciplinary team might all decide on different courses of action for particular given issues concerning someone with a learning disability. Perhaps an ethical framework which assists us with decision-making might be useful? Singer (1995) thought so. He developed a tool for encouraging ethical decision-making which emphasised the fundamental point that humans are at the 'centre of the universe' and decisions/actions should be made in view of this and therefore are made in the best interests of those persons. Singer's 'commandments' were from a bygone era, society and healthcare are ever-changing, but Jackson (2006) very nicely took them and applied them to the field of medical ethics. We will now be as bold and apply them to the field of learning disability practice, adapting them slightly where necessary and exploring their significance when encouraging person-centred, lawful, ethical and just decision-making with someone with a learning disability. The person with learning disabilities is the key person within the health and social care setting. Therefore, Singer's (1995) commandments seem a very appropriate tool to use.

- Commandment 1. *Treat all human life as of equal worth* (Singer, 1995).
- To be replaced by the new commandment: *Treat others as you would wish to be treated*.

Respect everyone as equal when making decisions. You might, at some point, have played the ethical dilemma game whereby you have to imagine you are one of the occupants of a hot air balloon. The balloon is deflating and to keep it afloat, someone has to be thrown out! The decision has to be made about who is the best person to go. How does one choose? Who is deemed to have the least worth? It needs to be made lighter so that the *most valued* people can therefore survive. Maybe you think you should stay in, maybe a good footballer, politician or favoured singer might be more likely to be kept in the balloon. What makes one person more valuable than another? A politician may have felt to have lied; maybe one of the group did something illegal. Maybe you think you have achieved nothing? Would you be less valuable than these people? Or would a member of your family be less valuable? Is someone with a learning disability less valuable? They may have never lied or broken the law but may not have achieved anything deemed of any value or importance either. Is someone with a learning disability unworthy of just treatment? Some of the care that Chrissy received appeared unjust. No one deserves to be treated unjustly. To avoid unacceptable treatments of someone with a learning disability, ask yourself, would you or members of your family want to be treated this way? We cannot judge the quality or the value of other people's lives until we have actually walked in their shoes. All life should be considered therefore equal and just treatment offered to all; the treatment that you would wish for yourself or members of your family.

- Commandment 2. *Never intentionally take innocent human life* (Singer, 1995).
- To be replaced by the new commandment: *Take responsibility for the consequences of your decisions.*

The above new commandment is the one that Jackson (2006) chose for medical ethics, and it is also appropriate for learning disability practice. Health and social care should be evidence-based. A practitioner should keep up-to-date with contemporary issues and initiatives and be appropriately educated. Be aware of relevant documentations, good practice policy and evidence and be able to reflect upon it. Subsequently, they should reflect upon client need and decide if findings are relevant to the person and apply their research findings to the role if applicable. By doing so, it is likely that effective practice will be achieved. A practitioner who uses evidence within their role is more likely to feel that they have done their best and worked in the best interests of that individual and will be more confident in their approach. We may, as practitioners, make mistakes; being ethical and moral does not preclude human error. But by being knowledgeable, well read, reflective and person-centred, we are better placed to be able to take more responsibility for the consequences of the decisions we make as they were well-intentioned and well-informed.

- Commandment 3: *Never take your own life and always try to prevent others from taking theirs* (Singer, 1995).
- To be replaced by the new commandment: *Respect others' choices.*

People with a learning disability should have choices and have a right to be heard and listened to (DH, 2001, 2009). The Mental Capacity Act (2005), as discussed, states that all people are presumed competent, until it is found that they are not and that where capacity exists, people should be supported to make choices. If a competent person makes what is felt to be a bad decision, it is right to discuss the possible outcome of this decision, but coercion cannot occur. He/she should be supported in whatever is chosen, no matter what those around the person think about the decision made. Autonomous choices should be encouraged from people competent to make decisions on all manner of things, for example, in relation to healthcare, finances, housing issues, daily living issues, and so forth. Some people may need support to make choices, they may need accessible information or explicitly detailed information given in a bid to ensure their understanding, but once understanding is gained and consequences of choices understood, then all decisions made by autonomous individuals should be upheld. Encouraging choices decreases the possibility of paternalism and generally promotes the rights of people with a learning disability, something that is very desirable.

The views of families are important; they are the experts in the care of those they care for. Their views and opinions should be sought when planning or delivering care. It is of paramount importance, however, to ask the person him/herself about what their views are first. A parent, as someone who is a relative and from a different generation, may not at times be the best person to advocate for the true feelings of someone with a learning disability. An independent advocate may, where appropriate, be of use if someone cannot articulate for themselves. They will speak out or give a voice to someone with a learning disability, while there is also the added benefit of them being independent of the health or social sector.

Reader activity 23.7 Capacity to make decisions

Which of the following decisions would you like your parents or siblings to make for you?

- how I can spend my money;
- whether I can have a sex life;
- whether I need emergency treatment;
- what contraception I use;
- how much alcohol I should drink;
- what I can wear;
- whether I can go to college or not;
- whether I should have an injection.

- Commandment 4: *Be fruitful and multiply* (Singer, 1995).
- To be replaced by the new commandment: *Communicate your actions and the rationale for them.*

Practitioners are not islands; they are members of a team. Multi-disciplinary working is essential when meeting the needs of people with a learning disability. Collaboration brings together the skills and perspectives of different professionals so that the service user is more likely to have his/her holistic needs met. Communication is essential for effective inter-professional working, but as discussed above, confidentiality must also be considered. Each role has boundaries, and as practitioners there are limitations within the remit of a role. Each professional should discuss their role, justify, clarify their perspective, so ensuring a seamless service. As well as encouraging effective team working, good communication can be a forum for ironing out ethical and moral issues.

- Commandment 5: *Treat all human life as always more precious that non-human life* (Singer, 1995).
- To be replaced by the new commandment: *Treat the needs of people with a learning disability as always more important than the needs of the establishment.*

Institutional care has been the history of many people with a learning disability. Goffman (1961) illustrated how institutional care was often concerned with putting the needs of the institution before the needs of the people residing there. He highlighted how it involved depersonalising people, how individuals are treated en masse, mealtimes were set. People queued and waited for all aspects of healthcare including personal care, medication and toileting, with the time span of their wait set at the discretion of care-givers. Such actions occurred to ensure the smooth running of the facility, people's individual needs were very much seen as an inferior concern. The Community Care Act (1990) and the move from long-stay institutions did not in some cases, see the end of the institutional care of people with a learning disability. The systems, their smooth running, the following of procedures, the needs of care staff and adhering to managerial rules and outcomes can all be relevant considerations for practitioners. The needs of the people using the service should be the priority. Person-centred approaches (DH, 2001, 2009) are essential; people's needs shaping the nature of services rather than the service, its policies and philosophies being something the person has to fit into.

Conclusion

This chapter has discussed the ethical and legal principles and considered in turn many aspects of the ethical considerations involved in the decision-making process. While it may be true to say that hard cases make bad laws, you have considered in detail the relevant key points in complex circumstances. Through personal reflection on each of the themes and debating the issues, you may now be in a more informed position to assist a person who has a learning disability to live a full and valued life. Which is not asking a lot for most of us, but one which we all deserve.

Points to remember

- All people deserve just treatment.
- The law and ethics should be used to consider if just treatment is being used.
- An ethical framework and reflective practice will help to ensure just treatment.

References

Beauchamp, T.L. and Childress, J.F. (2008) *Principles of Biomedical Ethics*. 6th edn. Oxford: Oxford University Press.

Burkhardt, M. and Nathaniel, A. (2008) *Ethics and Issues in Contemporary Nursing*. Albany, NY: Thomson Delmar Learning.

Care Quality Commission (2012) *The Operation of the Deprivation of Liberty Safeguards in England 2010/11*. London: CQC.

Centre for Developmental Disability Health (CDDHV) (2008) *Assessment of Sexual Knowledge Tool*. Victoria, Australia: Chimat.

DH (Department of Health) (2001) *Valuing People: A New Strategy for Learning Disabilities for the 21st Century*. London: HMSO.

DH (Department of Health) (2009) *Valuing People Now: A 3 Year Strategy for People with Learning Disabilities*. London: HMSO.

DH (Department of Health) (2011) *Safeguarding Adults: The Role of Health Service Practitioners*. London: HMSO.

DH (Department of Health) (2012) *Transforming Care: A National Response to Winterbourne View Hospital*. London: HMSO.

Department of Health and Social Security (1990) Community Care Act. London. DHSS.

Dimond, B. (2011) *Legal Aspects in Nursing*, 6th edn. Harlow: Pearson Education.

Flynn, M. (2007) *The Murder of Steven Hoskin: A Serious Case Review*, Executive Summary Cornwall Adult Protective Committee. Available at: www.pkc.gov.uk/CHttpHandler.askx?id=14720&P=O (accessed April 2013).

Goffman, E. (1961) *Asylums: Essays on the Social Situation of Mental Patients and Older Inmates*. New York: Doubleday.

Jackson, J. (2006) *Ethics in Medicine*. Cambridge: Polity Press.

Kraus, E. (2010) My decisions were taken quickly but turned out to be right. *Learning Disability Practice*. Available at: http//:learningdisabilitypractice.rcnpublishing.co.uk/students/clinical-placements/professionaldevement/growing-your-confidence (accessed November 2012).

Pinto, A. and Upshur, R. (2013) *An Introduction to Global Health Ethics*. London: Routledge.

Sexual Offenders Act (2003) www.legislation.gov.uk. (accessed November 2012).

Singer, P. (1995) *Rethinking Life and Death*. Oxford: Oxford University Press.

The Human Fertilisation and Embryology Act (1990) Available at: www.legislation.gov.uk. (accessed April 2013).

The Mental Capacity Act (2005) Available at: www.justice.gov.uk/protecting-the vulnerable/mental-capacity-act (accessed April 2013).

The Mental Health Act (2007) Available at: wwwlegislation.gov.uk (accessed April 2013).

Webster, C., Douglas, K., Eaves, D. and Hart, S. (1997) *Assessing Risk for Violence, HCR-20*. Northumberland: Ann Arbor Publishers.

William, L., Whitefield, E. and Carson, D. (2007) Questionnaire on attitudes consistent with sexual offending, *Legal and Criminal Psychology*, 12(1): 1–67.

Part V

Changing roles

Part V takes the reader on a long view of the development of professional services and statutory agencies working with people with learning disabilities both now and in the past. The key emphasis is on the change from custodial models of working with people with learning disabilities in the past which was reinforced and promoted by societal attitudes and care policy to the more contemporary approaches of health promotion, individualised and supported care, and the ideology of self-advocacy and self-determination in supporting people with learning disabilities to meet their needs with consultation and communication. This Part draws upon theory and practice examples to illustrate the variety of issues. In particular, the political agenda and historical contexts of the development and demise of stereotypical attitudes towards learning disability offer the reader useful background information and also an opportunity to analyse modern healthcare and social care practice.

The four chapters use Case studies, Reader activities and Practice alerts to engage the reader (who may or may not be a health or social care professional) in the challenging of ideas about the healthcare of people with learning disabilities in today's society. The traditional power relationships between 'carer' and 'cared for' are debated and the reader is encouraged to consider alternative ways to work within professional teams.

The chapters which make up Part V are:

Chapter 24 Inter-professional working
Chapter 25 Changing roles in meeting the needs of people with a learning disability
Chapter 26 Health promotion for people with a learning disability
Chapter 27 Public health and learning disability

24 Inter-professional working

Jo Lay and Stacey Atkinson

Learning outcomes

After reading this chapter you will be able to:

- explore the importance of inter-professional working through a case study approach
- reflect on your own experiences of inter-professional working
- be able to utilise good practice and guidelines in day-to-day working relationships
- feel empowered to challenge, support and develop an organisation's inter-professional working practices.

Introduction

> All of these people coming into my home asking me to do different things, sometimes its the same thing! Don't they ever talk to each other?.
>
> (The views of a parent whose child has a learning disability)

Much has been written about the importance of inter-professional work. In the health and social care literature different terminology is used to describe how different professionals work together, such as inter-professional; inter-agency; multi-professional and multi-disciplinary. These terms can refer to different professionals working in one team for one organisation but can also refer to professionals from different organisations working together for a common purpose. One example of this is adult safeguarding. There has been clear government directive since the publication of *No Secrets* (Department of Health and Home Office, 2000) towards partnership working in adult safeguarding (DH, 2010). Local areas have developed this guidance into joint working strategies. In Leeds, the Leeds Safeguarding Adult Partnership was established to determine a multi-agency procedure which protects adults who may need support to maintain their independence and well-being, and who are unable to protect themselves from harm (Leeds Safeguarding Adult Partnership, 2013). All local health and social care organisations across all sectors of provision (public, private and voluntary) are expected to follow the procedure and engage in the joint working strategy. The joint safeguarding procedure should be explicitly part of their own organisational policies and procedures.

The Department of Health (DH, 2003) identify that multi-professional working and good communication skills are essential in maintaining and improving standards of care; reducing stress for patients; giving staff greater job satisfaction and sharing skills and resources with staff, patients and families. It is accepted across child and adult services in health and social care that inter-professional collaboration is essential in improving services and this is reflected in legislation and frameworks for good practice. Reports of the failures in health and social care repeatedly identify difficulties in inter-professional working as a problem (House of Commons Health Committee, 2003). Often poor communication is caused by the different ways of working by different professionals with different goals and priorities. Doyle (2008) identifies that this can lead to duplication of care and a lack of confidence and trust in professionals.

Case study 24.1 Complex multiple impairment

Denzil is an 18-year-old young man of Nigerian origin who lives at home with his parents and younger sibling. He was referred to the complex multiple impairment (CMI) team by the School Nursing Service, to request support with his enteral feeding regime and his additional complex physical health needs. Denzil is in transition into adult education and required nursing support to access a local specialist college for people with a learning disability. Other than school, at which his attendance is sporadic, Denzil and the family have no other health and social care support. Denzil's parents have been advised to request an assessment for carer support and possible respite care for Denzil.

Denzil' s diagnosed conditions are:

- cerebral palsy caused by acquired brain damage due to anoxia (lack of oxygen) at 18 months;
- a severe learning disability;
- profound physical disabilities including kyphoscoliosis (abnormal curvature of the spine, both sideways and towards the upper back), hip dislocation and consequent right girdle-stones operation (hip replacement);
- gastrostomy and Nissen's fundoplication (an operation to treat gastro-oesophageal reflux). He currently has a G-button or Mic-key button (a 'button' which connects the stomach through which feeds and fluids can be given) and is nil by mouth; all nutrition, fluids and medications are given enterally.
- recurrent chest infections/pneumonia. Denzil has severely compromised lung function due to his profoundly abnormal body shape.
- recurrent styes (small lumps on the eyelids formed due to blocked eyelash follicles or glands);
- recurrent ear infections.

Denzil has a history of poor food tolerance and the resulting severe discomfort from trapped wind. He requires food to be delivered hourly with tube venting during feeds. This can result in the feeding being very slow and laboured, but it is imperative that he gets the correct calorific amount and a balanced diet needed in relation to his age and development, Denzil has low body weight, he presently weighs 26kg. Feeding intolerance is also exacerbated by episodes of anxiety, especially in relation to difficult relationships and arguments in the home. He requires regular positioning in his wheelchair and on equipment due to susceptibility to pressure sores. He has no specialist equipment at home and requires a full assessment of this postural management needs.

His current medication is:

- Lansoprazole 15mgs daily – for excessive stomach acid;
- Erythromycin 62.5mgs 4 times daily – for the prevention of recurrent infections;
- Baclofen 20mgs 4 times daily – to relax the muscles and to act as an anti-spasm agent;
- Diazepam 5mgs twice daily – a sedative used in this case as a muscle relaxant and for anxiety;
- Tizanidine 8mgs nightly – a muscle relaxant;
- Movicol 2 sachets daily – to prevent constipation;
- Salbutamol inhaler as required via an aero chamber – to open respiratory airways.

Social services have been involved due to parental disengagement regarding his health needs and subsequent concerns about his morbidity. For a definition of complex needs refer to Chapter 25.

Denzil has complex health needs and these need to be assessed from a holistic view point to incorporate the complexities and impact on him and his family. Holistic healthcare recognises the bio-psycho-social model of health which includes the impact of our feelings and belief systems on well-being (Llewellyn and Hayes, 2008).

Reader activity 24.1   Holistic healthcare

Denzil is clearly a young man with many very complex needs. Taking the importance of holistic healthcare into account, list the people you think would be involved in his care, specifying what role they might have and what their level of involvement might be.

Case study 24.1 refers to a complex multiple impairment (CMI) team. They are representative of many multi-disciplinary specialist teams (MDT) you might find throughout the United Kingdom, composed of different professionals possessing a variety of skills. Each will have specific roles in meeting service users' need but all will work together as part of a team to plan and prioritise nursing care with the service user, families and carers (Leeds and York Partnership Foundation Trust, 2013). Team working in this way has many advantages (Figure 24.1) but can also present its own range of problems.

Although members of the CMI team in the case study work within one organisation, they may have a variety of allegiances as individuals; to the team and to their professional groups (Firth-Cozens, 2001). Goodman and Clemow (2008, p. 44) took the *Oxford Dictionary*'s (2005) definition of a group to help them define what a multi-disciplinary team is and described it as a 'number of people allocated, gathered or classed together; regarded as belonging together, people with something in common'. What the CMI have in common is the shared goal of meeting the needs of a specific client group.

> • Inter-agency/professional understanding and awareness
> • Information sharing
> • Improved communication systems
> • Co-location (sharing environments)
> • Inter-agency/professional training and education
> • Shared record keeping and documentation
> • Partnership working and joint commitment to services.

Figure 24.1 Advantages of inter-professional team working

In 2007, the Department of Health published guidance on workforce planning (DH, 2007a). The guidance was principally concerned with the development of mental health teams but its philosophies can be applied more generally as it advocated good practice criteria for teams. The CMI team established as part of the Leeds and York Partnership NHS Trust adopted the approach recommended for community teams which suggests that 'the work and responsibility are distributed amongst the team based on individual members' competencies. Team members are responsible for their own clinical decision making, with each working at a level of complexity, commensurate with their ability' (ibid., p. 3). The specific aim of the service is to meet the needs of people of 18 or over who, like Denzil, have a severe or profound learning disability and 'life-limiting, chronic and long-term conditions' such as complex multiple disabilities and/or complex healthcare needs (Leeds and York Partnership NHS Foundation Trust, 2011). Service users may have one or more of the following difficulties: the need for enteral feeding, difficulties with swallowing or breathing, complex nutritional requirements, postural management needs, uncontrolled epilepsy, chronic constipation or other complex health criteria.

Currently the Clinical Team Manager (CTM; Band 7 role) in the CMI team in Leeds is a learning disability nurse. The manager is responsible for gate-keeping referrals to the team, ensuring they are appropriate for team involvement. The CTM provides clinical appraisal for the nurses within the group while other professionals seek appraisal from senior colleagues in their own disciplines. The CTM provides all staff with supervision, thus discouraging role overlap and duplication. The CTM is ultimately responsible for effective team working. The banding that each person has indicates the level of responsibility given within their role and is part of the Agenda for Change policy (NHS Employers, 2013). The Agenda for Change allocates NHS jobs to specific pay bands as part of a role evaluation scheme. The CTM should ensure that no one is given responsibilities they cannot or should not fulfil in their banding scale. In the Leeds team the CTM has a small caseload of clients, something which other managers may choose not to do, to maintain practice links and validate their knowledge. As a 'clinical' team leader it is important to maintain a clinical role as it gives visibility as a role model and manager and provides an opportunity to share expert knowledge.

The remit of the learning disability nurses in the team (Bands 5 and 6) is to meet the healthcare needs of the client group. Some nurses are based within City Council day services and further education provision and others work within the community. Learning disability nurses work holistically to address the five dimensions of health, thus addressing Denzil's physical, psychological, social, intellectual and spiritual needs (Hjelm, 2010). All nurses use the nursing process to assess, plan, implement and evaluate care (Orlando, 1972) (see Figure 20.3 on p. 397), thus ensuring that Denzil has the best care possible. The day service nurses provide some direct care but their role often is to guide others to provide care, making full use of their teaching skills to ensure the care staff or family members know what is required. Specifically Denzil's family need advice with regards to his feeding regime, positioning and health. People with complex needs frequently suffer very poor health compared to the general population, Mansell (2010) describes their healthcare needs as substantial, sustained, and complicated. A nurse would be involved where the person needs a health assessment, behavioural or psychological needs, has epilepsy, is in pain, has additional requirements such as gastrostomy care, tracheotomy or oxygen therapy, and so forth. All nurses must be professionally registered with the Nursing and Midwifery Council (NMC) and work to the NMC Professional Code (NMC, 2010).

Practice alert 24.1

According to the Department of Health guidance:

> Learning disability nurses provide a vital contribution to the well-being of people with learning disabilities. They work through providing direct care and support to those with complex needs and their family carers, and also through helping other health and social care workers respond appropriately.
>
> (DH, 2007b, p. 4)

The Occupational Therapists (OT: Band 6) within the CMI team support people with complex needs to have meaningful occupations and to have higher levels of engagement with others where desired. This might be in relation to someone with dementia who is unable to recall recent events or needs adaptations or equipment in the home.

Practice alert 24.2

According to NHS Careers (2013): 'Occupational therapy is the assessment and treatment of physical and psychiatric conditions using specific, purposeful activity to prevent disability and promote independent function in all aspects of daily life.'

In relation to Denzil's care, the OT may advise about specialist seating, positioning, pressure area or postural care. Elements of this support will be shared with other professionals such as physiotherapists in relation to postural care or Speech and Language Therapists (SLT) in relation to feeding issues and equipment needed (Lilywhite and Haines, 2010). The OT's role is essential in supporting individuals with a learning disability to develop competence, skills and, where possible, independence. Developing strengths through competence and skills is an important part of our personal development which gives us self-worth and belief and presents a more positive self-image. This positive image cannot be underestimated when supporting someone with a learning disability as historically low expectations have fostered negative attitudes about the learning disabled, which in turn have led to self-fulfilling prophesies. It must be recognised that independence is not always the goal as none of us lead completely independent lives.

Physiotherapists (Band 6) support individuals with a range of physical difficulties and provide support through manual therapy and advising on therapeutic exercise and the latest technologies/ techniques. In Denzil's case study the physiotherapist will be invaluable in providing support with postural management.

Practice alert 24.3

'Physiotherapists identify and maximise movement potential through health promotion, preventive healthcare, treatment and rehabilitation' (NHS Careers, 2013).

Many of those in the care of the CMI team have, like Denzil, complex body shapes and due to this may have respiratory problems and other healthcare deficits. The physiotherapists work with the other disciplines to provide a package of care which includes good postural care. They will, for example, teach parents and carers to passively move Denzil or to position him so that movement is maximised and further deterioration of posture does not occur. Physiotherapists also have an appreciation of psychological, cultural and social factors which influence their clients.

Speech and Language therapists (Band 6) are not only concerned with the acquisition of speech and language development, but are also specialists in assisting with the mechanics of eating (NHS, 2012).

Practice alert 24.4

According to NHS Careers (2013):

The role of a speech and language therapist (SLT) is to assess and treat speech, language and communication problems in people of all ages to enable them to communicate to the best of their ability. They may also work with people who have eating and swallowing problems.

Denzil now has a gastrostomy fitted to assist with meeting his nutritional needs but previously he has used the skilled of a speech therapist to help with swallowing and eating problems. It was only when his weight and health deteriorated badly that gastrostomy care was considered. A gastrostomy is an operation that makes an artificial opening in the stomach to provide direct nutritional support to the individual.

Dieticians (Band 5 and 6) are an essential part of the CMI team. People like Denzil, who have complex needs, have very specific dietary requirements in order to ensure a nutritional status which enables them to flourish.

Practice alert 24.5

'Dietetics is the interpretation and communication of the science of nutrition to enable people to make informed and practical choices about food and lifestyle, in both health and disease' (NHS Careers, 2013).

Dieticians have been involved in Denzil's care since early childhood when he experienced 'failure to thrive' due to his physical needs hindering his ability to eat sufficient food. Denzil now enjoys a balanced diet through intricate dietician involvement in his enteral feeding programme. Enteral feeding is where nutrition is provided via tubes directly into the stomach as opposed to food taken orally.

We have referred to healthcare professionals who work in a specific CMI team but in relation to Denzil's holistic health needs, you may have identified a broad range of other people. This may include roles such as a Social Worker or Care Manager. These professionals are dominant within social care and are essential members of inter-professional teams.

Practice alert 24.6

'Social work involves engaging not only with clients themselves but their families and friends as well as working closely with other organisations including the police, local authority departments, schools and the probation service' (NHS Careers, 2013).

As Denzil becomes older, he may need advice and support from social care agencies in order to access personal budgets; suitable housing and other facilities that will promote his independence. If professionals and services work together to support Denzil, there is a higher probability that his needs will be met in a timely and effective manner.

Reader activity 24.2 Family-centred care

Imagine that you are working within a team with someone with complex needs.

- How can you ensure that the care provided is both person- and family-centred?
- What are some of the issues you should consider in family-centred care?

Denzil has been referred to the local CMI team due to concerns that his complex health needs are not being met. At this stage this has not been identified as a safeguarding issue but it is important that members of the team engage with Denzil and his parents to assess what the difficulties are and ensure that future health needs are met. The team needs to use effective communication to support the family and avoid making assumptions about what difficulties there may be. Grant suggests it can be too easy for professionals to judge parents as 'aloof', 'difficult to deal with' or even as 'perpetrators of the difficulties faced by their disabled children' (2005, p. 224). Chapter 9 includes some detail on the importance of family-centred care when supporting adolescents but it is useful to consider how the inter-professional team may use this person-centred way of working to enable Denzil and his family to feel valued and included. The Royal College of Nursing (RCN, 2013) suggests a number of challenges in considering family-centred care but two that the CMI team could consider are:

1. Definitions of 'the family' have changed over the years and can be influenced by personal experience and individual belief systems. Who are Denzil's family? His parents have been mentioned but there may be other family members who contribute to his care. There may be other friends whom Denzil would like to be involved in decision-making with him. Are there cultural issues involved in his care? Do Denzil and his family understand what his specific needs are and who should be involved? Do they have expectations about the role of the CMI team?
2. Family-centred care can be an ambiguous concept and is dependent on definitions and subsequent understanding and interpretations of this.

How can Denzil be supported as an individual and young adult while appreciating the concerns and wishes of his family to support him in decision-making? We have recognised that members of the CMI team will have specific professional roles in Denzil's care and support but within their professional identities, individuals will need to develop skills as teacher, advocate and enabler. NHS Careers (2013) states that learning disability nurses require the following:

- excellent people skills;
- good communication and observation skills;
- the ability to answer questions and offer advice;
- ability to work happily as part of a team;
- ability to manage emotionally charged situations.

These are skills that are required by all the inter-professional team if family-centred care is to become a reality. These skills need to be underpinned by a shared values base that recognises an individual's rights. In the current NHS this is exemplified by the Six Cs of Care; Compassion; Competence; Communication; Courage and Commitment (DH, 2012). To work in partnership with families, the CMI team needs to foster openness and honesty; mutual respect and trust; and power sharing within a context of shared goals and realistic expectations (Lay and Kirk, 2012).

User and carer involvement

Despite pressure from service user groups, advocates and policy-makers, service user involvement and carer involvement have not always been achieved. Tait and Lester (2005) discussed how service user involvement has been a buzz word, something good to claim to follow, but not something that in reality often occurs, at least not to any truly meaningful degree. Effective service user and care involvement is concerned with placing the person with a learning disability in the driving seat, regarding their own care. This is very difficult when the person is someone with a severe or profound learning disability. It is a very skilled practitioner who can encourage involvement with this client group; but it should be achieved as far as possible, with the service user's wishes and preferences being taken into account throughout. In such cases, however, Mansell (2010) advocates also the need to include carers and their circles of support as they are vital sources of ideas and information, and as such should be treated as experts with regard to the needs of the person they care for. With this in mind, services should be delivered not only in a person-centred way but also be family-centred (ibid.). Circles of support encourage us to think about who the important people are in the life of the service user by inviting them to be part of their future plans. It challenges traditional thinking of including just health and social care professionals within care planning and prioritising. It places the balance of power with the service user and their families and friends. Sharing ideas and support for care with a larger group gives scope for creativity and innovation in meeting needs. Bringing ideas and discussion to the wider CMI team can also give an opportunity for the whole team to share knowledge and decision-making, as opposed to just those working directly with Denzil. Not all care interventions can be person-centred as ultimately professionals will have a duty of care to an individual. This has led to tensions between professionals and families where there are different opinions as to the best interests of the service user. This highlights the importance of user involvement where all parties should examine how they can promote active participation from the focus person. In Denzil's situation it is likely that a number of the team will be working with him. While undertaking specific assessments they can all contribute to developing a therapeutic relationship with Denzil by getting to know him as a person. Case study 24.1 provides succinct information relating to his health needs and it is likely that care plans will soon be developed that expand on these needs. To become more person-centred, these assessments and plans could be provided in different communication formats that encourage Denzil's participation, e.g. use of pictures or symbols. They could include information specific to Denzil, e.g. how he shows pleasure, distress, etc. These details help the team build a picture of the person Denzil is, not just his difficulties. Circles of support have another important feature of 'interdependence'. This is an important concept in the power dynamics between professionals and service users and families. It recognises that none of us are completely independent but rely on others at various times in our lives for a variety of functions. A circle of support for Denzil would not only provide a forum to help him plan and prioritise but would also build his confidence in recognising the importance he has in the lives of his family, friends and care workers. 'This interdependence is important as a means to recognise our own competence as it implies and expects reciprocity. We have to acknowledge where we rely on others in our lives as opposed to being completely independent' (Lay and Kirk, 2012). (See Reader activity 20.8).

Evaluation is a key part of service development in inter-professional working and should include listening to service users and carers and acknowledging what they have to say about the delivery of the service they have received. The Care Quality Commission, the regulators of all health and social care provision in England, recommend that quality assurance systems, appropriate complaints procedures, access to advocates to speak up especially for people like Denzil, should all be in place, be fully accessible, with methods taking into account people's developmental, language and literacy requirements (CQC, 2012).

The Department of Health (DH, 2001, 2009, 2012) advocate person-centred approaches to planning care for the person with a learning disability, to ensure they have as much autonomy as possible, given their mental capacity and while it is strongly encouraged that their needs are at the forefront of decisions made by the inter-professional team, it should be acknowledged that carers and families have needs too. They care often very profoundly about their loved ones and may at times be excluded by professionals, especially where there is team involvement. A team aiming desperately to get along with each other can often forget there are carers, who have cared for so long, who really need to be kept involved. Nolan *et al.* (2003) revised an extensive list of what is important to carers called the 'Senses Framework'. It captures the essence of what carers would like from their relationship with professionals involved in the care of their loved ones. They want the following:

- *A sense of security*: knowing that their needs are being recognised, that they have the right information and skills to meet the needs of their loved one. That they can feel secure that support will be available as required, should their own health or other needs deteriorate and that they can speak about or evaluate a service honestly without repercussions for themselves or the person they care for.
- *A sense of belonging*: That they do not have important decisions or control taken from them. That their relationships with their loved ones do not alter by having someone else helping. Carers do not want to feel isolated/alone in the care-giving situation and want to belong to a wider network, not just including other care-givers.
- *A sense of continuity*: To keep hold of things that matter and not to lose important links or routines because other help has become available. For care to be consistent, predictable and to still maintain active involvement in care processes for as long as possible.
- *A sense of purpose*: For carers to have their own goals acknowledged and valued and to be able to plan for the future.
- *A sense of achievement*: To know that the best care is being given to their loved one. To be able to develop new skills and knowledge so that carers do not need to stay dependent on care once it is no longer necessary, and being able to help other carers, so feeling that their care role is appreciated.
- *A sense of significance*: to feel that they as carers matter and are listened to.

Partnerships are essential within inter-professional working. The above provides a framework enabling services to more successfully meet carers' needs and for them to feel included in the inter-professional team.

Developing effectiveness in inter-professional working

Effective teams

Slevin *et al.* (2008) noted that when learning disability service teams such as the CMI team work well, they provide people like Denzil with highly effective specialist services. In effective teams, multi-professionals work together to provide seamless services; with professionals delivering their own specialist specific roles to the person but having an awareness of the role of others to refer to when necessary. The combined skills of the professionals enable the person's current holistic needs to be addressed but also support the development of the service, benefiting more people with a learning disability and their families and carers. In terms of the organisational and procedural workings of the team, an effective and motivated staff team is more likely to work through challenges or difficulties. They will tackle problems as they arise, making good use of the supportive environment to explore ideas and stimulate discussion about relevant issues. An effective team will find it easier to accept the challenges and opportunities of change. Services need to be well managed and resourced with staff who are committed to the shared goals of the team and the needs of people with a learning disability. Effective teams are ones who feel involved, included and share the same philosophy. Professionals should have professional respect for one another and the roles within the service, with staff trusting and supporting one another. This may sound like a utopian dream, but it is something that can be worked upon and achieved.

Barriers to effective team working

The diversity of different roles, the demands of different professional identities or sometimes merely the nature of being human can mean that problems do occur in teams. They might be in relation to one or more of the following areas:

- *Lack of clarity regarding the professional's role or the needs of the client.* This can result in service overlap, frustration and ineffective services for service users.
- *Professional difficulties among staff impacting upon team working.* An example might be prejudice about how certain groups of practitioners behave or professional rivalries.
- *Weak or unclear team focus,* resulting in a lack of understanding about the team philosophy, remit or how roles should be delivered.
- *Sparse resources within the team* which impacts on service delivery. Low staffing levels, the absence of a relevant staff member or high caseloads can impact on the effectiveness of the service and may result in staff burnout.
- *Professionals who are reluctant to accept change* which is needed to meet local contemporary need.

Reader activity 24.3   Professional rivalry

Consider the issue of professional rivalry:

- Why do you think it might occur?
- What might be done about it?

Leadership

In discussing the CMI team, we stated the manager also adopted a role as leader by being a role model and someone with expert knowledge. We also acknowledged that ultimately the CTM was responsible for effective team working. Leadership is important, but it equates often to responsibility and many within the social and healthcare settings prefer not to take on a leadership role for that reason. It is important to clarify our understanding of the terms 'leader' and 'manager' and the connotations within them. Levin (2005) suggests that in the absence of a named leader/manager, a key person in the life of someone with a learning disability can assume the leadership role, doing what needs to be done to ensure someone like Denzil has his healthcare needs met. A person-centred approach would advocate this development. In order to take on this role, the individual would need a support system that could involve professionals who could support Denzil's needs but also give advice on the different options and choices Denzil has in having those needs met. The individual would need the personal attributes to be an advocate for Denzil and assert his needs and wants.

Good management is essential within services and is necessary in ensuring good multi-professional working. Good managers do the following:

- *Organise regular multi-disciplinary meetings*: ideal situations whereby professionals can review care, explore previous roles and care plans and arrange future developments to meet clients' needs. Work can be shared with named professionals given responsibility for particular actions. All needs are very necessary matters when someone has complex needs. Such meetings can be the place for a review of the team processes and philosophies, can be an arena for team building, and the actions planned there can strengthen the teams' commitment to team working.

- *Provide clinical supervision* (Figure 24.2): Some supervision may be provided by the team manager who may be from a different professional group. The aim of this cross-disciplinary support is to monitor the service given to the client. Senior members of the professional's own group will also provide supervision which aims to address developmental issues such as the professional's skill base and knowledge as a practitioner, providing career and educational advice. During supervision, though a practitioner remains accountable for their own practice, the manager has the authority to ask for progress reports or care plans to ensure that the practitioner is meeting need in an effective manner. Øvretveit *et al.* (1997) discuss how the skill of a supervisor lies in balancing the nature of support for a supervisee between 'autonomy and controlling' what a practitioner does, thus ensuring the ethos of the service is adhered to while also guaranteeing the needs of the client group are being met.

- *Co-ordinate an evaluation of the service*: Specialist services such as nursing, social care services, occupational therapy services and medical services, etc. are expensive. It is the responsibility of a team manager/manager of care to ensure that there is effective use of such services. Objective evaluations need to occur in order to ascertain if successful outcomes are achieved. A good quality of life, carers who feel supported and carers knowing how best to meet the needs of the people they care for, are perhaps what professionals would hope for but they are not outcomes that can easily be assessed or quantified in an objective manner. What one person feels is a good quality of life or what someone feels is to be well supported is not necessarily what another feels. It is essential that following episodes of professional intervention objective outcomes are measured. For someone like Denzil, they might include:

  - increased episodes of sleep;
  - weight gain;
  - fewer ear and chest infections;
  - fewer episodes of pain/anxiety (measured by objective means);
  - increased happy episodes;
  - fewer pressure sores.

Evaluation of the wider service is relevant too. Knowing the patterns regarding the use of the service as a whole can show if the service is being used, if referrals are relevant or if service users/carers felt positively about the service they received.

Management mentoring/supervision: A manager mentors someone he/she has authority over. The manager is trained and experienced in the same field and can ascertain the support needed by the individual being mentored as he/she can see the direction their career may take.

Peer mentoring: A relationship of peers resulting in mutually beneficial support. Practice is reflected upon, shared and explored. The peers support each other at the stage they are both at. They have no professional responsibility with regards to each other's work loads but discuss ideas and issues.

Pool/group mentoring: A team openly discusses ideas and caseloads looking for advice and guidance. It is at the discretion of the professional if ideas are taken up but the team approach is helpful as ideas are 'pooled'.

Consultancy/professional supervision/mentorship: The offering of support, guidance or advice from someone who is another professional, maybe from the same field but not necessarily so. It is someone you trust professionally, who can offer objective support.

Figure 24.2 Models of supervision

Source: Cooper and Palmer (2000).

Team development

As discussed, the dynamics of the team can have an impact on group cohesion, affecting how different disciplines collaborate and work together. A new team or the introduction of a new team member causes unpredictability and unsettles the dynamics. Tuckman (1965) identified that there are certain processes that a newly established group must go through, stages that are natural, and therefore must be anticipated before a group works more proficiently as a team.

The stages are:

1. *Forming*: A stage of orientation where the group is busy getting to know each other both personally and professionally, learning about each other's personalities and roles. People may feel uneasy and unsure about each other; this can have an impact on the quality of the work produced.
2. *Storming*: This stage involves tension and arguments usually occur as people in the team or group start to compete. Competition may be around status or functions within the team. Individual team members may start to have conflicting ideas about processes and functions. They will seek to establish their place in the team but also contribute to the leadership and focus of the team. The team needs to learn ways of working that promote listening and involvement.
3. *Norming*: The group becomes more cohesive; members have become more familiar with each other on a personal level and understand the characters within the group, and professionally appreciate the boundaries of the professional roles.
4. *Performing*: Due to the sense of self and others within the group, actions can now be taken and more success is achieved. Individual members of the inter-professional team are comfortable in performing their role and have an expectation about the contribution of others.

Tuckman's model is fluid and there may be times, perhaps when a new task or a change of focus is presented, when previous stages of the model may be revisited. Knowing about the process equips practitioners with the insight to assess if new teams may be experiencing teething problems which in time may be resolved.

Think about a group you are a member of, maybe a leisure or a student group.

- How do you think Tuckman's ideas manifested in your group?
- Identify one aspect of this reflective activity where you feel you can develop your own practice and make an action plan which reflects SMART goals (Specific, Measurable, Achievable, Realistic and Timely).

On joining a new team or working with a new group of people, especially where members are from different professional perspectives, the norming stage is characterised by a period of making agreements, determining how things will be done. Staff who help to make such decisions will feel part of the team, will feel more valued, that they have contributed and been listened to. Øvretveit *et al.* (1997) provided a comprehensive list of what might need to be addressed in the early days of a group's amalgamation process.

- Deciding who is to receive the services of the team. It is difficult to decide who is eligible for services, as by the very nature of making such decisions, inevitably the decision is also being made about who is not eligible. It is difficult denying a service to people in need and concepts such as 'complex' or 'severe' make the process more burdensome. More objective determinants of eligibility need to be made, so that the criterion for input is clear. Services are not provided beyond the scope of expertise of a given service and gaps can be identified for people who fall outwith the remit for available provision.
- Considering how services will be provided. Roles will be identified and resources considered.
- Deciding upon where services will be provided or where a MDT will be based.
- Identifying the referral process or how access to the team will occur.
- Clarifying how decisions will be made, including how often team members will meet, how meetings will be managed, what paperwork, including care plans, will be completed and decisions made about information dissemination as applicable.
- Deciding how the delivery of services will be coordinated. This will include who the key workers are and an identification of their roles. The manager's role will also need to be clarified. A team who do not discuss this may later be disgruntled as they find the manager performs his/her role in a way they did not expect. How and when supervision occurs may be part of the agreement and how and when a service review occurs may also be agreed.

Targets will be agreed for work with service users and longitudinal targets made for the service as a whole, some of which may come from a higher authority, such as the Learning Disability Partnership Board of Health Authority.

Inter-professional education

In order to acknowledge the importance of shared learning and education in inter-professional working, it is useful to review the barriers to joint working arrangements. The following list identified some of the barriers to inter-professional working:

- the large numbers of professionals and agencies involved in health and social care;
- protectiveness about individual roles;
- lack of inter-professional knowledge as to others' roles and responsibilities;
- lack of knowledge about the benefits of working together;
- lack of opportunity for shared learning.

This last barrier deserves strong consideration because, if this one issue is addressed, there is the potential to positively impact on all the others. Commitment to shared learning is needed from individuals, teams, organisations and professional bodies. Education needs must be addressed through team assessment and service user feedback and be an explicit expectation within undergraduate pre-qualification education.

The Centre for the Advancement of Interprofessional Education (CAIPE) was founded in 1987 to respond to a recognised need for collaborative practice when a single profession is unable to respond to the complexities of user need alone. CAIPE is a registered charity funded through the membership fees of professionals and students. They describe interprofessional education thus:

> While doctors, nurses, social workers and allied health professions comprise the core, much of the challenge now lies in engaging others such as lawyers, police officers, probation officers and schoolteachers. Indeed, it is hard to conceive of any profession capable of exercising its public accountability without collaboration with others and opportunities to learn with, from and about them.
>
> (www.caipe.org.uk/about-us/)

Barr and Lowe (2011) identify specific learning outcomes which CAIPE expect Inter-professional education (IPE) to facilitate:

- engenders inter-professional capability (outcome-led);
- enhances practice within each profession (enabling);
- informs joint action to improve services and act as a catalyst for change when required (critical analysis);
- improves outcomes for the individual, family and communities (responsive);
- shares experiences through dissemination (contributes);
- engages in systematic evaluation and research (data collection).

These outcomes can be used as benchmarks for the development of inter-professional learning.

> ## Reader activity 24.5   Inter-professional learning
>
> Reflect on the last education or training event you attended that was multi-professional. Critically evaluate your experience based upon the following questions:
>
> - What was the learning objective of this event?
> - How did it develop your practice?
> - How did it address or impact on joint practice?
> - Was it responsive to service user need? How?
> - What opportunities were there to share experiences with others?
> - How was it evaluated?
>
> If you cannot identify a recent experience of IPE, you may find it useful to identify an area from practice where you believe IPE would improve care. Using the questions, consider how you might plan a teaching event.

Dr Joan MacLean and Anne-Marie Henshaw have been project leaders for developing inter-professional education in the School of Healthcare at the University of Leeds. They say:

> In the School of Healthcare the inter-professional education agenda is supported by way of the Transdisciplinary First Year (TFY) project. Implementation of this extensive project has been staged, with the ultimate aim of involving seven pre-registration undergraduate programmes in inter-professional learning (IPL) by 2013. Two new IPL modules, one focused on biological knowledge and the other on working inter-professionally, were piloted in the 2010/11 academic session with a group comprising 53 students from two programmes. The delivery of these modules was then extended to over 300 students from four programmes in the 2011/12 session; additional programmes joined in the 2012/13 session, increasing the numbers.
>
> Health and social care students must develop core competencies to enable them to become employable graduate practitioners in a relatively short period, normally three years. Many will seek jobs in the National Health Service, whose focus on improved healthcare by way of effective inter-professional teamwork is well documented (DH, 2007a, 2010). Despite the vocational element of these undergraduate programmes, employment is not assured, and job competition is increasing as health and social care services are subjected to financial constraints. A principal aim of the TFY project is to develop competent graduates with well-developed skills in inter-professional learning and working and to support them as they reach qualified status. One major objective, therefore, is to instil in our undergraduates a collaborative attitude towards inter-professional working, and to develop the skills which will help them deliver health and social care in the 21st century. A research study to evaluate the impact of this IPL is in progress.

A lack of awareness of the needs of the client group can affect inter-professional working. Those working within the team may fail to engage with the client's needs, not recognising the role they have to play. A Yorkshire and Humberside Strategic Health Authority-funded initiative led by

Kilminster *et al.* (2004), involving the Universities of Leeds, Huddersfield, Bradford and Leeds Metropolitan University, aims to address this situation for people who have an Autistic Spectrum Disorder (ASD) and used the following scenario.

Case study 24.2   Jane's story

Jane is a 17-year-old young woman with Asperger's, a milder form of autism. She is attending hospital overnight for a pre-admission visit but her admission is fraught with difficulties which include:

- specific communication needs which are attributed to ASD (see Chapter 15);
- a need for sameness/routine;
- sensory hypersensitivity which causes the sights and sounds of the hospital to be painful to her. This problem is increasing her anxiety as she tries to adjust to the environment.
- a need to have all information about her imminent hospital procedure communicated in a very graphic way. Jane has also researched the procedure on the internet but it is difficult to ascertain how much she has understood.
- issues around her mental capacity and consent.

Jane is accompanied by her mother, Rose. Rose is anxious about her daughter's pending admission.

Soon to be qualified, third-year student practitioners from all four fields of nursing (learning disabilities, child, adult, and mental health), physiotherapy, dietetics, speech and language therapy, medicine, social work, podiatry, occupational therapy, pharmacy and medicine regularly take part in this training programme. Through the use of patient simulation, therefore with actors playing the parts of Jane and Rose, the students are encouraged to engage and meet the needs of the patients. For some students this was the first time they had encountered someone with a learning disability, but the training provides a safe environment to meet patients' needs, practising skills but not hurting anyone! Feedback was provided to students using the 'Spanner' approach (Morris, 2006; Morris *et al.*, 2009). This is a student-centred model of providing feedback which also encourages the involvement of the wider group, including the simulated patients who also reflected upon how it had been for them. A multi-professional approach to feedback encouraged a sharing of ideas and discussion of roles.

The programme consistently evaluates well. Student feedback has been consistently positive, 99 per cent would recommend attendance to their peers, 98 per cent felt the teaching and learning methods were entirely or mostly effective, and 94 per cent felt the workshop was entirely or mostly relevant to their work – these perceptions are shared equally across the professions and figures have remained stable each year since the project began in 2005. This shows the junior staff's perceptions about the importance of interdisciplinary working, something which is very encouraging to see at such an early stage in their careers.

In this particular case no follow-up research has occurred to ascertain if learning had a long-standing positive effect on inter-professional working but due to the very positive comments seen above, it is hoped that a long-term impact is likely to occur.

Conclusion

Inter-professional working is widely accepted as crucial to the complexities of current health and social care services. As services continue to change rapidly in response to the economic market, user involvement, public health and professional development, it becomes even more essential to develop systems and ways of working that enhance communication between professionals and organisations. In 2010, the Coalition government in the UK published a White Paper entitled *Equity and Excellence: Liberating the NHS*. This White Paper again addressed the importance of inter-professional working but also stated that it was the government's intention to simplify and extend powers so that it would be easier for the NHS and Local Authorities to work together. CAIPE (2010) responded positively to this, recognising the essential areas for inter-professional education as:

1. Putting patients and the public first.
2. Patient safety.
3. Empowering professionals in improving service delivery and health outcomes.
4. The multi-disciplinary and partnership approach.
5. Equity and fairness.

These are essential if the proposed framework for service quality and improvement is to become a reality.

Points to remember

- MDT working is necessary to meet the needs of people with complex needs.
- Time, effort and skills are needed to encourage effective team working.
- Service users and carers are an essential part of the team.

Acknowledgements

Case study 24.2 was provided by collaboration between representatives from the Universities of Leeds, Huddersfield and Bradford (2008).

Thank you also to Julie Howard, CMI Team, Leeds & York Partnership Foundation Trust.

Resources

CAIPE Centre for the Advancement of Inter-Professional Education
www.caipe.org.uk/

Children Act 2004
www.legislation.gov.uk/ukpga/2004/31/contents

Children's Workforce Development Council
www.cwdcouncil.org.uk

Davis, J. and Smith, M. (2012) *Working in Multi Professional Contexts. A Practical Guide for Professionals in Children's Services*. London: Sage.

Department for Education
www.education.gov.uk

Social Care Institute for Excellence (SCIE)
www.scie.org.uk

References

Barr, H. and Lowe, H. (2011) *The Definition and Principles of Interprofessional Education*. Available at: www.caipe.org.uk/about-us/the-definition-and-principles-of-interprofessional-education/ (accessed 31 Oct. 2012).

CAIPE (2010) Response to the NHS White Paper July 2010 'Equity and Excellence: Liberating the NHS'. Available at: www.caipe.org.uk (accessed 25 April 2014).

CQC (Care Quality Commission) (2012) *Learning Disability Services Inspection Programme: National Overview*. Newcastle upon Tyne: CQC.

DH (Department of Health) (2001) *Valuing People: A New Strategy for Learning Disability for the 21st Century*. London: HMSO.

DH (Department of Health) (2003) *Patient Focus Benchmarks: Essence of Care*. London: TSO.

DH (Department of Health) (2007a) *Mental Health: New Ways of Working for Everyone. Developing and Sustaining a Capable and Flexible Workforce*. York: CSIP/NIMHE.

DH (Department of Health) (2007b) *Good Practice in Learning Disability Nursing*. London: TSO.

DH (Department of Health) (2009) *Valuing People Now: A New Three-Year Strategy for People with Learning Disabilities 'Making It Happen for Everyone'*. London: HMSO.

DH (Department of Health) (2010) *A Vision for Adult Social Care: Capable Communities and Active Citizens*. London: TSO.

DH (Department of Health) (2012) *Compassion in Practice: Nursing, Midwifery and Care Staff. Our Vision and Strategy*. NHS Commissioning Board. London: TSO.

Department of Health and the Home Office (2000) *No Secrets: Guidance on Developing and Implementing Multi-Agency Policies and Procedures to Protect Vulnerable Adults from Abuse*. London: TSO.

Doyle, C. (2008) Barriers and facilitators of multi disciplinary team working: a review, *Paediatric Nursing*, 20(2).

Fielden, S. (2012) *Interprofessional Education Programme*. Leeds: University of Leeds

Firth-Cozens, J. (2001) Multidisciplinary teamwork: The good, bad and everything in-between, *Quality in Healthcare*, 10: 65–66.

Goodman, B. and Clemow, R. (2008) *Nursing and Working with Other People*. Exeter: Learning Matters.

Grant, G. (2005) Experiences of family care: bridging discontinuities over the life course, in G. Grant, P. Goward, M. Richardson and P. Ramcharan (eds) *Learning Disability: A Life Cycle Approach to Valuing People*. Maidenhead: Open University Press.

Hjelm, J. (2010) *The Dimension of Health: Conceptual Models*. London: Jones and Barlett International.

House of Commons Health Committee (2003) *The Victoria Climbié Inquiry Report*. London: TSO.

Howkins, E. and Barr, H. (2010) *Response to the NHS White Paper July 2010 'Equity and Excellence: Liberating the NHS'*. London: CAIPE.

Kilminster, S. and Fielden, S. (2009) Working with the patient voice: developing teaching resources for interprofessional education, *The Clinical Teacher*, 6: 265–268.

Kilminster, S., Hale, C.A., Lascelles, M.A. *et al.* (2003) Can interprofessional education workshops affect interprofessional communications? *Journal of Interprofessional Care*, 17(2).

Kilminster, S., Stark, P., Hale, C. *et al.* (2004) Learning for real life: patient focussed inter-professional workshops do offer added value, *Medical Education*, 38(7): 717–726.

Lay, J. and Kirk, L. (2012) Person-centred strategies for planning, in H. Atherton and D. Crickmore (eds) *Learning Disability: Toward Inclusion*. Oxford: Elsevier.

Leeds and York Partnership NHS Foundation Trust (2011) Eligibility assessment for access to the Learning Disabilities Complex Multiple Impairment Team (CMI MDT). Draft document. Unpublished.

Leeds and York Partnership NHS Foundation Trust (2013) Available at: http://www.leedspft.nhs.uk/_documentbank/Community_Learning_Disability_Team_A4.pdf?phpMyAdmin—3W4e1cy%2CYXWyzbOphZOEVmy5x3 (accessed 29 Jan. 2013).

Leeds Safeguarding Adult Partnership (2013) Available at: http://www.leedssafeguardingadults.org.uk/ (accessed 20 Jan. 2013).

Levin, P. (2005) *Successful Teamwork! Student Friendly Guides*. Maidenhead: Open University Press.

Lilywhite, A. and Haines, D. (2010) Occupational Therapy and people with learning disabilities. Available at: www.COT.org.uk (accessed August 2012).

Llewellyn, A. and Hayes, S. (2008) *Fundamentals of Nursing Care: A Textbook for Students of Nursing and Healthcare*. Exeter: Reflect Press.

Mansell, J. (2010) *Raising Our Sights: Services for Adults with Profound Intellectual and Multiple Disabilities*. Kent: Tizard Centre.

Morris, P. (2006) Preparing for patients in the 21st century, in J. Thistlethwaite and P. Morris (eds) *The Patient-Doctor Consultation in Primary Care: Theory and Practice*. London: Royal College of General Practitioners.

Morris, P., Dalton, E., McGovern, A. and Symons, A. (2009) Preparing for patient-centred practice: delivering the patients' voice in health professional learning, in H. Bradbury, N. Frost, S. Kilminster and M. Zukas (eds) *Beyond Reflective Practice*. London: Routledge.

Morton-Cooper, A. and Palmer, A. (2000) *Mentoring, Preceptorship and Clinical Supervision: A Guide to Professional Roles in Clinical Practice*. Oxford: Blackwell.

NHS Careers (2013) Available at: www.nhscareers.nhs.uk/explore-by-career/allied-health-professions/careers-in-the-allied-health-professions/physiotherapist/ (accessed 29 Jan. 2013).

NHS Employers (2013) Available at: www.nhsemployers.org/PayAndContracts/AgendaForChange/Pages/Afc-AtAGlanceRP.aspx (accessed 29 Jan. 2013).

NMC (2010) *The Code: Standards of Conduct, Performance and Ethics for Nurses and Midwives*. London: NMC.

Nolan, M., Lundh, U., Grant, G. and Keady, P. (2003) *Partnerships in Family Care. Understanding the Caregiving Career*. Maidenhead: Open University Press.

Orlando, I. J. (1972) *The Discipline and Teaching of Nursing Process: An Evaluative Study*. New York: G.P. Putnam's Sons.

Øvretveit, J., Mathias, P. and Thompson, T. (1997) *Interprofessional Working for Health and Social Care*. Basingstoke: Palgrave Macmillan.

Oxford English Dictionary (2005) Compact edn, 3rd edn. Oxford: Oxford University Press.

Royal College of Nursing (RCN) (2013) *Section One: Users and Carers – Definitions and Perceptions*. Available at: http://www.rcn.org.uk/development/learning/transcultural_health/multiagency/sectionone (accessed 12 Jan. 2013).

Slevin, E., Truesdale Kennedy, M. *et al.* (2008) Community Learning Disability Teams: composition and good practice. *Journal of Intellectual Disabilities*, 12(1): 59–79.

Tait, L. and Lester, H. (2005) Encouraging user involvement in mental health services. *Advances in Psychiatric Treatment*, 11: 168–175.

Tuckman, B. (1965) Developmental sequence in small groups, *Psychological Bulletin*, 63(6): 384–399.

25 Changing roles in meeting the needs of people with a learning disability

Sheena Kelly and Lyndsey Charles

Learning outcomes

After reading this chapter you will be able to:

- demonstrate how the learning disability professional has adapted their role to the new requirements over recent years to how the person with a learning disability is supported
- emphasise the importance of the learning disability health professional having a significant role within the whole healthcare system
- emphasise the importance of embedding person-centred planning in the model of service delivery
- provide guiding principles through the case study and exercises on the importance of multi-disciplinary working
- demonstrate the clear unique role of the learning disability health professional and community learning disability team.

Introduction

Nobody can go back and start a new beginning but anyone can start today and make a new ending.

(Robinson, 2011)

This chapter will demonstrate how health professionals in learning disability services have transformed their working practices and learned to adapt their skills over recent years to more effectively meet the needs of people with learning disabilities. The chapter shows how the health professional does not work in isolation of other health professionals and how, through a systematic process of care delivery, he/she ensures the person with learning disabilities receives the healthcare required. It will also provide some contextual background on the cultural shift and changes in how learning disability services are delivered in response to significant reports regarding access to healthcare services.

Case study 25.1   Jane's story

Jane is 45 years old, she used to live with both her parents until her mother died. Due to her father's ill health she then moved into 24-hour accommodation. Since her father's death, there is no other family involvement. Jane has now lived in her current home for the last five years with two other service users. Jane has mild/moderate learning disability and, other than epilepsy, has no other associated diagnosis.

Her epilepsy is now well controlled through medication, though due to her seizures in the past, she was required to wear a helmet, which she still chooses to wear. Jane's mobility has recently deteriorated, she now uses a wheelchair, but still assists with standing transfers.

Jane can have simple conversations with staff on topics that interest her. She attends day services but when there will often choose not to engage with other service users. Jane can be perceived as 'difficult to get on with'. She quite often shouts at other service users in the home who become upset. Jane is uncooperative in helping herself and as a consequence over recent months, she has become deskilled and increasingly more dependent on staff.

Jane's skin condition on her legs has deteriorated recently, to the degree that it is quite fragile and susceptible to damage and infections. She has had several episodes of cellulitis, (infection of the deep dermis of the skin caused by haemolytic streptococci which is a bacterial infection) and this has resulted in repeated hospital admissions.

Factors that influence changing roles

Why have the roles of healthcare professionals changed when working with people with learning disabilities? What influenced the need for these roles to change? And why does this affect the care that the health professional delivers on a daily basis? By exploring these key questions, healthcare professionals are able to identify the contributions and boundaries of their role within current healthcare delivery as well as considering what may influence future role change.

In the first half of the twentieth century people with learning disabilities were referred to as being 'mentally handicapped' and were largely forgotten by the wider society, while they lived in hospital institutions, sometimes for many years. A major turning point, the White Paper, *Better Services for the Mentally Handicapped* (DH and Social Security, 1971) proposed the idea of moving people with learning disabilities back into the community, thus eliminating block treatment and poor living conditions within a hospital setting. It was not until the 1980s and the Community Care Act (1990) that the major task was identified for the closure of mental handicap hospitals to enable people to live in their own homes wherever possible.

The closing of large institutions saw a significant shift in how healthcare services were provided to people with learning disabilities. The change of healthcare service delivery, along with healthcare policies, culture and attitudes, saw the balance start to shift from the healthcare professional 'doing to' to 'working alongside' people with learning disabilities. Thus, empowering people with learning disabilities in relation to decision-making around their own individual care.

The model for healthcare delivery now shifted towards a social model of care which put increasing emphasis on consumer involvement in healthcare and placed the individual at the centre of decisions regarding their care. Within learning disability services there was also a move from the professional silo approach of care delivery where care staff worked separately and physically apart from each other, to multi-disciplinary teams where care staff work alongside one another to form integrated healthcare teams. These fundamental shifts in delivery and culture have had a significant impact on the way in which healthcare professionals' roles, skills and knowledge have developed.

The concept of reasonable adjustments within mainstream health services made in order to encourage the use of community health and other resources is illustrated widely within this book. Special consideration needs to be made, however, especially for those with complex health needs. While such people have compounded difficulties, with reasonable adjustments made, their specific requirements can be met within mainstream society.

What is complex health?

There are many definitions, but, on the whole, there are some guiding key principles:

- People with complex needs may in their life span be confronted with any number of different issues that require interventions from health and/or social care.
- People with learning disabilities are recognised as a vulnerable group who may experience a combination of medical/health needs.
- On occasions the health need may require input delivered by specialist learning disability services both in the community and in hospital.

Complex health may be defined as a range of impairments based on severity and frequency of the health need. The range of impairments includes:

- mental health/mental disorder needs: such as, for example, dementia, autistic spectrum disorder, depression;
- challenging behaviour needs: such as, for example behaviours that may harm the individual or others and cause damage to the environment;
- physical health needs: these require advice/interventions in primary healthcare for people who have chronic conditions described as life-limiting or technology-dependent, e.g. tube feeding/ gastrostomy feeding, respiratory suctioning, complex epilepsy which requires holistic management from the multi-disciplinary team;
- sensory needs: such as, for example, hearing loss or visual impairments or sensory processing disorders which may manifest in someone experiencing problems in one or more of the sensory systems that may occur at any point in the sensory integration process. As a result, the individual may experience difficulties in producing adaptive responses in order to meet the demands of the physical and social environment in which they live.
- communication needs: including determining the appropriate type and level of communication support and intervention required.

The essential fundamental philosophy is that the learning disability health professional should be working proactively with service users to improve health where possible, or in the case of long-term or degenerative conditions, to slow the rate of deterioration and maintain health and function for as long as possible. By working in this way, healthcare services aim to reduce the risk of, or prevent service users entering into crisis – the most costly outcome both to the service in terms of finance and to the service user and their carers in terms of quality of life. Health maintenance cannot be underestimated, especially in people with learning disabilities who have chronic long-term conditions. It is key to the person's quality of life to prevent deterioration.

The role of a specialist learning disability health professional

This can be categorised into three areas:

- direct care delivery role;
- indirect care delivery role;
- consultative role.

The direct care role

The health professional directly delivers the treatment that is required. In the learning disability service, if a person is admitted to an inpatient assessment/treatment service with an acute episode, then the multi-disciplinary team would deliver the care directly. In the community setting, the different professions in the community learning disability teams commence the assessment, planning and delivery of treatment and care packages and may deliver this directly in the home setting, whether it is a family home or a care provider.

The indirect care role

Learning disability health professionals have seen a significant increase in the indirect care role over recent years. The health professional delivers care interventions through others, such as family carers and paid carers in provider organisations. Carers are able to spend more time with people with learning disabilities in a supportive capacity on a more regular basis than a health professional from community learning disability teams and are therefore an essential resource in the consistent and regular delivery of treatment programmes. From the community learning disability team perspective, professionals provide a range of community-based interventions by giving advice, training and support to family carers or care providers. Health professionals monitor the implementation of the care delivery and treatment to ensure that the health need that requires intervention is improving, stabilised or has reduced the risk of further health loss. The learning disability professional is very active in signposting and ensuring that the service user gains access to the most appropriate mainstream services to meet all their specific health requirements. The role of carers is crucial in recognising and monitoring and reporting ill health as well as implementing any necessary health treatment programmes.

The consultative role

The consultative role of the learning disability health professional is paramount. Its primary aim is to raise the skills and awareness of professionals who are not trained specifically to meet the needs of people with learning disabilities. Health professionals aim to educate, encourage, support and empower them to make 'reasonable adjustments' within their practice. This will enable them to have confidence to communicate, interact and include people with learning disabilities, thereby ensuring safe and equal access to healthcare for people with a learning disability. One benefit of this work is that mainstream healthcare professionals become less reliant on learning disability specialist services, thereby enabling the learning disability specialist to deliver care for people who have more complex needs.

Multi-disciplinary working

The concept of the multi-disciplinary team, including community learning disability teams, is not new in learning disability services. The structure and make-up of these community learning disability teams can differ but the principle remains that their primary aim is to deliver care and treatment to people with a learning disability within the community. Variations within team structure and team workings can be influenced by a number of factors, including the clinical need of the local population, the economic or financial position of the organisation, and the skills or knowledge of local services. Despite some idiosyncrasies which make teams and services unique, there are a number of shared fundamental aims including the delivery of direct care, treatment and interventions, the effective co-ordination of care delivery, liaison and partnership working with other services. One of the key roles and functions of the community learning disability team is to support collaborative working. The intricacies of inter-professional working are detailed in Chapter 24, however, for discussion here, specifically concerning working relations when working with people with complex needs, some points must be explicitly emphasised. A team may share an organisational identity and culture, however, if the roles of each professional within the team are not correctly understood and acknowledged, then problems can arise. Macadam and Roger (1997, p. 194) identified this issue, and stated that healthcare professionals:

> are trained to practice distinctive skills, which can be important to their status and identity. If these skills are not recognised, or if they overlap with the expertise of another professional then conflicts can result . . . the skills and roles of each professional need to be known to everyone concerned, and equally valued.

In considering the changing roles of healthcare professionals in meeting the needs of people with a learning disablity, it is important to consider the impact of these roles. They must be clearly communicated, not just to the service user and their carers, but also within the team and its members. Failure to do so can have significant impact on the type and quality of services delivered. Mathias and Thompson (2001) recognised the importance of multi-disciplinary teams in providing an example in which multi-professional care is not just confined to the learning disability specialists but also within mainstream services.

Structured approach of care delivery for meeting the needs of people with a learning disablity

As the previous section outlined the merits of multi-disciplinary integrated teams, it is important for the health professionals to have a co-ordinated structured approach to deliver a service.

Practice alert 25.1

The following four-part approach is essential in ensuring the comprehensive and effective delivery of high quality care:

- Assessment
- Formulation
- Care Intervention/Treatment
- Review/evaluation of the episode of care from referral to discharge.

The case study will be used to illustrate this structured approach in practice and will also demonstrate the role of health professionals working with people with learning disabilities and the function of the community learning disability team.

Assessment

For people with complex needs, assessment is the cornerstone to ascertaining the essential information pertaining to the individual's current and historical needs. A good assessment is vitally important and should not be rushed, not should corners be cut, as thoroughness is needed in order to ensure all needs have been identied. This information enables the health professional to fully understand the individual's requirements. The assessment involves carers and significant people involved in the individual's life, but it is also important also to ascertain what the person with a learning disability feels are their own needs. All this information is invaluable in creating a picture of the person's quality of life in relation to health needs. Assessments can take place in a variety of settings, for example, in the service user's own home, their day activity centre, and so on. Due to the complex needs of people with learning disabilities, Vlaskamp (2005) stated that large numbers of different disciplines need to be involved in assessment to ensure the best interventions and support are offered.

Each discipline is trained differently so they will offer a different perspective on what is required for the service user's care package. Vlaskamp also highlighted that assessment should be looked at as a process rather than a set rigid procedure. This cannot be over-emphasised as the care that is delivered requires continual evaluation and re-assessment.

Jane was referred to the community learning disability team by the general hospital physiotherapist. The physiotherapist identified that Jane required continued rehabilitation for her mobility following repeated admissions for cellulitis.

Based on the information received so far, which discipline/s do you consider appropriate to be involved in the initial assessment?

Case study 25.2   Jane's initial assessment

The physiotherapist visited Jane in her home. The purpose of the visit was to gather information on Jane's current presenting needs in order to determine what appropriate actions or interventions should be taken and by whom. The usual method for a physiotherapy assessment includes the 'hands on' physical assessment of the individual which may involve: observing the person mobilising and transferring, for example, moving from sitting in a chair to a standing position. Jane would not respond or tolerate physical prompts to engage in a 'hands on' assessment and would only tolerate minimal physical touch. She was non-compliant with verbal instructions and attempts to engage her in the assessment process doing this intial stage of the assessment failed. The physiotherapist needed therefore to identify alternative methods for collecting the assessment information required to accurately identify Jane's needs. On observation, however, the following information was noted:

- Jane's wheelchair was a poor fit and did not have any elevating foot rests that would have supported the elevation of her legs. These are needed in order to help reduce her lower leg oedema.
- As well as poor skin condition on Jane's legs, the physiotherapist also noted tissue viability concerns on Jane's buttocks and lower back, her skin condition was compounded by her nocturnal urinary incontinence.
- Jane's feet and lower legs where swollen and ulcerated as a result of her infected cellulitis and lack of mobility. Her legs were heavily bandaged causing her to be unable to wear shoes.

The physiotherapist liaised with Jane's support staff and gathered the following additional information:

- Jane's mobility had significantly reduced over the last year.
- Jane sits in her wheelchair all day and refuses to sit in an armchair.
- Support staff were experiencing difficulty in encouraging Jane to elevate her legs.
- Jane spent prolonged periods within the house which support staff felt was affecting her mood.
- As part of Jane's treatment for cellulitis, she had been prescribed diuretics, which contributed to her becoming incontinent at night.
- Support staff reported that she had difficulties transferring out of bed at night and would become verbally and racially abusive to staff when they made attempts to meet her personal care needs. This behaviour was disturbing other service users' sleep.

(continued)

(continued)

- Support staff reported a slow and steady deterioration of Jane's activities of daily living, particularly at mealtimes as Jane was unable to sit at the table and had difficulty with her hand motor control. This was a particular issue when Jane was trying to feed herself.
- Support staff reported that Jane was not prescribed any pain-relief medication.

Reader activity 25.2   Any additional information?

From the initial assessment information above, summarise what you feel are Jane's needs:

- Does this initial assessment provide you with enough information?
- Do you need additional information, if so what information do you need?
- Are there questions that remain unanswered from the initial assessment?
- How would you go about assessing this and collect further information?

The initial assessment did not provide all the information that the physiotherapist required to effectively begin to treat Jane. The physiotherapist recognised that she needed the skills and expertise of other members of the team to support her in completing a holistic assessment of Jane's needs specifically in relation to the following questions:

- How to better engage and communicate with Jane and gain her trust?
- Why was Jane not mobilising?
- What was contributing to Jane's verbal and racial abuse of support staff?
- What was Jane's capacity to understand her condition and the options for how these needs could be met?
- What was the root cause of Jane's incontinence?
- What was the root cause of Jane's skin integrity problems and cellulitis?

Practice alert 25.2

In order to elicit the above information the physiotherapist requested further assessments from:

- *Speech and language therapy*: to advise on how to present information to Jane in a way that she could understand, so as to support them to develop a trusting, therapeutic relationship with Jane as well as to support Jane to engage in treatment and interventions.

- *Learning disability nursing*:

  - to provide care co-ordination and liaise with all disciplines involved in Jane's care, including mainstream services such as district nurses, continence nurses and tissue viability nurses;
  - to complete a behavioural assessment and develop a behavioural management plan.

- *Psychology*:

  - to complete a capacity assessment to ascertain if Jane could understand her condition and options for how these needs could be met.
  - To provide advice regarding behaviour.
- *Occupational therapy*: to complete a functional assessment regarding eating and drinking.
- *GP*: referral for appropriate regular analgesia for pain relief.

Formulation

Although there is no universally agreed definition for the term 'formulation', Johnstone (Johnstone and Dallos, 2006, p. 1) describes formulation as a way in which '[to] synthesize information and explanatory ideas into working hypotheses which are then used to suggest appropriate and effective ways of working to relieve problems'. From this definition it can be seen that formulation helps the healthcare professional to establish a hypothesis or set of hypotheses about an individual's needs and the risks that arise as a result of these needs. More specifically, a formulation draws on theory and professional frameworks and uses information gained from a range of assessment data to provide a hypothesis that helps the healthcare professional to understand:

- the causes of the individual's needs;
- what precipitates these needs;
- the factors that prevent these needs from occurring;
- the factors that are protective for the individual.

Formulation provides the healthcare professional and clinical teams with a guide for determining clinical interventions that identify effective ways of working with the individual to address their needs. Formulations are not static, they evolve and develop in line with the changing needs of the individual and as more information is gained. They require regular review and evaluation to ensure that they continue to accurately reflect the individual's needs and their current circumstances and presentation.

Reader activity 25.3   Formulation

Using the assessment information provided, formulate Jane's needs by considering the following:

- List Jane's needs.
- What do you feel are the causes of Jane's needs?

- What do you think made Jane vulnerable in the first place?
- What could be potential triggers for the most recent problems?
- Are there any factors that are making things worse?
- Are there any factors that are maintaining these needs for Jane?
- Using the answers that you gave for the above questions, begin to formulate a plan of action to meet Jane's needs.

Table 25.1 summarises the hypothesis that the team formulated for Jane's main presenting needs. Perhaps you can identify others.

Care intervention/treatment

From formulation and having a structured plan of action, whether under the framework of Care Programme Approach, or a written treatment/care plan, the health professional can then implement the plan.

The interventions will take the form of one or more of the three roles outlined earlier in the chapter, either direct care delivery, indirect through the individual's carer support network, or consultative work. The health professional will consider time schedules and outcomes for the different aspects of care interventions estimating when the episode of care may be completed. The written care plan provides instructions for all staff responsible for the person's care package, giving guidance on how best to meet the identified health need. This ensures continuity of care especially in supported living environments, where there may be more than one carer delivering the person's package of care.

When considering care interventions and evaluating the care package, the health professional needs to know when goals are achieved. There are a host of outcome measures that health professionals can use which have either been developed by their own profession or tools that are specific to a unique health condition or diagnosis. What is important is that the outcome measure should be relevant, validated and reliable. Many learning disability services will adopt specific outcome measurement tools to monitor care under their respective clinical governance frameworks. Outcome measures are taken at the start of care to gain a baseline picture before care interventions take place and at the end of the episode of care to establish what has been the health benefit. On longer treatment schedules it would also be appropriate to have an intermittent measurement to review if progress is being made.

Reader activity 25.4 The care plan

- How would you begin to plan the care required to meet Jane's needs?
- How would you engage Jane in this process?
- What other actions would you take to make this plan of care as successful as possible?
- From your care plan, consider the roles of the health professionals, are they carrying out a direct, indirect or consultative role?

Table 25.1 Formulation of Jane's needs

	Cellulitis	Low mood	Challenging behaviour
Causes	Factors that may have impacted on Jane developing and continuing to suffer from cellulitis may include: • Lack of mobility which is compounded by the dressings on Jane's lower limbs. • Jane's poor compliance with treatment programme has affected her rehabilitation progress. • Jane's poor compliance with leg elevation to reduce the oedema.	Factors that may impact on Jane experiencing low mood may include: • Pain. • The vulnerability of Jane's skin integrity and the risk that further skin damage may result in a further infection has led to social isolation. As she was unable to access her usual activities in her community this contributed to her low mood which led to her becoming withdrawn in her home.	Factors that may have impacted on Jane having behaviours that challenge: • Pain. • Poor therapeutic relationships with staff not having the skills to communicate and understand Jane's needs. • Jane may be experiencing anxiety through lack of understanding of her condition & treatment package.
Precipitants	Factors that may give rise to these issues occurring may include: • Jane may be experiencing pain which will affect her motivation to engage in her treatment programme. • Lower leg oedema makes it difficult for Jane to mobilise, Jane's urinary incontinence is exacerbating her tissue viability risk which increases the likelihood of further infection. • Jane is spending long periods sat in her wheelchair, reluctant to sit in other chairs affecting her ability to elevate her legs.	Factors that may give rise to these issues include: • Continued non-compliance with treatment programmes resulting in the risk of developing further infection leading to increased isolation. • Poor management of pain.	Factors that may give rise to these issues include: • Support staff lack the skills and knowledge to know how to communicate and appropriately support Jane. • Repeated occurrence of cellulitis and poor tissue viability leading to pain. • Jane's capacity to understand her treatment programme.

(continued)

Table 25.1 *(Continued)*

	Cellulitis	Low mood	Challenging behaviour
Protective	Factors that may protect Jane from these issues arising may include: • Jane has trained support staff that can monitor and support her health needs and treatment programmes. • Jane has active engagement from mainstream services (e.g. district nursing) and specialist health, Learning Disability services, both of which are working in partnership to address Jane's health needs.	Factors that may protect Jane from these issues arising may include: • Jane has access to 24-hour support staff. In addition Jane's care package is monitored by CLDT Inc psychiatry. • Jane lives with other people, although her motivation to engage with them is much reduced, they are around should Jane choose to engage.	Factors that may protect Jane from these issues include: • Support staff are motivated to being trained on how to effectively work with Jane, to understand how Jane's needs affect her behaviour. • Training is available through the Community Learning Disability Team.
Maintenance	Factors that may continue to maintain the above issues for Jane: • No access to appropriate equipment to support her health needs. • Jane's continued non-compliance with her treatment programme. • Support staff have ineffective engagement and communication techniques that are necessary to motivate, encourage, support, understand and communicate with Jane. • Support staff lack the skills, knowledge and confidence to effectively support Jane and deliver her treatment programme.	Factors that may continue to maintain the above issues for Jane : • No access to appropriate equipment. • Repeated infections and poor skin integrity. • Absence of an appropriate care package.	Factors that may continue to maintain the above issues for Jane: • Lack of understanding of Jane's needs. • Staff intolerance negative perceptions and attitudes towards supporting and understanding Jane. • No training available to develop support staff's skills and understanding.

The team used the Therapy Outcome Measures (TOMs) tool (Enderby *et al.*, 2006). It is a cross-disciplinary method of gathering information on a broad spectrum of issues and was developed to provide a practical method of measuring outcomes in routine clinical practice. The following healthcare professionals worked simultaneously to meet Jane's needs each considering outcome measures to determine the success of their interventions.

Speech and Language Therapy (SandLT)

A one-to-one assessment was completed with Jane. The assessment identified that Jane had a difficulty understanding higher-level aspects of language and her verbal reasoning skills were poor. Jane also had difficulties retaining information. She responded well to visual aids and praise and encouragement, so staff were encouraged to communicate with her in a positive manner and used praise where necessary.

A training session was held by the SandLT therapist; its aim was to inform all those involved how to engage with her and to give general advice regarding the need to follow instructions. The aim for this intervention was to ensure a consistent approach when communicating with Jane in order to meet her health needs. This included the use of pictures for Jane, and for staff, written communication and monitoring charts to record times when Jane had been able to follow advice. Staff were encouraged to remind Jane of treatment advice by referring her back to the visual aids.

This assessment information was essential; it ensured the efficient and effective success of subsequent interventions. Without effective communication, healthcare professionals might struggle to develop therapeutic relationships with Jane and secure her engagement, and co-operation with subsequent treatment delivery. It also ensured that Jane remained at the centre of all planned care and afforded her greater involvement.

Physiotherapy

The moving and handling assessment ascertained some contributory factors for Jane's decreased mobility. There was a reduction in Jane's mobility due to swelling of her feet and legs, which were very painful on weight bearing. This also led to weight gain. Jane's seating and wheelchair were therefore no longer suitable. The following actions therefore followed:

- A new wider wheelchair with elevating foot plates was acquired to support Jane in elevating her legs.
- A rise and recline chair was recommended and provided to support Jane with sitting comfortably when out of her wheelchair. The chair was functional for two reasons, it assisted to make transfers easier and to elevate her legs to reduce the oedema.
- The doorway into Jane's bedroom was widened to accommodate her new wider self-propelling wheelchair, so maintaining her independence at home.
- The GP prescribed appropriate analgesia for Jane's pain.
- Staff were shown how to assist Jane to complete safe standing transfers. These specific moving and handling techniques were necessary in order to maintain her current skin integrity.

Occupational therapy

Jane was unable to sit at the dining table to eat her meals, as the existing table did not accommodate her wheelchair. This was affecting social interaction with other service users and staff at mealtimes. Through an observation, assessment was made that Jane had hand tremors that made fine motor control and grip difficult. The tremor prevented the successful manipulation of utensils while eating her meals. The outcome of the occupational therapist's assessment was:

- Large grip adaptive cutlery was provided.
- The provision of built–up plates and matting to secure crockery while Jane ate. This not only helped avoiding plates slipping off the table but helped Jane conserve energy as she wasn't 'chasing' the food round the plate.
- A more appropriate table was acquired to accommodate Jane's wheelchair.

All the above encouraged Jane to maintain her independence while eating and drinking, and supported her social inclusion at mealtimes.

Psychology

The psychologist spent time observing and assessing Jane's interactions and behaviours to enable the completion of a capacity assessment. The assessment ascertained that Jane did not have the capacity to understand the complexities of her treatment package and the implications of her non-engagement. In particular, she was found not to understand the importance of elevating her legs during the day, a procedure needed to increase lymphatic drainage, thus helping to decrease the amount of urine passed at night. This was crucial in order to ensure Jane had undisturbed sleep. Importantly less urine production would also improve the skin condition to her buttocks and groin area, so improving her skin integrity and reducing pain.

The support staff were asked by the psychologist to complete behavioural monitoring forms for behaviour analysis. The analysis aimed to understand the reasons for her behaviour and what the behaviour communicated. This enabled the psychologist to ascertain if the staff understood Jane's communication patterns. This information was essential for the development of the behavioural management plan that was required to improve Jane's compliance with health interventions.

Nursing

A behavioural assessment was completed with support staff in conjunction with the psychologist's observations and analysis. At this point consideration was given to the outcome of the capacity assessment. The nurse wished to improve Jane's quality of life and promote her health and well-being. It was clear that Jane did not have the capacity to consent to some aspects of her care treatment. A Best Interest meeting was therefore convened by the nurse because Jane lacked capacity for certain decisions. As highlighted by the DH (2001, p.12), the meeting was to ensure that 'Ideally decisions should be made which both those close to the person and the healthcare team agree are in the best interests.'

Health professionals and support staff met to discuss and agree aspects of care delivery. The care package and behavioural plan were discussed to gain consensus and to check this was in Jane's best interest. The behavioural plan was written and explained to support staff with clear instructions on how to implement it, using the communication methods of engagement recommended by SandLT. This was to reduce the verbal and racial abuse towards staff and encourage greater compliance and engagement from Jane.

A care plan was devised to encourage Jane to sit with her feet raised for set periods several times a day. The staff were asked to complete a monitoring form to record, where Jane sat and to note if Jane had co-operated with her feet being elevated. The nurse took on the role of care co-ordinator under the framework of Care Programme Approach (CPA). This framework was felt to be essential as Jane had a number of significant health needs which required many professionals. The role of the CPA incorporates monitoring the care and liaising with all professionals to ensure that they are fulfilling the requirements of the package of care. The care co-ordinator also ensures the individual is fully involved and the care package delivered is person-centred.

The nurse liaised with the primary care continence nurse who prescribed new continence pads which were larger and more absorbent than her previous ones. The aim was to reduce the need to transfer Jane out of bed at night, due to the need to change soiled bed linen which subsequently disturbed her sleep pattern. The pads also would be of benefit as they reduced the risk of further skin infections and concerns with tissue viability.

The learning disability nurse liaised with the tissue viability nurse and the district nurse. Their advice and recommendations about the management of the skin on Jane's feet and lower limbs were incorporated into the care plan. The nurse liaised with Jane's GP and psychiatrist regarding a review of medication for pain relief, for suspected depression and made some enquiries about Jane's hand tremors. Jane was prescribed appropriate pain relief with a proactive schedule of administration. At this point it was felt inappropriate to prescribe an anti-depressant, but the nurse was asked to continue monitoring Jane's mood. The GP made a referral to neurology regarding the tremors.

Given the presenting health needs, as the care co-ordinator, the nurse considered the need to review Jane's care with the Adult Social Care Management team to determine if the current support package was appropriate.

Reader activity 25.5   Professional roles

Reflecting on the information above, identify for each profession what role they undertook with their interventions:

- Direct
- Indirect
- Consultative.

Much of the care that was provided was 'hands on' care. The psychologist directly observed Jane's interaction with the support staff and the community learning disability team in order to understand Jane better. This helped to inform the staff how to enable Jane to have more control over her care interventions. This was done in conjunction with the SandLT who also demonstrated appropriate communication strategies. The physiotherapist and occupational therapist advised on the purchase of new equipment and demonstrated the safe and appropriate use of them.

Other care was more indirect, for example, the behavioural management plan was developed by the nurse in collaboration with other members of the multi-disciplinary team. This was delivered by the support staff in Jane's home on a day-to-day basis. The health aspects were also being delivered indirectly on behalf of the community learning disability team. The health professionals need to regularly monitor and review the care package. This is done in a variety of ways; by analysing the monitoring forms provided by direct care staff, through direct observation, and by gaining feedback from Jane and the staff involved in her care. Health staff played an essential consultative role in instructing the support staff in the home. They consulted with social care staff through 'hands on' demonstrations, but provided rationale for the interventions and educative advice on the importance of the care being offered. This helped the staff to achieve a better understanding of the care delivery, leading to a more successful outcome

Review and evaluation

Reviewing the care interventions is aimed at ensuring that the treatment and intervention have worked and that there is health gain or health maintenance.

Reviews should be conducted at regular intervals, focusing on changes in need. If the care package is not effective, the health professional needs to re-formulate. This may require re-assessment, while reviewing the care to see if it has been consistently delivered and identifying factors that may have hampered the expected health outcomes. If the individual has experienced a problematic complex health need over a long period of time, it may be that the changes in their health status are less obvious or improvement is slower, and if this is the case, timescale adjustments may be required.

Reader activity 25.6   Outcomes

Consider what outcomes you would like to see if you were the care co-ordinator to demonstrate the care package has been successful.

As a result of the implementation of the multi-disciplinary team care plans the following outcomes were achieved:

- Jane became increasingly more tolerant and compliant with hoisting. This, along with the provision of appropriate continence aids, reduced the impact of Jane's urinary incontinence on her tissue viability and skin integrity. Jane's increased tolerance towards hoisting meant that there was a reduction in the challenging behaviours that she exhibited, reducing disturbance to other people within Jane's home.
- Jane now safely completes safe standing transfers with staff and spends increasing amounts of time out of her wheelchair. She sits in her armchair in the lounge, resulting in her spending less time

isolated in her bedroom, thereby increasing her opportunity to socialise with the people she lives with.

- Jane now elevates her legs, thus reducing her lower leg oedema. This supported Jane in reducing her risk of developing cellulitis. Six months after this care package was developed, Jane has still had no re-occurrence of cellulitis and has not been admitted to the general hospital.
- Jane's tissue viability risks has reduced and she no longer has any skin integrity issues or pressure sores on her lower back, buttocks or lower limbs. This has reduced the amount of pain and discomfort that Jane is experiencing. The reduction in pain and risk of infection means that Jane had now greater opportunity to leave her home and engage in a wider variety of activities within her local community. This had a positive impact on her mood.
- Jane's relationships with the staff and the other residents have improved. The staff provided examples of Jane engaging more with other people and described a reduction in the amount of time that she wished to spend in her bedroom. The staff also reported an increase in Jane's motivation to engage in more activities which was another indication of her change of mood.
- It was evidenced through the monitoring charts that there was a reduction in Jane's verbal abuse.

One of the key factors of success for this care package was the integrated and multi-disciplinary approach and partnership working.

The role of the multi-disciplinary team for people with a learning disability in the future

The largest shift of roles for learning disability health professionals in the last 20 years, as highlighted earlier, is from that of custodian in institutions, to empowerment of the service user primarily in the community. The learning disability health professional has developed an educative and advisory role, advising other agencies on how the needs for people with a learning disability may be best met. It is envisaged that equally dramatic changes could take place in the next 5–10 years as the health needs of people with a learning disability evolve further and cultural attitudes change. Emerson and Hatton (2008) acknowledged the difficulty of planning services for people with a learning disability as there are no accurate records of the number of people with learning disabilities in England. However, based on current prevalence and incidence rates of the population of England predicted to rise, it may be assumed that the numbers of people with a learning disability will equally increase. Emerson and Hatton argued there are factors which are likely to lead to an increase in the prevalence rates for individuals with learning disabilities in England over the next two decades, these include:

1. Increase in survival rates among young people with severe and complex disabilities.
2. Reduced mortality among older adults with learning disabilities.

DH (2009) estimated 65,000 children and 145,000 English adults have a severe/profound learning disability, and 1.2 million English adults have a mild/moderate learning disability. Factors which may lead to a change in incidence and prevalence include:

- access and uptake of screening and selective termination of pregnancy;
- increased life expectancy;
- access and uptake of interventions that may prevent learning disability, e.g. gene therapy.

For effective management of need, resources should be matched against predicted prevalence rates. A failure to increase professional recruitment where necessary would result in the learning disability health professionals being too stretched to deliver services effectively. This could result in the needs of people with a learning disability being unmet. Effective managers, however, in the meantime might review learning disability health professionals' roles, again, encouraging their creativity, using the skills professionals have in more effective ways. This, however, should never be done at the detriment of client care.

Relevant government policies and reports continue to be the driving force in changing and developing learning disability services. Similarly, ongoing exposure by the media of shocking and neglectful practices continue to work as a spur to improving services. It remains the case that healthcare professionals need support and encouragement to make reasonable adjustments for patients with learning disabilities. This is where community learning disability teams, in their consultative role, are in a strong position to work in partnership with mainstream health services, encouraging the facilitation and monitoring of health needs for people with learning disabilities, thus ensuring parity of service to those without a learning disability.

The Parliamentary and Health Services Ombudsman's report (2009, p. 3) illustrated: 'Some significant and distressing failures in service across both health and social care, leading to situations in which people with learning disabilities experienced prolonged suffering and inappropriate care.' The inspectorates are a driving force for inproving care. The Care Quality Commission continue to highlight failings as a result of care not being person-centred, where the person was fitted into services rather than services being tailored to meet individual needs. Community care continues to be recommended in place of institutional long-term care. It is envisaged that the Ombudsman's report, which raises issues around future commissioning requirements, will lead to greater prominence being placed on specialist community learning disability teams. This enables people with a learning disability to receive services that supports their place with the home and community environment.

The CQC Report (2012) and major national campaigners such as Mencap continue to evidence that we are still not adequately meeting the needs of people with learning disabilities. The Health and Social Care Act (2012), which emerged as a result of national debates and controversy, is one of the biggest influences on contemporary health services and focuses on a key policy shift towards clinically-led commissioning: 'Clinical commissioners have a crucial role to play in ensuring that care is integrated and delivered in the community with maximum input of local people and patients' (Health and Social Care Act 2012 Fact sheet B1, p. 1).

Fast facts 25.1 Clinical Commissioning groups

Clinical Commissioning groups (CCGs) will reflect the wider involvement of health professionals other than GPs in NHS decision-making. The key responsibilities of the NHS Commissioning Board and CCGs are to directly help reduce health inequalities and to promote better integration of health services within health and social care. In addition, Health and

Wellbeing Boards are to be established by local authorities. The purposes of these boards are to bring everyone together to work in an integrated manner, 'to encourage health and care commissioners to work together to advance health and wellbeing of the people in its area' (Health and Social Care Act 2012 fact sheet C3, p. 1).

This does sound like good news for people with learning disabilities and similar vulnerable groups. CCGs are responsible for reducing inequalities between patients with respect to their ability to access health services and to ensure that better health outcomes are achieved.

Future debates on specialist services are required as mainstream health services strive to be more receptive and to make reasonable adjustments to support inclusion and equal access. This could mean different role expectations for the learning disability health professional, as is often the case, when organisational changes occur within the NHS. There continues to be anxieties within learning disability services that the powers that be do not understand the complexities of the learning disability population, and a greater uncertainty regarding how resources are allocated. Upholding the presence of people with a learning disability within community settings will encourage greater public and political understanding of their needs.

Reader activity 25.7 Understanding needs

What are the risks to the people with learning disabilities if CCGs do not understand the complexities of their needs?

It is vital that specialist learning disability services have good communication with the CCGs and with local Health and Wellbeing Boards in their area to ensure service specifications reflect local needs.

Conclusion

The case study demonstrates the importance and contribution of different health professional roles and the concept of multi-disciplinary team working. It is essential that the most appropriate package of care is delivered in order to meet the needs of the person with learning disabilities, thus encouraging them to lead a full active life within the community. Learning disability services have developed. The future, as in previous times, however, is still unclear. It is imperative that health professionals continue to be flexible in their roles. Future advancement is inevitable, by adapting roles it will be ensured that the specialist skills of learning disability professionals continue to be effectively used by the future population of people with learning disabilities. This chapter highlights the importance of community learning disability teams in having a pivotal role in co-ordinating more complex care packages and drawing together the expertise of different professions to deliver a person-centred, holistic and effective care package.

Point to remember

- The services offered to people with a learning disability must develop in order to meet the changing needs of the population and to reflect societal norms and influences.

Resources

Health Action Plans and Health Facilitation Good Practice Guide.
www.dh.gov.uk

Health and Social Care Act Explained. Fact sheets for an overview and the key policy areas in the Act.
www.dh.gov.uk

Person-centred approaches.
www.careuklearningdisabilities.com

Sensory integration
www.sensoryintegration.org.uk

References

Care Quality Commission (2012) *Learning Disability Services Inspection Programme: National Overview.* London: CQC.

DH and Social Security (1971) *Better Services for the Mentally Handicapped*, White Paper. London: HMSO.

DH (2001) *Seeking Consent: Working with People with Learning Disabilities.* London: HMSO.

DH (2009) *Valuing People Now: A New Three Year Strategy for People with Learning Disabilities.* London: HMSO.

Emerson, E. and Hatton, C. (2008) *People with Learning Disabilities in England.* Lancaster: Centre for Disability Research, Lancaster University. Available at: http://eprints.lancs.ac.uk/9515/1/CeDR_2008-1_People_with_Learning_Disabilities_in_England.pdf.

Enderby, P., Alexandra, J. and Petheram, B. (2006) *Therapy Outcome Measures for Rehabilitation Professionals*, 2nd edn. Chichester: John Wiley and Sons Ltd.

Johnstone, L. and Dallos, R. (2006) *Formulation in Psychology and Psychotherapy: Making Sense of People's Problems.* London: Routledge.

Macadam, M. and Roger, J. (1997) The multi-disciplinary and multi-agency approach, in J. O'Hara and A. Sperlinger (eds) *Adults with Learning Disabilities.* Chichester: John Wiley and Sons Ltd.

Mathias, P. and Thompson, T. (2001) Interprofessional and multiagency working, in J. Thompson and S. Pickering (eds) *Meeting the Health Needs of People Who Have a Learning Disability.* Edinburgh: Baillière Tindall.

NHS and Community Care Act (1990) London: HMSO.

Parliamentary and Health Services Ombudsman (2009) *Six Lives: The Provision of Public Services to People with Learning Disabilities. Part One :Overview and Summary Investigation Reports.* London: HMSO.

Robinson, M. (2011) The most inspiring quotes on change. Available at: http:exploreforayear.com (accessed April 2013).

Vlaskamp, C. (2005) In J. Hogg and A. Langa (eds) *Assessing Adults with Intellectual Disabilities.* Oxford: Blackwell and BPS.

26 Health promotion for people with a learning disability

Stacey Atkinson and Sheena Miller

Learning outcomes

After reading this chapter you will be able to:

- explore the concept of health
- understand what health promotion is
- consider how person-centred approaches enable effective health promotion activities
- appreciate the role of a therapeutic relationship with a person with a learning disability and how vital this is within health promotion work
- consider individualised programmes of health promotion for people with a learning disability.

Introduction

> The physical health and well-being of people with intellectual disabilities have not been promoted to the same extent as with non-disabled people. Internationally there is a growing recognition of the many health problems found among this population and the difficulties they experience in accessing appropriate health services. Their uptake of health screening is low and few health promotion campaigns are targeted at their needs.
>
> (Marshall *et al.*, 2003)

Consider this quote in relation to the lady you are about to meet and decide for yourself if it is ethical or right, what are you going to do about it?

Before reading this chapter and embarking on health promotion work, consider the following advice and adhere to it but don't let it deter you from health promotion work unless you are specifically advised by a health professional not to do it.

Practice alert 26.1   Health promotion programme

A word of warning: a health promotion programme should always be undertaken following collaboration with a doctor or health professional.

If you are worried about someone who has a learning disability, who is excessively overweight, is behaving erratically or appears unwell, always refer them to a healthcare professional.

Remember as clearly outlined in the Introduction of this book, there is a lot of research that tells us that people with a learning disability often suffer from undetected health problems. Your role in health promotion and in working to meet the needs of people with a learning disability will help to address this situation.

Health is a dynamic concept. A changeable, sometimes subjective perception that can mean different things to different people. At 16, health is something that enables us to perhaps to run in the school cross-country, dance all night long in the club, meet friends and shop till you drop! At 70, health enables us to perhaps socialise at the older person's club, take the dog for a short walk, and stay independent. For someone with a learning disability, depending on the person's developmental level, health will help the person to do some of the above that others do but also may enable a person to, for example, drive one's own motorised wheelchair, perhaps work on reception at the day centre, stay out of hospital having avoided yet another chest infection due to one's unusual body shape and to keep smiling!

Health isn't just physical and it is concerned with the interconnection of different influences such as social, psychological, intellectual and spiritual well-being. If someone has no social life, for example, they may be lonely, and this can impact upon their mental and psychological health. Mental ill-health, if untreated, can lead to isolation and depression. A depressed person may not self-care as they should and may not attend health appointments. In time physical well-being may be affected, a vicious circle.

This chapter will, with the use of a case study, explore further what health is and will consider how health can be promoted for Morag and other people with learning disabilities. Health promotion is a key role for health and social care professionals. This chapter will provide an overview of the key points in addressing health promotion for people with a learning disability, but it will not explore health promotion as a key concept in its own right. The authors recommend therefore that deeper exploration of health promotion as a concept is undertaken. Health promotion is something that research tells us is very beneficial for the client group but as the quote above shows, it often does not occur. It takes skill and careful consideration to promote health for someone with a learning disability. This chapter will address how the health needs of people with a learning disability can be effectively identified and promoted. We have discovered already that health is individual and due to its individuality, each person requires their health to be promoted in different ways. Hints and advice will be given on how best to promote health for people so that individual needs are met. The rest, the getting on with promoting health, from here on will then be up to you!

Case study 26.1   Morag's story

Morag is 45 and has a severe learning disability. She has Prader-Willi Syndrome (PWS) and lives with her sister. Morag is severely overweight and will, due to PWS, eat excessively, seemingly without the need to stop. She will also, given the opportunity, eat anything that is vaguely edible such as soap and soil.

Morag's sister Steph appreciates Morag's 'love of food' and will use it as a behavioural reinforcement; giving her Mars Bars for positive behaviour. At other times Steph tries to curb Morag's intake as she knows she is overweight. So the messages Morag receives about food are erratic. Morag's obsession with food has resulted in many quite violent behavioural outbursts. They have occurred when Steph has tried to prevent her eating. Her weight is now 21 stone (approximately 133 kgs), she is 5 feet 4 (162.56 cms). Morag's weight impacts on her health.

Reader activity 26.1   What is health?

What do you think health is and how would you define it?
What do you think are Morag's health needs? Don't forget the different dimensions of health (the physical, mental and social, etc. dimensions).

The World Health Organisation defined health in 1948 as 'a state of complete physical, mental and social well-being and not merely an absence of disease or infirmity.' The definition is felt to be so good it has not changed since 1948! It enables us to perceive health as a desirable commodity that can enable us to lead the lives that we as individuals choose.

Reader activity 26.2   Your own health

Consider your own life, what do you like to do that ill health might prevent you from doing?

Fast facts 26.1   Prader-Willi Syndrome

As discussed, Morag has Prader-Willi Syndrome (PWS). This is a rare, complex genetic disorder, present from birth and continues throughout life. In early life, poor muscle tone causes many problems, including not being able to eat well throughout infancy. In later life PWS causes those affected to have an untreatable, insatiable appetite, resulting in almost constant feelings of hunger, together with other physical and emotional symptoms (Prader-Willi Syndrome Association, 2013). Most people with PWS also have a learning disability. As

(continued)

(continued)

their lives continue, due to the desire to over-eat, if not addressed, people with PWS often can become excessively over-weight at which point they often also develop health problems associated with obesity.

The priority for Morag is for her to lose weight and her food must meet her nutritional, rather than behavioural or social needs. No one finds losing weight easy, but for Morag it is very difficult indeed. The symptoms of PWS cause her to crave food, she also like most of us, enjoys the physical pleasure of eating something tasty. She feels full but only for a short time, before another craving begins and this is of course, reinforces her need to eat. Food also has become a social reinforcement for positive behaviour and she associates having tasty treats as an indication that her sister is pleased with her. This is doubly reinforcing as we all like to know we are in favour, especially with the people we love and if food is an indication of this. Wow, for Morag, life doesn't get much better!

Health promotion for Morag will be concerned with what is important to her and her well-being, and what will improve her quality of life. Health promotion will be primarily concerned with her weight reduction and the maintenance of a healthier weight and lifestyle. Morag may not recognise at present that a reduction in her weight is in her best interests and, as discussed, due to the symptoms of PWS weight reduction will be difficult for her. Health promotion activities will therefore centre on teaching her and her family about the benefits of weight loss and will support the management of Morag's weight in ways that are accessible and meaningful to her.

Health promotion is:

A process of enabling people to increase control over and to improve their health. Health promotion represents a comprehensive social and political process, it not only embraces actions directed at strengthening the skills and capabilities of individuals, but also actions directed towards changing social, environmental and economic conditions so as to alleviate their impact on public, and individual health.

(WHO, 1998)

The above quote is interesting, as it highlights how health promotion is relevant for individuals, but it is also the concern of communities and it is a political issue. If someone is over-weight, then potentially this can lead to health service costs, should obesity-related illnesses occur. The health service is everyone's business, it is something shared by society yet its management and organisation are affected by political agendas. The distribution of health service resources often cause societal and political unrest. One person's illness can impact on other people, through our taxes we pay for each other's healthcare. Should the extreme happen and Morag becomes unwell, she will need more health resources to re-establish good health.

Reader activity 26.3   Inclusion

Consider the quote by Marshall, McConkey and Moore (2002) at the start of the chapter. It highlights the fact that many people with learning disabilities are not included in health promotion. What do you think would be the benefits if they were more included?

Many models of health promotion have been explored by other authors. You will meet these when you research this topic more comprehensively. For the purposes of this chapter, which is concerned with promoting the health of someone with a learning disability, person-centredness will be explored as a model to use in promoting the health of Morag. Assessments are needed in order to ensure a truly person-centred approach to care.

The role of assessment in health promotion work

The role of assessment has been discussed in other chapters. Chapter 24 outlines the role of assessment within a multi-disciplinary team when working with someone with complex needs. Some of the principles discussed there apply here, but when considering assessment in this context, the role of the assessment is to identify how best to do health promotion work with Morag and for this reason an in-depth knowledge of the person is required. Defined by Anderson in 1998, assessment is identification of the needs, preferences and abilities of a person. In all cases, if a holistic, more generalised and thorough assessment is used, more detailed information is obtained about a person's background, health status, cognitive understanding, personal goals and aspirations. Assessment is the means by which the practitioner gathers, organises and analyses information (Lloyd *et al.*, 2007), guiding the practitioner to greater understanding of the person's needs and perspectives. It is generally a health professional such as a learning disability nurse or physiotherapist, who would undertake a holistic assessment to meet the health needs of someone with a learning disability. The person with a learning disability is central to it and must be involved so their perspective is sought, and carers, either paid or family carers, also have a vital role in contributing to the assessment.

In Morag's case, the assessment should be used to gain:

- an overview of her holistic needs, in particular, the assessment should focus on providing a picture of Morag's present health needs and the ramifications of these needs;
- an appreciation of Morag's developmental needs. This is essential for health promotion work to be successful. Her level of learning disability should be understood with a detailed insight into how her disability impacts on her. It is important to comprehend Morag's communication needs, finding out both how Morag communicates and how others relate best to her. It is imperative also to discover how she learns best, her literacy levels and motivation for change will all have a bearing on her interest in the health promotion programme and indeed her ability to learn and advance from it.
- an insight into Morag's family situation. The dynamics within this situation and an overview of how they might assist with the health promotion activities.
- a précis of the resources, emotional, physical, and perhaps monetary resources required for the health promotion work. These may include family time to support the work, the energy levels of family members. Those members more involved in a daily caring role might have less energy available for educational activities. Other items are: the availability of healthy food and money

available for purchasing such foods, family members' understanding of the needs for the health promotion work and the need for the required resources. Other resources such as educational tools will be available through local health authority health education services.

There are many kinds of assessments available. The choice of which to use should be made by considering which best meets the needs of the person with whom you are working, which will be more focused towards the needs of that individual and will help you as a practitioner to learn the most about the person's present needs and their situation. While assessments are always necessary, the tools available may be sometimes felt to be restrictive or may be felt not to be sufficiently person-centred. If this is the case, sometimes it is just as valid to create something truly individual. An overview of some key assessments is given in Table 26.1. This list, however, is not exhaustive and merely shows the variety of holistic assessments available.

Table 26.1 Key assessments

Assessment	What is assessed	Uses
Roper, Logan and Tierney (2002)	This is principally a nursing assessment, but has uses within social care too. It provides a framework for assessing the 12 'activities of living' which are maintaining a safe environment, communicating, breathing, eating and drinking, eliminating, personal cleansing and dressing, controlling body temperature, mobilising, working and playing, expressing sexuality, sleeping and dying.	It is used to gather holistic information about a person's life and how they perform aspects of each activity. It has been criticised as having limited use for people with a learning disability as it does not cover social aspects such as community participation and housing (Brittle 2004) but these can be covered within the twelve activities if the person is assessed by a skilled, insightful practitioner.
Aldridge (2004)	The individual is assessed holistically with consideration of the person as a social being who interacts with society. Psychological aspects are covered. The model was designed for learning disability practice and pays attention to the ever changing needs of people with a learning disability.	Used for holistic assessment when a more learning disability focussed assessment is required and health promotion needed due to someone's learning disability and the impact of their health upon their daily living skills.
Maps and person-centred plans (see Figure 26.1)	Tools for person-centred planning. Planning and mapping focuses on what is important to the person and helps to develop the plans people wish to follow. Doing maps and plans with a shared understanding and mutual commitment to the action (Winney, 2012).	They are drawn with the service user so their motivation, cognitive understanding and communication needs can all be learnt whilst the maps and plans are being developed. Little or much information can be included; maps and plans can be revisited as they can be dynamic and ever-evolving.

One-page profiles See Figure 26.2	This is a way of collecting essential information about a person on one page. It could include likes and dislikes, strengths and talents, good day and bad day information and anything the person feels or wishes others to know about him	It is used as a communication tool to enable the individual to share his chosen information with those who support him in order to for them provide the best service possible.
Initial baseline assessments	Different assessments perhaps used locally in different health and social care environments which are matched to the needs of people with a learning disability. It provides a baseline or an outline of the person's needs	More in-depth assessments are often needed in addition to the baseline in order to gain further information regarding additional needs.

Further assessment tools should also be used to gather specific information specific to the person. For example the OK health checklist (Matthews and Hegarty, 1997) to review health needs, nutritional, sleep, continence, sexuality assessments and so forth used to gather information about a specific health or social care need.

Person-centred approaches within health promotion work

'Person-centred care' is the name given to a model of working with and supporting people with a learning disability that puts the emphasis on what each supported person wants in their lives. The White Paper for learning disabilities, *Valuing People*, tells us that a person–centred approach starts with the individual (not with services), and takes account of their wishes and aspirations (DH, 2001). So you can see it is a much bigger idea than traditional service provision. It is often referred to as Person-centred Planning; or PCP, to reflect the importance of finding out what someone wants and helping them to make it happen.

It might seem like common sense to work with people in a way that is meaningful to them; however, this has not always been the case. Sadly there is a long history of people with a learning

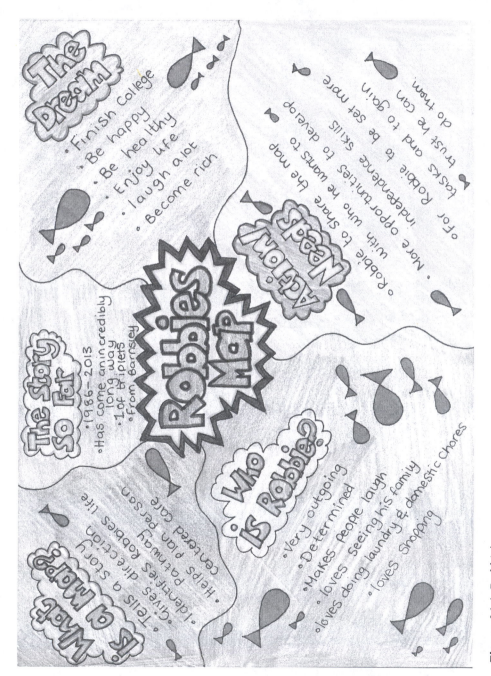

Figure 26.1 Robbie's map

Source: Lara Brewer (student learning disability nurse)

Morag's one page profile

Things people like and admire about me...

☺ Sociable
☺ Kind and caring
☺ I enjoy a joke
☺ Good swimmer
☺ Love animals

How to support me well...

① Help me to structure my day with plans and tell me ahead of any changes.
① Give me clear boundaries and guidelines.
① Keep food out of sight and don't eat in front of me.
① Stick to meal time routines.
① When I'm annoyed you can help me by keeping calm, helping me to laugh or focus on something else.
① Encourage me to be more active and move about more.

Things that are important to me...

✓ food
✓ my sister, Steph
✓ my friends
✓ people around me understanding my feelings about food and helping me with them
✓ Regular meals

Figure 26.2 Morag's one-page profile

disability being viewed very negatively by society, where they were, at best, seen as unimportant or a burden to their families and society and at worst, they were seen as mad, bad, deviant or dangerous. This history has been covered elsewhere in the book, but it would be helpful to review this now.

Person-centred planning has its roots in normalisation and social role valorisation; and these ideas, were about providing a normal everyday life and socially valued roles (Nirje, 1969; Wolfensberger, 1971). As these ideas developed and momentum grew, hospitals closed and services in the community began to increase, such as nursing and residential homes; day centres and training centres; and respite care. Initially, services focused on the goals that *they* should be achieving to demonstrate that they were providing care in keeping with the new values of normalisation and community care. One example is O'Brien and Lyle who developed a service model that was very influential in the 1980s and 1990s called the Five Service Accomplishments (O'Brien and Lyle, 1987). Of course, this model helped these new services to provide value-based support to people; however, it wasn't long before people began to recognise that truly valuing people with a learning disability meant that service-led care would have to give way.

O'Brien and Lyle, along with others, saw that a more meaningful approach should be used, where the person with a learning disability who needed support should be asked what kind of support they wanted, how it should be given, and who should give it. This was a radical shift in thinking and asked a fundamentally different question; from 'What can we offer' to 'What do you want?' It opened up a world of possibility for people who had previously had very limited access to life's opportunities, raising their aspirations. Person-centred approaches had arrived and they are still very relevant in health and social care work, including health promotion work with people with a learning disability today.

O'Brien and Lyle (1988) recommend five principles for person-centred planning:

1. The person is at the centre.
2. Family members and friends are full partners in planning.
3. The plan shows what is important to the person, both now and in the future:

    1. their strengths, gifts and talents;
    2. their rights and choices;
    3. identifying what support they need.

4. The plan helps the person to be a part of their community and helps the community to welcome and include them.
5. The plan is a promise by everyone involved to continually:

    1. listen;
    2. learn;
    3. make things happen.

Person-centred working is not without its challenges. It is easy to see that it is ethically the right thing to do, but practically there are often barriers such as communication, expectations and attitudes in the person themselves or in others around them such as family, paid staff and friends. Fortunately, however, there is much you can do to overcome these barriers.

So how could we work with Morag to develop a person-centred plan of health promotion work which takes account of her wishes, needs and aspirations? The first step is often to draw up a circle of support, which you have seen in Chapter 20. Building this circle with Morag helps her, and us, as facilitators, to see who is important in her life and invite them to be part of the planning process, if indeed that is what Morag wants.

It is important to note here that anyone can be Morag's person-centred planner; the essential point is that Morag should choose whom she wants to facilitate her plan. Some people in her life might have specialist skills and knowledge, or have better planning skills and be good at drawing up person-centred plans, but if Morag does not choose them to be her facilitator, then they are not the right person. Their expertise, however, should not be wasted, they can provide valuable support and advice and this would be an entirely appropriate way to use the knowledge and skills of the people in Morag's life. The only skill really necessary to be a person-centred planner is person-centred thinking (Sanderson and Smull, 2003) A student nurse for example drew up the map (Figure 26.1) for Robbie, a person she was working with.

Morag may already have a person-centred plan to address important issues in her life, so how could we, as health and social care practitioners, support Morag to address her health needs and make these a part of her PCP? In 2008, O'Brien famously said that without our health we cannot do the things that we want to do. This has been explored somewhat at the beginning of this chapter. It is vital therefore that health is integrated into PCPs. As we have heard, Morag's biggest health need is her obesity. As person-centred planning is about an attitude shift, it is worth remembering that we do not start with problems, we start with what is important to the person. In this case the health promotion work will commence by discovering how Morag feels about her weight and health promotion advice. This will ensure that Morag can make a fully informed choice about her lifestyle.

The therapeutic relationship within health promotion work

Sensitive personal discussions with service users require good communications skills and a client/practitioner relationship. The therapeutic relationship is vital and it is totally unique. It is based on 'trust, respect and the appropriate use of power. It is the means by which we can enter someone's world, a relationship which is based solely upon meeting the health and social care needs of the client' (UKCC, 1999). In other relationships you gain something for yourself, you may gain love, security or a sense of belonging. Within the therapeutic relationship, practitioners give more than they gain. You will gain a sense of positivity or pride in the fact that you are doing all you can for the person you are working with but the client is able to gain so much more. They benefit from the skills and caring arena you provide and by using your skills by being in the relationship, they are able, in collaboration with you, to develop their health or social care needs. The person-centred approach complements the therapeutic relationship. It also puts the person at the heart of care. Without a therapeutic relationship, health promotion work would be very difficult.

Carl Rogers, who was perhaps the founder of person-centredness within therapeutic relationships, said in 1961: 'If I can provide a certain type of relationship, the other person will discover within himself the capacity to use that relationship for growth and change and personal development will occur.' Therapeutic relationships are important in order for a person with a learning disability to develop through health promotion activities. The facets of this relationship as identified by Rogers are unconditional positive regard, empathy and genuineness.

- Unconditional positive regard is important within the relationship with Morag when promoting her health. She needs to be aware that there is an acceptance of her as a lady with specific needs and her needs should be considered when health promotion work is being delivered. If the health promoter was a practitioner who was judgemental or negative, he would have struggled to meet the needs of someone like Morag. There is no place for such negativity within a therapeutic relationship, and such traits are detrimental to progress.
- Empathy, defined often as 'walking in the shoes of someone else', is needed to gain a sense of how it feels from the other person's perspective. It aids a practitioner in gaining an understanding of another person's situation and encourages their flexibility and person-centred support during health promotion work.
- With genuineness comes honesty, closely followed by someone's trust. If the practitioner is genuine within their caring role, this encourages genuineness from those with whom they care. Such replicated honesty aids a mutual understanding whereby Morag, for example, would be able to honestly talk about her difficulties. Again, this relationship aids the health and social care role. Mutuality, or a mutual understanding of needs, can be gained through the development of genuineness. The practitioner and client are able to honestly discuss the direction and expectations of care, making mutually agreed plans and goals for how care will be developed.

Confidentiality is important within a therapeutic relationship. Being confidential about someone's needs communicates respect for the person with whom we are working. Their personal details should not be divulged without the expressed permission of the person him/herself. Confidentiality includes the prevention of:

- Unauthorised release of information about the person to other people.
- Discussions about people with others who are not involved in the person's care.
- Taking pictures/using photographs of the client without the client's consent.
- Data production about the client, without the client's consent (Arnold and Boggs, 2003).

The client must be given information about the reasons why an action is necessary, what the process will be and the potential outcomes of the action or process. All information should be communicated in an accessible format for that individual so their full understanding is gained and consent is informed.

The Mental Capacity Act (2007) is important within health promotion work, it provides guidance in relation to any actions which need to be taken when someone's capacity is questioned. In short, it is a practitioner's role, in the first instance, to always assume that Morag is able to give consent. If her capacity appears limited at any stage of the health promotion work, best interest decisions will need to be made by those best placed to make a person-centred decision for Morag. This should be done in a way that is respectful of Morag, so as not to damage the therapeutic relationship or the health promotion work. Presuming Morag's capacity in the first instance is beneficial to the development of the therapeutic relationship.

> ### Reader activity 26.4 Therapeutic relationship
>
> Why do you think that unconditional positive regard, empathy, genuineness and confidentiality are important within a therapeutic relationship?

Health promotion plans

By providing a care plan healthcare practitioners show what they intend to do both with and for the person with whom they are working. They create a visual representation of how work with a patient, client or service user will be delivered, in what time frame and specifically by whom, while identifying precisely what the goals will be. The care plan is, when drawn up with a service user and their family, often seen as a contract, which is viewed as being binding, both for the practitioner and the client. This is useful, as it encourages mutual commitment. The care plan provides details of how care will progress and as it shows intended outcomes. It gives some indication of when involvement will possibly end. If a practitioner is working with someone and liaising also with their staff team, when distributed, it ensures the team is aware of the intended care processes, so all have been provided with a consistent message and it encourages the staff team to work with the practitioner, all aiming and working towards the same outcomes, instead of perhaps acting in ways which are detrimental to care.

Reader activity 26.5   Care plan for Morag

Based on what you know about Morag and the need for her to lose weight, consider a plan which encourages her weight loss and weight maintenance. It should include:

- Long-term goals. How much weight will be lost over what length of time? Be realistic about the aims of the programme.
- Short-term plans on how to achieve the long-term goal.
- A plan of the strategies to be used.
- An indication of who will be involved and the role they will have.
- Details of how the programme will be evaluated, e.g. measurement of Morag's knowledge, weighing Morag every two weeks, etc.
- Details of any exercise/leisure programmes
- Anything else you feel is relevant, it's your programme!

This care plan feels like a very complicated thing to do, but it's worth doing. It encourages consistency and that is vital to the success of the programme!

Individualised health promotion and meeting Morag's needs

Health promotion for Morag will be involved ultimately in reducing her body mass and encouraging this reduction to be maintained. Educating Morag and the family about the health benefits of this weight loss programme is essential while looking at measures also to ensure weight reduction is reinforced. This all needs to done in an accessible manner for both Morag and her family.

Fast facts 26.3   Benefits of losing weight

The benefits of losing weight are that you lower the risk of:

- blood pressure or prevent high blood pressure.
- heart disease
- stroke
- type 2 diabetes
- some kinds of cancers
- infertility
- osteoporosis
- back pain
- depression

(NHS direct, 2013)

Someone with Prader-Willi Syndrome who is excessively overweight will be at risk of these health concerns.

Morag may not understand many of the health terms listed in the Fast facts box 27.2, but it is essential that both her and her family are aware of the risks of obesity. This is done by giving facts, leaflets, statistics, research data and very factual information, depending on their cognitive levels. The information given to Morag might need to be broken down and made much more accessible, the level it will be aimed at will depend on Morag's cognitive understanding and information about this is collected at the assessment stage.

Strategies for health promotion can be as wide as a practitioner's imagination. They may involve using a varying array of resources, but must be tailor-made for the individual. What works best may only be discovered through trial and error but there must be close monitoring of the progress made. As highlighted in Chapter 18, in the assessment of sexual awareness, here also a baseline assessment of what the person knows already might be helpful as it provides a picture of what knowledge needs to be given and can be used later when evaluating the health promotion work. Strategies for health promotion may include:

- Use of specific health resources designed for people with a learning disability. (See the resource list at the end of the chapter.)
- Role play
- Games
- Rhymes and songs
- Drawing, artwork or collages
- Use of magazines and books
- Use of video/audio recording
- The creation of wall posters
- Encouragement of healthy eating strategies reinforced by parents/carers
- Reinforcement of positive/healthy lifestyles
- Reward systems for reinforcement
- Exercise and leisure programmes
- Social stories (The National Autistic Society, 2013).

The list is endless!

Reader activity 26.6 Health promotion strategies

Can you think of other health promotion strategies which might be used for Morag or someone you know who has a learning disability?

Consistent reinforcement is essential, all family members and carers should reinforce the health promotion programme, by adhering to the plans made.

Morag has agreed that her community learning disability nurse, Omar, can help her develop a plan to address her weight. Morag and Omar draw a circle of support to find out who else Omar feels should be included and Morag wants her sister, Steph, to be involved. Omar talks to Morag and Steph about Prader-Willi Syndrome, the effect it has on Morag's life and her weight. Omar uses easy to read information on obesity, healthy lifestyles and nutrition from the local hospital to explain the health risks of being overweight. It is really helpful to have Steph on board as she is very influential in Morag's life, especially where food is concerned. Omar helps Morag to decide what her goal is and Morag thinks that she would like to be healthy so that she can dance. This goal is written down on a large sheet of paper.

This is a very practical starting point for Morag in her PCP journey. Omar helps her to develop this further by using his communication skills to talk to Morag and her sister about the kind of emotional and psychological support that Morag might need. They are developing a therapeutic relationship. Omar explains to Steph that supporting Morag might be difficult at times as her PWS makes her food cravings intensely difficult to resist. Omar supports Morag to tell her sister how she would like to be supported during these difficult times; and Omar makes suggestions based on his nursing knowledge about interventions that might help. Morag and Steph agree that Mars Bars are no longer a helpful reward and together they come up with the following ideas, which are recorded on the paper so that everyone can remember what they are:

- Making sure that Morag has available healthy snacks of her liking, for example:

  - fruit
  - vegetable sticks
  - yoghurt

- Finding distractions from the cravings:

  - watching the TV or a DVD
  - listening to music
  - having bubble baths

- Meeting her friends for support
- Meeting with the learning disability nurse regularly for weight monitoring, support and advice
- Getting regular exercise including:

  - swimming/aqua aerobics
  - dancing
  - a walk in the park.

Morag loves to dance, so this is included in her personalised health promotion plan. Omar asks Steph to find local dance groups and Morag tries some out. Another great idea is for Morag to go to a club night for people with learning disabilities. Here Morag may feel less vulnerable and more able to make new friends. Steph wonders if Morag might like aqua aerobics as this combines her love of dancing with swimming and exercise. You might have noticed that these ideas are very holistic in their nature and Morag's specific interests have been used. Through her interest in dance Morag will increase her chances for social contact and maybe friendships. Special relationships may develop, these will help to nurture and help her in the future. This in turn improves her likelihood of feeling good about herself and raising her self-esteem. A better self-concept might provide her with personal strength for the inevitable tough times in her journey. So, at the end of the meeting with Omar, Morag's plan looks like Figure 26.3.

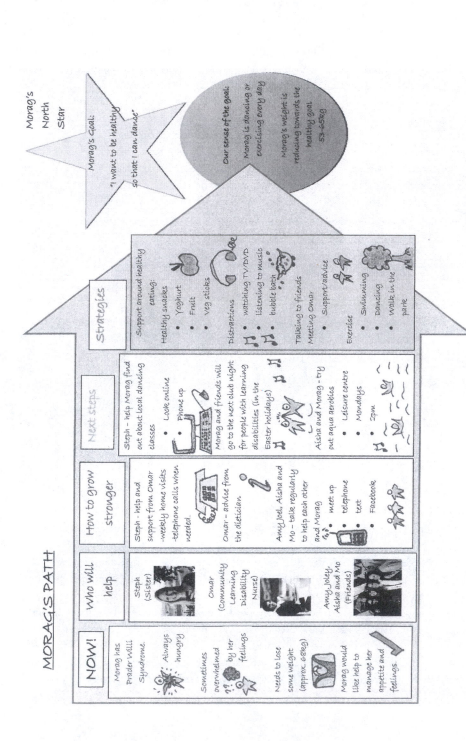

Figure 26.3 Morag's plan

A learning disability nurse assisted here with the development of health promotion work, other health or social care providers can also develop skills which enable effective health promotion work. Untrained staff must seek healthcare support. Working together with someone, such as a learning disability nurse, can raise a member of staff's skill base and together health promotion work can be achieved. As O'Brien (2008) stated in his summary of person-centred planning, the key skill needed in person-centred planning is to 'imagine better'. This is certainly the starting point for a better tomorrow.

Evaluation of health promotion work

Having a comprehensive assessment of the baseline and a detailed health promotion plan enables a practitioner to reflect more easily on the progress made. Intermediate or final results can be mapped against the client's original needs. If more detailed analysis has occurred, perhaps specific measurements were made about pain or symptoms, these measurements can be used and a reduction in symptoms or improvement in the condition can more accurately be ascertained.

Should improvement be slow or results not as expected, one must question if the health promotion plan was acceptable or sufficiently person-centred. The care plan may have been unrealistic, maybe steps were too large or goals difficult to achieve. Motivation may have not been accurately considered, cognitive levels or the individual's understanding may have been inaccurately assessed. Evaluation often leads to re-assessment (Hogston and Marjoram, 2007). This may be necessary if the outcomes are undesirable. This should not be seen as a failure. It perhaps shows the complexity of many health situations and therefore the need for more intricate assessments and implementation of plans of care. Discuss the progress in these circumstances again with other members of the multi-disciplinary team, so interprofessional collaboration occurs regarding how best to proceed. Progress in many cases is slow and this can cause the health needs of people with a learning disability to remain unmet for longer time spans, however, continued perseverance is the key to successful outcomes.

Conclusion

This chapter has explored how health and social care practitioners may undertake a health promotion role with someone with a learning disability. While it is a role which requires multi-professional, client and carer involvement, it has its challenges. The challenges in this area are perhaps the reason why previous health promotion work has been limited for people with a learning disability, one key challenge is knowing how best to do health promotion work with someone with a learning disability, approaches are detailed here. Systematic working, including thorough assessments, detailed care planning and meticulous attention to person-centred approaches can enable success. People with learning disabilities, carers and practitioners should celebrate successes when meeting the health needs of people with a learning disability.

Points to remember

- People with learning disabilities need accessible information which communicates how health and other needs are going to be met.
- They should direct the care they receive.
- On-going therapeutic relationships, skill and flexibility ensure the effectiveness of care.

Resources

This list is given as suggested reading only, and it shows the variety of resources and tools available. There are many more resources which might be useful to the specific health promotion work you are doing and the specific needs of the person you are working with.

Bellis K (2008) *A Healthy Mouth, Oral Healthcare for People with PMLD.* www.pmldnetworking.org/resources/Oral_healthcare_PMLD_factsheet.pdf

Welcome to easyhealth! A webpage with lots of health advice and resources for people with learning disabilities. There are health leaflets, videos, information on food and exercise. www.easyhealth.org.uk.

Supporting People with Learning Disabilities to Take Care of Their Breasts: A Guide for Supporters. With practical hints and help for supporting someone with breast care and examinations. www.breastcancercare.org.uk/upload/pdf/Guide_for_supporters.pdf.

Down's Syndrome Association and Down's Syndrome Scotland have lots of resources designed for people with learning disabilities to learn from, they cover topics such as diet, health and exercise, getting older, puberty, periods, menopause, keeping well, dementia.

Cancer Research UK has many books on cancer for people with learning disabilities in their 'Books Beyond Words' series. www.cancerresearchuk.org.

References

Aldridge, J. (2004) Intellectual disability nursing: a model for practice, in J. Turnbull (ed.) *Learning Disability Nursing.* Oxford: Blackwell Publishing.

Anderson, K.N. (ed.) (1998) *Mosby's Medical, Nursing and Allied Health Dictionary*, 5th edn. London: Mosby.

Arnold, E. and Underman Boggs, E. (2003) *Interpersonal relationship professional Communications Skills for Nurses.* Philadelphia. PA: Saunders Elsevier.

Brittle, R. (2004) Managing the needs of people who have a learning disability, *Nursing Times*, 100(10): 28–29.

DH (Department of Health) (2001) *Valuing People: A New Strategy for Learning Disability for the 21st Century.* London: HMSO.

Hogston, R. and Marjoram, B.A. (eds) (2007) *Foundations of Nursing Practice*, 3rd edn. Basingstoke: Palgrave Macmillan.

Lloyd, H., Hancock, H. and Campbell, S. (2007) *Vital Notes for Nurses: Principles of Care*. Oxford: Blackwell Publishing.

Marshall, D., McConkey, R. and Moore, G. (2003) Obesity in people with intellectual disabilities: the impact of nurse-led health screening and health promotion activities, *Journal of Advanced Nursing*, 41(2): 147–153.

Matthews, D. and Hegarty, J. (1997) The OK Health Checklist: a health assessment checklist for people with a learning disability, *British Journal of Learning Disabilities*, 25(4): 138–143.

Nirje, B. (1969) The normalization principle and its human management implications, in R. Kugel and W. Wolfensberger (eds) *Changing Patterns in Residential Services for the Mentally Retarded*. Washington, DC: President's Committee on Mental Retardation.

O'Brien, J. (2008) From progress to transformation: the contribution of person-centred planning. Lecture, Manchester.

O'Brien, J. and Lyle, C. (1987) *Framework for Accomplishment: A Workshop for People Delivering Services*. Lithonia, GA: Responsive Systems Associates.

O'Brien, J. and Lyle, C. (1988) *A Little Book about Person-Centred Planning*. Toronto: Inclusion Press.

Prader–Willi Syndrome Association UK (2013) Available at: http://www.pwsa.co.uk. (accessed July 2013).

Rogers, C. (1961) *On Becoming a Person*. Boston: Houghton. Mifflin.

Roper, N., Logan, W. and Tierney, A. (2002) *The Elements of Nursing*, 4th edn. Edinburgh: Churchill Livingstone.

Sanderson, H. and Smull, M. (2003) *Person-Centred Thinking and Planning*. Available at: http://www.helnsandersonassociates.co.uk. (accessed October 2013).

The National Autistic Society (2013) Social stories. Available at: www.autism.org.uk/living-with-autism/stratgies-and-appraoches/social-stories-and-comic-strip-conversation/how-to-write-a-social-story.aspx.

UKCC (1999) *Practitioner-Client Relationships and the Prevention of Abuse*. London: UKCC. Available at: www.nmc.org.uk.

WHO (World Health Organisation (1948) *International Health Conference*. New York: WHO.

WHO (World Health Organisation) (1998) *Ottowa Charter for Health Promotion*. Geneva: WHO.

Winney, F. (2012) *Factsheet Person-Centred Planning*. Care UK. Available at: www.careuklearningdisabilties (accessed September 2013).

Wolfensberger, W. (1971) *The Principles of Normalization in Human Services*. Toronto, National Institute of Mental Retardation.

27 Public health and learning disability

Alex McClimens

Learning outcomes

After reading this chapter you will be able to:

- understand public health and its relationship to learning disability
- deliver a public health agenda to individuals in care
- explain the history of the state's involvement in public healthcare.

Introduction

Those who cannot remember the past are condemned to repeat it.

(Santayana, 1905)

For our purposes, both public health and learning disability can be understood to have developed into a shape we recognise today in response to nineteenth-century medical science. As such, a fuller understanding of the connections between public health and learning disability needs to accommodate some appreciation of the economics, the history, the guiding philosophical influences and competing ideologies because these have had an impact on policies and practice today. The chapter will therefore begin with some explication of the background which clears the way for a later focus on the more practical and 'how to' aspects associated with delivering a public health agenda to the individuals in our care.

To do this I want to create a narrative that begins with reference to some well-known examples of nineteenth-century social engineering and end with an examination of contemporary approaches to public health. Between times the reader should refer to the case study. This should provide a reference point for the debate. Exercises occur throughout the chapter to assist understanding and prompt reflection.

If we accept that public health is defined by the twin concepts of universal access and early intervention and can therefore be summarised crudely as 'prevention is better than cure', then we must

Table 27.1   Official state responses to public health and learning disability issues in the nineteenth century

Public health issue	State concern	State response	Learning disability issue	State concern	State response
Cholera epidemics	Widespread illness and death in populations	Using scientific enquiry (e.g. 'germ theory' and antisepsis) Engineering works: J.Bazalgette building sewers Policies (e.g. 1848 Public Health Act)	Low intelligence	Moral panic at growing numbers Worry over the health of the population Concern that low intelligence is hereditary	Segregation Asylum building Establish colonies Eugenics–inspired policies

ask why it is that the state took a controlling interest in public health. If we know why that happened, it might give us a clue about why the state later took a controlling interest in learning disability too (Table 27.1). It is on that action and its consequences that we focus in the beginning of the next section. Later, as we approach the conclusion, the chapter will consider whether this state control is being eroded in favour of a more individual approach to maintaining public health and whether this is also reflected in the care of people with learning disability.

Case study 27.1   Yasmin's story

Meet Yasmin Akram. She is 16 and she lives in Rotherham, S. Yorks with her mum and two younger brothers in rented accommodation they share with their extended family. They are originally from the Kashmir region of Pakistan. Yasmin's grandfather came to the area in the late 1950s and got work in the local steel industry. Her father was born here and he married her mother as part of an arranged marriage.

Yasmin has Down's Syndrome and moderate/severe learning disability. She also has epilepsy. Due to an accident when on an outing with the day centre staff when she fell from climbing equipment, she also uses a walking frame to assist mobility.

Recently she has started to put on a lot of weight and she is being assessed by physiotherapists. They think she may need to use a wheelchair eventually. Her congenital heart disease (which is a common medical phenomenon for people with Down's Syndrome) means that she tires very easily and finds exercise difficult (Robertson *et al.*, 2010).

Yasmin understands English better than she can speak it. Her communication is mostly through the signs she makes up herself. Her family prefer her to be cared for in a way that reflects her Muslim faith.

At her most recent assessment a psychologist queried whether she may be exhibiting some autistic tendencies.

The choice of a young Pakistani/Kashmiri woman as a case study has two main reasons. We know from the literature that this ethnic group are more prone to exhibit certain health conditions (Emerson, 2009). We know too that the ethnic population with disability in the UK is growing and ageing (Parrot *et al.*, 2008). Taken together, this means that services must be prepared to meet the needs of groups and individuals who have different cultural and spiritual aspects to their lives, as well as presenting with some difficult health needs. These factors may well impact directly on the care provided in terms of the gender of carers, preparation of food and the timing of some events and practices. This will also affect the provision of short breaks and respite services (Buckner *et al.*, 2009). Depending on which part of the country you live in and work in, this may be a more or less pressing issue. But population projections suggest that all areas of the country will experience more ethnic diversity in their populations over the next generations (Wohland *et al.*, 2010).

As the chapter progresses, ask yourself how the topics discussed will impact on Yasmin, her care and her family.

Consider the information in Table 27.1. At the time of the cholera epidemic, learning disability and its causes were poorly understood. Early work on intelligence testing by Alfred Binet (1857–1911) was later used by eugenecists to 'prove' that low intelligence needed to be controlled by the same techniques that were applied to the public health management of disease. An extract from the Stanford–Binet manual suggests that intelligence testing could bring about 'the elimination of an enormous amount of crime, pauperism, and industrial inefficiency' (White, 2000: 7).

This might seem very reactionary today but in its own time it was a highly respected perspective. The disease metaphor is plain to see. And this is one of the reasons that learning disability populations today are sometimes cared for by nurses. It can be traced directly to the powerful influence of medicine in the nineteenth century and its part in combatting infection and so promoting public health. It also offers an answer to why the state wanted to control both public health initiatives and the shape of policy regarding those with low intelligence: the state was in both instances doing its duty by the people by protecting them from disease.

The current scene

Reader activity 27.1 Eugenics

Can you see any traces of eugenics in contemporary policies?

The 'Big Society' and 'nudge theory' are currently popular ways of addressing public health issues. How effective are these with the population of people with learning disabilty? What factors might influence their uptake?

People with learning disability generally live with poorer health status than the rest of the population. Why should this be? Can Health Action Plans improve this situation? Check out Howatson (2005) for a neat example of how these might work.

Reader activity 27.2 Universal healthcare for all?

In providing a health service for the population, the state has to consider the distribution of resources. Should the NHS attempt to provide universal healthcare for all, when all really means ALL?

- Make a list of groups in society you think absolutely should receive free healthcare. Now are there any groups who you think might reasonably be asked to pay for their healthcare?
- And are there any groups or individuals you think could or should be refused certain treatment or therapies?
- Why?

Reader activity 27.3 Cultural values

How much do you know about the cultural values of people from different ethnic backgrounds? Do you know what food groups Muslims avoid? What is the main religion of Chinese people? Are Travellers classed as a distinct sub-catgegory? What's the difference between being British and belonging to the UK?

If you have to administer medication to Yasmin which states that it needs to be taken every four hours *after food*, how do you do this during Ramadan? And, yes, you do need to know what Ramadan means.

Public health: what is it and where did it come from?

The work of McKeown (1976) is often cited as helping to explain the reduction in mortality during the eighteenth and nineteenth centuries. He argues, in crude summary, that it was largely through improved nutrition that the population prospered. And he was sceptical that medical intervention in the shape of public health initiatives could take much credit for the healthier population. He argued that better sanitation, for example, would have been effective only in curbing the spread of water- and food-borne diseases.

In the nineteenth century, cholera was thought to be an airborne disease. John Snow was a London doctor who thought otherwise. In 1853, he observed a pattern of deaths in his practice and he suggested to the local authority that they remove the pump handle from a particular well in Broad Street in Soho. They did so and the deaths from cholera soon stopped.

Sretzer takes up the story:

By dividing London into districts according to the different companies supplying water, the problem was narrowed down to the East London Waterworks Company, who were illegally supplying water from the Old Ford reservoir in Bethnal Green, which was contaminated by the recently completed West Ham sewage system.

(1988, p. 22)

The death rates from diseases like cholera and smallpox prompted the government to enforce vaccinations when the mechanics became available. However, the 1853 Vaccination Act, which made vaccinations compulsory in England and Wales, was opposed by mass protests and many individual acts of non-compliance occurred. In 1971, vaccination against smallpox was abandoned in the UK (Salmon *et al.*, 2006). The application of scentific discoveries like germ theory meant that medical science did have a big part to play in protecting the health of the population. One way of doing this is through programmes of inoculation. Jenner's early work with cowpox proved that inoculation could be effective and from this the idea of 'herd immunity' was derived. Bear with me, this is all very relevant to Yasmin!

Fast facts 27.1   Herd immunity

Herd immunity refers to the indirect protection offered to people susceptible to disease by the high levels of inoculated individuals. This reduces background levels of the disease and so the likelihood of becoming infected is greatly reduced (Brisson and Edmunds, 2003).

Reader activity 27.4   Vaccination choice

Should vaccination be compulsory? Is it better for the state to control public health or should individuals decide for themselves what is good/bad for them?

Now consider the population of people with a learning disability. What assistance might they need in deciding about vaccination? Who should be involved in that decision-making process?

They shoot horses, don't they? Or how eugenics influenced ideas on 'mental deficiency'

A public health policy for people with what was once termed 'mental deficiency' and now referred to as intellectual or learning disability, has been available for some time. When first mooted, it had many adherents though its appeal has lessened somewhat since the early days of the twentieth century. In 1904, Sir Francis Galton drew up this definition of eugenics. He had coined the term to suggest that a 'good life' could be biologically engineered by selective breeding. He said: 'Eugenics is the science which deals with all influences that improve the inborn qualities of a race; also with those that develop them to the utmost advantage' (1904, p. 1). This way of thinking was very unsympathetic to any individual or group who were deemed to 'deviate' from the norm.

It is axiomatic that providing care costs money. So consider this: if it costs the state X million to provide care for Yasmin over a lifetime, and if Yasmin, due to the nature of her condition, is never going to make a direct contribution to the state (i.e. get a job and pay taxes), what would be the financial savings to the state if we take the cost of caring out of the equation? And in doing the sums you should consider the savings made by removing the salaries of nurses, therapists and social carers.

Now ask yourself this: could the money saved be better spent on improving public health for future generations? If you cannot argue an economic case for caring, then you may find it very difficult to justify your role in an environment where services increasingly have to account for their spending.

Eugenics was a very popular idea in the late nineteenth and early twentieth centuries. There was a real concern that low intelligence was hereditary and that if those people with low intelligence were allowed to breed, they would dilute the overall well-being of the nation. At the same time in the United States, the same segregation was in place but it was complemented by a mass sterilisation programme of people with what was referred to as 'mental retardation'. Type 'Buck vs Bell' into your favourite search engine for an insight into how this affected people. This kind of thinking has not entirely gone away. Today pregnant women are routinely screened for a variety of 'abnormalities'. If a woman discovers that her foetus has an 'abnormality',' she will be advised or counselled about her choices. One of the options offered to women in this situation is abortion.

Fast facts 27.2   Abortion

The latest guidance available from the Royal College of Obstetricians and Gynecologists (RCOG, 2010) states that in 2008 (the most recent year for which figures are available) just under 2000 abortions were performed under Section 1(1)(d) known as Ground E of the Abortion Act. This applies to cases where there is a substantial risk that, if the child were born, it would suffer physical or mental abnormalities that would result in serious handicap. And 'handicap' is their word, not mine.

Is the situation just described an example of contemporary eugenics in action?

Then ask yourself this: if you are caring for a young man or woman with mild/moderate LD and they tell you that they and their girl/boyfriend are 'trying for a baby', how would you handle this?

What rights do they have? And if they have the right to start a family, then what responsibilities do they have to care for the child? And how will they enact those responsibilities?

Now think about Yasmin. Her family is very keen that she be 'protected' and they mean from any contact with men. They cite religious and cutural differences but the support staff who work with Yasmin believe that it's about sex. They have seen Yasmin looking at men. So, should Yasmin receive 'sex education'?

Sex and drugs and sausage rolls: or does everything really give you cancer?

The chapter has so far had a theoretical or conceptual focus that has borrowed from history to explain how we have arrived at where we are today. In this section we turn to the up-to-date scene and consider how ideas continue to dominate policy and so shape public health practice. We will also move to considering the more practical aspects of public health and learning disability. In short, what are YOU going to do about it?

The ideas may be different but still some parallels with earlier times remain. To begin with, we look at an extract from a contemporary work of fiction that asks questions about individual responsibility. The character Renton inhabits a novel called *Trainspotting*. Maybe you read the book or saw the film. There was even a poster with the following quotation. He lives what a social worker might describe as a 'chaotic lifestyle'. In plainer language, Renton is a smackhead. But he's not stupid. This is his take on the public health agenda and its efforts to guide people's lifestyle choices. He has a Scottish accent!

> Society invents a spurious convoluted logic tae absorb and change people whae's behaviour is outside its mainstream. Suppose that ah ken aw the pros and cons, know that ah'm gaunnae huv a short life, am ay sound mind etcetera, etcetera, but still want tae use smack? They won't let ye dae it. They won't let ye dae it, because it's seen as a sign ay thir ain failure. The fact that ye jist simply choose tae reject whit they huv to offer. Choose us. Choose life. Choose mortgage payments; choose washing machines; choose cars; choose sitting oan a fuckin couch watching mind-numbing and spirit-crushing game shows, stuffing fuckin junk food intae yir mooth; choose rotting away, pishing and shiteing yersel in a home, a total fuckin embarrassment tae the selfish, fucked-up brats ye've produced. Choose life. Well, ah choose no tae choose life.
>
> (1993, p. 188)

It's a bleak assessment. And at odds with the central messages in documents like *Choosing Health: Making Healthier Choices Easier* (DH, 2004). Maybe Renton wouldn't get away with this if his social worker used motivational interiew techniques, noted by Martins and McNeil to have 'been applied to a number of areas of behavioural change and best known for applications in the realm of substance abuse' (2009, p. 283).

Renton, however, makes a good point when he asserts his own rights as an individual even when these run contrary to the law. Rose (2001) identifies what he calls 'bio politics' as an extension of eugenics. He argues that governments, when they try to manage risk and risk behaviours (think over-eating or smoking) by implementing policies designed to exert control over individuals' lifestyle choices, can be argued to be acting in a discriminatory manner against 'those found biologically abnormal or defective' (ibid., p. 2).

Rose means that if everyone has their body mass index (BMI) measured, for example, it is then possible to calculate a mean figure. When we know what the average is, we can then put policies and interventions in place to deal with those who are above or below average. The same thing happened with intelligence. The difference here is that people with above average intelligence are not subject to state controls advising them to lose intelligence, as they might be if they were overweight. People with below average intelligence, however, assessed as having an IQ score below 70, for example, will immediately be subject to state interventions. The first sign of this is that they will be labelled as having 'learning disability'.

In the rest of this chapter we will look at contemporary health and social care policy and the thinking behind it to see if there is any merit in the perspectives offered by Rose and Renton. There are two main ideas to consider here: the so-called 'Big Society' and 'nudge theory'. As ever, keep thinking about Yasmin and the people you care for and ask how this will affect their lives.

The Big Society

> The hallmark of a truly 'big' society should be its willingness and capacity to develop public and social policies that are sufficiently generous and resource-rich to embrace those who are most marginalised.
>
> (Ellison, 2011, p. 57)

When governments take over the provision of some services or pass laws that require universal observance, they are sometimes criticised for being 'paternalistic', which in this context means, literally, acting like a parent. This is sometimes referred to as the 'nanny state' by people who believe that the state is interfering too much in how they live their lives. They argue that individuals, groups, communities and societies are mature enough to secure their own needs and make decisions about matters that affect them. The Prime Minister, David Cameron apparently agrees because he wants local groups to be involved in running things like parks, post offices, libraries and local transport services (Cameron, 2010).

Reader activity 27.7 Running a group

Take a moment to reflect on which groups and individuals this might work well for. Now think about where this may not work so well. Who might want to run an activity group for people with severe learning disability who have little access to the outdoors? What qualifications would such people need to have?

Some people might have the time and energy to contribute to this. But would they need any training? Would they need any level of security clearance, like criminal record checks? Would they need communication skills for things like BSL or Makaton? Would they be able to issue medication in emergency or even routinely? Would they have the attitudes and values necessary to provide care for people with high support needs and who are from a different cultural background?

For some activities, and running a post office might be one of them, it seems that there is some degree of training necessary to carry them out successfully. To look after Yasmin, even for half an hour, would be very demanding. In fact, you might need to be a nurse, social worker or very skilled social carer to do this properly. If that is the case, then is this an argument for removing health and social care provision for people with more profound needs from charities, volunteers or third sector agencies?

One of the reasons for the emphasis on individuals taking responsibiity for their own health is apparent in the values or ideologies to which the main political parties adhere. These must be seen within the context of the need to reduce costs incurred by public services where possible because of the global economic situation. One immediate result of this is that the NHS is committed to save money. This means that hospital managers are considering whether or not to offer treatment to some groups of people whose lifestyle choices have contributed to their poor health. Hence smokers and obese people may find that they are asked to lose weight or reduce their nicotine intake before they are considered for some non-emergency procedures.

Campbell's (2012) article posits the idea that if people want to take risks with their health behaviour, then it is within their human rights so to do and that the NHS, if it truly is national in its reach and universal in its principles, should not be allowed to ration services on the basis of judging individual lifestyles.

There are two points to consider here. The first is an example of the 'slippery slope' argument. The second is a point of principle. Both have consequences for you, me and Yasmin too.

So, point one: People who are seen to behave 'irresponsibly' by over-eating or smoking and drinking excessively to the point where it becomes a health issue, are now being targetted for behaviour change regimes prior to receiving certain health interventions.

Is this reasonable? If you agree, then this is where the slope starts to get very slippery. So, ask yourself, should people who play sport expect to receive free treatment if they present at A&E with broken limbs as a result of an accident incurred while rock climbing, cycling, or skiing backwards down the Matterhorn for charity?

Point two: how responsible is Yasmin for her overall condition? What control does she have over her lifestyle choices? How responsible is any of us for what we eat? And consider the power of advertisng, the choice and price of 'value' products in supermarkets and the availability of fresh fruit and vegetables. It wasn't the British Salad Growers Association who sponsored the London Olympics.

Reader activity 27.8   The Big Society

If we really are 'all in it together', then surely it must be right that people with learning disability also take their share of the burden? Yes? No? And whichever answer you favour, then ask yourself how someone with learning disability might opt in or out of the Big Society.

The nudge theory

The Public Health Responsibility Deal, effective as of 2011, is a collaboration between the Department of Health and the private sector designed to influence public health. It follows up on the then Secretary of State, Andrew Lansley's, description of government thinking when he said that they want to 'guide people's everyday decisions' by 'nudging people in the right direction rather than banning or significantly restricting their choices' (DH, 2010, para 2.34).

Nudge theory (Thaler and Sunstein, 2009) is an an examination of the potentials of psychological approaches to influencing health behaviour. To pursue this on a public health level, the Department of Health has instigated the creation of a 'behavioural insights team' within the Cabinet Office. This team comprises academics and civil servants who apply their thinking to areas like smoking cessation where it is felt that the population can be 'nudged' towards making better lifestyle choices. This then obviates the need for costly treatment further down the line (Wanless, 2004). Better lifestyle choices means a healthier society. Everybody is a winner. Or so the theory goes.

Rationing

Just before we think about resources, consider this. The NHS was set up in 1948 under the principle of universal healthcare for all, free at the point of delivery. How does this square with denying some procedures to people unless they can conform with targets set by hospitals, such as reducing their weight or their alcohol and/or tobacco intake? How do you explain to Yasmin that she has to lose weight before she can get treatment?

You may have heard of 'postcode lotteries' when applied to the availability of treatment. This is explained neatly in the NHS *Atlas of Variation*, 2011. Essentially some areas spend more than others on, say, cancer treatment. So, if you have cancer and live in area A where they spend a lot of money on cancer treatment, then you may get a good service. On the other hand, someone living in area B where the spend is less, may not get such a good deal. The difference can only be explained by location, hence the 'postcode lottery'.

Now let's get back to Yasmin. We know that she has congenital heart disease as part of her overall condition. And according to the RCN, 'heart disease is the second highest cause of death for people with learning disabilities' (2011, p. 7). How likely is she to get treatment?

Part of the answer is in where she lives. But we know where she lives, she lives in Rotherham. The next part of the answer lies in health economics, specifically the Quality Adjusted Life Years (QALYs). According to Weinstein *et al.*, the QALY is 'a widely used measure of health improvement that is used to guide health-care resource allocation decisions' (2009, p. S5). It means that there is a calculation that can be performed to discover whether someone, in this case, Yasmin, is economically worth treating. You'll have noticed we're already a long way from the founding principles of the NHS.

Because the calculation involved does not take account of subjective and personal factors we enter into 'Alice in Wonderland' territory. Weinstein again says, 'States worse than dead can exist and they would have a negative value and subtract from the number of QALYs' (ibid.). So it is apparently possible to be arithmetically better off dead. Remember that the next time you have a bad hangover. The calculation goes something like this. And I speak here as someone who regularly uses their fingers to count. Here goes . . .

Fast facts 27.3   QALY

The QALY is assumed to be one year of life in perfect health and = 1. So it follows that a year of life with less than perfect health (I count myself here, how about you?) is < 1. So QALYs are expressed in terms of perfectly healthy years, such that six months = 0.5 QALYs. Or to look at it another way, one year of life in imperfect health might also equate to 0.5 QALYs.

It's a fairly rigid system that takes no account of the effects of a variety of disability. And that's why Disability Adjusted Life Years (DALYs) have been introduced. According to the World Health Organisation: 'The DALY combines in one measure the time lived with disability and the time lost due to premature mortality' (2006). And remember, people with learning disability have a much reduced lifespan when compared to the general population.

Reader activity 27.9   Choosing a candidate

Here's a nice parlour game to test your understanding of the QALY/DALY debate. You are an NHS manager and you have £10, 000 to spend on *one* heart operation only. You have three candidates for surgery. You can assume that clinically/surgically they are all pretty much alike.

1. Candidate A is Alison White, aged 23, from Sheffield. Alison is the mother of one 6-month-old child and is married to Tom, an architecture student. Alison has congenital heart disease.
2. Candidate B is Joe Black. Joe is 23 and from Barnsley. Joe is unemployed, steals cars for a living and is currently residing at Her Majesty's pleasure in HMP Lindholme, near Doncaster. Joe has congenital heart disease.
3. Candidate C is Yasmin Akram.

So, who gets the operation? The thing about applying the QALY/DALY formula is that it takes the heartache (no pun intended) out of decision-making. All things being equal the decision lies somewhere between Alison and Joe. Yasmin doesn't make the cut because her life expectancy is lower to begin with, as Emerson (Robertson *et al.*, 2010) has pointed out, so any investment in her health now will quickly diminish as she ages. Under this application of arithmetic, Yasmin's life is less valued than that of Alison or Joe. Is that fair?

Now here's a thing. Hirsky (2007) points out that professional bodies such as the Nursing and Midwifery Council expect standards of care from their members. He says:

> The emphasis on the promotion of the interests of patients can be linked to patient care and the level of resources that are allocated, which in turn inevitably results in the level of resources being linked to the standard of care.
>
> (ibid., p. 79)

It's hard to argue against. How then can any individual, irrespective of their health status, be morally or legally denied treatment, even on an economic basis?

The future now

At the beginning of this chapter Table 27.1 contrasted the official government responses to public health issues (with cholera as an example) with responses to learning disability. We saw there that the same actions were applied to both areas as they were both understood to be disease processes. In Table 27.2 we consider a more up-to-date sitiuation. Here I've used 'obesity' as the contemporary

Table 27.2 Official state responses to public health and learning disability issues in the twenty-first century

Public health issue	State concern	State response	Learning disability issue	State concern	State response
Obesity epidemic	Widespread and growing ill health (diabetes, heart disease, some cancers)	Spending cuts			
		Rationing of care/services			
		Health promotion via 'nudge theory'			
	Pressure on resources (particularly NHS and public sector)				
		Policy retreat on the universal aspects of health and social care			
	Lack of funds				
	Loss of faith by some of the electorate	Emphasis on personal responsibility for lifestyle choices			

epidemic (James *et al.*, 2004). You could substitute smoking or drinking without damaging the argument.

Reader activity 27.10   Policy choices

Note that the sections on learning disability are empty. That's because *Valuing People Now* (DH, 2009) was the last government White Paper on learning disability and it had a three-year shelf life. So, you have a blank sheet of paper. What should the policy look like?

Today, for example, the emphasis is less on state intervention to secure better health for the population and more on promoting individual responsibility through motivational interviewing techniques (Tappin *et al.*, 2000).

Motivational interviewing (MI) was first described by Miller (1983) who worked with 'problem drinkers'. It employs psychological techniques to get people to think about why they indulge in certain health behaviours. It doesn't try to get people to stop or to convert them to other regimes. It is very much about giving people the time and space to reflect on their behaviour and its consequences. Rollnick and Miller put it this way. MI is a 'directive, client-centred counselling style for eliciting behaviour change by helping clients to explore and resolve ambivalence' (1995, p. 325). Its success in helping people to overcome some potentially dangerous health behaviours has two immediate flaws that I can see if it is to be applied to people with learning disability. The clue to the first is apparent in the name: 'interviewing'. It is a talking kind of therapy and for people with communciation difficulties, this might be a barrier to its efficacy. The second flaw that I can see is in the nature of the relationship between the 'counsellor' and the 'client'. In Rollnick and Miller's version, they emphasise the autonomy of the client. Again, for someone with learning disability, this might be a contested notion.

Reader activity 27.11 MI

- So how would you adapt a motivational interview to discuss weight loss with Yasmin?
- Would you open the interview up to other people?
- What communication methods or techniques might you use?

In 2013, Public Health England will be launched as an executive agency of the Department of Health. This body will have oversight of the public health agenda. It is premised on one overall aim which is to improve and protect the nation's health and to improve the health of the poorest, fastest. Given the close associations of poverty and disability (Emerson, 2005), this should be good news for the learning disability population.

Out of this overall aim there are five specific objectives described as 'domains'. These are:

- *Health protection and resilience*: Protecting the population's health from major emergencies and remaining resilient to harm.
- *Tackling the wider determinants of health*: Tackling factors which affect health and well-being and health inequalities.
- *Health improvement:* Helping people to live healthy lifestyles, make healthy choices.
- *Prevention of ill health*: Reducing the number of people living with preventable ill health.
- *Healthy life expectancy and preventable mortality*: Preventing people from dying prematurely.

To conclude this chapter we need to consider how the past has influenced the present and how the present is likely to impact on the future. In doing so we need also to keep our population in mind and ask how we can best guide them as the public health agenda unfolds.

From the wealth of the nation to the health of the nation

Today, with a clean water supply, good sanitation and improved nutrition, the focus of public health is much more about education, awareness and lifestyle. People in the UK no longer die of smallpox in their thirties; they die of cancer and heart disease in their old age instead.

This trend is starting to affect people with learning disability too. In one way it's a good thing but only if we can make sure they incorporate a healthy lifestyle into their later years. Cockerham (2005) points out that, as we have seen, the change in disease patterns means that many more people are living longer. But this 'epidemiological transition' (ibid., p. 52) is not enough on its own to explain why people live longer. Another kind of transition might help to explain.

The NHS and Community Care Act (1990) was a significant move towards ending institutionalisation as the default care setting. For many people with learning disability this meant that for the first time in their lives they could have their own room, in their own home and, with support, become part of their own communities. One of the biggest changes was in the organisation of their domestic routines. No longer reliant on a centralised system to provide the basic amenities, these people were very quickly introduced to the 'consumer society' (Bauman, 2005).

Care in the community had obvious benefits. But it also introduced people to some of the risks of a contemporary consumer society. These risks were not always well managed as organisations and staff invoked the principle of 'choice' in determining how people should live their new lives.

Along with 'rights', 'independence' and 'inclusion', choice is one of the key ideas in learning disability policy for the twenty-first century (DH, 2001, 2009). Choice is, coincidentally, also a key idea associated with consumerism (McClimens and Hyde, 2012). So the move from institutions to communities allowed former 'patients' to become 'consumers' and that had some unfortunate consequences as they were introduced to a contemporary 'lifestyle'.

Lifestyle is a recent expression and usually attributed to Max Weber, a German sociologist ([1922] 1978). Cockerham has elsewhere redefined the term as 'collective patterns of health-related behaviour based on choices from options available to people according to their life chances' (2005, p. 162). In technical terms, this refers to structure and agency. In less technical terms this means that we need to consider what opportunities our clients have to direct their own activities (what to eat, where and when to exercise, who with), what knowledge they have about those activities and their consequences (pudding tastes good but too much is bad for you) and how we can improve their lifestyle choices.

Reader activity 27.12   Lifestyle

Is this starting to sound like nudge theory? Again, it might be useful to consider your own 'lifestyle' and then to contrast this with Yasmin or someone you know and care for. Do you go to a gym? Do you go swimming? How much does that cost? And how do you get there? Do you smoke or drink? How much? And how much does that cost?

Fast facts 27.4   Health economics

If you ask a health economist, they might tell you that in 2006/07 smoking and drinking cost the NHS £6.6 billion. If you add diet-related ill health, that's another £5.8 billion. Add physical inactivity and it's £0.9 billion more. Obesity on its own cost £5.1 billion (Scarborough et al., 2011). Go back to the section on the Big Society. How much of that saving could be made right here?

Smokers and drinkers might point to the revenue they contribute through the taxes they pay for their pleasures. The Institute for Alcohol Studies did some calculations. They count the cost of alcohol harm to the NHS in 2008 at £2.7 billion. Then there are other less calculable costs like absence from work, lost productivity and family distress.

So the entire population needs to be careful about its lifestyle, but where should we go for advice? Your GP should be a good resource. But just before we move on, here's a question . . . are you registered with a GP? Of course you are. Now are all the people with learning disabilities also registered? *Valuing People* (DH, 2001) set out a timetable. All people with a learning disability were to be registered with a GP by June 2004. And all people with a learning disability were to have a Health Action Plan and have an identified health facilitator to help them access primary care services by June 2005 (ibid., p. 61). The IHAL (2012) does not provide exact numbers but they do report that more people with learning disabilities are being counted on GP practice lists at 4.2 in every thousand in 2009–2010.

The Annual Health Check

There has been plenty of government guidance on public health-related issues. Four major policy statements cover the past twenty years: *Health of the Nation* (1992), *Saving Lives: Our Healthier Nation* (1999), *Choosing Health: Making Healthier Choices Easier* (2004) and *Health Lives, Healthy People: Our Strategy for Public Health in England* (2010).

In addition, there have been reports and recommendations which prompt the policy-makers. From the Black Report (1980) through Acheson (1998), Wanless (2002, 2004), *Our Health, Our Care, Our Say* (DH, 2006) to *Fair Society, Healthy Lives* (DH, 2011), the core message has been that health inequalities exist and that people in the lower-income groups live shorter lives and have more illness.

What are the implications for our client population? There have been specific reports and enquiries.

- *Equal Rights: Closing the Gap*: a report from the Disability Rights Commission (DRC, 2006). This examined the disparity between the levels of healthcare on offer to the general population and the population of people with learning disability.
- Mencap's report *Death by Indifference* (2007), discussed elsewhere, but it must be mentioned here also was a damning indictment of hospital and local authority care that took the deaths of six people with learning disability as a case study and exposed the lack of training and understanding shown by staff.
- *Healthcare for All*: The findings of the independent inquiry into the health inequalities of people with learning disabilities (Michael, 2008). This was the government response to the fallout from *Death by Indifference*. The first recommendation was that more training was needed in learning disability matters for non-specialist staff. And that, where possible, this should include input from people with learning disability and their families.
- *Six Lives: The Provision of Public Services to People with Learning Disabilities* (Parliamentary and Health Services Ombudsman, 2009). A vindication of Mencap's report.

These documents are discussed in *Improving Health and Lives* (2012) which is a dedicated survey of the health of people with learning disability in England. The report makes it plain that the differences in healthcare between people with and without learning disability are avoidable and preventable. To put this into some perspective, consider this angle on the report from Parish (2012) who sums it up with some neat arithmetic.

Fast facts 27.5   About 25 years earlier

On average, a person with learning disability will still die about 25 years earlier than someone born on the same day who does not have such a disability (Parish, 2012, p. 3).

There are many legitimate responses to this, including outrage and letters to the editor but let's stick to the main avenues and consider, to begin with, what m'learned friends might say if asked to pass judgement. The NHS has a legal obligation described in the Equality Act (2010) to make 'reasonable adjustments' when caring for people with a variety of disabilities so that they are not disadvantaged when accessing services and receiving treatment or therapy. This needs to beconsidered against the figures for the uptake of Annual Health checks. At the time of writing, this has just been released and stands at just 53 per cent of the possible population (ldtonline.co.uk).

Health checks for people with learning disability are not new. First, Howells (1986) indicated they might be necessary. Subsequently, Matthews (Matthews and Hegarty, 1997) developed the 'OK' Health Check while Cassidy *et al.* (2002) report on an attempt to promote good practice by involving GPs and community learning disability teams. More recently, Marsh and Drummond (2008) have issued a reminder for the 'OK' Health Check. Felce *et al.* (2008) demonstrate their worth in terms of detecting and treating unmet health needs while Romeo *et al.* (2009) are the first to have attempted a cost-benefit analysis which suggests that they are also economically justified.

The idea was first proposed in legislation in *Valuing People* (DH, 2001). However, it was only after the events that led to the publication of *Death by Indifference* (Mencap, 2007) and *Health Care for All* (Michael, 2008) that the Department of Health instigated the Direct Enhanced Service (D.E.S) (Learning Disability) which contained the framework for annual health checks. The health check itself is based on the Cardiff Health Check. However, GP practices are not obliged to undertake to provide DES but there are financial incentives available to persuade them. This amounts to approximately £100 per patient. I know a GP and I asked them if their practice implemented the in full first annual health checks. They said no, because looking at their practice purely as a business, it wasn't worth their while. So if you want to know where to begin to make improvements in the overall health of the population with learning disability, then I suggest you start right here and see if Yasmin has had a health check.

Health and Health Action Plans

In the introduction to their article, Marshall, McConkey and Moore (2003) highlight the poor overall health status of the people with learning disabilities when compared to the rest of the population. They refer to a relative lack of health promotion, difficulties in accessing healthcare settings and low uptake of screening services (2003, p. 147). In pointing out that obesity is a growing concern for this population, they list the potential dangers as 'cardiovascular disease, diabetes, hypertension and various cancers' (ibid., p. 148). In addition, a third of the people who had a pin-prick test (n = 284) were found to have raised cholesterol levels while 42 individuals or 9 per cent of the total sample (n = 407) were smokers (ibid., p. 150).

One way to address this, and this was the tactic adopted by the studies reported above, was to instigate nurse-led clinics to screen for health problems and then signpost the individuals as necessary to appropriate treatment or interventions. A similar scheme could be envisaged for any number of health-related issues where people with learning disability seem to have poorer than average outcomes. Kerr *et al.* (2003) report on a large-scale health screening of hearing and visual problems. Of just over 500 individuals, only four had no vision problems. Of the 490 individuals who had their hearing tested, 52 had no hearing problems. And as the authors point out, 'sensory defects impact directly on quality of life and hinder early detection of other health problems with potentially serious consequences' (ibid., p. 143).

The oral and dental care of people with learning disability is also sub-optimal (Tiller *et al.*, 2001). And Robertson *et al.* (2000) calculate that most adults with learning disability do not have good knowledge of healthy eating and in particular do not get enough fresh fruit and veg.

Emerson (2005) focuses on exercise/activity. He uses figures derived from Bennett *et al.* (1995) and calculates that when comparing the learning disability population to the general population, 92 per cent of the learning disabilities population are not getting enough exercise.

So, what to do? In their guidance, the Department of Health (2008) frame health action planning as a means by which to combat the health inequalities typically suffered by the population of people with learning disability and summarised in the examples above. Health Action Plans, first introduced in *Valuing People* (DH, 2001) are seen as a way of personalising support. *Action for Health* (DH, 2002) outlined the part to be played by Partnership Boards who are to be key stakeholders, responsible for bringing all parties together.

A key policy paper which informed this initiative was *Choosing Health: Making Healthy Choices Easier* (DH, 2004) which delivered three principles of working:

- informed choice for all;
- personalisation of support to make healthy choices;
- partnership working.

The template is there, all it needs now is for some enthusiastic and dedicated individuals to make this happen. That means YOU.

The end?

> Economics is all about how people make choices. Sociology is all about why they don't have choices to make.
>
> (Duesenberry, 1960, p. 232)

Duesenberry might as well have been talking about learning disability and public health. In the nineteenth century the state began to take control of public health issues. It did this through improved engineering works that were based on an increased understanding of medical science. The success of these interventions was such that similar methods were used with the growing population of the 'feeble-minded' who were subject to segregation and physical removal from the community.

The focus of twenty-first-century public health concern is now very much on the individual as the state retreats from providing universal healthcare. This is partly an economic argument and partly ideological. We are all now encouraged through health promotion and education to take more care of ourselves by attending to our lifestyle choices. These have been shown to inflict a huge financial burden on the state when they lead to increased levels of ill health and impairment.

Meanwhile, people with learning disability are encouraged to join the consumer society, to look for work, to manage their own care through individualised financial schemes and to become part of the community. There is an economic argument to say we cannot afford to look after people with learning disabilities. The counter-balance to this is that as a civilised society we cannot afford not to either. This brings in the notion of advocacy and that requires people to choose their allegiance. Now, whose side are you on?

Reader activity 27.13 Learning outcomes revisited

Q: Can you see any traces of eugenics in contemporary policies?

A: All through history there is evidence of negative social reactions to impairment and disability (http://langdondownmuseum.org.uk/four-box-headings/the-history-of-learning disability/idiots-imbeciles-and-intellectual-impairment/). We don't throw deformed babies into rivers any more so maybe it's progress of a sort.

Q: Nudge theory is currently popular for addressing public health issues. How effective is this with the population of people with learning disabilty? What factors might influence uptake?

A: Communication might be an issue.

Q: People with learning disability generally live with poorer health status than the rest of the population. Why should this be? Can Health Action Plans improve this situation?

A: If GPs are not required to undertake Annual Health Checks, then somebody else has to. Who that will be in a vanishing NHS is anybody's guess. It might have to be you.

Points to remember

- The health of all of us, including people with learning disabilities, is influenced by governmental policies and agenda.
- It is important to be politically aware.
- Advocating on behalf of people with a learning disability is essential if you see barriers which prevent people from having their health needs met.
- Person-centred planning is vital.

References

Acheson, D. (1988) *Public Health in England*. Report of the Committee of Inquiry into the Future of the Public Health Function, Cm 289. London: HMSO.

Bauman, Z. (2005) *Work, Consumerism and the New Poor*. New York: McGraw-Hill.

Bennett, N., Dodd, T., Flatley, J., Freeth, S. and Bolling, K. (1995) *The Health Survey for England 1993*. London: The Stationery Office.

Black, D. (1980) *Inequalities in Health: Report of a Research Working Group*. London: HMSO.

Brisson, M. and Edmunds, W.J. (2003) Varicella vaccination in England and Wales: cost–utility analysis, *Archives of Disease in Childhood*, 88: 862–869.

Buckner, L., Fry, G. and Yeandle, S.C. (2009) *Carers in the Region: A Profile of Yorkshire and The Humber*. Leeds: University of Leeds.

Cabinet Office Behavioural Insights Team (2010) Applying behavioural insight to health. Available at: www.cabinetoffice.gov.uk/resource-library/applying-behavioural-insight-health (accessed June 2012).

Cameron, D. (2010) 'Big society' speech, Liverpool, 19 July 2010. Available at: http://www.number10. gov.uk/news/speeches-and-transcripts/ 2010/07/big-society-speech-53572) (accessed June 2012).

Campbell, D. (2012) Doctors back denial of treatment for smokers and the obese. *The Observer*, Sunday 29 April.

Cardiff Health Check (n.d.) Available at: http://www.easyhealth.org.uk/sites/default/files/Cardiff_ Health_Check.pdf (accessed Nov. 2012).

Cassidy, G., Martin, D.M., Martin, G.H.B. and Roy, A. (2002) Health checks for people with learning disabilities, *Journal of Learning Disabilities*, 6(2), 123–136.

Cockerham, W.C. (2005) Health lifestyle theory and the convergence of agency and structure, *Journal of Health and Social Behaviour*, 46: 51–67.

DH (Department of Health) (1980) *Inequalities in Health Report of a Research Working Group*. London: DHSS.

DH (Department of Health) (2001) *Valuing People: A New Strategy for Learning Disability for the 21st Century*. London: TSO.

DH (Department of Health) (2002) *Action for Health: Health Action Plans and Health Facilitation*. London: TSO.

DH (Department of Health) (2004) *Choosing Health: Making Healthy Choices Easier*. London: TSO.

DH (Department of Health) (2006) *Our Health, Our Care, Our Say: A New Direction for Community Services*. London: TSO.

DH (Department of Health) (2009) *Valuing People Now: A New Three Year Stratgey for People with Learning Disabilities* London: TSO.

DH (Department of Health) (2010) *Healthy Lives, Healthy People: Our Strategy for Public Health in England*. London: Department of Health.

Disability Rights Commission (2006) *Equal Treatment: Closing the Gap*. London: DRC.

Duesenberry, J.S. (1960) Comment. In Universities National Bureau Committee for Economic Research, *Demographic and Economic Change in Developed Countrie*. Princeton, NJ; Princeton University Press, pp. 231–234.

Editorial (2010) The UK Public Health White Paper: 'just words', *The Lancet*, 376, December 11, p. 1959.

Ellison, N. (2011) The Conservative Party and the Big Society, in C. Holden, M. Kilkey and G. Ramia (eds) *Social Policy Review 23: Analysis and Debate in Social Policy*. [online] The Policy Press.

Emerson, E. (2005) Underweight, obesity and exercise among adults with intellectual disabilities in supported accommodation in Northern England, *Journal of Intellectual Disability Research*, 49(2): 134–143.

Emerson, E. (2009) *Estimating Future Numbers of Adults with Profound Multiple Learning Disabilities in England*. CeDR Research Report. Lancaster: CeDR.

Felce, D., Baxter, H., Lowe, K., Dunstan, F., Houston, H., Jones, G. *et al.* (2008) The impact of repeated health checks for adults with intellectual disabilities, *Journal of Applied Research in Intellectual Disabilities*, 21: 585–596.

Galton, F. (1904) Eugenics: its scope and aim, *American Journal of Sociology*, 10(1): 1–25.

Hirsky, P. (2007) QALY: an ethical issue that dare not speak its name, *Nursing Ethics*, 14: 72–84.

Howatson, J. (2005) Health action plans for people with learning disabilities, *Nursing Standard*, 19(43): 51–57.

Howells, G. (1986) Are the medical needs of mentally handicapped adults being met? *Journal of the Royal College of General Practitioners*, 36: 449–453.

Improving Health and Lives Observatory (2012) *People with Learning Disabilities in England in 2011: Services and Supports*. Lancaster: IHAL.

James, P.T., Rigby, N. and Leach, R. (2004) The obesity epidemic, metabolic syndrome and future prevention strategies, *European Journal of Cardiovascular Preventative Rehabilitation*, 11: 3–8.

Kerr, A.M., McCulloch, D., Oliver, K., McLean, B. *et al.* (2003) Medical needs of people with intellectual disability require regular reassessment, and the provision of client- and carer-held reports, *Journal of Intellectual Disability Research*, 47(2): 134–145.

Langdon Down Museum (n.d.) Available at: http://langdondownmuseum.org.uk/four-box-headings/the-history-of-learning disability/idiots-imbeciles-and-intellectual-impairment/ (accessed July 2012).

Ldtonline (n.d.) Available at: http://www.ldtonline.co.uk/2012/07/only53-of-people-with-learning-disabilities-receive-health-check (accessed July 2012).

Marmot Review (2010) *Fair Society, Healthy Lives: Strategic Review of Health Inequalities in England Post-2010*. London: The Marmot Review.

Marsh, L. and Drummond, E. (2008) Health needs in people with learning disabilities: using the 'OK' Health Check, *Learning Disability Practice*, 11: 16–21.

Marshall, A. (1885) Theories about facts and wages, in *Principles of Economics*, 9th edn. London: Macmillan.

Marshall, D., McConkey, R. and Moore, G. (2003) Obesity in people with intellectual disabilities: the impact of nurse-led health screenings and health promotion activities, *Journal of Advanced Nursing*, 41(2): 147–153.

Martins, R.K. and McNeil, D.W. (2009) Review of Motivational Interviewing in promoting health behaviors, *Clinical Psychology Review*, 29(4): 283–293.

Matthews, D. and Hegarty, J. (1997) The OK Health Check: a health assessment checklist for people with learning disabilities, *British Journal of Learning Disabilities*, 25: 138–143.

McClimens, A. and Hyde, M. (2012) Intellectual disability, consumerism, identity and choice: to have and have not? *Journal of Intellectual Disabilities*, 16(2): 132–141.

McKeown, T. (1976) *The Modern Rise of Population*. London: Edward Arnold.

Mencap (2007) *Death by Indifference*. London: Mencap.

Michael, J. (2008) *Healthcare for All: Report of the Independent Inquiry into Access to Healthcare for People with Learning Disabilities*. London: TSO.

Miller, W. R. (1983) Motivational interviewing with problem drinkers, *Behavioural Psychotherapy*, 11: 147–172.

Muntaner, C., Lynch, J. and Smith, G.D. (2001) Social capital, disorganized communities, and the third way: understanding the retreat from structural inequalities in epidemiology and public health, *International Journal of Health Services*, 31(2): 213–237.

NHS *Atlas of Variation* (2011) Available at: http://www.rightcare.nhs.uk/index.php/atlas/atlas-of-variation-2011/ (accessed Nov. 2012).

Nunkoosing, K. and John, M. (1997) Friendships, relationships and the management of rejection and loneliness by people with intellectual disabilities, *Journal of Intellectual Disabilities for Nursing, Health and Social Care*, 1: 10–18.

Orme, J., Powell, J., Taylor, P. and Grey, M. (eds) (2007) *Public Health for the 21st Century: New Perspectives on Policy Participation and Practice*. Maidenhead: McGraw-Hill.

Parish, C. (2012) Small changes, big benefits, *Learning Disability Practice*, 15(6): 3.

Parliamentary and Health Services Ombudsman (2009) *Six Lives: The Provision of Public Services to People with Learning Disabilities*. London: TSO.

Parrott, R., Wolstenholme, J., and Tilley, N. (2008) Changes in demography and demand for services from people with complex needs and profound multiple learning disabilities, *Tizard Learning Disability Review*, 13(3): 26–34.

Pressman, S.D. and Cohen, S. (2005) Does positive affect influence health? *Psychological Bulletin*, 131: 925–971.

Public Health Responsibility Deal (2010) Available at: http://responsibilitydeal.dh.gov.uk/ (accessed June 2012).

Putnam, R. (2000) *Bowling Alone: The Collapse and Revival of American Community*. New York: Simon & Schuster.

RCN (2011) *Meeting the Health Needs of People with Learning Disabilities*. London: RCN.

RCOG (2010) *Termination of Pregnancy for Fetal Abnormality in England, Scotland and Wales*. London: RCOG.

Robertson, J., Emerson, E., Gregory, N. *et al.* (2000) Lifestyle-related risk factors for poor health in residential settings for people with intellectual disabilities, *Research in Developmental Disabilities*, 21: 469–486.

Robertson, J., Roberts, H. and Emerson, E. (2010) *Health Checks for People with Learning Disabilities: A Systematic Review of Evidence*. Lancaster: IHAL Learning Disabilities Observatory.

Rollnick, S., Butler, C.C., McCambridge, J. *et al.* (2005) Consultations about changing behaviour, *British Medical Journal*, 331: 961–963.

Rollnick, S. and Miller, W.R. (1995) What is motivational interviewing? *Behavioural and Cognitive Psychotherapy*, 23: 325–334.

Romeo, R., Knapp, M., Tyrer, P., Crawford, M. and Oliver-Africano, P. (2009) The treatment of challenging behaviour in intellectual disabilities: cost-effectiveness analysis, *Journal of Intellectual Disability Research*, 53(7): 633–643.

Rose, N. (2001) The politics of life itself, *Theory, Culture & Society*, 18: 1–30.

Rotherham Ethnic Minority Association (2010) *Aiming High for Disabled Children and Young People in Rotherham*. Rotherham.

Salmon, D.A., Teret, S.P., MacIntyre, C.R. *et al.* (2006) Compulsory vaccination and conscientious or philosophical exemptions: past, present, and future, *Lancet*, 367: 436–442.

Santayana, G. (1905) *The Life of Reason*, vol. 1. *Reason in Common Sense*. New York: Charles Scribner.

Scarborough, P., Bhatnagar, P., Wickramasinghe, K.K. *et al.* (2011) The economic burden of ill health due to diet, physical inactivity, smoking, alcohol and obesity in the UK: an update to 2006–07 NHS costs, *Journal of Public Health*, 33(4): 527–535. DOI:10.1093/pubmed/fdr033

Sennet, R. (2006) *The Culture of the New Capitalism*. New Haven, CT: Yale University Press.

Sim, F. and McKee, M. (eds) (2011) *Issues in Public Health*. Maidenhead: McGraw-Hill.

Simmons, H.G. (1978) Explaining social policy: the English Mental Deficiency Act of 1913, *Journal of Social History*, 11(3): 387–403.

Simpson, J.H. (2010) 'What do you expect? She is mentally retarded!' On meeting the health challenges of individuals with intellectual disability, *The Internet Journal of Health*, 11(1). DOI: 10.5580/e9 (accessed July 2012).

Smith, A. (1776) *An Inquiry into the Nature and Causes of the Wealth of Nations*. London: W. Strahan and T. Cadell.

Snow, J. (1855) *On the Mode of Transmission of Cholera*. London: John Churchill.

Sretzer, S. (1988) The importance of social intervention in Britain's mortality decline c.1850–1914: a re-interpretation of the role of public health, *Society for the Social History of Medicine*, 1: 1–41.

Stapleton, D., O'Day, B., Livermore, G. and Imparato, A. (2006) Dismantling the poverty trap: disability policy for the twenty-first century, *The Milbank Quarterly*, 84(4): 701–732.

Tappin, D.M., McKay, C., McIntyre, D. *et al.* (2000) A practical instrument to document the process of motivational interviewing, *Behavioural and Cognitive Psychotherapy*, 28: 17–32.

Thaler, R. and Sunstein, C. (2009) *Nudge: Improving Decisions about Health, Wealth and Happiness*. New Haven, CT: Yale University Press.

Tiller, S., Wilson, K.I. and Gallagher, J.E. (2001) Oral health status and dental service use of adults with learning disabilities living in residential institutions and in the community, *Community Dental Health*, 18: 167–171.

Topley, W.W.C. and Wilson, G.S. (1923) The spread of bacterial infection: the problem of herd immunity, *Journal of Hygiene*, 21: 243–249.

Wakefield, A.J., Murch, S.H., Anthony, A., Linnell, J., *et al.* (1998) Ileal lymphoid nodular hyperplasia, non-specific colitis, and pervasive developmental disorder in children, *Lancet*, 351: 637–641 [retracted *Lancet* 2010 375].

Wanless, D. (2002) *Securing Our Future Health: Taking a Long-term View, Final Report*. London: HM Treasury.

Wanless, D. (2004) *Securing Good Health for the Whole Population, Final Report*. London: HM Treasury.

Weinstein, M.C., Torrance, G. and McGuire, A. (2009) QALYs: the basics, *Value in Health*, 12(1): 5–9.

Welsh, I. (1993) *Trainspotting*. London: Secker & Warburg.

White, S. (2000) Conceptual foundations of IQ testing, *Psychology, Public Policy, and Law*, 6(1): 33–43.

Wohland, P., Rees, P., Norman, P., Boden, P. and Jasinska, M. (2010) Working Paper 10/02l: Ethnic population projections for the UK and local areas, 2001–2051. Leeds: School of Geography, University of Leeds. Available at: http://www.geog.leeds.ac.uk/fileadmin/downloads/school/research/projects/migrants/WP_ETH_POP_PROJECTIONS.pdf (accessed May 2012).

Woodham-Smith, C. (1950) *Florence Nightingale, 1820–1910*. London: Constable.

World Health Organization (2006) *Disability Adjusted Life Years*. Available at: http://www.who.int/healthinfo/boddaly/en/print.html (accessed June 2012).

Index

Please note that page numbers relating to Figures or Tables will be in italics.